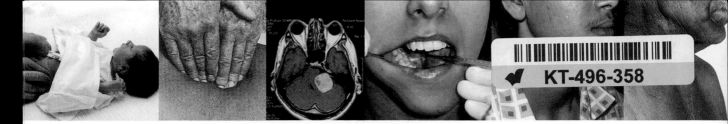

HUTCHISON'S CLINICAL METHODS

An integrated approach to clinical practice

EDITED BY

MICHAEL SWASH MD FRCP FRCPath

Honorary Consulting Neurologist
St Bartholomew's and the Royal London Hospital
Emeritus Professor of Neurology
Queen Mary's School of Medicine and Dentistry
London, UK

MICHAEL GLYNN MA MD FRCP ILTM

Consultant Physician and Gastroenterologist,
Clinical Director for Medicine and Deputy Medical Director,
St Bartholomew's and the Royal London Hospitals,
London, UK

TWENTY-SECOND EDITION

SAUNDERS

ELSEVIER

EDINBURGH LONDON NEW YORK OXFORD
PHILADELPHIA ST LOUIS SYDNEY TORONTO 2007

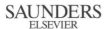

An imprint of Elsevier Limited

© Harcourt Publishers Limited 2002
© 2007, Elsevier Limited. All rights reserved.

First edition 1897
Twenty-second edition 2007

ISBN-13: 978 0 7020 2799 4
ISBN-10: 0 7020 2799 5
 Reprinted 2007

IE ISBN-13: 978 0 7020 2798 7
IE ISBN-10: 0 7020 2798 7
 Reprinted 2007

British Library Cataloguing in Publication Data
A catalogue record for this book is available from the British Library

Library of Congress Cataloging in Publication Data
A catalog record for this book is available from the Library of Congress

Note
Knowledge and best practice in this field are constantly changing. As new research and experience broaden our knowledge, changes in practice, treatment and drug therapy may become necessary or appropriate. Readers are advised to check the most current information provided (i) on procedures featured or (ii) by the manufacturer of each product to be administered, to verify the recommended dose or formula, the method and duration of administration, and contraindications. It is the responsibility of the practitioner, relying on their own experience and knowledge of the patient, to make diagnoses, to determine dosages and the best treatment for each individual patient, and to take all appropriate safety precautions. To the fullest extent of the law, neither the Publisher nor the Editors assume any liability for any injury and/or damage to persons or property arising out of or related to any use of the material contained in this book.

The Publisher

Working together to grow
libraries in developing countries

www.elsevier.com | www.bookaid.org | www.sabre.org

ELSEVIER   BOOK AID International   Sabre Foundation

ELSEVIER   your source for books,
journals and multimedia
in the health sciences
www.elsevierhealth.com

The
publisher's
policy is to use
**paper manufactured
from sustainable forests**

Printed in China

Preface to the twenty-second edition

With this edition Hutchison's Clinical Methods is well into its second century of production, and the core clinical skills of history and examination remain as relevant as ever. We live in an era in which, at first sight, there appears to be a test for every disease and, indeed, in which many patients expect a diagnosis to be made just from a few blood tests or an all inclusive scan. While for some patients this is technically possible, for the majority, a set of symptoms, or a long illness, represents a complex interaction between the underlying cause and its pathology, and the patient's individual bodily and psychological make-up. For this reason a doctor can only be in the position to give the best help and advice if the whole process and development of the patient's illness and disease is understood. In turn, this can be achieved only by highly skilled and sensitive history-taking and clinical examination. For many patients diagnosis by history and examination alone is far preferable, saving both the patient and doctor time, saving the cost of tests, saving some patients from the potential adverse effects of some of these tests, and being universally applicable; both in developed and less-developed areas of the world. Complex or expensive tests clearly have an increasing role in modern medical and surgical practice. They will often reveal new complexities and subtleties to old-established clinical methods, and their role must be absorbed into clinical methodology. Every clinical test and investigation has its own relevance, and any test, whether an old-established clinical method, or a complex modern investigation, should be applied when it is likely to yield trustworthy information, and not in other circumstances. The clinical teacher and the clinical student must work thus ever harder to ensure that core clinical skills are taught, learned, and practised skilfully and appropriately.

Hutchison's Clinical Methods emphasizes this approach to clinical medicine, beginning with chapters that describe the overall approach to a patient, and the general, initial clinical assessment. There follows a group of chapters describing the assessment of the core bodily systems – respiratory, cardiovascular, gastrointestinal, locomotor and nervous. We have provided 17 chapters, many of them new, describing clinical methods in particular patient groups (e.g. the old, the young, the unconscious), in relation to specific areas (e.g. eyes, ears, face, jaws), specific diseases (e.g. cancer, sexually transmitted infections), and in special situations (e.g. intensive care, pain management). This forms a logical sequence if read straight through, but also allows study of each section separately. Overall, the organization of the book still follows the aims set out by Hutchison with his colleague, Rainy, in the first edition, published in 1897.

The plan of this new edition continues to emphasize that teaching the medical history and examination in isolation from the process of diagnosis and planning management, is illogical and likely to lead to error. Therefore, each chapter describes both the process of history-taking and examination in a particular situation and, also, how the information gained is integrated into the process of diagnosis and planning of care. This makes the book an essential adjunct to a standard textbook of medicine, surgery or a specialty.

As in all past editions of Hutchison's, all the authors have existing or past links with 'Barts and the London', now consisting of The Royal London Hospital, St Bartholomew's Hospital and The London Chest Hospital. The editors acknowledge gratefully the work of all the current authors, as well as previous authors who have not contributed to this new edition. In particular we pay tribute to the work of two recently deceased friends and colleagues, Professor Gerry Bennett (Older people) and Dr Ivor Levy (Eyes).

Michael Swash and Michael Glynn
Royal London Hospital

Sir Robert Hutchison MD FRCP (1871–1960)

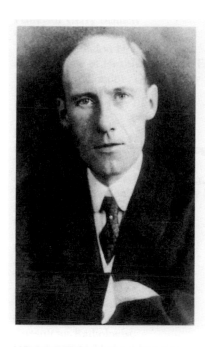

CLINICAL METHODS

A GUIDE TO THE PRACTICAL STUDY
OF MEDICINE

BY

ROBERT HUTCHISON, M.D., M.R.C.P.
DEMONSTRATOR IN PHYSIOLOGY, LONDON HOSPITAL MEDICAL COLLEGE

AND

HARRY RAINY, M.A., F.R.C.P.Ed., F.R.S.E.
UNIVERSITY TUTOR IN CLINICAL MEDICINE, ROYAL INFIRMARY, EDINBURGH

WITH 132 ILLUSTRATIONS AND 8 COLOURED PLATES

CASSELL AND COMPANY, LIMITED
LONDON, PARIS & MELBOURNE
1897
ALL RIGHTS RESERVED

Clinical Methods began in 1897, three years after Robert Hutchison was appointed Assistant Physician to The London Hospital. He was appointed full physician to The London and to the Hospital for Sick Children, Great Ormond Street, in 1900. He steered *Clinical Methods* through no less than 13 editions, at first with the assistance of Dr H. Rainy and then, from the 9th edition, published in 1929, with the help of Dr Donald Hunter. Although Hutchison retired from hospital practice in 1934 he continued to direct new editions of the book with Donald Hunter, and from 1949 with the assistance also of Dr Richard Bomford. The 13th edition, the first produced without Hutchison's guiding hand, was published in 1956 under the direction of Donald Hunter and Richard Bomford. Dr A. Stuart Mason and the present author joined Richard Bomford on Donald Hunter's retirement to produce the 16th edition, published in 1975, and following Richard Bomford's retirement prepared the 17th, 18th and 19th editions. Each of these editions was revised with the help of colleagues at The Royal London Hospital, in keeping with the tradition that lies behind the book.

During the many years of its continuous publication *Clinical Methods* has been translated into many languages. Indeed it is one of the great pleasures of association with the book to receive letters from far parts of the world, offering friendly advice, criticism and correction. Students have often noted errors that have escaped the eye of the editors.

Sir Robert Hutchison died in 1960 in his 90th year. It is evident from the memoirs of his contemporaries that he had a remarkable personality. Many of his clinical sayings became, in their day, aphorisms to be remembered and passed on to future generations of students. Of these the best known is his petition, written in his 82nd year:

'From inability to let well alone;
from too much zeal for the new and contempt for what is old;
from putting knowledge before wisdom, science before art, and
cleverness before common sense;
from treating patients as cases;
and from making the cure of the disease more grievous than the
endurance of the same, Good Lord, deliver us.'

Michael Swash and Michael Glynn
The Royal London Hospital

Contributors

Trevor Beedham MB BS BDS MIBiol FRCOG
Consultant Obstetrician and Gynaecologist,
St Bartholomew's and the Royal London
Hospitals; Honorary Senior Lecturer,
Queen Mary's School of Medicine and Dentistry,
London, UK

Margaret Browne MSc PhD FRCPath
Consultant Clinical Biochemist,
St Bartholomew's and the Royal London
Hospitals, London, UK

John Carter FRCS FDSRCS
Consultant Oral and Maxillofacial Surgeon,
St Bartholomew's and the Royal London
Hospitals, London and Princess Alexandra
Hospital, Harlow; Honorary Senior Lecturer,
Queen Mary's School of Medicine and Dentistry,
London, UK

Rino Cerio BSc MB BS FRCP(Lond) FRCP(Edin) FRCPath
Consultant Dermatologist, St Bartholomew's
and the Royal London Hospitals; Professor in
Dermatopathology, Queen Mary's School of
Medicine and Dentistry, London, UK

Tahseen A. Chowdhury MD FRCP
Consultant Physician in Diabetes and Metabolic
Medicine, St Bartholomew's and the Royal
London Hospitals, London, UK

John Coakley MD FRCP
Consultant in Intensive Care Medicine,
Homerton University Hospital, London, UK

Timothy Coats FRCS FFAEM
Professor of Emergency Medicine,
University of Leicester, Leicester, UK

Andrew Coombes BSc MB BS FRCOphth
Consultant Eye Surgeon,
St Bartholomew's and the Royal London
Hospitals; Honorary Senior Lecturer,
Queen Mary's School of Medicine and Dentistry,
London, UK

Frank Cross MS FRCS(Eng)
Consultant Surgeon, St Bartholomew's and the
Royal London Hospitals; Honorary Senior
Lecturer, Queen Mary's School of Medicine and
Dentistry, London, UK

David D'Cruz MD FRCP
Consultant Rheumatologist, The Louise Coote
Lupus Unit, St Thomas' Hospital, London, UK

William Drake DM MRCP
Consultant Physician and Endocrinologist,
St Bartholomew's and the Royal London
Hospitals, London, UK

Adam Feather MB BS MRCP
Consultant Geriatrician, Newham University
Hospital; Senior Lecturer in Medical Education,
Queen Mary's School of Medicine and Dentistry,
London, UK

Jayne Gallagher MB BS FRCA
Consultant Anaesthetist, St Bartholomew's and
the Royal London Hospitals, London, UK

Michael Glynn MA MD FRCP ILTM
Consultant Physician and Gastroenterologist,
Clinical Director for Medicine and Deputy
Medical Director, St Bartholomew's and the
Royal London Hospitals, London, UK

Beng Goh MB BS FRCP FRCP(I) Dip Derm Dip Ven
Consultant Physician in Genito-urinary
Medicine, St Bartholomew's and the Royal
London Hospitals and Moorfields Eye Hospital,
London, UK

Roger Harris MD FRCP FRCPCH DCH
Senior Lecturer in Child Health, Queen Mary's
School of Medicine and Dentistry, London, UK

Graham Hitman, MD FRCP
Consultant Physician in Diabetes and Metabolic
Medicine, St Bartholomew's and the Royal
London Hospitals; Professor of Molecular
Medicine, Queen Mary's School of Medicine
and Dentistry, London, UK

John McAuley MA MD FRCP
Consultant Neurologist, St Bartholomew's,
the Royal London Hospital and King George's
Hospitals; Honorary Senior Lecturer, Queen
Mary's School of Medicine and Dentistry,
London, UK

Michael Millar MB BCh MD FRCPath
Consultant Microbiologist, St Bartholomew's
and the Royal London Hospitals, London, UK

John Monson MD FRCP FRCPI
Clinical Centre for Endocrinology, London;
Emeritus Professor of Clinical Endocrinology,
Queen Mary's School of Medicine and Dentistry,
London, UK

John Moore-Gillon MA MD FRCP
Consultant General and Respiratory Physician,
St Bartholomew's and the Royal London
Hospitals, London, UK

Serge Nikolic MD FRCA
Clinical Lecturer in Anaesthesia, Queen Mary's
School of Medicine and Dentistry, London, UK

Nicholas Plowman MA MD FCRP FRCR
Consultant Clinical Oncologist,
St Bartholomew's and the Royal London
Hospitals and The Hospital for Sick Children,
London, UK

Jeremy Powell-Tuck MD FCRP
Consultant Gastroenterologist, St Bartholomew's
and the Royal London Hospitals; Professor of
Clinical Nutrition, Queen Mary's School of
Medicine and Dentistry, London, UK

Drew Provan MD FRCP FRCPath
Consultant Haematologist, St Bartholomew's
and the Royal London Hospitals, London, UK

Howard Ring MD MRCPsych
Consultant Psychiatrist, Cambridge and
Peterborough Mental Health NHS Trust;
Lecturer in Psychiatry, University of Cambridge,
Cambridge, UK

Michael Swash MD FRCP FRCPath
Honorary Consulting Neurologist,
St Bartholomew's and the Royal London
Hospitals; Emeritus Professor of Neurology,
Queen Mary's School of Medicine and Dentistry,
London, UK

Raj Thuraisingham MD MRCP
Consultant Nephrologist, St Bartholomew's and
the Royal London Hospitals, London, UK

Adam Timmis MA MD FRCP
Consultant Cardiologist, London Chest and the
Royal London Hospitals; Professor of Clinical
Cardiology, Queen Mary's School of Medicine
and Dentistry, London, UK

Michael Wareing MB BS BSc FRCS(ORL-HNS)
Consultant Otolaryngologist, Head and Neck
Surgeon, St Bartholomew's and the Royal
London Hospitals, London, UK

Contents

Section 5   Ethics   495

Appendices   507

SECTION 1

The approach to the patient

Section contents

Doctor and patient: General principles of history taking

M. Swash, M. Glynn

1

INTRODUCTION

The word 'patient' is derived from the Latin *patiens*, meaning sufferance or forbearance. The overall purpose of medical practice is to relieve suffering. In order to achieve this purpose, it is important to make a diagnosis, to know how to approach treatment, and to design an appropriate scheme of management for each patient. It is therefore essential to understand each person as fully as possible, whatever their social class or ethnic and cultural background. The thorough doctor will not only elucidate the problems posed by disease, but also apply his or her skill to advise patients and families how to manage these problems. The distinction between cure of disease and relief of symptoms remains as valid today as in the past. No patient should leave a medical consultation feeling that nothing can be done to help them, even when the disease is incurable.

Clinical methods – the skills doctors use to achieve this aim of excellence in clinical practice – are acquired during a lifetime of medical work. Indeed, they evolve and change as new techniques and concepts arise, and as the doctor develops in experience and maturity. Clinical methods are acquired by a combination of study and experience, and there is always something new to learn.

The initial aims of any first consultation are to understand the patient's own perception of their problem and to start or complete the process of diagnosis. This double aim requires a knowledge of disease and its patterns of presentation, together with an ability to interpret a patient's symptoms and signs. Appropriate skills are needed to elicit the symptoms from the patient's description and conversation, and the signs by observation and physical examination. Difficulties posed by assessing the patients themselves, or by the variety of cultural and ethnic backgrounds found in modern life, must be accepted and factored into the interpretation of the data acquired during the consultation. This requires not only experience and considerable knowledge of people in general, but also the skill and interest in people to strike up a relationship with a range of very different individuals.

There are two main steps to making a diagnosis:

- To establish the clinical features by history and examination – this represents the clinical database
- To interpret the clinical database in terms of disordered function and potential causative pathologies, whether physical, mental, social, or a combination of these.

This book is about this process. This chapter introduces the basic principles of history and examination; more detail about the history and examination of each system (cardiovascular, respiratory and so forth) is set out in the individual succeeding chapters.

SETTING THE SCENE

Most medical encounters or consultations occur not in the wards but in an outpatient or primary care setting. Stability to the context of the consultation, including the consulting room environment itself, the waiting area and all the associated staff, makes the process of clinical diagnosis easier. Although the environment may be unfamiliar for the patient, the doctor needs to be able to make an assessment against a constant background. Patients are less often assessed in their own home than in the past, and when a doctor is asked to do this considerable skill may be needed.

Meeting the patient in the waiting room allows the doctor to make an early assessment of their demeanour, their hearing, their walking and any accompanying persons. Offer a greeting and make an introduction. Observe the response unobtrusively, but with care. Patients are easily confused by medical titles and hierarchies. All of the following questions should be quickly assessed: Does the patient smile, or appear furtive or anxious? Do they make good eye contact? Are they frightened or depressed? Are posture and stance normal? Is the patient short of breath, or wheezing? In some conditions (e.g. congestive heart failure, uraemia, Parkinson's disease, stroke, severe anaemia, jaundice) the nature of the problem is often immediately obvious. It is very important to identify the patient correctly, particularly if they have a name that is very common in the local community. Carefully check the full name, date of birth and address. Make sure any previous records you have are those of the correct patient, not of someone else with a similar name.

Pleasant surroundings are very important. It is essential that both patient and doctor feel at ease, and especially that neither feels threatened by the encounter. Avoid having patients full-face across a desk. Note taking is important during consultations, while being able to see the patient and establish eye contact, and to show sympathy and awareness of their needs during the discussion of symptoms, many of which may be distressing or even embarrassing. Arrange the seating so that it is clear the patient is the centre of attention, rather than any others present.

HISTORY TAKING

Having overcome the strangeness of meeting and talking to a wide variety of people that they might not ordinarily meet, the new medical student usually feels that history taking ought to be fairly simple but that physical examination is full of pitfalls, such as unrecognized heart murmurs and confusing parts of the neurological examination. However, the experienced doctor comes to realize that history taking is immensely skilled and fascinating. The extent to which history-taking skill increases with experience is much greater than that for clinical examination.

BEGINNING THE HISTORY

The process of information gathering may actually begin by reading any referral documentation and with the immediate introduction of doctor and patient. However, once the social introductions are achieved the doctor will usually begin with a single opening question. Broadly, there are two ways to do this.

A single open-ended question along the lines of 'Tell me what has led to you coming here today' gives the patient the chance to begin with what they feel is most important to them, and avoids any pre-judgement of issues, or the exclusion of what at first may seem less important. However, at this stage the patient may be very anxious and nervous, and still making their own assessment of how they will react to the doctor as a person. Therefore, a beginning that focuses on issues that may be more factual and less emotive can be more rewarding and lead to a more satisfactory consultation. Box 1.1 lists some of the areas of questioning that can be usefully included at the beginning of the history. It is important to inform the patient that this is going to be the order of things, so that they do not feel that their

> **Box 1.1   Areas of questioning that can be covered at the beginning of history taking**
>
> - Confirm date of birth and age
> - Occupational history
> - Social history
> - Past medical history
> - Smoking
> - Alcohol consumption
> - Family history

pressing problems are being ignored. A statement along the lines of 'Before we discuss why you have come today, I want to ask you some background questions' should inform the patient satisfactorily.

There is a particular logic in taking the past medical history at this stage. For many conditions that patients may bring to a new doctor, the distinction between what is a current problem and what is past history is unclear and arbitrary. A patient presenting with an acute exacerbation of chronic obstructive pulmonary disease may have a history of respiratory problems going back many years. Therefore, taking the history along a 'time line' will often build up a much better picture of all of the patient's problems, how they have developed, and how they now interact with their life and work. Many doctors find out about the social background and family history at this point, as this information then stands on its own, unaffected by the context of the patient's own symptoms, which are as yet unspoken.

Once these preliminaries have been completed, the doctor should use a simple and open-ended question to encourage the patient to give a full and free account of the current issues. Encourage the patient – at least initially – to tell their own story without interruption from spouse, carer, or anyone else present: they can have their say later. Use a phrase such as 'Tell me what has led to you coming here today', or 'What's the problem today?'. This leaves as open as possible any question about the cause of the patient's problems and why they are seeing a doctor, and could give rise to an initial answer, beginning with such varied phrases as 'I have this pain...', 'I feel depressed...', 'I am extremely worried about...', 'I don't know but my family doctor thought...', 'My wife insisted...', or even 'I thought you would already know from the letter my family doctor wrote to you'. All these answers are perfectly valid, but each gives a different clue as to what are the real issues for the patient, and how to develop the history-taking process further for that patient. Try to understand the patient's mood: sometimes the response to your initial question will be vague or concrete, or even hostile; the latter suggests emotional conflict and needs to be talked through.

This initial part of the history is particularly important and highly dependent on the skill of the doctor. It is very tempting to interrupt too early, but once interrupted the patient rarely completes what they were intending to say. Even when they appear to have finished giving their reasons for the consultation, always ask if there are any more broad areas that still need discussion, before beginning to discuss each in more detail.

DEVELOPING THEMES

This stage of the history is likely to see the patient continuing to talk much more than the doctor, but it remains vital for the doctor to steer and mould the process so that the information gathered is complete, coherent and, if possible, logical. Some patients will present a clear, concise and chronologically perfect history with little prompting, although these are in a minority. For most patients the doctor will need to do a substantial amount of clarifying and summarizing, with statements such as 'You mean that…', 'Can I go back to when…', Can I check I have understood…', So up to that point you…' , 'I am afraid I am not at all clear about…', and ' I really do not understand; can we go over that again?'. If a patient clearly indicates that they do not wish to discuss particular aspects of the history, this wish must be respected and the diagnosis based on what information is available. Always try to have a conversation with your patient. Never interrogate unless it is absolutely necessary.

NON-VERBAL COMMUNICATION
During any consultation non-verbal communication is as important as what the patient says. There may be obvious contradictions, such as a patient who does not admit to any worries or anxieties but who clearly looks as if they have many. Particular gestures during the description of pain symptoms can give vital clinical clues (Box 1.2). While concentrating on the conversation with the patient, the doctor should remain aware of other clues.

VOCABULARY
It is very important to use vocabulary the patient will understand and use appropriately. This under-standing needs to be at two levels: they must understand the basic words used, and their interpretation of those words must be understood and clarified by the doctor. Box 1.3 lists words and phrases that may be used and which the doctor needs to be very careful to clarify with the patient. If the patient uses one of the ordinary English words listed, their meaning must be clarified. A patient who says they are dizzy could be describing actual vertigo, but could just mean light-headedness or a feeling that they were going to faint. A patient saying that they have diarrhoea could mean liquid stools passed hourly throughout the day and night, or could mean a couple of urgent soft stools passed first thing in the morning only. Therefore, the doctor needs to use words that are almost certainly going to be clearly understood by the patient, and must clarify any word or phrase the patient uses, to avoid any possibility of ambiguity.

Box 1.3 Words and phrases that need clarification

Ordinary English words
- Diarrhoea
- Constipation
- Wind
- Indigestion
- Being sick
- Dizziness
- Blackouts
- Headache
- Double vision
- Pins and needles
- Rash
- Blister

Medical terms that may be used imprecisely by patients
- Arthritis
- Sciatica
- Migraine
- Fits
- Stroke
- Palpitation
- Angina
- Heart attack
- Diarrhoea
- Constipation
- Nausea
- Piles/haemorrhoids
- Anaemia
- Pleurisy
- Eczema
- Urticaria
- Warts
- Cystitis

Box 1.2 Particular gestures useful in analysing specific pain symptoms

- A squeezing gesture to describe cardiac pain
- Hand position to describe renal colic
- Rubbing the sternum to describe heartburn
- Rubbing the buttock and thigh to describe sciatica
- Arms clenched around the abdomen to describe midgut colic

INDIRECT AND DIRECT QUESTIONS

Broadly, questions asked by the doctor can be divided into indirect or open-ended and direct or closed. Indirect or open-ended questions can be regarded as an invitation for the patient to talk about the general area that the doctor indicates is of interest. These questions will often start with phrases such as 'Tell me more about…', 'What do you think about…', 'How does that make you feel…', 'What happened next…' or 'Is there anything else you would like to tell me…'. They inform the patient that the agenda is very much with them, that they can talk about whatever is important, and that the doctor has not prejudged any issues. If skilfully used, and if the doctor is sensitive to the clues presented in the answers, a series of such questions should allow the doctor to understand the issues that are most important to the patient. The patient will also be allowed to describe things in their own words. Always listen carefully, and maintain eye contact. Do not take too many notes!

Many patients are in awe of doctors and have a conscious or subconscious need to please and agree. If the doctor prejudges the patient's problems and tends to direct the conversation to fit the diagnosis that they have assumed too early, the patient can easily go along with this and give simple answers that do not fully describe their situation. Box 1.4 illustrates this extremely simple, common and important pitfall of history taking.

Box 1.4   Example of a history that leads to a poor conclusion

A general practitioner (GP) is seeing a 58-year-old man who is known to be hypertensive and a smoker. The receptionist has already documented that he is coming with a problem of chest pain. The GP makes an automatic assumption that the pain is most likely to be angina pectoris, because that is probably the most serious possible cause and the one that the patient is likely to be most worried about, and starts taking the history with the specific purpose of confirming or refuting that diagnosis.

GP:	I gather you've had some chest pain?
Patient:	Yes, it's been quite bad.
GP:	Is it in the middle of your chest?
Patient:	Yes.
GP:	And does it travel to your left arm?
Patient:	Yes – and to my shoulder.
GP:	Does it come on when you walk?
Patient:	Yes.
GP:	And is it relieved by rest?
Patient:	Yes – usually.
GP:	I'm afraid I think this is angina and I will need to refer you to a heart specialist.

The GP has only asked very direct and closed questions. Each answer has begun with 'Yes'. The patient has already been quite firmly tagged with a 'label' of angina, and anxiety has been raised by the specialist referral.

Alternatively, the GP keeps an open mind and starts as follows:

GP:	Tell me why you have come to see me today.
Patient:	Well, I have been having some chest pain.
GP:	Tell me more about what it's like.
Patient:	It's in the centre of my chest and tends to go to my left arm. Sometimes it comes on when I've been walking.
GP:	Tell me more about that.
Patient:	Sometimes it comes when I am walking and sometimes when I'm sitting down at home after a long walk.
GP:	If the pain comes on when you are walking, what do you do?
Patient:	I usually slow down, but if I'm in a hurry I can walk on with the pain.
GP:	I am a little worried that this might be angina but some things suggest it might not be, so I am going to refer you to a heart specialist to make sure it isn't angina.

The GP has asked questions which are either completely open-ended or leave the patient free to describe exactly what happens within a directed area of interest. Clarifying questions have been used. While being reassuring, the GP expresses some concern about angina and is clear about the exact reason for the specialist referral (for clarification).

PATIENT-CENTRED

An interview that uses lots of direct questions is often 'disease-centred', whereas a 'patient-centred' interview will contain enough open-ended questions for the patient to talk through all their problems, as well as providing sufficient time. This will help to avoid the situation in which the doctor and the patient have different agendas. There can often appear to be a conflict if the patient complains of symptoms that are probably not medically serious, such as tension headache, while the doctor is focusing on some potentially serious but relatively asymptomatic condition such as anaemia or hypertension. In this situation a patient-centred approach will allow the patient to air all of their problems, and allow a skilled doctor to educate the patient as to why the other issues are also important and must not be ignored. The doctor needs to grasp the difference between the *disease framework* (what is the diagnosis?) and the *illness framework* (what are the patient's experiences, ideas, expectations and feelings?), and to be able to apply both to a clinical situation, varying the degree of each according to the differing demands.

JUDGING THE SEVERITY OF SYMPTOMS

Many symptoms are subjective and their severity will depend on the patient's personal reaction and how the symptoms interact with their life. A tiny alteration in the neurological function of the hands and fingers will have a huge impact on a professional musician, whereas most others might scarcely notice the same dysfunction. A mild skin complaint might be devastating for a professional model, but cause little worry in others.

Trying to assess how the symptoms interact with the patient's life is an important aspect of history taking. A simple question such as 'How much does this bother you?' might suffice. It may be helpful to ask specific questions about how daily life is affected and in what way, with comparison to events that many patients will experience. Box 1.5 illustrates some of the relevant areas.

Medical symptomatology often involves pain, a symptom that is inevitably subjective. Many patients are stoical and bear severe pain uncomplainingly, whereas others seem to complain much more about apparently less severe pain. A simple pain scale can be very helpful in assessing the severity of pain. The patient is asked to rate their pain on a scale from 1 to 10, where 1 is pain that is barely noticeable and 10 is the worst pain they can imagine, or the worst pain they have ever experienced. It is also useful to clarify what is their reference point for '10', which for many women will be the pain of labour. The pain scale assessment is useful in diagnosis, and in monitoring disease, treatment and analgesia. Assessing a patient with pain is discussed in more detail in Chapter 24.

WHICH ISSUES ARE IMPORTANT

A problem to doctors who wish to take the history in chronological order – 'Start at the beginning and tell me all about it' – is that people usually start with what they regard as most important to them. This is, of course, entirely relevant and is also important to the doctor, as the issue that most bothers the patient is then brought to attention. Sometimes the history actually begins long before the patient recognizes. It is important to be aware of the most important symptoms, as, for example, pain may be relieved even though the underlying cause is still present. It is very common for a doctor to be pleased that a condition has been resolved, but the patient still complains of the main symptom that they originally presented with.

Unrelated information, introduced by the patient apparently out of context, is often of particular importance. When presented with another, apparently disparate point, the doctor should note it carefully and come back to it later. It may fall naturally into place, but it may also be a clue to the nature of the underlying disorder. For example, the patient with fatigue may describe a fleeting rash or joint pain that suggests systemic lupus erythematosus as the underlying cause.

A SCHEMATIC HISTORY

A suggested schematic history is detailed in Box 1.6. There will be many clinical situations where it will be clear that a different scheme should be followed. An important part of learning about history taking is that each doctor develops their own personal scheme that works for them in the situations that they generally deal with. Nevertheless, it is useful to start with a basic outline in mind.

Box 1.5 Areas of everyday life that can be used as a reference for the severity, importance or clarification of symptoms

Exercise tolerance: 'How far can you walk on the flat going at your own speed?' 'Can you climb one flight of stairs slowly without stopping?' 'Can you still do simple housework, such as vacuum cleaning or making a bed?'

Work: 'Has this problem kept you off work?' ' Why exactly have you not been able to work?'

Sport: 'Do you play regular sport, and has this been affected?'

Eating: 'Has this affected your eating?' 'Do any particular foods cause trouble?'

Social life: 'What do you do in your spare time, and has this been restricted in any way?' 'Has your sex life been affected?'

Box 1.6 Suggested scheme for basic history taking

- Name, age, occupation, country of birth, other clarification of identity
- Main presenting problem
- Past medical history – 'Before we talk about why you have come I need to ask you to tell me about any medical problems you have had in the past'.
- Specific past medical history – e.g. diabetes, jaundice, TB, heart disease, high blood pressure, rheumatic fever, epilepsy
- History of main presenting problem
- Family history
- Occupational history
- Smoking, alcohol, allergies
- Drug and other treatment history
- Direct questions about bodily systems not covered by the presenting complaint

Box 1.7 Bodily systems and questions relevant to taking a full history from most patients. If the specific questions have been covered by the history of the presenting problem they do not need to be included again. If the answers are positive then the characteristics of each must be clarified

Cardiorespiratory
- Chest pain
- Intermittent claudication
- Palpitation
- Ankle swelling
- Orthopnoea
- Nocturnal dyspnoea
- Shortness of breath
- Cough with or without sputum
- Haemoptysis

Gastrointestinal
- Abdominal pain
- Dyspepsia
- Dysphagia
- Nausea and/or vomiting
- Change in appetite
- Weight loss or gain
- Bowel pattern and any change
- Rectal bleeding
- Jaundice

Genitourinary
- Haematuria
- Nocturia
- Frequency
- Dysuria
- Menstrual irregularity – women
- Urethral discharge – men

Locomotor
- Joint pain
- Change in mobility

Neurological
- Seizures
- Collapse or blackouts
- Dizziness and loss of balance
- Vision
- Hearing
- Transient loss of function (vision, speech, sight)
- Paraesthesiae
- Weakness
- Wasting
- Spasms and involuntary movements
- Pain in limbs and back
- Headache

DIRECT QUESTIONS ABOUT BODILY SYSTEMS

Many disease processes have features that occur in several bodily systems that at first may not seem to be related to the patient's main complaint. For example, a patient presenting with back pain may have had some haematuria from the renal cell carcinoma that has spread and is causing pain. For this reason, any thorough assessment must include questions about all bodily systems, and not just areas that the patient perceives as problematic. This area of questioning should be introduced with a statement such as: 'Now I am going to ask you some extra questions'. A list of such question areas is given in Box 1.7.

In addition, during any medical consultation, however brief, the doctor must be alert to all aspects of the patient's health and not just the area or problem with which they have presented. For example, a general practitioner would not ignore a high blood pressure reading in a patient presenting with a rash, even though the two are probably not connected. This function of any consultation can be regarded as 'screening' the patient. Screening a whole population for a disease is a different issue, but once the patient has attended a doctor, a simple screening process can be incorporated into the consultation with little extra time or effort. The direct questions (and full routine examination) encompass this screening function as well as contributing to solving the patients' presenting problems.

CLARIFYING DETAIL

One of the basic principles of history taking is not to take what the patient says at face value but to clarify it as much as possible. Almost all of the history will involve clarification, but there are specific areas where this is particularly important.

PAIN

Whenever a patient complains of pain there should follow a series of clarifying questions as listed in

Box 1.8. Of all symptoms, pain is perhaps the most subjective and the hardest for the doctor to truly comprehend. A simple pain scale has been described above. The other characteristics are vital in analysing what might be the cause of pain. Some painful conditions have classic sites for the pain and the radiation (myocardial ischaemia is classically felt in the centre of the chest, radiating to the left arm). Pain from a hollow organ is classically colicky (such as biliary or renal colic). The pain of a subarachnoid haemorrhage is classically very sudden, 'like a hammer blow on the head'. Some pains have clear aggravating or relieving factors (peptic ulcer pain is classically worse when hungry and better after food). Colicky right upper quadrant abdominal pain accompanied by jaundice suggests a gallstone obstructing the bile duct; headache accompanied by preceding flashing lights suggests migraine. Some of these points will come out in the open-ended part of the history taking, but others will need specific questions.

DRUG HISTORY

At first glance, asking a patient what drugs they are taking would seem to be one of the simplest and most reliable parts of taking a history. In practice this could not be further from the case, and there are many pitfalls for the inexperienced. This is partly because many patients are not very knowledgeable about their own medications, and also because patients often misinterpret the question, giving a very narrow answer when the doctor wants to know about medications in the widest sense. The need for clarification in the drug history is given in Box 1.9. This part of the history, almost more than any other, benefits from being repeated at another time and in a slightly different way. For example, in trying to define a possible drug reaction as a cause of liver dysfunction it is not unusual to find that the patient has taken a few relevant tablets (such as over-the-counter non-steroidal analgesics) just before the onset of the problem, and only remembered or realized it was important when asked repeatedly in great detail.

FAMILY HISTORY

Like the drug history, the family history would seem at first glance to be simple and reliably quoted. In general this is true, but it can be dissected into sections that will uncover more information if covered in detail. These are set out in Box 1.10.

OCCUPATIONAL HISTORY

It is always useful to know the patient's occupation, if they have one, as it is such an important part of their life and one with which any illness is bound to interact. In some situations their occupation will be directly relevant to the diagnostic process. Other problems, such as asbestos exposure or silicosis, produce effects many years after exposure, and a careful chronological occupational history may be required to elucidate the exposure. For patients with non-organic problems the work environment can often trigger the development of the problem.

ALCOHOL HISTORY

The detrimental effects of alcohol on health cause a variety of problems, and the frequency of excess alcohol usage in western countries means that up to 10% of adult hospital inpatients have a problem related to alcohol. To accurately estimate alcohol consumption and any possible dependency, it is essential to enquire carefully and not to take what the patient says at face value, but to probe the history in different ways (Box 1.11). For documentation purposes, the reported amount should then be converted into units of alcohol per week (Box 1.12). If the reported amount seems at all excessive then an assessment should be made of possible dependency, for which the CAGE questions are very useful (Box 1.13).

RETROSPECTIVE HISTORY

The concept of retrospective history taking is a refinement of taking the past medical history and develops the theme of never taking what the patient says at face value. Many patients will clearly say that they have had certain illnesses or previous symptoms using medical terminology. This may not be accurate, either because the patient has misinterpreted the information, or because they were given the wrong information or diagnosis in the first place. This area becomes particularly important if any new diagnosis is going to rely on this type of information. For instance, in assessing a patient with chest pain a past history of angina will be considered a risk factor for ischaemic heart disease and increase the likelihood of that being the current diagnosis. However, on closer questioning it might become clear that what the patient was told was angina (perhaps by a relative and not even a doctor) was in fact a vague chest ache coming on after a period of heavy work, and not a clear central chest pain coming on during exertion. The degree to which past history is re-examined in detail will vary according to the case being analysed.

PARTICULAR SITUATIONS

It is true to say that although there are many themes, patterns and common areas to history taking – and some areas might seem routine – the process of history taking in no two patients will be identical. There are some particular and often challenging situations that deserve further description

GARRULOUS PATIENTS

A new medical student will meet a patient who says a huge amount without really revealing the information that goes towards a useful medical history. This will be in marked contrast to others, who from the first introductory question (e.g. 'Tell me about what has led up to you coming here today') will reveal a perfect history with virtually no prompting. A fictitious but typical history from the former type of

Box 1.11 Probing the alcohol history

Doctor: Do you drink any alcoholic drinks?
Patient: Oh yes, but not much – just socially.
Doctor: Do you drink some every day?
Patient: Yes.
Doctor: Tell me what you drink.
Patient: I usually have two pints of beer at lunchtime and two or three on my way home from work.
Doctor: And at the weekend?
Paitent: I usually go out Saturday nights and have four or five pints.
Doctor: Do you drink anything other than beer?
Patient: On Saturdays I have a double whisky with each pint.

The first answer does not suggest a problem. Based on the figures in Box 1.12, however, the actual amount adds up to 70 units per week, which clearly confers a considerable health risk to this patient.

Box 1.12 Units of alcohol (1 unit contains 10 g of pure alcohol)

Standard-strength beer – 1 pint = 2 units
Very strong lagers – 1 litre can = 4 units
Spirits (whisky, gin etc.) – 1 UK pub measure (approx 30 ml) = 1 unit
Wine – 1 standard glass = 1 unit

The upper weekly limit to avoid any health problems related to alcohol is 21 units for a man and 14 for a woman.

Box 1.13 The CAGE assessment for alcohol dependency

C – Have you ever felt the need to Cut down your alcohol consumption?
A – Have you ever felt Angry at others criticising your drinking?
G – Do you ever feel Guilty about excess drinking?
E – Do you ever drink in the mornings (Eye-opener)?

patient is given in Box 1.14. When faced with such a patient the doctor will need to significantly alter the balance of open-ended and direct questions. Open-ended questions will tend to lead to the patient giving a long recitation with little useful content. The doctor will have to use many more clear, direct questions which may just have yes/no answers. The overall history will inevitably be less

Doctor: 'Tell me what has led to you coming here today.'

Patient: 'Well Doctor, you see it was like this, I woke up one day last week – I'm not quite sure which day it was – it might have been Tuesday – or no, I remember it was Monday because my son came round later to visit – he always comes on a Monday because that's his day off College – he's studying law – I'm so pleased that he's settled down to that – he was so wild when he was younger – do you know what he did once…'

Doctor (interrupting):   'Can you tell me what did happen when you woke up last Monday?'

Patient: Oh yes – it was like this – I am not sure what woke me up – it may have been the pain – no – more likely it was the dustmen collecting the rubbish – they do come so early and make such a noise – that day it was even worse because their usual dustcart must have been broken and they came with this really old noisy one…'

Doctor (interrupting):   'So you had some pain when you woke up then?'

Patient: Yes – I think it must have been there when I woke up because I lay in bed wondering where on earth there might be some indigestion remedy – I knew I had some but I am one of those people who can never remember where things are – do you know what I managed to lose last year…'

Doctor (interrupting):   'Was the pain burning or crushing?'

Patient: 'Well that depends on what you mean by…'

Doctor (interrupting):   'Yes but did you have any crushing pain?'

The doctor gradually changes from very open-ended to very closed questions in order to try and get some information that is useful to building up the diagnostic picture – eventually a question is asked that just has a yes/no answer. The information may not be reliable.

satisfactory, but it is never possible to get the 'perfect' history in every patient.

ANGRY PATIENTS

Not many patients are overtly angry when they see a doctor, but anger expressed during a consultation may be an important diagnostic clue while at the same time getting in the way of a smooth diagnostic process. Some patients will be angry with the immediate circumstances, such as a late-running clinic.

Others will have longer-term anger against the surgery, department or institution, which will be more difficult to address. It is always important to acknowledge anger, try and discover what underlies it, and apologise for simple things such as late running.

In some patients anger may be part of the symptomatology, or expressed as a reaction to the diagnosis or treatment. This will be particularly true in patients with a non-organic diagnosis who insist that there is 'something wrong' and that the doctor must do something. Many types of presentation will fall into this grouping, including tension headache, irritable bowel and back pain. There may be obvious secondary gain for the patient (such as staying off work and claiming benefits), and challenging this pattern of behaviour may provoke anger.

Occasionally it may be best to acknowledge that the doctor–patient relationship has broken down and that facilitating a change to another doctor may be in the best interests of the patient.

THE WELL-INFORMED PATIENT

Twenty or more years ago doctors often looked after patients for a long time without really explaining their illness to them, and patients were reasonably happy about this, taking the attitude that 'the doctor knows best'. This approach is now unacceptable, and the doctor must give the patient as much information about their illness as possible, particularly so that they can make informed choices about treatments. This change of approach has led to many patients seeking information about their problems from other sources, particularly the Internet.

The doctor must take all this in their stride, go through the information with the patient, and help them by showing what is relevant and what is not. In general it is much easier and more rewarding to look after well-informed patients, provided they do not fall into the very small group who have such fixed and erroneous ideas about their problems that the diagnostic and treatment process is impeded.

ACCOMPANYING PERSONS

Some people come to consultations alone, others with one or more friends or family members. Always spend time during the initial exchange of greetings to identify who is present and to get some idea of the group dynamics. There is always a reason why people come accompanied, but if there appear to be too many people present, or if the presence of others might threaten the relationship with the patient at any time in the consultation, it is appropriate to consider asking the others to leave, even if only briefly. It is reasonable to ascertain why others wish to be present, and, certainly, whether this is also the patient's wish. This is particularly difficult if the doctor does not speak the patient's language but can speak to those accompanying. Consider whether specific questions about history should be asked of those accompanying, either with the patient or separately, with specific consent.

Beware of a situation where the accompanying people answer all the questions, even if there is no language difficulty. Reasons for this may include embarrassment in front of those accompanying, such as a teenager accompanied by parents. In such circumstances it may be necessary to leave parts of the history until those accompanying can be reasonably asked to leave – for example during the physical examination. Occasionally it is clear that the patient will not talk for themselves, in which case the history from those accompanying will have to suffice.

USING INTERPRETERS/ADVOCATES

In the inner cities of western countries there are often large immigrant populations who do not speak the language of the country, even if they have been resident for some years. It is impossible for all such patients to be looked after by health professionals who speak their language, and the consultation has to be undertaken with the help of an interpreter. The most immediate solution may be to use a family member, but if the issues are private or embarrassing this often does not work well, and it is generally unwise to use an underage family member as an interpreter. The best solution is to have available an independent interpreter/advocate for the consultation, although in areas where many patients are not native speakers, many such interpreters may be needed for a range of languages. Another solution for infrequently encountered languages is a telephone interpreting service.

The history taken via an interpreter or advocate may be quite limited in subtlety by the exigencies of the double translation, and the doctor therefore often utilizes a much more direct style of questioning for which the answers will be unambiguous. Unfortunately, it is not unusual for the interpreter/advocate and the patient to have a few minutes of conversation following an apparently simple question from the doctor, but then a very short answer is returned to the doctor. This leaves the doctor bemused as to what is really going on. Finally, history taking via an interpreter/advocate usually takes much longer than when the doctor and the patient speak the same language.

NEGATIVE DATA

With experience, the analysis of the history and the process of diagnosis will begin as soon as the doctor meets the patient, and certainly as soon as the history is commenced. This means that during the initial process, and without the need for so much later review, questions can be asked for which a negative answer is as important as a positive one. These questions are usually very specific and direct, often

with a yes/no answer. A patient presenting with exertional chest pain can immediately be asked if the pain is worse on increased exertion, and how long a period of rest is needed to relieve it. Pain that is not predictably produced by exertion and is not reliably relieved by rest may well not be angina pectoris.

WHAT DOES THE PATIENT ACTUALLY WANT?

If a patient comes to a doctor with a long history it is always worth trying to find out why they have come and what they actually want from the consultation. There may be various scenarios, as listed in Box 1.15. It is always worth trying to find out which might apply to the current patient, because this sets the scene for advice and treatment, particularly if an exact diagnosis or a complete treatment cannot be provided. It is often much easier to reassure a patient that there is nothing seriously wrong, than to give them an exact diagnosis or relieve their symptoms fully.

RETAKING THE HISTORY

It is clear that history taking is an inexact process heavily influenced by the interaction between doctor and patient. The logical conclusion of this is that no two histories taken from the same patient about the same set of symptoms will be identical, even if the same doctor repeats the process. Given two slightly or significantly different histories, it may be hard to know on which one to base the diagnosis, or whether to regard history taking for that patient as so unreliable as to be useless. The main message is that a single attempt at the history may not suffice, and that repeated histories, taken at different times, by different people and in different ways, may provide just as much extra information on which to base a diagnosis as more and more detailed special investigations. When a patient is seen for a second

---

Box 1.15 General reasons for patients to come to doctors when they do (other than for a severe or acute problem)

- Cannot tolerate ongoing symptoms
- Someone else noticing specific problems (e.g. jaundice)
- Another doctor noticing specific problems (e.g. high blood pressure)
- Worry about underlying diagnosis (often induced by relatives, friends, books, media or Internet)
- Spouse or relative worried about patient
- Cannot work with symptoms
- Colleagues/bosses complaining about patient's work or time off
- Requirement of others (insurance, employment benefit, litigation)

Box 1.16   Duties of doctors registered with the UK General Medical Council

- Make the care of your patient your first concern
- Treat every patient politely and considerately
- Respect patients' dignity and privacy
- Listen to patients and respect their views
- Give patients information in a way they can understand
- Respect the right of patients to be fully involved in all decisions about their care
- Keep your professional knowledge and skills up to date
- Recognize the limits of your professional competency
- Be honest and trustworthy
- Respect and protect confidential information
- Make sure that your personal beliefs do not prejudice your patients' care
- Act quickly to protect patients from risk if you have good reason to believe that you or a colleague may not be fit to practise
- Avoid abusing your position as a doctor
- Work with colleagues in the ways that best serve patients' interests

In all these matters you must never discriminate unfairly against your patients or colleagues, and you must always be prepared to justify your actions to them.

or alternative opinion the doctor usually spends more time on retaking the history than on repeating the examination.

CONCLUSION

History taking is the essence of medical practice. It combines considerable interpersonal skill and diversity with the need for logical thought, based on a wealth of medical and general knowledge about society, and is the beginning of treating and caring for patients in the widest sense. Almost all the attributes of good medical practice as set out by the UK General Medical Council (Box 1.16) are encompassed in good history taking. Taking a detailed history while getting to know a patient and arriving at a likely diagnosis is as rewarding in itself as performing a technical procedure for a patient, or seeing them get better in the end.

2 Physical examination: General principles

M. Swash, M. Glynn

The physical examination is a time-honoured technique in medical practice. For example, methods of medical examination are described in Egyptian papyri, in the classical world of ancient Greece and Rome, and in Vedic medicine in India. Indeed, people expect their doctor to examine them as part of a medical consultation. The physical examination, as currently used, was developed in the early 19th century as a method to evaluate symptoms in relation to recognized pathologies, in order to facilitate diagnosis and treatment. It was then the only method available for assessment of patients and therefore became highly formalized – and also highly sophisticated – as early editions of this book illustrate. As modern technologies for assessment and diagnosis have become generally available, especially medical imaging, biochemical and immunological methods, and more recently, genetic testing, the features sought by the clinician during the physical examination have become more focused and more specific. None the less, the classical methods of physical examination remain valid. In particular, modern imaging methods are adjunctive to classical clinical methods and do not replace them.

The techniques for examination of the different bodily systems are described in the system specific chapters of this book. It is important to develop a routine of physical examination that combines speed with thoroughness, sensitivity and alertness, but which disturbs the patient no more than necessary. The examination must be carried out as gently as possible, without tiring the patient needlessly. In severely ill patients it may be necessary to postpone a routine examination and to perform only that required for provisional diagnosis and treatment.

Different doctors use different routines in different circumstances. Start the examination in a manner that is relevant to the patient's symptoms. For example, if the presenting symptom is sciatica, start with the legs and the spine. However, a systematic approach to each functional system is essential in order to obtain information that is both *complete* and *relevant*. This serves to remind the clinician of any omissions. Always try to be thorough. With experience you will become more confident in looking directly for certain signs suggested by the history, and then conducting a systematic examination in this context.

GENERAL APPROACH

A physical examination requires a cooperative patient and a quiet, warm and well-lit room equipped with a couch, a chair and some steps to help disabled people get on to the couch. Ideally, the couch should be capable of being raised or lowered, and of being broken at one end to provide a backrest. Daylight is better than artificial light, which may mask changes in skin colour, for example the faint yellow tinge of slight jaundice. Remember that the physical examination starts from the moment you meet the patient – you will be able to notice aspects of their general demeanour, stance, nutrition and personality at first acquaintance which will be important in your approach to the history, and, later, to the examination itself. Every moment of your contact with the patient, every gesture and every communication is full of information.

For a thorough examination the patient should be asked to undress completely, or at least to their underclothes, and to lie or sit on the couch or bed partially covered with a sheet or dressing gown. For more restricted examinations such complete exposure is not necessary. None the less, always resist the temptation to conduct an examination through clothing, which will obscure a full inspection of the part affected. Ideally a chaperone should be present when a male doctor is examining a female patient, both to reassure the patient and to protect the doctor from subsequent accusations of improper conduct. A chaperone is essential when conducting an intimate examination such as vaginal or rectal examination.

In considering the patient's general appearance, it is important to make a rapid assessment of the degree of illness. This is not making a diagnosis. Simply consider the question: 'Does this patient look well, mildly ill or severely ill, thus needing urgent attention?'. Experienced nurses are often highly skilled in this kind of assessment and their opinion should never be ignored.

Every moment of the consultation is important. Certain abnormalities may sometimes be recognized

Box 2.1 The physical examination: summary of plan of general physical examination

- Mental and emotional state
- Physical attitude
- Gait
- Physique
- Face
- Skin
- Hands
- Feet
- Neck
  - lymphatic and salivary glands
  - thyroid gland
  - pulsation
- Breasts
- Axillae
- Temperature
- Pulse
- Respiration
- Odours

as soon as you meet the patient, and you may well notice things about them during history taking. For example, shortness of breath, pallor, jaundice, parkinsonism, stroke, skin rashes and other features may be recognized immediately. Watching the patient getting undressed or dressed is often especially revealing of neurological and rheumatological disorders, and may also reveal the degree of any pain, or shortness of breath. The examination 'begins on meeting the patient, and continues until the consultation ends'. An abnormal finding on examination may indicate the need for further questions – do not hesitate to revisit the history in the light of such findings at the end of the examination. Box 2.1 shows a summary plan for the general physical examination. This should be followed when it is necessary to check the various bodily systems. Such a routine may have to be modified according to the needs of the patient – for example, the minimum necessary examination in an acutely ill patient, the examination of the nervous system in a patient with cardiac symptoms, or simply according to the circumstances.

The object of a routine examination is to check the different bodily systems to exclude abnormality. In considering symptoms related to the patient's presenting complaint a more focused and detailed examination is often necessary.

MENTAL AND EMOTIONAL STATE

Try to make some initial assessment of the patient's intelligence and mental and emotional state, but recognize that this initial impression may be inaccurate. As well as the history, observation is important in assessing the emotional state. Thus an anxious person may be restless, with wide palpebral fissures and sweating palms. Is the anxiety reasonable in the circumstances, or is the patient overanxious? In depression, the lowered mood, inability to concentrate or make decisions, mental retardation, apathy or even obvious misery may be clearly evident; however, these features may not be obvious, although they are important and lead to physical symptoms.

PHYSICAL ATTITUDE

Consider the patient's posture. Severely ill patients slip down the bed or chair into uncomfortable attitudes they are unable to correct. Patients with heart failure sit up because they may become dyspnoeic if they lie flat (*orthopnoea*). Patients with abdominal pain due to peritonitis lie still, whereas patients with colic are restless or may even roll about in a futile attempt to find relief. People with painful joint diseases often have an attitude of helplessness. Various neurological disorders produce characteristic abnormal postures (see Chapter 10).

GAIT

Always observe the gait in patients able to walk (Chapters 9 and 10). Remember that simple things such as a painful corn, an ill-fitting shoe or a strained muscle may produce a temporary limp. The gait is best observed as the patient walks into the consulting room, before the formal assessment commences, because at this time the patient usually feels unobserved and this is their natural gait. Under formal examination the gait may appear more abnormal, as the patient may then try to demonstrate certain subjective abnormalities to the physician.

GENERAL APPEARANCE

Much can be learned from a general inspection of the patient's physique. Is the appearance consistent with the patient's chronological age? Is he or she tall, short, fat, thin, muscular or asthenic? Are there any obvious deformities, and is the body proportionate? Height should be roughly equal to the fingertip-to-fingertip measurement of the outstretched arms, and twice the leg length from pubis to heel. Obesity is mostly a problem of developed countries. In some parts of the world signs of malnutrition, such as wasting, apathy, anaemia and skin changes, may be encountered; they should also be looked for in neglected elderly patients in developed countries. A history of weight gain or loss can be checked by observation, remembering that fluid retention (*oedema*) will increase weight. Obvious weight loss, even when food intake has increased, is a feature of thyrotoxicosis and diabetes mellitus.

15

Psychogenic loss of appetite usually affecting girls (*anorexia nervosa*) causes extreme emaciation while physical activity remains unimpaired.

FACIAL APPEARANCE

Observe the patient's face. The expression, and particularly the eyes, indicates real feelings better than words. Some diseases, for example Parkinson's disease, depression, hypothyroidism, thyrotoxicosis, acromegaly, third and seventh cranial nerve palsies and paralysis of the cervical sympathetic nerve (Horner's syndrome), produce characteristic facial appearances. *Parotid swellings* are obvious on inspection of the face. The cheeks give information regarding the patient's health: in anaemia and hypopituitarism they are pale; in the nephrotic syndrome they are pale and puffy; in cases of mitral stenosis there is sometimes a bright circumscribed flush over the malar bones; in many persons who lead an open-air life they are red and highly coloured; in congestive heart failure they may also be highly coloured, but the colour is of a bluish tint which cannot be mistaken for the red cheeks of weather-beaten people. In some cases of systemic lupus erythematosus there is a red raised eruption on the bridge of the nose that extends on to the cheeks in a 'butterfly' distribution. *Telangiectases*, minute capillary tortuosities, or *naevi*, may be seen on the face in liver disease and, rarely, as a hereditary disorder.

THE SKIN

The detailed examination of the skin is described in Chapter 11. The most important abnormalities in the skin relevant to general examination are *pallor, yellowness, pigmentation* and *cyanosis*. In dehydration the skin is dry and inelastic so that it can be pinched up into a ridge. The skin is atrophied by age, and sometimes after treatment with glucocorticoids. In acromegaly it is thickened, greasy and loose.

Pallor depends on the thickness and quality of the skin, and the amount and quality of the blood in the capillaries. Pallor occurs in persons with thick or opaque skins, who are always pale; in hypopituitarism; in states where the blood flow in the capillaries is diminished, such as shock, syncope or left heart failure; locally in a limb deprived of its blood supply; or in the fingers or toes when arterial spasm occurs on exposure to cold, as in Raynaud's disease. Generalized pallor may also occur in severe anaemia. Anaemia, however, is a feature of 'the colour of the blood rather than that of the patient' and the colour of the skin may be misleading. The colour of the mucous membranes of the mouth and conjunctivae gives a better indication, as does the colour of the creases of the palm of the hand.

Yellowness is usually due to jaundice. A pale lemon-yellow tint is characteristic of haemolytic jaundice; in obstructive jaundice there is a dark yellow or orange tint. In obstructive jaundice there may be scratch marks from itching evoked by bile salts. In rare cases yellowness may be due to carotenaemia.

Pigmentation (see Chapter 11) is most commonly racial. The pigmentation of Addison's disease affects the buccal mucous membranes as well as exposed skin and parts subject to friction. In von Recklinghausen's disease (neurofibromatosis type 1) patches of café au lait (milky coffee) pigment, ranging from freckling of the axillae to large (>5 cm in length) areas on the limbs, trunk or face, are a characteristic feature.

Cyanosis is a bluish colour of the skin and mucous membranes owing to the presence of reduced haemoglobin in the blood. A similar bluish or leaden colour rarely may be produced by methaemoglobinaemia or sulphaemoglobinaemia, usually due to the taking of certain drugs, such as phenacetin. This should be considered in any patient who is cyanosed but not breathless. Carbon monoxide poisoning produces a generalized cherry-red discoloration, owing to the presence of carboxy-haemoglobin.

Oedema is an excess of fluid in the subcutaneous tissue causing swelling of the tissues. In *dependent oedema*, which is typically present in congestive heart failure, and in conditions associated with a low plasma protein level, the swelling first appears at the ankles and over the dorsum of the foot, and only gradually involves the legs, thighs and trunk. In local venous obstruction the oedema is confined to the parts from which the return of blood is impeded. Oedema of the whole upper part of the body may result from intrathoracic tumours. Oedema can be recognized by the pallid and glossy appearance of the skin over the swollen part, by its doughy feel, and by the fact that it pits on finger pressure. In bed-bound patients oedema often appears first over the sacrum. To recognize pitting oedema it is important to press firmly and for a sustained period, and the 'pit' is as easily felt as seen. The oedema of lymphatic obstruction does *not* pit on pressure.

Subcutaneous emphysema is uncommon, but if present can be recognized by the crackling sensation produced by lightly compressing the part affected.

THE HANDS

The patient's hands should be carefully examined. A range of abnormalities may be present in the structure and function of the hands, including evidence of arthritis, neurological disease, liver disease anaemia and acromegaly. Classic appearances that should always be sought include finger clubbing, nailbed 'splinter' haemorrhages, Dupuytren's contracture, and *koilonychia*, which occurs in long-standing iron-deficiency anaemia. *Tremor* should be assessed carefully, distinguishing between a fine tremor such as that due to thyrotoxicosis and the coarse jerky tremor of metabolic encephalopathy. In *hypertrophic pulmonary osteoarthropathy,* besides clubbing of the fingers there is tender thickening of the periosteum of the radius, ulna, tibia and fibula.

THE FEET

The feet must not remain obscured under bedclothes or socks during the examination. *Pitting oedema* may be recognized only in the ankles and dorsal surfaces of the feet. The condition of the skin of the feet is especially important in diabetics and the elderly. *Peripheral vascular disease* will make the skin shiny, and hair does not grow on ischaemic legs or feet. The dorsalis pedis and posterior tibial pulses may be reduced or absent. If the toes of an ischaemic foot are compressed their dull purple colour will blanch and only slowly return. Passive elevation of an ischaemic leg will cause marked pallor of the foot as perfusion against gravity falls. Painless trophic lesions, often with deep ulceration, on the soles are seen frequently in diabetic peripheral neuropathy (the diabetic foot).

THE NECK

The neck should be inspected and palpated. Swellings in the neck are usually best felt from behind. Careful note should be taken of lymph glands (see Chapter 19) and the thyroid (see Chapter 12). Carefully assess the major arteries and veins palpable in the neck (see Chapter 7).

THE BREASTS

The chance of finding a treatable cancer should make a full examination of the breasts a necessary feature of every general examination of a woman over 30 years of age (see Chapter 25). Any swelling of the male breast is likely to be seen at a glance. The swelling can be distinguished as breast tissue rather than pectoral fat by palpating when the patient's hands are behind his head. At some stage of puberty the majority of normal boys will have a palpable disc of breast tissue beneath the areola.

In women, start with the patient sitting to assess asymmetry, a visible mass, distortion or skin tethering (Fig. 2.1). Involvement of the deeper fascia causes dimpling of the overlying skin of the breast. Nipple discharge or ulceration, and oedema and erythema of the skin (*peau d'orange*) all suggest carcinoma of the breast. Lymphadenopathy in the axilla may be visible, or cause oedema of the arm from obstruction of lymphatic drainage. Next *palpate* the

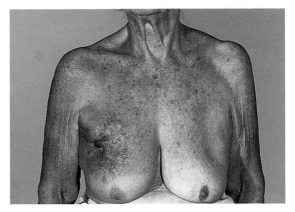

Figure 2.1 Breast cancer: right breast mass with skin invasion causing tethering and incipient ulceration.

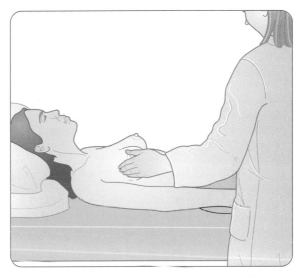

Figure 2.2 Palpation of the breast in the supine position.

breasts. The patient should lie in a near-supine position, so that the breast can be easily examined between the flat of the examiner's hand and the chest wall posteriorly (Fig. 2.2). A semi-decubitus position, with the patient's arm raised and the hand behind her head, is helpful if the breast is large. The normal lobular consistency of the breast tissue varies during the menstrual cycle, becoming more pronounced during the oestrogenic phase. After the menopause the breast parenchyma is replaced by fatty tissue, which retains a less-marked lobular consistency. Gently palpate the four quadrants of the breast, including the axillary tail (Fig. 2.3), and then, using the thumb and forefinger, define any suspected mass in relation to its size, consistency, fixation to skin or deep fascia, and relationship to the nipple and areolar complex. Remember to examine the axillary and cervical draining nodes, and the abdominal organs for metastatic involvement.

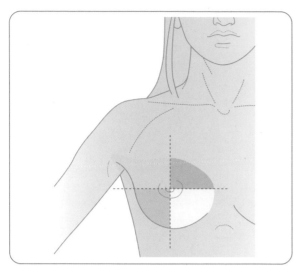

Figure 2.3 The four quadrants of the breast should be carefully and systematically palpated.

AXILLAE

Examine the axillae. It is difficult to feel enlarged lymph glands unless the patient's arm is raised to allow the examining fingers to be pushed high into the axilla. The arm is then lowered in the flexed position to rest across the examiner's arm, and palpation is continued downwards along the chest wall.

TEMPERATURE

When taking the temperature, remember the following points:

- Before inserting the thermometer, make it an invariable rule to wash it in antiseptic or in cold water and see that the mercury is well shaken down. Afterwards, wash it before replacing it in its case.
- The thermometer must be accurate. The centigrade (Celsius) scale is in general use in the UK (normal <37°), but many people are still more familiar with the Fahrenheit scale (normal <98.4°).
- It must be kept in position long enough to allow the mercury to reach body temperature. It is advisable to exceed the period the instrument professes to require. The ordinary 'half-minute' thermometer should be left in position for a full minute. Collapsed, comatose and elderly patients should have their rectal temperature taken with a special 'low-reading' thermometer.

Accidental hypothermia is common in the elderly in winter.

In conscious adults the temperature is taken in the mouth or the axilla. In young children the thermometer should be placed in the fold of the groin and the thigh flexed on the abdomen; or it may be inserted into the rectum. The temperature of the mouth and rectum is generally at least half a degree higher than that of the groin or axilla. When the temperature is taken in the mouth, the patient must breathe through the nose and keep the lips firmly closed during the observation. An electronic thermometer is now often used in the ear, and provides a fast and accurate reading.

PULSE

Count the pulse for a full half-minute when the patient is at rest and composed. Abnormalities due to cardiovascular causes, such as disturbances of the normal rhythm (*arrhythmia*), are described in Chapter 7. The rate in health during the stress of a medical examination varies from about 60 to 80 beats/minute, but people who are physically very fit may have a resting pulse as low as 45.

RESPIRATION

Count the patient's respirations for a full half-minute, starting when their attention is directed elsewhere. It is convenient to do this when the patient thinks you are still counting the pulse. The normal rate in an adult is about 14–18 respirations/minute, but wide variations occur in health. Respiratory rate is a useful sign that many doctors ignore, and when examining the patient on a bed can be the main sign of a significant chronic obstructive pulmonary disease.

ODOURS

The odour of *alcohol* is easily recognizable on the breath, although patients may try and mask it by sucking a mint, but it does not necessarily mean the patient's condition is due to alcohol intoxication. The odour of *diabetic ketosis* has been described as 'sweet and sickly'; that of *uraemia* as 'ammoniacal or fishy'; and that of *hepatic failure* as 'mousy', but too much reliance on such delicate distinctions is unwise. *Halitosis* (bad breath) is common in patients whose dental hygiene has been poor, and is associated especially with *chronic gingivitis* (periodontal or gum disease).

Differential diagnosis: The beginning of a management plan

M. Swash

3

INTRODUCTION

The purpose of each clinical assessment is to establish reliable data from the history and the physical examination in order to facilitate diagnosis and plan treatment. This may require further investigation, which will itself be suggested by the clinical data. Thus clinical assessment defines both diagnosis and management. *Management* is a word that is used in clinical practice to include diagnosis, definition of the major symptoms, and making a plan for further investigation and treatment. Clinical management therefore includes specific medical, surgical and psychiatric treatments and, importantly, management of the whole problem, as seen by the patient.

It is therefore essential that clinical information be organized in such a way that it can be easily accessed and utilized. Clinical data should be recorded in a standard format, using accepted abbreviations that can be interpreted by other doctors. Usually, clinical data are recorded in more detail for patients admitted to hospital than for those seen only in an outpatient clinic, if only because inpatients are likely to require more complex investigations and treatments, and generally to be more sick than people seen in clinics.

ORGANIZING THE DATA

Clinical information is obtained through the history and examination, and must be considered in a number of logical steps so that an appropriate and efficient path to management can be planned and followed. The following questions need to be considered:

- Is the patient seriously ill, or is there risk, either to life or of permanent disability?
- Is there an immediately evident diagnosis? If a diagnosis is not apparent, consider first whether there is an organic abnormality.
- Which system is mainly affected?
- Are multiple organ systems involved?
- Is urgent assessment necessary?
- What investigations are likely to be informative?
- What is the differential diagnosis?
- What is the patient's understanding of the illness?

This path to diagnosis and management can be followed in several different ways, but all depend on a logical presentation and ordering of the clinical database. For this reason the clinical data should be recorded ('written up') in a standardized format. This orderly presentation will allow other medical and non-medical staff, such as physiotherapists and nurses, to understand the management plan. Information related to the course of the illness and its treatment should be recorded under headings derived from this initial assessment. It is a prime objective of care and treatment to anticipate future events, complications and the effects of therapy, so that the outcome of the disorder can be controlled as far as possible. When a serious complication develops unexpectedly, the situation becomes potentially uncontrolled. Decisions may then have to be made rapidly. It is better if a plan already exists to deal with any such anticipated complication, however unlikely this might seem. This 'risk assessment' is always worth thinking through at the beginning; (that is, at the time of the initial diagnostic assessment). Always consider *what might go wrong?*

SEVERITY OF THE ILLNESS

Ill patients deserve special attention. Accident and emergency department staff are skilled at such assessments as part of their triage or initial assessment of the patient, but doctors in their consulting rooms or outpatient clinics should remember that their patient may be more sick than appearances may at first suggest. The patient may not recognize the importance of certain symptoms, such as tight pain in the anterior chest radiating to the left arm, a symptom that the doctor will consider as suggestive of myocardial ischaemia or incipient myocardial infarction. On the other hand, haemorrhage – a dramatic symptom – is often thought by the patient to be more important than it necessarily is. For example, coughing blood, even in small quantities, is likely to have a serious cause, but blood in the stools is most likely to be due to bleeding haemorrhoids, although it might also indicate an underlying carcinoma of the rectum. These possibilities will pass through the mind of the physician as the patient tells their story.

Acutely ill patients show signs of illness, especially fever, shock, circulatory collapse, disturbed consciousness, confusion, severe pain, or evidence of metabolic failure – for example ketosis, jaundice or uraemia – or abdominal pain and distension with vomiting. Lay people generally recognize these signs as features of serious illness, but the patient may not present until the disorder is relatively advanced, largely because the change in function has progressed slowly over time. Some serious features, such as an acute petechial rash with drowsiness and fever, the presenting signs of meningococcal septicaemia, are easily neglected until, within a few hours, the patient has become shocked, confused and stuporous.

Slowly progressive conditions, although also serious, are particularly difficult to recognize. The progressive pallor and skin haemorrhages of aplastic anaemia, often due to a myeloproliferative disorder, may be neglected until pointed out by an acquaintance who has not seen the person for a few weeks and who therefore notes the change. Similarly, the slow onset of primary hypothyroidism or pituitary failure will often go unremarked by those in close contact with a person – even by the patient's own GP.

People vary in their ability to cope with illness. Some will say nothing until the illness has become well developed and obvious, whereas others will present with 'unbearable' symptoms very early in the natural history. It is much more difficult for the physician to interpret and recognize illness in patients who have a low threshold for symptoms, as there may be no abnormalities on examination, leading to a suspicion that the patient is anxious, overly concerned, depressed, or simply exaggerating. Thus, it is the suspicion that there might be an underlying organic cause for a patient's symptoms that should lead to the decision to investigate further. Any investigation planned must be definitive. It is not satisfactory to plan an investigation that has poor sensitivity and specificity and then to rely on this unsatisfactory information.

The most satisfactory and sensitive tool in the hands of the physician is the history and examination. The experienced physician will continually be thinking of possible physiological and anatomical explanations for the patient's symptoms *as they are described*.

PATTERN RECOGNITION AND LOGIC IN DIAGNOSIS

Diagnosis is often accomplished by a process of *intuitive pattern recognition* based on experience and formal knowledge. Many disorders present in characteristic ways, with a sequence of developing symptoms and with confirmatory signs on examination. Certain key negative aspects of the history and examination can be used to exclude other conditions. This pattern recognition strategy can be very efficient in planning further investigation and management, but the clinician must be alert for any anomalous features that do not readily fit the diagnostic hypothesis.

The diagnostic process is sometimes summarized in flowcharts for *decision analysis*, which provide steps in the diagnostic process that lead to, validate or invalidate a diagnosis. Such charts are useful as learning tools, but are rarely followed exactly by clinicians because they fail to take account of the importance of establishing certainty in the history and in the examination. Only the individual clinician can know how reliable the clinical data are in any individual case. Of course, it is the essence of clinical methods to establish a reliable database of clinical information. The clinician therefore weighs up the reliability of the evidence upon which the diagnostic assessment is to be made, and then follows a logical diagnostic path in thinking through the possible diagnosis and considering which investigations will be helpful. This logic must take account of the relative strength of the data available. The diagnosis can only be as good or reliable as the data on which it is based. More mistakes are made from basing a diagnosis on inaccurate clinical data than from making an error in reasoning.

There have been many attempts to formulate mathematical concepts of sensitivity and specificity in relation to clinical data, in order to improve the accuracy of clinical decision-making and diagnosis by computer analysis, but so much depends on the interpretation of the symptoms themselves, and on the validity of the signs elicited, that these methods are not yet useful in practice. None the less, algorithms for the diagnosis of certain common symptoms, for example chest or abdominal pain, are available and can be helpful.

The student will sometimes notice an experienced clinician make an immediate diagnosis based on a few seconds' acquaintance with a patient. The consultant then uses the remainder of the consultation to explore other possibilities, to exclude other disorders and to consider various diagnostic investigations and the plan of management. Such skill comes with experience, requiring constant practice and knowledge. Knowledge can be acquired from medical texts and from the literature, but it needs to be based on clinical experience and clinical method in order to be usable; the two skills of clinical method and medical knowledge work together to inform medical practice.

The diagnostic process is a complex mental task in which clinical data are weighed in the clinician's mind against previous experience and formally acquired medical knowledge. There is no substitute for knowledge, but knowledge can only be used appropriately when its significance is understood in relation to everyday clinical experience. A clinician will arrive at a diagnosis because it is clear that certain aspects of the patient's history or physical signs have especial significance. The way in which a patient describes upper abdominal pain may be more important than the precise characteristics of the pain in suggesting a diagnosis of cardiac or oesophageal disease. On the other hand, it is possible to be misled by over-reliance on clinical intuition. A legitimate use of investigative techniques is to check diagnostic accuracy, as well as to quantify an abnormality for planning management. The role of computerized imaging cannot be overestimated in this regard.

Clinicians constantly update their own personal database (i.e. their memory of patients and of the clinical features of particular disorders) in relation to the acquisition of factual knowledge derived from textbooks, medical journals, conferences and the Internet. There is always something new to be learned in medicine, even for the most experienced doctor. Computer-based diagnostic systems and reference databases have become useful tools in this process of informing clinicians, but they are not substitutes for learning, for wisdom and, above all, for clinical skills and easy patient relationships.

MULTIPLE CAUSATION

Although it is axiomatic that one should try to account for all of a patient's symptoms by one disease process (the principle of Occam's razor), a surprising number of patients in fact have more than one overt diagnosis, for example coronary artery disease and hiatus hernia, both of which may produce central chest pain; and still more have a disease process which either does not explain the symptoms at all or does not explain all the symptoms, for example weakness and tiredness in a patient with mild angina pectoris or mild anaemia. Moreover, an apparently simple event may have a complex medical background. For instance, an old lady gets out of bed, trips and breaks her wrist. It is possible that she was hurrying to the lavatory as she had cystitis, that she tripped because her vision was impaired by cataracts, and that the wrist fracture occurred because her bones were weakened by osteoporosis.

In making a diagnosis one should try to account for a person's total disability, and one should not be dismayed if this involves more than one item. Thus the diagnosis in an old woman with multiple symptoms might be:

- Loneliness
- Depression
- Mild degenerative osteoarthritis.

or, in a young man with dyspepsia:

- Impending marriage
- Anxiety state
- Duodenal ulcer.

A diagnosis of this kind, which lists the patient's problems and is not confined to labelling organic disease, gives a true picture of the state of affairs. The symptomatic complaint forms but one part of the patient's problems. Always view the patient as a whole. Will they be restored to full mental and physical health when this symptom has resolved? Note that a mental adaptation to illness features in this diagnostic set, a component of the illness that is arguably that part most susceptible to influence by the physician and nurse.

WRITING UP THE NOTES

Carefully organized clinical notes will indicate the database with clarity, and will also reveal errors and missing data. Did you forget to take the blood pressure? Or to examine the neck for enlarged cervical lymph nodes? If you follow a rigid and stereotyped note-keeping system (Box 3.1) as you write up the clinical notes, you will notice any omissions and any data that are incompatible with your initial diagnostic hypothesis will also be revealed.

Begin with *basic social data* – name, age, address, marital status, dependent family members and children, occupation – and then proceed to describe the *family history* and the *past medical history*. Note the *social history* and any relevant past *occupational history*, together with a note about *drugs* taken regularly, *alcohol* ingestion and the *smoking history*. Make a note of any doctors who have previously attended, and if there is information about previous investigations and treatments or psychiatric interventions describe these also.

Box 3.1 Recording the clinical findings
- Basic personal and demographic data
- Occupational history
- Marital and sexual history
- Past history
- Social history
- Family history
- Drug history
- Alcohol, smoking and substance abuse?
- Presenting problems
- History of current problems
- Examination
- General features
- System findings
- Summary
- Plan of investigation and management
- Follow-up notes (signed and dated)

Indicate the *major presenting symptom* or symptoms and their duration, and then record the *current history* (history of present condition), not necessarily as given by the patient but interpreted as a conceptual and coherent narrative, starting at the beginning and running through to contemporary events. With experience it is often possible to write notes that fulfil this aim as the patient describes the problems, simply by categorizing the events and symptoms in relation to their main headings, for example headache, dizziness and shortness of breath. Each of these would justify a separate paragraph including what the patient said and what the responses were 'on direct questioning' (ODQ). Unrelated *direct questions* designed to exclude other conditions or problems should be noted separately at the end of the narrative history. A short note about the mental state and intellectual level is often useful, particularly in retrospect as the illness progresses, complications develop or recovery occurs.

Sometimes the past history has relevance to the present history; for example, a patient may have had a congenital heart disorder operated on in infancy and is now presenting in adult life with an aortic aneurysm. In this case it is reasonable to run together the relevant past history with the current complaint, as it will be clear that the one has led to the other.

The *physical examination* should be recorded quite rigidly, as abnormal findings may be found in more than one bodily system. There are also often abnormal features on *general examination*, such as pallor, jaundice, a rash, clubbing of the fingers or lymphadenopathy. The initial statement should describe the patient briefly, without any hint of judgement, to try and give a picture of the person, for example 'well nourished, muscular man', or 'emaciated, frightened', or 'jaundiced, breathless, cooperative', or 'confused, agitated and restlessly wandering'. Significant general abnormalities and features of systemic illness, such as abnormalities in the skin (e.g. nailbed infarcts, ecchymoses, vitiligo etc.), should be noted.

The physical examination, whatever the order in which it is carried out, should be written up separately for each *major bodily system*. Thus there will be separate brief descriptions of the findings in the gastrointestinal system (often termed the abdomen), the cardiovascular system, the respiratory system, the nervous system, the skin, and the limbs and joints. The absence of signs can be as important as their presence. Simple line drawings can often convey more information than much writing. The minimum statement about a patient's cardiovascular system, for example, might read as in Table 3.1.

The case notes should conclude with a brief *summary* of the history and the main abnormalities found on examination, followed by a tentative diagnosis, a list of *investigations* planned and arranged,

Table 3.1   Example of a CVS statement

Pulse 76 regular, peripheral pulses normal
Neck veins not distended. No peripheral oedema
BP 130/80
Apex beat not displaced
Heart sounds I and II heard in all areas
No murmurs, lungs clear

and a *differential diagnosis*. The *plan of management* should be outlined, and those features to be used as an index of progress should be indicated. These might be clinical findings or might be derived from various investigations, for example the chest X-ray or the results of blood tests.

PROBLEM-ORIENTED RECORDS

The distinction between the patient's problem and the diagnosis, discussed earlier, is sometimes stressed by the adoption of a format of case-recording in which these problems are enumerated at the conclusion of the record and used to derive a notation in each follow-up note, by ascribing a number to each problem. Attention is then given to treatment and management of each problem individually. Although inclined to repetition, this *problem-oriented* method of medical record-keeping serves to remind the clinician to attend to all of a patient's problems individually. Certainly, it is relevant to distinguish the patient's *subjective symptoms* from the *diagnosis* at the outset, as the former must be relieved if at all possible, even if the diagnosis is such that cure is not feasible. It is sometimes helpful to combine this approach with the traditional diagnosis-related case record in order to remind the doctor that the patient's problems are the symptoms the medical or surgical treatment is designed to relieve.

IDENTIFICATION

All medical notes should be *dated* and *timed*, *signed* or *initialled*, so that the examiner can be identified. Every note must be signed. Every page of the record should have the patient's name and identifying number clearly written in the top corner, in order to avoid confusion with other patients.

PROGRESS NOTES

The progress notes should discuss the diagnosis, the patient's symptoms and signs, the results of investigations and any changes in management. Progress notes should clearly state the results of investigations, the development of the management plan, the treatment plan and the clinical progress. The nature of information given to the patient and to their family and friends must be documented, and special instructions or plans noted. If any discussion has occurred with the patient or family concerning resuscitation or decisions related to this, should it prove necessary, this should be carefully and frankly noted (see discussion of ethical issues, Chapter 28). If the patient has been visited or examined by doctors other than the physician signing the note, these physicians should be identified in writing and their opinions or advice carefully noted.

WRITING LETTERS AND REPORTS

It is important to communicate your findings clearly to other doctors. Any doctor receiving a referral letter from you should have a clear idea what question requires his or her advice. A doctor receiving the result of your consultation, on the other hand, wants to know what you have found, and what plans there are for further investigation and treatment. The patient also wants this information.

You will probably dictate your letters and reports – this requires some skill and practice. Try to visualize the sentences as you speak them, and use the more formal grammatical constructions typical of written, rather than spoken, language. Above all, *be brief*. Letters that occupy two or three sheets of paper may well not be read with great care, and probably contain uncertain advice! Set out the positive findings, the questions and the answers as you see them. Discuss any particular problems or difficulties. Be clear on your recommendations, or what you think is the nature of the underlying medical problem. State the patient's expectations and fears.

Medical reports are written as formal documents, usually for lawyers, courts, insurance companies, or statutory bodies such as social security agencies. A medical report should fully identify the patient, the doctor, and the source of the information used to provide the report, including a list of documents

studied, and the date and place of any examination carried out. Your instructions concerning the report should be clearly set out at the beginning. The data should be reviewed under appropriate headings, including conventional headings such as past medical history, current history, description of any accident etc., and the results of the examination set out fully. The report should conclude with a discussion of the relevant findings and a clear opinion or list of conclusions. If necessary, references to textbooks or other medical literature should be given. In the case of medicolegal reports, the courts in Britain and in many other countries require a declaration of any conflict of interest, and of the doctor's overriding duty to the court. Remember that your report may be used as the basis for detailed discussion and questioning in the event that its contents are disputed.

DISABILITY AND HANDICAP

It is useful when dealing with someone with poor physical or mental function to consider whether they suffer from an impairment, a disability or a handicap. These terms have separate meanings (Box 3.2). Essentially, a *disability* is a lack of a normal functional ability, and a *handicap* is a disadvantage resulting from a disability. Handicap can therefore be modified by attention to the social and behavioural environment of the patient. Disability is a biologically determined dysfunction that may not be treatable. In other words the handicap suffered by a patient with the disability of impaired walking can be managed by the provision of a wheelchair, resulting in a measurable improvement in quality of life.

PLANNING INVESTIGATIONS

Investigations are useful in defining the nature and extent of any disease process. They may also be used to monitor the progress of a disease during treatment. When planning investigations keep in mind the issues listed in Box 3.3.

Box 3.2 Impairment, disability and handicap: definitions

- An *impairment* is the absence or abnormality of a basic biological function, for example hand movement or vision.
- A *disability* is a lack of a normal functional ability, whether physical or psychological, and represents a lack of normal interaction between a person and the environment. Disability is easier to assess than impairment.
- A *handicap* is the disadvantage resulting from a disability. It thus often consists of dependency on others, or on some piece of equipment, and can be modified or even overcome by suitable manipulation of the environment. Measurement of handicap may not always be relevant, as it can be modified by social changes.

Box 3.3 Issues underlying the choice of investigations

- What investigations will be informative?
- What discomforts and risks attach to each investigation?
- What information does the laboratory require?
- What specimens are required? How should they be obtained and preserved?
- What is the cost?
- Are there any risks to laboratory staff?
- How will the results be used in the patient's management?

CHOOSING THE INVESTIGATION

The result of any investigation should have a value in management. It should complement the clinical findings from the history and examination, as in the case of blood counts in anaemia or myeloproliferative disease, or new information, as in the case of physiological data such as an ECG recording or chest X-ray. Some investigations can be used to follow the progress of a disease, for example the ESR (erythrocyte sedimentation rate) in some autoimmune disorders such as giant cell arteritis. Automation has led to the production of 'screening tests', as for example from an autoanalyser of blood biochemistry. These automated results should be studied with care, as not all the test results will at first be thought relevant to the patient, although the discovery of unexpected abnormalities (e.g. in liver function tests) may reveal unsuspected problems such as subclinical alcoholic liver disease or hypercalcaemia due to metastatic cancer. Tests can be repeated at selected intervals, determined by clinical need in relation to treatment or the expected outcome of a disorder.

DISCOMFORT AND RISKS

Discomfort and risk should be kept to a minimum. Discomfort can usually be alleviated by good technique, for example during invasive angiography, venepuncture or lumbar puncture. Risk may be minimized by good technique, but some risk will accompany any test, even venepuncture, when, for example, a small cutaneous nerve may sometimes be damaged, causing pain. The risk should be assessed before the test, and fully explained to the patient in the context of the benefit expected from the information to be obtained. If the information is not useful in clinical management, or its usefulness is considered to be less than the risk, the test should not be performed.

WHAT THE LABORATORY NEEDS TO KNOW

The laboratory or imaging department needs to be fully informed as to the reasons for the test. If in any doubt, consult with laboratory staff about the value of the test – there may be other ways of approaching the problem. The laboratory ought to be informed about any possible risks (e.g. infectivity with HIV or other pathogens). Special problems, such as a bleeding tendency, should be made known to the phlebotomist or interventional radiologist, or to a surgeon carrying out a biopsy. Any allergies to local anaesthetic agents must be recognized. The timing of the blood sample, its arrival in the laboratory (usually required during working hours, so that it can be processed properly and not stored), and the preservative medium in which it is kept are all important. In bacteriological work these can be particularly important issues.

Every specimen must be clearly labelled with the patient's name and hospital number, the ward or clinic, and the date and time it was collected. The container should also state clearly the nature of the specimen and the storage medium used for blood and bacteriological specimens. In the case of pathological specimens requiring frozen section or electron microscopy, special methods are used for storing and processing and these must be followed precisely.

SPECIAL PROCEDURES

Venepuncture and the collection of bacteriological specimens are described in Appendix 2.

MAKING THE BEST USE OF RESULTS

The interpretation of any laboratory test will depend on the relevance of the test to the presumptive diagnosis and the doctor's knowledge of pathology, biochemistry and physiology. The task of a clinical laboratory is to put these disciplines to work in the solution of a diagnostic problem. All tests are subject to errors of performance. Fortunately these are rare, but the clinician will help the pathologist if any 'rogue' result that does not accord with other data is reported back to the laboratory. Results depend on the precision of the method used and the variability of the measurement in a healthy population.

In non-quantitative tests, as in cytology, there may be false positives and false negatives. The laboratory should be able to say with what frequency these may occur. For example, in bronchial carcinoma malignant cells are often detected in the sputum; however, in a very small proportion of examinations apparently malignant cells in the sputum will be reported when there is no bronchial carcinoma. Abnormal results are therefore often checked in the laboratory by a second observer to ensure, as far as possible, their accuracy. The clinician can give some weight to such findings by considering the clinical context. If the patient is a middle-aged man who smokes heavily the report of malignant cells would be likely to be a true positive, as bronchial carcinoma is prevalent in such patients. Conversely, if the patient is a non-smoking young girl, the positive sputum report would be likely to be false and should be reassessed.

For quantitative tests, as in biochemistry and much of haematology, the *sensitivity* and *specificity* can be determined statistically in relation to their value in diagnosis. The *accuracy of the assay* must also be monitored within the laboratory and in cooperation with other laboratories. The accuracy of the assay is expressed as the variance around the mean value of multiple determinations carried out on the same specimen. The normal range of the assay is the mean value of the measurements in a population of normal subjects plus or minus two standard deviations; 95% of the results in a normal population will fall within this range, but 1 in 20 of these normal subjects will show results just outside the normal range. Therefore, a value just outside the normal range does not necessarily indicate relevant abnormality. It should also be remembered that normal ranges have to be established for the sex and age of the groups studied, and also for the method as performed in each laboratory.

Good clinical management depends on wise analysis and understanding of the clinical data as a whole.

SECTION 2

General assessment

Section contents

Psychiatric assessment

H. A. Ring

4

INTRODUCTION

Because psychiatric disorders are common, every doctor must be able to carry out a psychiatric assessment. Psychiatric disorders may present with primary psychiatric complaints or with physical symptoms, and physical and psychiatric illness often coexist. In psychiatry, information is obtained by interview and observation and from witnesses such as family members and friends. Specific psychological investigations, including tests of the cognitive state and, less frequently, structured questionnaires to assess aspects of personality and mood, are also used. Laboratory tests and neuroimaging are used in some cases.

THE PSYCHIATRIC HISTORY

INTERVIEW TECHNIQUE

Always put the patient at ease, establish a positive, friendly relationship, and use words they can understand. As in any specialty, the quality and accuracy of the information gathered will determine the adequacy of the diagnostic formulation. The experience of the interview itself may be therapeutic for the patient, and good communication and interviewing skills are especially important as psychiatric patients, by the very nature of their disturbances, may find communication difficult. Even for the most well-adjusted person the interview may involve the discussion of potentially embarrassing or even distressing issues. Be aware of these. The psychiatric history should be approached systematically (Box 4.1). Several interviews may be required, depending on the needs of the individual patient.

HISTORY OF THE CURRENT ILLNESS

Encourage the free expression of symptoms and thoughts. This requires the doctor to be relaxed, sympathetic and, above all, a good and unhurried listener. Patients must feel that their problems are respected. Initially, let the patient do most of the talking. Clarify things later, if necessary, by asking leading questions. It is often useful to write down a

---

Box 4.1   The psychiatric history: what topics to cover

- Reason for referral
- Presenting complaints
- History of current illness
- Family history
- Personal history
  - childhood
  - schooling
  - occupation
  - psychosexual and marital experiences
  - forensic history
  - past medical history
  - past psychiatric history
  - drug and alcohol abuse
  - premorbid personality
  - social circumstances
- Witness account (with patient's permission)

---

patient's complaints word for word, but generally keep eye contact with the patient. Try to analyse each symptom as in Box 4.2.

ASSOCIATED SYMPTOMS

Sleep disturbance of recent onset is usually highly significant, whereas chronic sleep impairment, although distressing to the patient, is usually less important in diagnosis. Disturbances of sleep have many causes:

- Difficulty sleeping
  - physical problems, e.g. pain or breathlessness
  - psychological disturbance, e.g. anxiety, drug withdrawal
- Early morning waking and nightmares, with depression
- Excessive sleep: drugs, substance abuse or organic illness
- Reversed sleep pattern (sleepiness during the day and wakefulness at night) in acute confusional states
- Broken sleep in affective disorders or organic illness.

Appetite is decreased in anorexia nervosa but may be increased in bulimia and in anxious patients who 'eat for comfort'. In depression, appetite may alternate between reduced and increased. Loss of appetite leads to loss of weight in depression, anorexia nervosa or self-neglect. Cycles of weight gain and weight loss sometimes occur in eating disorders. Weight gain is a feature of treatment with some psychotropic and other drugs.

FAMILY HISTORY

The family background is always relevant (Fig. 4.1). *Environmental factors* are important in determining the outcome in many psychiatric illnesses, and are often complex. For example, the death of a mother in the patient's early life predisposes to depression in later life, and failure of bonding may lead to difficulty in establishing relationships in adult life. The family history must be considered in detail, including information about parents and siblings and also, when relevant, members of the extended, non-nuclear family. *Genetic factors* are important in schizophrenia and the affective psychoses.

Find out the *age* and the *physical* and *psychiatric health* of each parent. If necessary ask about the causes of death and the patient's age and reaction to any *bereavement*. The *occupations* and *personalities* of both parents, and their relationship with each other and with the patient, including any separations from the patient in childhood, are all relevant. People whose parents had a bad marriage are themselves vulnerable to the development of psychosexual and marital difficulties. Find out about each sibling, including marital status. Some idea of the family relationships and the position of the patient within the family will have been gained through this enquiry. Finally, enquire about *alcoholism* and *suicide*. An unexplained death in the family may hint at suicide.

PERSONAL HISTORY

A structured enquiry will ensure that important areas are not omitted, though the emphasis placed on different aspects of the personal history may differ from patient to patient. However, do not constrain the history by fixing the order in which the patient wishes to talk about their problems. The self-defined story tells you about the significance attached to various features of the illness. Display the information on a life chart (Fig. 4.2) to clarify the relationships between different areas of the patient's life and to illuminate the cause of the current symptoms.

CHILDHOOD

Begin with questions about the *patient's birth*. Was it planned? What was the length of gestation? Find

---

Box 4.2   What to consider for each complaint

The symptom itself
The date and circumstances of onset of the symptoms
- Consider any precipitating factors or recent stresses. The illness may have commenced before the onset of the current symptoms. When was the patient last well?

Relieving and aggravating factors
- What factors in the family, at work or elsewhere, seem relevant?

Consistency
- Is there diurnal or day-to-day variation? Depression is often worse in the morning.

Severity
- How does the symptom interfere with normal life?

Definition
- Be clear what the patient means. Confusion may mean one thing to the layman and another to the doctor. Abnormal beliefs or experiences may not be clearly described, but the doctor must be absolutely sure about them if the correct diagnosis is to be reached.

Effect of the complaint on the patient
- Assess the effect of the experience of each symptom on the patient's emotional state. Some patients find auditory hallucinations unimportant, whereas others find them terrifying.

Site
- This is mostly relevant when the patient complains of physical symptoms. Hearing voices outside or inside the head may have a different significance.

Associated symptoms
- Ask in detail about other somatic symptoms, especially sleep, appetite and weight (see text).

---

out about the mother's health during pregnancy, and whether the delivery was difficult. Note the infantile and childhood milestones. Most people are only aware of these if their parents have told them of any difficulties.

Neurotic traits, such as recurrent fears, or periods of physical or emotional disorder at times of stress, may only become apparent in later childhood. Consider these in the light of relationships with peers and family members, the home atmosphere, and any bereavement or other *major life event*. The possibility of *child abuse*, whether physical, sexual or psychological, should be discussed tactfully and sympathetically when appropriate – usually when asking about childhood, the family history or the psychosexual history.

ADOLESCENCE

Assessment of adolescence arises from the enquiry about childhood, and overlaps with the psychosexual history. Adolescence is also interrelated with schooling and occupation.

SCHOOLING AND HIGHER EDUCATION

Details of starting, leaving and changing schools, the level of academic achievement, relationships

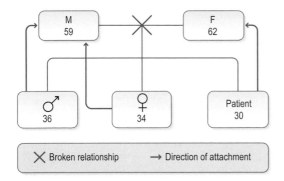

| X Broken relationship | → Direction of attachment |

Figure 4.1 Diagram of personal relationships. The patient was aged 30 years. The older two siblings, aged 34 and 36 years, were closer to their mother, and the patient was closer to her father. The parents were separated.

with peers and teachers, difficulties in learning or behaviour, and any periods of non-attendance may all be relevant. Non-attendance includes *truancy*, in which the child – usually without the parents' knowledge – indulges, often with others, in more enjoyable pastimes instead of going to school, and *school refusal*, in which the child stays at home with the knowledge of the parents because of a fear of leaving home or of going to school. *Enforced absence* is usually due to illness, although it must be remembered that illness may also be a manifestation of school refusal. Agoraphobic parents may keep children off school to help them cope with their own anxieties.

OCCUPATIONAL HISTORY

A comprehensive work history can be tedious. Use a shortened approach by asking about the number of jobs, the length of time unemployed in total and in the last five years, the longest job, the highest level of achievement, any difficulties at work, including being dismissed from a job, general relationships with colleagues and employers, and the general work record, while asking in more detail about the current job. Where relevant, military service can be dealt with in much the same way as any other occupation.

Date	Age	Social history	Family history	Psychosexual history	Medical history	Psychiatric history
1962	0					
1967	5					
1972	10	School	Parents' divorce		Pain in chest	Difficulties at school
1977	15					
1982	20	Secretary		Marries (leaves home)	Pain in back	Relieved by diazepam
1987	25			First child born		Puerperal depression
1992	30	Part-time work		Second child born	Pain in back	Sleep and appetite impaired, lethargy
2002	40			Marital stress	Head- ache	Sleep disturbance, anxiety, feelings of inability to cope

Figure 4.2 Life chart of a 40-year-old married mother of two from a broken home referred to the orthopaedic department with backache, for which no cause could be found. Associated symptoms included sleep disturbance, poor appetite and lethargy. Given this patient's background, in particular the divorce of her parents, one would not be surprised if she were vulnerable in psychosexual areas, and this is shown clearly in the chart to be the case by the development of emotional disturbance at the time of her marriage and the birth of her first child. One would therefore anticipate that the birth of her second child would also be a traumatic time for her. The presentation with physical symptoms – pain in the back – as a manifestation of psychiatric disorder is consistent both with her symptomatology after her parents' divorce and at the time of her marriage, and the presence of the associated symptoms of sleep and appetite disturbance and lethargy, all common manifestations of emotional upset. The life chart clearly displays these links.

PSYCHOSEXUAL HISTORY

Although sometimes difficult or even embarrassing, this is essential in understanding the patient and the illness. It may be necessary to leave some of the questions to later interviews, although sensitive interviewing usually enables adequate exploration of this area at the first interview, and this is usually the best time to deal with sexual matters. Lead from easy to difficult issues by asking questions in such a way as to reassure patients, for example: 'How old were you when you had your first sexual experience?' rather than 'What sexual experiences have you had?'. It may be tactful to use less emotionally laden wording, such as 'physical' rather than 'sexual' relationship. Remember that the social, religious and cultural background will influence the patient's approach to these issues. A full *sexual history* should consider all aspects of sexual experience, including any same-sex experiences (Box 4.3). The

---

Box 4.3   The sexual history

- Puberty
- Menstrual history
- Sex education
- Masturbation and fantasies
- Relationships with members of the opposite sex, especially the duration and intensity of sexual contact and enjoyment
- Engagement and marriage (see below)
- Any homosexual feelings and experiences
- Any deviant sexual experiences and fantasies, including sexual abuse in childhood or adolescence

---

Box 4.4   The marital history (the same questions should be asked concerning stable non-marital relationships)

- Parental attitudes to the marriage
- Quality of marriage: disagreements, separations
- Current sexual relationship, including frequency and quality of sexual intercourse
- Extramarital affairs, if any
- Pregnancies, terminations and miscarriages
- Stillbirths and live births
- Ages and behaviour of children
- Was child rearing delayed? If so, why?
- Is there difficulty conceiving?
- Are both partners employed? Is this necessary financially? Or are there other reasons?
- Have there been previous marriages? Divorce or death of partner?
- If not married or in a stable relationship is there a reason for this?

---

marital history includes the relationship with the spouse from the time of meeting through the development of their relationship, engagement and marriage. Note the age and occupation of the spouse (Box 4.4).

FORENSIC HISTORY

This includes all confrontations with the law at any time in life. Details of offences committed and punishment received should be noted.

PAST MEDICAL HISTORY

Ask about:

- Illnesses or operations in childhood or during adult life
- Periods of hospitalization or incapacity and any resulting disability and interference with the patient's life
- The reaction of the patient and family to these episodes
- The frequency and nature of contact with the family doctor.

It is illuminating to find out that the patient who now presents with physical symptoms has had a number of previous episodes of similar symptoms at times of stress, and has recovered when the stress was resolved.

PAST PSYCHIATRIC HISTORY

Include any episodes of emotional upset, even those thought not severe enough to need medical attention. Note any minor symptoms treated by the family doctor, as well as severe psychiatric disorders needing expert psychiatric treatment. Record whether outpatient, day-patient or inpatient care was arranged, on a voluntary or a compulsory basis. Ask about circumstances, precipitating factors, place of treatment, duration of and response to treatment, and any continuing symptoms or medications. Ask if the patient has taken psychotropic medication in the past, whether prescribed by the family doctor or obtained in other ways, for example from other family members. Finally, ask about contact with voluntary organizations, such as the Samaritans, or with social services.

ALCOHOL ABUSE

Alcohol abuse is common (Box 4.5) and may have physical, psychiatric and social consequences, yet it may not be recognized. Where there is any suspicion of alcohol-related problems, a thorough and systematic drinking history must be obtained.

Questions about the content, time, place, type and usual circumstances of first and all subsequent drinks in a day, and whether the patient drinks alone or in company, are often revealing. Find out about the speed at which the first drink is consumed (people with physical dependence often gulp rather

---

> **Box 4.5   Features that suggest alcohol abuse**
>
> - Excessive weekly intake
> - Inability to stop drinking
> - Craving for alcohol
> - Primacy of drinking behaviour
> - Secret drinking and drinking alone
> - Morning drinking
> - Withdrawal symptoms
> - Drinking to avoid withdrawal
> - Amnesia for events during a drinking binge
> - Conviction for drunken driving, or other alcohol-related crime
> - Violent behaviour
> - Marital problems
> - Employment problems
> - Alcohol-related physical illness

than sip their first drink). Find out how much money the patient spends on drink, and relate it to their income. Is there a family history of heavy drinking? At what age did the patient start drinking? Have there been any personal difficulties caused by drinking in the family? Any drink-related physical or psychiatric illness? Any problems at work? Does the patient recognize they might have a problem with alcohol?

A history of serious medical or social complications, such as alcoholic hallucinosis, delirium tremens, any antisocial behaviour resulting in encounters with the police, or alcohol-related marital problems is especially significant.

SUBSTANCE ABUSE

This term implies not only drugs of addiction, whether major (e.g. morphine, heroin, cocaine, amphetamines) or minor (e.g. cannabis), but also so-called 'recreational drugs' such as Ecstasy, prescribed drugs (mainly benzodiazepines) and non-prescribed drugs not normally considered addictive (e.g. cough linctus, analgesics). Information concerning the route of drug intake should be obtained. An assessment similar to that outlined above for alcohol abuse should be used. Note any psychiatric symptoms that have developed at times of drug use. The financial consequences of the substance abuse are an important indication of its importance in the patient's life.

PERSONALITY

The personality is the *sum of those characteristics that make a person into the individual he or she is* (Box 4.6). Personality may change with brain lesions, or with severe illness: for example, disinhibition occurs with frontal lobe damage. The premorbid personality is most reliably assessed from an informant familiar with the patient before the onset of the illness. Ask the patient how others see them. Some features of personality, such as histrionic behaviour, will be obvious during the interview; others will already have been elicited in the history. The personality is illustrated by *relationships to others, attitude to authority, level of independence, usual mood, religious beliefs, interests or hobbies, and fantasy life* (Box 4.6). Personality determines behaviour.

BEHAVIOUR

Think of behaviour in terms of *actions* and *reactions*. *Actions* include level of achievement, deliberate self-harm or aggression towards others, disinhibition, obsessional behaviour (e.g. excessive tidiness, being overly houseproud, perfectionist, over-conscientious or obsessionally checking) and dependence on alcohol or drugs. *Reactions* occur in response to stressful life events, such as illness, bereavement and other losses, or to examinations, promotion at work, failure and disappointment, and inability to cope with change. Reactions are often rather stereotyped, including being panicky or unflappable, placid or short-tempered.

SOCIAL FACTORS

Ask about home and relationships with other members of the household, neighbours and social contacts. Are there any financial problems or other stressors?

SUMMING UP

At the end of the history, sum up with the patient. Ask whether you have grasped the problem fully, or left out any important areas. Besides clarifying the history, this discussion will also show that you have been listening and have understood.

WITNESS ACCOUNTS

It is often very helpful to get an account of the patient's present and past mental state from someone who knows them well, such as a partner. However, always obtain the patient's permission first. Patients with severe psychiatric illnesses may be unable to give a coherent history. In psychotic illness there is no insight into the abnormal nature of the mental state, and so these experiences may not be disclosed. If there is a persecutory delusional state the patient may choose not to disclose the experience. In depression, the present and the past may be so coloured by the current prevailing mental state that no hint of any previous happiness may be presented.

THE PSYCHIATRIC EXAMINATION

This should include a physical examination, although this may be deferred until the initial psychiatric assessment has been completed.

Box 4.6   Points to consider when assessing personality

Attitude to self
- Self-interested or thoughtful about others
- Level of self-esteem and self-criticism
- Self-consciousness and sensitivity
- Self-confidence, whether high, or low and constantly needing reassurance

Social relationship to others
- Ease of making and keeping social relationships
- Introverted or extroverted
- Suspiciousness
- Assertiveness
- Warm and affectionate or cold and undemonstrative
- Tolerant or authoritarian and intolerant
- Relationships at work and with the family

Sexual relationship to others
- Level and nature of psychosexual development, especially the capacity to make sexual relationships
- Direction of sexual attraction
- Areas of difficulty

Attitude to authority
- Anxious and uncertain
- Generally tolerant or intolerant

Level of independence
- Has the patient left home?
- Still living with parents?

- Accepting of responsibility for own actions?
- Capable of making decisions?

Usual mood
- Prone to anxiety, and if so, about what (e.g. illness, work, family)?
- Pessimistic or optimistic?
- Cyclothymic (i.e. swinging from elation to depression without reaching illness proportions)?
- Calm or irritable?
- Bottles up or shares feelings and emotions?
- Easy-going, or short-tempered and easily angered?

Religious beliefs and moral attitudes
- Which religion, and whether practising or not
- Whether tolerant of beliefs and attitudes of others
- Ability to show regret or remorse and limit actions according to conscience

Interests or hobbies
- What types?
- Time spent on them?
- Passive spectator or active participant?
- Social or solitary pastimes?

Fantasy life
- Sexual fantasies
- Non-sexual fantasies

PHYSICAL EXAMINATION

Note general features as you talk with the patient. Acutely anxious patients may show signs of thyrotoxicosis. Evidence of liver disease may suggest alcoholism. Needle marks in the arms point to drug abuse; scars of slashed wrists or other signs of self-mutilation may point to psychiatric illness. Confusion is usually due to organic disease. Visual hallucinosis often has an organic cause, but auditory hallucinosis rarely does.

PSYCHIATRIC OR MENTAL STATE EXAMINATION

This should be approached systematically (Box 4.7).

APPEARANCE AND BEHAVIOUR

The patient's appearance and behaviour are revealing of the underlying psychiatric disorder. Note especially *dress*, *personal hygiene* and general grooming. Self-neglect is often due to depression, dementia or psychotic illness. Observe the gait and demeanour as the patient walks into the interview room. Ataxia suggests organic brain disease, drug

---

Box 4.7   How to examine the mental state

Use the following headings
- Appearance and behaviour
- Speech
- Mood
- Thought content
- Abnormal beliefs
- Abnormal experiences
- Cognitive state
- Intelligence
- Insight and rapport
- Specific tests of cerebral function
  - questionnaires
  - structured interview schedules

---

effects or alcoholism. The breath may smell of alcohol. There may be signs of *hysterical ataxia* that improves with suggestion or exhortation, or *malingering* or *simulation*, in which the limp varies from moment to moment and is most marked when the patient knows they are being watched.

The *facial expression* is an outward sign of a person's mood. Tearfulness or poverty of expression occur in depression, elation in mania, tenseness in anxiety, perplexity in schizophrenia. The *affect* may be inappropriate, such as the schizophrenic patient who laughs when relating upsetting material. It must be remembered none the less that anxious people may also laugh in similar circumstances. The emotional expression may be abnormally labile, as in mania or organic brain disease.

Posture

The way the patient sits gives important clues:

- Is the patient relaxed and at ease, or sitting tensely and fidgeting?
- The agitated depressive or the excited manic or schizophrenic may be so agitated that they get up from their seat and pace up and down the room.
- The demented or confused patient may wander around uncomprehendingly.
- Delusions of persecution may cause the patient to feel threatened and become angry, or to terminate the interview.
- The patient with retarded depression may show little movement during the interview.
- The patient who drifts off to sleep repeatedly may be confused, with fluctuating levels of consciousness. Consider oversedation and remember subdural haematoma.

There may be involuntary movements, many of which may also occur in organic neurological disease:

- Dystonia is a common feature of treatment with older major antipsychotic drugs.
- Choreiform movements are a feature of Huntington's chorea. They are common with L-dopa therapy for Parkinson's disease.
- Tic-like mannerisms, odd postures or other bizarre disorders of movement occur in patients with schizophrenia or in organic brain disease, or may represent psychogenic disturbance. Tics are also quite frequent in normal adolescence during periods of emotional stress.
- *Catatonia*, a perseveration of posture in which the patient's limbs can be moved into an abnormal position, is a feature of schizophrenia; there is *waxy flexibility* of muscle tone.
- In *negativism*, the patient opposes the examiner's intention.
- In *echopraxia* the interviewer's actions are copied.
- Voluntary movements may be *retarded*, i.e. slowed, especially in depression.
- *Stupor* is commonly caused by organic disorders but may also be a result of functional psychoses such as schizophrenia and depression. Stupor may also occur in hysteria, or in uncontrolled anxiety following extreme stress; or it may be simulated by malingerers.

Behaviour

During the interview behaviour may be *disinhibited*, as in the manic patient who strips, or the patient with frontal brain disease who starts to urinate or masturbate. *Manipulative, seductive* or *violent behaviour* may be seen if the patient's wishes are not met. There may be verbal *aggression* or physical violence, the latter against either the interviewer or objects in the room. On the other hand, the patient may appear to be unduly submissive or self-critical, or may show little or no eye contact with the interviewer. A *suspicious* attitude is a pointer to an underlying personality disorder or paranoid illness. A patient apparently *preoccupied* with internal thoughts should suggest auditory hallucinations (i.e. hearing voices). The patient may even be talking to or arguing with these voices. *Fear* without any obvious cause, or attempts to touch or shoo away non-existing objects, is often due to visual hallucinations. Remember that unusual behaviour or inability to relate to the interviewer may represent learning disability, not psychiatric illness.

SPEECH AND ITS CONTENT

Consider the flow of speech. If the patient appears *mute*, is this deliberate, hysterical, or part of a depressive or catatonic stupor? In the mute patient it is important to assess all aspects of language production, including the ability to produce sounds and communicate non-verbally. Most patients speak: is this spontaneous, or only in answer to questions? With monosyllabic or more elaborate replies? Is speech slow and expressionless, as in depressive illness, or so quick and continuous, with *flight of ideas*, that it is impossible to interrupt, as in hypomania and mania? Are there long pauses before the patient replies, or are there arrests of speech in mid-sentence (e.g. in schizophrenia)?

Are the words normal or are there neologisms, as in some types of schizophrenia or organic brain disease? Is there evidence of dysphasia or dysarthria? When the words themselves are normal, are the phrases and sentences normal and do they fit together, or does the patient seem to jump from topic to topic? If the latter, is there a link between topics, as in *flight of ideas* in mania, or is there no recognizable link, as in the *thought disorder* of schizophrenia? Is the link, if present, not one of content but of form, as in rhyming or punning (usually features of mania)? Is there *echolalia*, in which the patient repeats what the interviewer says, or *perseveration*, when the patient continues with the same theme even if this is no longer appropriate? For example, a 60-year-old man replying to the question 'How old are you?' answers '60, 61, 62, 63, 64, 65, 66' and so on; when asked the subsequent question 'What year were you born?' he answers '1960' and to the next question, 'What year is it now?', also answers '1960'. Both echolalia and perseveration occur in organic brain disease and in some types of schizophrenia.

When speech is abnormal, write some of it down verbatim, as this is the only reliable way of recording the abnormality for future assessment. Two doctors may differ in what they call formal thought disorder, and therefore writing in the case notes: 'There was evidence of formal thought disorder' is not helpful. A recorded sample of the patient's speech gives much less room for disagreement.

MOOD

Mood has both a subjective component, which is reflected in the way someone describes their emotional state, and an objective component, i.e. what the interviewer sees, for example, tears. The subjective and objective components of mood are usually – but not always – congruent. An example of incongruence is the smiling face of some severely depressed patients. Ask the patient how they feel, or how are their spirits (subjective mood). If necessary, leading questions such as 'Are you anxious or depressed?' may be used. Abnormal mood most commonly includes depression and anxiety, but also elation, irritability, anger and perplexity. In affective disorders the content of any hallucinations or delusions are generally mood congruent: depressed patients may think they are evil, whereas manic patients may believe that they are God.

Depression

This may be mild and influenced by daily activities, or severe. The clinical features are characteristic (Box 4.8). In severe depression, symptoms may be worse in the morning. There may also be ideas of worthlessness, self-deprecation, poverty, guilt, persecution, bodily ill-health or nihilism. These may sometimes be delusional in intensity. The patient may be agitated or retarded, sometimes even to the point of stupor, and may be mute or, in lesser cases, show retardation of speech.

Box 4.8 Features supporting a diagnosis of depression

- Loss of interest/enjoyment in life
- Lethargy
- Poor concentration
- Early-morning waking
- Appetite and weight disturbance
- Ideas of worthlessness, guilt, persecution, nihilism
- Self-deprecation
- Retardation, leading to depressive stupor
- Retardation of speech, or muteness
- Paradoxical agitation and delusional state

Suicidal thoughts

The depressed patient feels despairing and hopeless, and sees no future. Suicidal ideation must always be considered in depressed patients; often it is also relevant in other psychiatric disorders, such as schizophrenia, alcohol dependence, hypomania and severe anxiety disorders. Discussing suicide does not encourage patients to kill themselves, but failure to discuss it may lead to tragedies that could have been prevented (Box 4.9). It can be approached directly or through a series of questions, such as: 'How do you see the future?' 'Have you felt it would be nice to escape, or be able to sleep and not wake up?' 'Do you feel at times that you would rather be dead, or that you are such a burden to others that they would be better off if you were dead?' 'Have you had thoughts of suicide, however fleeting?' 'Have you made any plans?'. Where it is felt that the patient is suicidal but denies it, it is worth asking 'What stops you killing yourself?' or 'What do you have to live for?'. Some patients admit to having suicidal thoughts but deny that they would do anything because of the impact it would have on the family, or because it is against their religion or they do not have the courage. Suicide, however, is not a respecter of family feelings, religious beliefs or personal bravery. Homicidal thoughts may also be present.

Sometimes patients report that they have thought about suicide but that they would not actually kill themselves because things are not quite bad enough. In this case it is appropriate to enquire as to what would need to happen in order for things to become that bad. Occasionally only very small changes would lead to the risk of suicide.

Anxiety

Anxiety states often present with somatic symptoms related to autonomic nervous system arousal or

Box 4.9 Features suggesting increased risk of suicidal behaviour

- Previous self-harm, especially
  - poison
  - stabbing
  - hanging
  - jumping from heights
  - falling under vehicles
- Continuing suicidal thoughts
- Current depressive or schizophrenic psychosis
- Male sex, aged over 40 years
- Social isolation, especially in adolescence or the recently bereaved or divorced
- Chronic painful illness
- Alcoholism and drug abuse
- Family history of suicide

hyperventilation (Box 4.10), or to psychic symptoms (Box 4.11) or both. The anxiety may be free-floating or situation dependent, as in phobic disorders, e.g. agoraphobia, and other phobias. Panic attacks consist of sudden surges of extreme anxiety, with physical symptoms, sometimes with a desire to run away, or coupled with an inability to move.

Elation

A feeling of being on top of the world, feeling happier than ever before, is a feature of *hypomania*. In *mania* it is associated with overactivity, pressure of speech, flight of ideas, inability to sleep, irritability and grandiose ideas. In mixed affective states the mental state may show signs of both depression and elation.

Other abnormal mental states

Irritability occurs in anxiety states and hypomania, and in situational and relationship disturbances, such as marital problems. It may also be part of the usual mood in some personalities. *Anger* may be related to a specific person or situation, or may be part of an underlying psychiatric disturbance, particularly when ideas of persecution are present. Irritability and anger are common after closed head injuries with frontal contusions. *Perplexity* is usually

---

Box 4.10 Somatic symptoms of anxiety

- Headaches and other muscular aches and pains
- Palpitations
- Tremor
- Breathlessness
- Chest pain
- Urinary frequency
- Faintness and lightheadedness
- Fatigue
- Pins and needles
- Diarrhoea
- Dry mouth
- Abdominal discomfort
- Flushes
- Sweating

Box 4.11 Psychic symptoms of anxiety

- Feelings of anxiety
- Irritability
- Inability to relax
- Inability to concentrate
- Initial insomnia – difficulty getting off to sleep
- Feeling of impending doom
- Depersonalization

---

found in schizophrenic patients, who are suspicious that something is going on but cannot quite put their finger on what it is.

THOUGHT FORM

This refers to disturbance in the ability to maintain a coherent, directed train of thought. In schizophrenia, thoughts may be joined one to another with no apparent link, and in hypomania and mania, as noted above, thoughts may flow very rapidly from one to the next based on a variety of links, for instance the sound of words ('who are you, I'm one hundred and two, how are you?').

THOUGHT CONTENT

Use an open question about the patient's main concerns, and then ask if they are preoccupied by any thoughts. In *severe depression* there may be preoccupation by thoughts of suicide. In *obsessive–compulsive disorder* obsessional thoughts predominate (e.g. 'If I do not fold my clothes every night then something bad will happen'). The patient recognizes these thoughts as their own, realizes they are foolish and may try to resist, but is unable to do so. There is a compulsion to carry out the act, despite recognizing its absurdity. Hand-washing is a common compulsive ritual, associated with obsessional thoughts about contamination; the patient may wash his or her hands 40 or 50 times a day until they are raw. Obsessional checking is another common manifestation: for example, the woman who switches off her bedroom lights before leaving the house, gets to the bottom of the stairs and repeatedly has to go back up again to check that the lights are off. If these obsessional rituals are not followed exactly, the thoughts leading to them cause extreme anxiety.

ABNORMAL BELIEFS

These range from *delusions* (Box 4.12), in which the patient has false and unshakeable beliefs which are out of keeping with their social milieu, to *over-valued ideas*, in which the patient has false beliefs which, although of major concern to him or her, are

---

Box 4.12 Examples of abnormal beliefs

- Delusions
  - of persecution (paranoid delusions)
  - of grandeur
  - of poverty (depressive delusions)
  - of reference
  - of love
  - of infidelity
  - of interference (passivity)
  - nihilistic (e.g. that the internal organs are dead and rotten)

not completely unshakeable. These abnormal beliefs include misinterpretations, in which the patient concocts false explanations for various normal events which may or may not be delusional in extent. Record abnormal ideas verbatim. Not all abnormal beliefs denote psychiatric illness, as they may also occur in normal people, such as ideas of reference, in which people can feel that what others are saying refers to them, or that other people are laughing at them behind their back. This is common in sensitive people, especially in anxiety-provoking situations, such as parties where most of the other guests are strangers.

Delusions may be *primary* or *secondary*. *Primary delusions* are fully formed delusions that suddenly enter the patient's mind, as in the person who for no reason suddenly believes that their food is being poisoned. This is often preceded by a delusional mood, in which the patient feels that there is something going on and that things are not quite right, but is unable to elaborate this feeling. In delusional perceptions the object is perceived normally but is interpreted in a delusional way, for example the man who sees an ashtray on the table, recognizes it as an ashtray, but believes that it has been put there to show people that he is a spy. This is not understandable in terms of the rest of the patient's psychopathology. *Secondary delusions* are understandable in terms of the rest of the patient's psychopathology, as in affective psychoses.

Paranoid delusions or delusions of persecution are common. They may occur alone or with other abnormal mental signs, as in organic psychoses such as confusional states, dementia, alcohol- and drug-induced psychoses, stress-induced psychogenic psychoses, and in some people with paranoid personalities. They also occur in some endocrine disorders and in cerebral vasculitis, such as systemic lupus erythematosus. *Delusions of grandeur* are characteristic of the now uncommon syphilitic general paralysis of the insane, but also occur in mania and schizophrenia. Patients may believe they are on a special mission, or that they are Napoleon or Christ. Depressed patients may insist that they are destitute and have no clothes (*delusions of poverty*). Other common false beliefs include self-deprecation, worthlessness and guilt: 'I have done something terrible and should be in prison and not in hospital'. Delusions of ill-health may occur and persist despite every assurance of the patient's physical health. Some people with sensitive personalities develop isolated abnormal ideas about their own appearance which may sometimes be delusional in intensity, for example that their nose is too long, or their hair is falling out. These symptoms may precede the onset of depression or schizophrenia. *Nihilistic delusions*, in which the patient says that they or a body part is dead, occur mainly in severe depressive illnesses. *Delusions of love (erotomania)* occur

---

Box 4.13   How to diagnose schizophrenia

Are there any of Schneider's first-rank symptoms of schizophrenia?
- Hearing voices in the third person arguing or commenting on what the patient is doing
- Hearing one's own thoughts spoken out loud
- Thought alienation (insertion, withdrawal or broadcast)
- Delusional perceptions (a primary delusion)
- Passivity phenomena – everything in the spheres of feeling, sensations, volition and actions experienced as being imposed on the patient or influenced by others

---

mainly in schizophrenia and other organic psychoses. Morbid jealousy *(delusions of infidelity)* involves a belief that a patient's spouse is having an extramarital affair, sometimes leading to extreme violence. These delusions occur in people with suspicious personalities, especially when associated with alcohol abuse, in schizophrenia and in affective psychoses.

DELUSIONS OF INFLUENCE

The *phenomenon of passivity* or *alienation* is one of Schneider's first-rank symptoms in the diagnosis of schizophrenia – those symptoms which, in the absence of organic brain disease, suggest schizophrenia (Box 4.13). The patient says that their mind or body is being controlled (*influenced*) by outside forces, such as laser beams or microchips. Thoughts are forced either into or out of their head. Another form of *thought alienation* is thought broadcast, in which the patient's thoughts leave his or her head, travel through the air and enter into other people's heads, so that when the patient thinks something everyone else thinks the same. *Alienation*, or *passivity*, may also affect perception, as in patients who experience somatic hallucinations that they say are being caused by other people or by external forces. These may be divided into abnormal perceptions and abnormal experiences of the self or the environment.

Abnormal perceptions

Abnormal perceptions may occur in any of the sensory modalities – hearing, vision, smell, taste and touch (Box 4.14). Objects may be distorted while remaining recognizable or misperceived, as in illusions or hallucinations. Distortions in *intensity*, either increased or decreased, may be due to functional or organic disorders; distortions in *quality* (e.g. colour) are often due to toxic substances; distortions in *form* (e.g. *micropsia*, when the object appears smaller or further away, or *macropsia*) may be due to organic lesions of the visual pathway.

> **Box 4.14 Examples of abnormal perceptions**
>
> - Distortions – an abnormally perceived object
> - Illusions – a disturbance of perception of a real object
> - Hallucinations – an apparent perception: the object does not exist (the patient may be aware of the unreality of the perception)

Illusions

Illusions occur when the object is real but mis-perceived. Illusions are usually related to unusual features of the perceptual environment of the object, coupled with a state of high emotion in the perceiver. A common example is the experience of walking through a lonely alley on a dark night and perceiving a tree in the distance to be the figure of a man. Vision is impaired by the poor illumination and the lonely alley induces a feeling of fear, thereby leading to the illusion. However, illusions are common in psychiatric illness, particularly acute confusional states.

Hallucinations

Hallucinations occur in the absence of a perceived object. The commonest hallucinations are auditory and visual but, as with normal perceptions, they can occur in all sensory modalities. They may be due to organic disease of the nervous system or to extreme environmental disturbances, as in sensory deprivation. In certain instances they may be non-pathological phenomena, as in *hypnagogic* and *hypnopompic* hallucinations experienced by a person going to sleep or waking up. Hypnogogic hallucinations also occur in narcolepsy.

In psychiatric practice, hallucinations occur both in organic and functional psychoses, including schizophrenia and affective illnesses, when there is marked anxiety, in grief reactions and in hysterical illnesses. They may be linked to certain places or contexts, as in hallucinations with a religious content, or paranoid hallucinations of neighbours plotting heard through the walls of the house.

Auditory hallucinations

These may be undifferentiated noises, music, unidentifiable distant mumbling, words, phrases, or more elaborate speech. When patients hear voices rather than sounds they may sometimes be able to recognize them as belonging to people they know. The voices may be talking to the patient, or talking about him or her (see below). They may be persecutory, neutral or pleasing. The patient may talk back to the voices, or may appear to be listening to them intently. In some cases the voices direct the patient to certain actions that they may feel they must follow.

Second-person voices

Second-person voices with distressing content – 'You stink, you're horrible, go kill yourself' – are found in severe depressive illnesses. Third-person voices, which discuss or argue about the patient or comment on what he or she is doing, are suggestive of schizophrenia in the absence of organic brain disease (see Box 4.13), as is hearing one's own thoughts spoken out loud (*écho des pensées*). In grief reactions the bereaved person may hear the footsteps or other stigmata of the dead person.

Visual hallucinations

These vary in complexity from simple flashes of light to sophisticated 'visions' of people or animals. They are more common in organic psychoses, especially acute confusional states, than in functional psychoses. Visual hallucinations may be frightening, as in the hallucinations of spiders, insects and rats that occur especially in delirium tremens, or pleasing, as with Lilliputian hallucinations, in which the patient sees tiny people. They may coexist with auditory hallucinations, as in temporal lobe epilepsy.

Hallucinations of smell and taste

In temporal lobe epilepsy unpleasant *olfactory hallucinations* may be the initial symptom of the attack. They are frequent in schizophrenia and in depressive illnesses. *Hallucinations of taste* are rare in psychiatric practice but may occur in temporal lobe epilepsy.

Tactile and somatic hallucinations

In cocaine psychosis patients may complain that insects are crawling over them (formication). Other patients insist that they are experiencing odd sensations in various parts of their body which are produced by other people, as in the man who complained that his neighbour's laser gun was producing a cold feeling that travelled up his legs. In the absence of organic brain disease tactile hallucinosis is a first-rank symptom of schizophrenia (see Box 4.13). These hallucinations may have a sexual content, as in the patient who insisted that someone was having intercourse with her and she could feel it happening all the time.

Other hallucinations and illusions

Some people complain that, when alone, they feel the presence of someone else beside them. This may occur in grief reactions; when the patient is frightened; as a manifestation of hysteria; or in organic brain disease and schizophrenia. *Vestibular hallucinations* may occur in acute organic brain disease, such as the patient with delirium tremens who has the sensation of flying through the air.

ABNORMAL EXPERIENCES OF SELF AND ENVIRONMENT

DÉJÀ VU
This may occur in normal people but is often associated with temporal lobe epilepsy, and is characterized by the patient feeling that they have been in their current situation before.

CAPGRAS' SYNDROME
In this syndrome, which occurs most commonly in schizophrenia but may also occur in dementia, the patient asserts that people are not who they claim to be, but are their double.

DEPERSONALIZATION
This is often a manifestation of heightened anxiety levels. The patient does not feel his or her normal self, and may describe this unpleasant experience as if floating above their own body looking down on it. The patient may also complain of losing the capacity to feel at an emotional level. This may be one of the most marked symptoms in depressed patients.

DEREALIZATION
This often accompanies depersonalization. Patients say that their surroundings feel unreal, or grey or colourless.

ASSESSMENT OF THE COGNITIVE STATE

In elderly people, or when organic brain disease is suspected (e.g. in acute confusional states), assessment of cognitive state is extremely important. Semi-quantitative tests of cognitive function are often used, for example the *Mental Status Questionnaire* (MSQ) (Table 4.1) and the *Mini-mental State Examination* (MMSE) (Table 4.2). The MSQ consists of 10 simple questions that relate to alertness, orientation for time and space, and recent and long-

Table 4.1   Mental Status Questionnaire

1. What is the name of this place (where are we now)?
2. What is the address of this place?
3. What is the date?
4. What month is it?
5. What year is it?
6. How old are you?
7. When is your birthday?
8. What year were you born?
9. Who is the Prime Minister?
10. Who was the previous Prime Minister?

Each question is scored 0 for incorrect, and 1 for a correct response.
Normal subjects score 9 or 10; scores less than 8 imply a degree of mental confusion.

term memory. Normal subjects achieve 9 or 10 correct answers; scores less than 8 imply some degree of mental confusion. Patients with severe confusion score less than 3. The MMSE (Table 4.2) differs from the MSQ in that it is more detailed, and scores are to some extent dependent on educational level. The test has subcategories related to orientation, registration, attention, recall and language. The maximum score is 30, and scores lower than 21 are associated with cognitive impairment. Neither the MSQ nor the MMSE is capable of differentiating multifocal from diffuse organic brain disease, but both provide useful baseline assessment of a patient's cognitive performance.

LEVEL OF CONSCIOUSNESS
The patient's level of alertness or, if they are unconscious, the level of unconsciousness may be assessed. Some patients have fluctuating levels of consciousness; the mental state may then fluctuate between lucidity and gross abnormality. This is a manifestation of an acute organic confusional state. For a full account of the examination of the unconscious patient see Chapter 21.

ORIENTATION
The patient's orientation in time, place and person should be formally assessed by direct questioning and the patient's answers written down verbatim. Disorientation is an important sign of organic brain disease, whether chronic or acute, but may also occur in chronic institutionalized schizophrenics and in hysterical dissociative states.

TIME
Ask about the day, date, month, year and time of day. If the patient does not know the month, ask about the season. All patients should know the year, and either the month or season and the approximate time of day (e.g. morning, afternoon, evening or night). Long stays in hospital, where one day is much like the next, however, are not conducive to an awareness of which particular day it is or the exact date of the month.

PLACE
Patients should know where they are (e.g. home or hospital) and approximately where it is situated (e.g. what town or part of the town). They should know the way to places such as the bathroom or toilet. Some patients with acute confusional states may say they are in hospital, but that the hospital is part of their own home.

PERSON
If disorientation is suspected the patient should be asked his or her name and address.

ATTENTION AND CONCENTRATION

The patient's behaviour during the interview will have shown whether they are easily distracted or have been paying attention to and concentrating on the questions you have asked. This can be tested more formally by asking the patient to subtract serial sevens from 100 or, as this may be difficult even for normal people, serial threes from 20. Tasks such as recounting the months of the year and days of the week backwards and repeating a sequence of digits (digit span) forwards are also useful. Repetition of digits backwards (e.g. the doctor says 165 to which the patient should reply 561) is dependent not only on attention and concentration but also on the ability to register the numbers 165 and remember them long enough to reverse them, and is thus a test of immediate memory. Normal people should be able to manage seven digits forward and five backwards; telephone numbers in most large cities consist of seven digits. Another useful test is to ask the patient to spell 'world' backwards: the impaired patient often transposes the central letters of the word. Remember that literacy is implied in this test.

MEMORY

In chronic organic brain disease *memory for recent events* is diminished, whereas early in the illness the patient often remains able to remember events that have happened in the past and is thus able to give a coherent account of the family and early personal history. Some patients with memory impairment – as in Korsakov's psychosis, which is usually due to thiamine deficiency following poor nutrition or associated with heavy drinking – may confabulate. For example, a long-hospitalized patient may state that he had been at work the day before, and then describe in great detail what he had for his lunch that day. Confabulation is not deliberate invention. It most frequently consists of the inappropriate recall of recent or distant past experiences, illustrating a defect in the process of recall of memories.

In the case of head injuries or in epileptic attacks an attempt should be made to assess the presence of

---

Table 4.2 Mini-mental State Examination

Orientation
1 point for each correct answer
What is the:

time	
date	
day	
month	
year	**5 points**

What is the name of this:

ward	
hospital	
district	
town	
country	**5 points**

Registration
Name three objects
1, 2, 3 points according to how many are repeated
Resubmit list until patient word perfect in order to use this for a later test of recall
Score only first attempt .... **3 points**

Attention and calculation
Have the patient subtract 7 from 100 and then from the result a total of five
  times; 1 point for each correct subtraction .... **5 points**

Recall
Ask for three objects used in the registration test, 1 point being
  awarded for each correct answer .... **3 points**

Language
1 point each for two objects correctly named (pencil and watch) .... **2 points**
1 point for correct repetition of 'No ifs, ands and buts' .... **1 point**
3 points if three-stage commands correctly obeyed: 'Take this piece of paper in
  your right hand, fold it in half and place it on the floor' .... **3 points**
1 point for correct response to a written command, such as 'close your eyes' ... **1 point**
Have the patient write a sentence. Award 1 point if the sentence is meaningful,
  has a verb and a subject .... **1 point**
Test the patient's ability to copy a complex diagram of two intersecting pentagons ... **1 point**

Total score 30

retrograde and anterograde amnesia, if any, in some detail. Memory impairment may be simulated for gain by some manipulative patients, some of whom may give approximate answers. For example, if the date is Monday 20 September 2004 they may say it is Tuesday 14 October 2003, and then correct themselves to Sunday 16 December 2004. Hysterical amnesia may occur in dissociative states in which there is a sudden total loss of memory. In contrast, in organic amnesia, even in dementing illnesses, long-term memory and personal identity are usually spared until the later stages of the disorder. Patients who are apathetic or depressed may appear to have memory impairment, in the latter case called *depressive pseudodementia*. This may only become apparent when the depression lifts and the memory improves.

Past memory will already have been assessed while asking about the family and personal history, but recent memory will need more specific testing. A useful approach is to ask the patient about recent television programmes, such as the events in a popular soap opera, or the fortunes of a favourite football team. Other recent events will include details about the hospital itself, and how the patient got there. Current affairs should also be asked about, such as the names of top politicians and details of any recent happenings of major importance. A less direct approach is to ask the patient what has been going on in the world or in this country recently. A more systematic approach to testing of recent memory is to ask the patient to repeat a name and address, immediately and again after about 5 minutes. Or give the patient a sentence – for example 'The one thing a nation needs in order to be rich and great is a large, secure supply of wood' – and see how many repetitions are necessary for accurate reproduction. Where relevant, visual as well as auditory memory should be tested. This can be done by giving the patient a picture depicting a series of objects and a few minutes later asking them to recall as many of them as they can.

The patient's answers to all specific questions about memory should be recorded. Where there is evidence of potentially significant memory impairment, formal assessment using detailed tests, often performed by a neuropsychologist, is indicated.

INTELLIGENCE

An assessment of the patient's intelligence is one objective of the interview. Not only will this help to determine suitable treatment, it will also affect the interpretation of the mental state examination itself. In the patient with intelligence below the normal range bizarre behaviour and abnormal ideas may occur as part of a normal fantasy life or as a result of stress or conflict, and may not represent psychiatric illness. An approximate assessment of intelligence can be obtained from the educational and occupational history and from an assessment of general knowledge. Alternatively, this can be tested more formally especially by using the National Adult Reading Test (NART), as reading ability correlates closely with intelligence in the absence of other disabilities (see below). If in doubt, enquire whether the patient can read and write, and see whether they are able to solve simple mathematical problems, especially where these are related to daily activities, such as shopping. In patients in whom organic brain disease is suspected, a more detailed assessment of cerebral function should be carried out. In addition to the above, this includes an assessment of speech, both verbal and written; spatial, visual, motor and numerical abilities; awareness of body image; and the presence of released primitive reflexes. These comprise part of the neurological examination (see Chapter 10).

INSIGHT

Patients show varied levels of insight. First, insight may be lacking altogether, so that illness is denied. This lack of contact with reality is a hallmark of psychotic illness. Other patients accept that they are ill but perceive their illness as a physical rather than psychiatric problem; this is a feature of hysterical disorders and some anxiety states. Discussion of the illness may not lead to full insight. Some patients accept their need for psychiatric help but fail fully to unravel the complexities of their problems.

RAPPORT

The rapport established between doctor and patient depends not only on the interview technique but also on the personality and mental attitude of the participants. The doctor must not force his or her own personality and attitudes on to the patient. The way the patient relates to the doctor (see section on behaviour, p. 33–35) offers an insight into the patient's internal psychological state, enabling the doctor to make an evaluation of points such as dependence, relationships to others, especially those in authority, mood and paranoid ideation. With psychotic patients the doctor may feel that meaningful contact has never really been achieved. The doctor–patient relationship is a most important element in treatment. Psychotherapeutic insights suggest that a patient may displace on to the doctor feelings directed to other important people in his or her own life. For example, anger more appropriately directed towards a spouse or parent may instead manifest itself in the interview setting, with the doctor the recipient of this displaced emotion. Finally, patients may project their feelings on to the doctor. An angry patient may not overtly show this anger but may leave the doctor feeling angry; similarly, depression and elation may be transmitted to the doctor in the interview. Thus noting how you feel during the interview may give valuable added information for the assessment of the patient's mental state.

FURTHER INVESTIGATIONS

Extended information gathering during further interviews, continuing assessment of the mental state, some laboratory investigations, psychological testing, brain imaging, social enquiry and occupational therapy assessment are all important.

MENTAL STATE EVALUATION

The evaluation of the mental state is a continuous process and should be carried out at each interview. The behaviour on the ward of patients admitted to hospital should be observed and documented. This includes the way they relate to other patients, to staff and visitors, and whether there are any signs of sleep or appetite disturbance or other abnormal behaviour. Questionnaires and structured interview schedules may aid quantitative assessment of the mental state and in evaluating progress.

NEUROPSYCHOLOGICAL TESTING

Psychological tests can be used to quantitatively assess the patient's cognitive state, behaviour, personality and thinking process. Tests can be given to assess the level of intelligence, either briefly with the Mill Hill test or Raven's Progressive Matrices, or in more detail with the Wechsler Adult Intelligence Scale (WAIS). In behavioural disorders it is useful to carry out a thorough behavioural analysis; this must be designed to be relevant to the individual problem. These investigations require the specialized skills of a clinical psychologist. If there is a question of localized organic brain dysfunction, neuropsychological tests that aim to explore specific cognitive processes or the functions of individual brain regions will be employed by the clinical neuropsychologist. A detailed neuropsychological assessment may be indicated to establish the presence of current cognitive functioning when cognitive decline is suspected. By comparing performance against expected premorbid levels and against comparable population norms, the abnormality may be defined. Repeat testing after an interval of several months may help to clarify an unclear diagnosis or support a more detailed prognosis when a diagnosis of a dementia has been reached. Repeat testing may also help to distinguish the relatively static cognitive deficits arising from chronic depression in the elderly from the deteriorating scores in dementing illness. Patients with schizophrenia, at least in the acute stage, do not normally have cognitive decline, so if there is some clinical evidence of disturbed cognition then formal cognitive assessment may help to establish whether a condition other than schizophrenia is present.

BRAIN IMAGING

EEG, CT and MRI are sometimes appropriate when exploring the possibility of a demonstrable organic cause for behavioural signs and symptoms, such as epilepsy or a space-occupying lesion. Indications for these techniques include periodicity to the behavioural changes, the presence of an altered level of consciousness, or the finding of abnormalities on neurological examination. In the absence of any of these, and in the presence of a typical psychiatric presentation, the chances of finding any contributory structural brain anomalies are small. However, if a clinical presentation is atypical, if the course of the illness does not proceed as expected, or if a diagnosis of dementia is questioned, then structural brain imaging may be helpful.

5 Nutritional assessment

J. Powell-Tuck

INTRODUCTION

The prevalence of obesity in the developed world is increasing. Weight loss is often a consequence of illness, and disease-related undernutrition is common in our hospitals and nursing homes, though it tends to be underdiagnosed and inexpertly treated. Malnutrition, whether over- or undernutrition, has implications for the prevention and optimal management of disease (Box 5.1). It must be recognized and quantified as part of the routine history and examination of every patient, as a prelude to correct nutritional and metabolic management.

HISTORY

Enquiry should be made as to the patient's 'usual weight' in health. If this is variable then it is important to determine the trends in weight. How much did the patient weigh before the illness weight loss commenced, and how much do they weigh now? The estimated timing of weight loss should be elicited, and whether or not it was intentional. Similarly, the timing of weight gain should be elicited in the obese.

Patients at risk of malnutrition are those with reduced food intake because of a poor appetite or inability to eat. Malnutrition can also develop in patients with gastrointestinal failure and when metabolic demands exceed energy needs, as in thyrotoxicosis.

Reduced food intake can be due to inability to eat (loss of consciousness), inability to swallow (oropharyngeal or oesophageal disorders), poor appetite, early satiety or vomiting. Appetite is the desire for food, whereas early satiety is the feeling of abdominal distension and fullness after eating small meals. Poor appetite can accompany any severe illness, such as malignancy, chronic renal or cardiac failure, in which nausea or vomiting are often accompanying symptoms. Other common causes of decreased appetite include depression, viral illness, and chronic drug and alcohol abuse.

Is the patient short of breath and unable to eat? Abdominal pain or diarrhoea made worse by eating may also limit intake. Enquire about the frequency and volume of bowel movements, as water/electrolyte

deficiency is likely with increased frequency. An enquiry into everyday life will give an indication of daily activities, sport and quality of life, and reveal limitations as a result of disease, physical handicap or undernutrition. The amount of alcohol a patient drinks in units per week should be determined in the history. Remember that glasses of wine tend to be larger these days than the standard single unit, especially if poured at home. A 250 ml glass of 12.5% wine is 3 units. Some beers are much stronger than the usual 4.5%.

Early satiety can be due to gastric ulcer or malignancy, pressure from surrounding organs on the stomach (pancreatic cancer or cardiomegaly), or non-ulcer dyspepsia. Gastrointestinal disorders such as coeliac disease, bacterial overgrowth syndromes or inflammatory bowel disease can cause steatorrhoea, which may result in weight loss, and in particular expose the patient to the risk of specific deficiencies of vitamins and minerals (Table 5.1). Weight loss due to malabsorption without reduced intake, or even with increased intake, can occur in short bowel syndrome or severe pancreatic insufficiency.

Hypermetabolic states occur in severely ill patients, especially in those with fever, burns or cancers, or following major trauma, sepsis or burns, and may occur even during adequate nutrition. Increased exercise demands increased food intake for weight maintenance.

DIETARY HISTORY

A full dietary history is the province of a dietitian, but a simple dietary history is useful in the assessment of any patient and is invaluable in the malnourished. The frequency and times of meals and snacks throughout the day, the variety of foods eaten and a guide to quantity should be obtained. Does the patient put themselves at risk as a result of a poor diet? What foods does the patient enjoy eating, and what are their dislikes? Is the patient eating as much as before, or as much as their spouse or siblings?

Is the patient unconscious, or is consciousness impaired? Are they able to swallow? If not, is there an oropharyngeal problem? Is swallowing safe

Box 5.1 Health penalties of malnutrition

Obesity

- Insulin resistance, hyperglycaemia, type II diabetes mellitus, hepatic steatosis, non-alcoholic steatohepatitis (NASH) and impaired polymorph function
- Hypertension, heart failure and cerebrovascular disease
- Abnormal lipid metabolism, atheroma, coronary heart disease (CHD), myocardial infarction and gallstones
- Increased operative risk, increased risk of cancer, increased mortality
- Poor mobility and fitness, osteoarthritis, poor quality of life, low self-esteem, poor social integration and depression
- Hiatus hernia and gastro-oesophageal reflux disease

Undernutrition

- Impaired muscle function, poor respiratory and cardiac function, reduced exercise tolerance, reduced mobility, delayed convalescence
- Reduced plasma volume
- Psychological problems – fatigue, apathy, depression
- Poor immune function, depressed, delayed hypersensitivity, poor wound healing, increased operative risk
- Osteoporosis, fractures, poor fracture healing
- Specific deficiency syndromes (see Table 5.1)
- Risk of refeeding syndrome

(coughing/spluttering after swallowing)? Is there difficulty swallowing (solids/liquids)?

Some patients avoid certain foodstuffs, and this should be sought in the nutritional assessment. Do they follow a strict diet, or avoid foods that relieve gastrointestinal symptoms? Some patients try these diets unadvised, which can confuse diagnosis. Patients with coeliac disease avoid products containing gluten, such as wheat-based products, and patients with intestinal lactase deficiency avoid milk. Vegetarians should be asked if they are on a strict vegan diet, and what are their sources of B_{12}. Excessive dietary fibre leads to flatulence, bulky stools, increased bowel frequency and uncomfortable distension. Low dietary fibre intake is associated with constipation or difficult defecation. In anorexia/bulimia, a disorder that usually affects young women, there are cyclic changes in appetite and food intake, and dietary fads develop in association with a pathological aversion to body habitus and self. These should be sought in the history.

EXAMINATION

In the general examination of nutritional status attention should be paid to anaemia, the presence and distribution of body fat, the muscle bulk and the presence of oedema. The hydration status of the patient should be assessed (tongue, skin turgor and postural hypotension, peripheral oedema (ankle and sacral), ascites, jugular venous pressure). Hypoalbuminaemia, which occurs in relation to an inflammatory response, may lead to oedema. A lying and standing (or sitting) blood pressure measurement is invaluable for nutritional assessment. A drop in systolic blood pressure on standing of more than 15 mmHg is described as postural hypotension, and if it is accompanied by the expected increase in pulse rate it indicates blood volume or saline depletion.

In malnutrition loss of muscle mass is common. Wasting of the temporalis muscle results in the gaunt appearance of the starved. The skeletal muscles of the extremities also serve as an indicator of malnutrition. Additional clues to malnutrition include a dry cracked tongue and skin, loss of scalp and body hair, and poor wound healing. The limb muscles are thin and the distal reflexes difficult to elicit, and subcutaneous fat is atrophic. A careful search should be made for the signs of specific deficiencies of minerals and vitamins (see Table 5.1).

Subcutaneous fat stores should be examined for losses in weight or for excess accumulation.

A clinical examination must include measurement of weight and height. Body weight must be expressed as a function of height (see BMI below).

At the end of the examination the patient should be classified as well nourished, moderately malnourished or severely malnourished. Use BMI, mid-upper arm circumference (MUAC), waist and waist:hip ratio, skinfold thickness, and especially the Malnutrition Universal Screening Tool (MUST) to support this classification.

BODY MASS INDEX (BMI)
OR QUETELET INDEX (QI) (Table 5.2)

Nutritional status is best quantified by comparing weight with height – the Quetelet (body mass) index.

$$\text{BMI or QI} = \frac{\text{Weight (kg)}}{(\text{Height in metres})^2}$$

In the UK, the range 20–25 is often regarded as desirable, but the lower level of 18.5 is more applicable internationally. Patients with an index of more than 30 need to lose weight. In malnourished children height retardation lags behind that of weight, and the relation between weight and height should always be compared with age using appropriate charts.

If height cannot be measured, there are nomograms that relate the length of the forearm (ulna) or knee height (knee to heel) to the true height.

MID-UPPER ARM CIRCUMFERENCE (MUAC)

If neither height nor weight can be measured or obtained, nutritional assessment can be estimated using the mid-upper arm circumference. The patient should be standing or sitting. The non-dominant arm should be used if possible, and the patient asked to remove clothing so the arm is bare. The top of the shoulder (acromion) is located together with the point of the elbow (olecranon process) (Fig. 5.1).

The distance between the two points is measured and the midpoint marked. The circumference of the arm at the midpoint is then measured (Fig. 5.2). The tape measure should not be pulled tight: it should just fit comfortably round the arm.

- If the MUAC is ≥25 cm the BMI is likely to be ≥20.
- If the MUAC is ≥23.5 cm and <25 cm, the BMI is likely to be ≥18.5 and <20.
- If the MUAC is <23.5 cm then the BMI may be <18.5.

The MUAC can be used to estimate weight change over a period of time and can be useful in

Table 5.1 Principal symptoms and signs due to vitamin and mineral deficiencies

Nutrients	Deficiency syndrome	Principal symptoms/signs
A, Retinol (carotenoids)		Night blindness, keratomalacia
B_1, Thiamine	Wernicke–Korsakoff, beri-beri	Nystagmus, sixth cranial nerve palsy, ataxia, acidosis, dementia, paraesthesiae, neuropathy and cardiac failure
B_2, Riboflavin	Ariboflavinosis	Angular stomatitis, glossitis, magenta tongue
Niacin, nicotinic acid	Pellagra	Dermatitis of sun-exposed areas, dementia, poor appetite, difficulty sleeping, confusion, sore mouth
B_6, Pyridoxine		Poor appetite, lassitude, oxaluria
Panthothenic acid		Nausea, abdominal pain, paraesthesiae, burning feet
Biotin		Dermatitis, depression, lassitude, muscle pains, ECG abnormalities, blepharitis
Folic acid		Macrocytic anaemia, thrombocytopenia and megaloblastic bone marrow
B_{12}		Subacute combined degeneration, macrocytic anaemia
C, Ascorbic acid	Scurvy	Poor wound healing, fatigue, limb pain, shortness of breath, difficulty sleeping, gingivitis, perifollicular purpura, hyperkeratosis
D, Ergo-/cholecalciferol	Rickets/osteomalacia	Bone pain, proximal myopathy
E, Tocopherol		Haemolysis, posterior column signs, ataxia, muscle wasting, retinitis pigmentosa-like changes, night blindness
K, Phylloquinone and other menaquinones		Bruising, purpura, nose and gastrointestinal bleeds
Trace elements		
Iron		Koilonychia, smooth tongue, anaemia, oesophageal web
Zinc	Acrodermatitis enteropathica	Peristomal/perinasal/perineal erythema, thin hair, diarrhoea, apathy, anorexia, growth failure, hypoglycaemia
Copper		Microcytic hypochromic anaemia, neutropenia, scurvy-like bone lesions, osteoporosis
Chromium		Peripheral neuropathy, hyperglycaemia
Selenium		Cardiomyopathy
Iodine		Goitre

patients in long-term care. It can be used in patients with ascites or leg oedema if the fluid accumulation does not involve the arms.

MUAC needs to be measured repeatedly over a period of time, preferably taking two measurements on each occasion and using the average of the two.

● If the MUAC changes by at least 10% then it is likely that weight and BMI have changed by approximately 10% or more.

SKINFOLD THICKNESS (Table 5.3)

The nutritional state can be measured at sites such as the biceps, triceps, infrascapular and suprailiac regions, using Harpenden calipers. This is designed so that the jaws of the device remain parallel and constant pressure is exerted between them at different skinfold thicknesses. The triceps skinfold (TSF), midway between acromion and olecranon, is the most commonly used site. The skinfold oppo-

site, on the flexor surface of the mid-upper arm, is termed the biceps skinfold. The skinfold thickness is measured in the vertical plane with the arm hanging relaxed by the side of the body. Sites just below the inferior tip of the scapular and above the iliac crest are also used sometimes, and are termed infrascapular and suprailiac, respectively. Percentage body fat, and hence given body weight – lean body mass – can be calculated from skinfolds if the patient's age and gender are known. Arm muscle circumference (AMC) is sometimes derived as follows:

$$AMC = MUAC - (4.18 \times TSF).$$

WAIST AND WAIST:HIP RATIO

Simple circumferences can provide useful measures of body fat. Strong correlations have been found between subcutaneous and intra-abdominal fat (on

Table 5.2 World Health Organization (WHO) classification of obesity

Category	BMI/Quetelet index
Underweight	<18.5
Healthy weight	18.5–24.9
Overweight	25–29.9
Moderately obese	30–34.9
Severely obese	35–39.9
Morbidly obese	>40

Table 5.3 Skinfold thickness: normal skinfold thickness measured by Harpenden callipers (mm). The 80% and 60% ranges are associated with nutritional depletion

	Standard	80%	60%
Adult males	12.5	10.0	7.5
Adult females	16.5	13.0	10.0
Nutritional state	Normal nutrition	Moderate depletion	Severe depletion

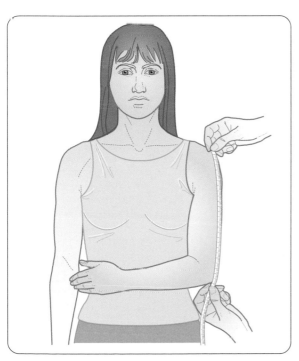

Figure 5.1 Measurement from top of the shoulder to point of the elbow.

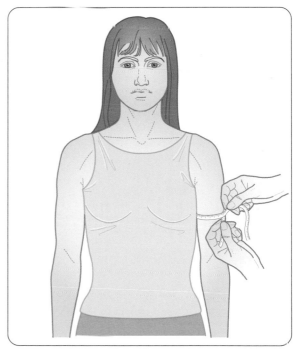

Figure 5.2 Measurement of circumference of arm to midpoint.

Table 5.4 Sex-specific waist circumferences for risk of obesity-associated metabolic complications

	Increased	Substantially increased
Men	>94 cm	>102 cm
Women	>80 cm	>88 cm

computerized tomography (CT) and waist and hip circumferences and waist ratios for both sexes. The circumference of the waist is a strong predictor of the degree of subcutaneous and intra-abdominal fat (Table 5.4). It is also a good indicator for the complications of obesity, such as coronary heart disease.

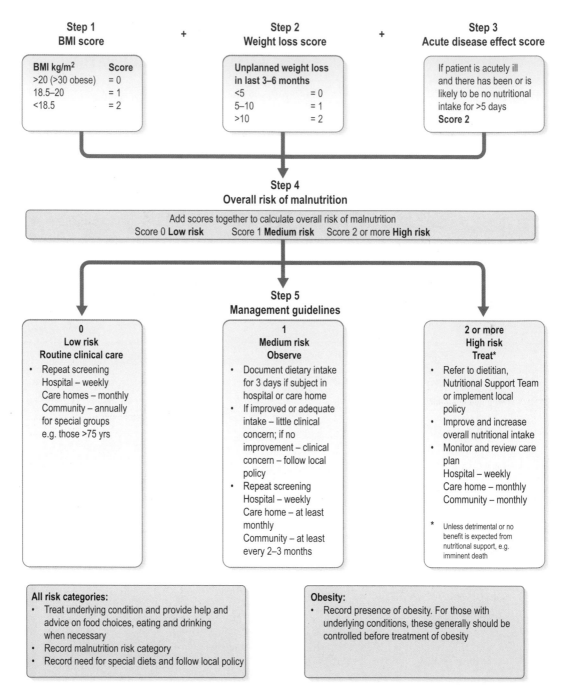

Figure 5.3 Malnutrition Universal Screening Tool (MUST) developed by the Malnutrition Advisory Group, a standing committee of BAPEN.

MALNUTRITION UNIVERSAL SCREENING TOOL (MUST)

The MUST is a five-step screening tool to identify adults who are malnourished, at risk of malnutrition (undernutrition) or obese. It has been developed by the British Association for Parenteral and Enteral Nutrition (BAPEN) for general use and incorporates management guidelines that can be used to develop a care plan (Fig. 5.3).

Step 1 Measure height and weight and calculate the BMI.

Step 2 determines unexplained weight loss over 3–6 months and is a more acute risk factor for malnutrition than BMI. The patient is asked if there has been any weight loss in the last 3–6 months, and if so, how much. The medical notes are often helpful in this respect. The current weight is deducted from the previous weight to calculate the amount of weight lost. Weight loss tables are used to calculate weight loss scores. If the subject has not lost weight this is taken as a score of 0 (Table 5.5).

Table 5.5 Step 2 – Weight loss scores

	Score 0 Wt Loss <5%	Score 1 Wt Loss 5–10%	Score 2 Wt Loss >10%		Score 0 Wt Loss <5%	Score 1 Wt Loss 5–10%	Score 2 Wt Loss >10%
34 kg	<1.70	1.70 – 3.40	>3.40	5st 4lb	<4lb	4lb – 7lb	>7lb
36 kg	<1.80	1.80 – 3.60	>3.60	5st 7lb	<4lb	4lb – 8lb	>8lb
38 kg	<1.90	1.90 – 3.80	>3.80	5st 11lb	<4lb	4lb – 8lb	>8lb
40 kg	<2.00	2.00 – 4.00	>4.00	6st	<4lb	4lb – 8lb	>8lb
42 kg	<2.10	2.10 – 4.20	>4.20	6st 4lb	<4lb	4lb – 9lb	>9lb
44 kg	<2.20	2.20 – 4.40	>4.40	6st 7lb	<5lb	5lb – 9lb	>9lb
46 kg	<2.30	2.30 – 4.60	>4.60	6st 11lb	<5lb	5lb – 10lb	>10lb
48 kg	<2.40	2.40 – 4.80	>4.80	7st	<5lb	5lb – 10lb	>10lb
50 kg	<2.50	2.50 – 5.00	>5.00	7st 4lb	<5lb	5lb – 10lb	>10lb
52 kg	<2.60	2.60 – 5.20	>5.20	7st 7lb	<5lb	5lb – 11lb	>11lb
54 kg	<2.70	2.70 – 5.40	>5.40	7st 11lb	<5lb	5lb – 11lb	>11lb
56 kg	<2.80	2.80 – 5.60	>5.60	8st	<6lb	6lb – 11lb	>11lb
58 kg	<2.90	2.90 – 5.80	>5.80	8st 4lb	<6lb	6lb – 12lb	>12lb
60 kg	<3.00	3.00 – 6.00	>6.00	8st 7lb	<6lb	6lb – 12lb	>12lb
62 kg	<3.10	3.10 – 6.20	>6.20	8st 11lb	<6lb	6lb – 12lb	>12lb
64 kg	<3.20	3.20 – 6.40	>6.40	9st	<6lb	6lb – 13lb	>13lb
66 kg	<3.30	3.30 – 6.60	>6.60	9st 4lb	<7lb	7lb – 13lb	>13lb
68 kg	<3.40	3.40 – 6.80	>6.80	9st 7lb	<7lb	7lb – 13lb	>13lb
70 kg	<3.50	3.50 – 7.00	>7.00	9st 11lb	<7lb	7lb – 1st 0lb	>1st 0lb
72 kg	<3.60	3.60 – 7.20	>7.20	10st	<7lb	7lb – 1st 0lb	>1st 0lb
74 kg	<3.70	3.70 – 7.40	>7.40	10st 4lb	<7lb	7lb – 1st 0lb	>1st 0lb
76 kg	<3.80	3.80 – 7.60	>7.60	10st 7lb	<7lb	7lb – 1st 1lb	>1st 1lb
78 kg	<3.90	3.90 – 7.80	>7.80	10st 11lb	<8lb	8lb – 1st 1lb	>1st 1lb
80 kg	<4.00	4.00 – 8.00	>8.00	11st	<8lb	8lb – 1st 1lb	>1st 1lb
82 kg	<4.10	4.10 – 8.20	>8.20	11st 4lb	<8lb	8lb – 1st 2lb	>1st 2lb
84 kg	<4.20	4.20 – 8.40	>8.40	11st 7lb	<8lb	8lb – 1st 2lb	>1st 2lb
86 kg	<4.30	4.30 – 8.60	>8.60	11st 11lb	<8lb	8lb – 1st 3lb	>1st 3lb
88 kg	<4.40	4.40 – 8.80	>8.80	12st	<8lb	8lb – 1st 3lb	>1st 3lb
90 kg	<4.50	4.50 – 9.00	>9.00	12st 4lb	<9lb	9lb – 1st 3lb	>1st 3lb
92 kg	<4.60	4.60 – 9.20	>9.20	12st 7lb	<9lb	9lb – 1st 4lb	>1st 4lb
94 kg	<4.70	4.70 – 9.40	>9.40	12st 11lb	<9lb	9lb – 1st 4lb	>1st 4lb
96 kg	<4.80	4.80 – 9.60	>9.60	13st	<9lb	9lb – 1st 4lb	>1st 4lb
98 kg	<4.90	4.90 – 9.80	>9.80	13st 4lb	<9lb	9lb – 1st 5lb	>1st 5lb
100 kg	<5.00	5.00 – 10.00	>10.00	13st 7lb	<9lb	9lb – 1st 5lb	>1st 5lb
102 kg	<5.10	5.10 – 10.20	>10.20	13st 11lb	<10lb	10lb – 1st 5lb	>1st 5lb
104 kg	<5.20	5.20 – 10.40	>10.40	14st	<10lb	10lb – 1st 6lb	>1st 6lb
106 kg	<5.30	5.30 – 10.60	>10.60	14st 4lb	<10lb	10lb – 1st 6lb	>1st 6lb
108 kg	<5.40	5.40 – 10.80	>10.80	14st 7lb	<10lb	10lb – 1st 6lb	>1st 6lb
110 kg	<5.50	5.50 – 11.00	>11.00	14st 11lb	<10lb	10lb – 1st 7lb	>1st 7lb
112 kg	<5.60	5.60 – 11.20	>11.20	15st	<11lb	11lb – 1st 7lb	>1st 7lb
114 kg	<5.70	5.70 – 11.40	>11.40	15st 4lb	<11lb	11lb – 1st 7lb	>1st 7lb
116 kg	<5.80	5.80 – 11.60	>11.60	15st 7lb	<11lb	11lb – 1st 8lb	>1st 8lb
118 kg	<5.90	5.90 – 11.80	>11.80	15st 11lb	<11lb	11lb – 1st 8lb	>1st 8lb
120 kg	<6.00	6.00 – 12.00	>12.00	16st	<11lb	11lb – 1st 8lb	>1st 8lb
122 kg	<6.10	6.10 – 12.20	>12.20	16st 4lb	<11lb	11lb – 1st 9lb	>1st 9lb
124 kg	<6.20	6.20 – 12.40	>12.40	16st 7lb	<12lb	12lb – 1st 9lb	>1st 9lb
126 kg	<6.30	6.30 – 12.60	>12.60				

Weight before weight loss (kg)

Weight before weight loss (st lb)

Table 5.6   Revised Schofield Equations Committee on Medical Aspects of Food Policy 1991

Revised Schofield equations COMA 1991		W = weight (kg)	
Males	**Kcal/day**	**Females**	**Kcal/day**
Age (years)		Age (years)	
10–17	17.1W + 657	10–17	13.4W + 692
18–29	15.1W + 692	18–29	14.8W + 487
30–59	11.5W + 873	30–59	8.3W + 846
60–74	11.9W + 700	60–74	9.2W + 687
75+	8.3W + 820	75+	9.8W + 624

Step 3 Acute disease can affect risk of malnutrition. If the patient is currently affected by an acute pathophysiological or psychological condition and there has been no nutritional intake or the likelihood of no intake for more than 5 days, they are likely to be at nutritional risk. This includes patients who are critically ill, who have swallowing difficulties (after stroke) or head injuries, or who are undergoing gastrointestinal surgery. This subset of patients receives a score of 2.

Step 4 The scores from steps 1, 2 and 3 are added together to calculate the overall risk of malnutrition.

Step 5 The overall risk of malnutrition can be incorporated into management guidelines to develop a care plan.

LABORATORY TESTS

Patients should have routine blood tests with a full blood count, prothrombin time, urea and electrolytes, liver function tests and serum haematinics. Serum haematinics should include serum iron, total iron-binding capacity, ferritin, serum B_{12} and red cell folate. Despite a wide appreciation of the value of regular intramuscular B_{12} in patients following total gastrectomy or resection of more than 50 cm of terminal ileum, other deficiencies are often overlooked. Specific deficiency syndromes are outlined in Table 5.1. Serum magnesium and zinc should be measured in patients with high intestinal output. Calcium, phosphate and alkaline phosphatase should be measured and vitamin D estimated in patients who are absorbing fat inefficiently, or those who are confined indoors out of the sun as a result of ill-health. Investigations can provide information about protein deficiency and can also indicate specific micronutrient deficiencies. Plasma albumin can be used to assess visceral protein depletion; however, hypoproteinaemia does not equate with protein malnutrition. Injury, inflammation and the presence of liver disease may all reduce the plasma albumin concentration. The ratio of C-reactive protein to albumin provides a better estimate of protein depletion. Plasma transferrin and prealbumin can be used as more sensitive parameters of visceral protein status. Urinary nitrogen (or urea nitrogen) reveals the degree of protein catabolism.

NITROGEN BALANCE

Most proteins contain about 16% nitrogen. Therefore 6.25 g of protein equates with 1 g nitrogen. Nitrogen balance is the difference between dietary nitrogen intake and excretion from the body. Protein intakes vary, but let us assume that in an adult 62.5 g is eaten, which is 10 g of nitrogen – a reasonable and convenient example. In the healthy person this is balanced by the loss of 8.5 g nitrogen in urine (mainly as urinary urea), 0.75 g in faeces, and a further 0.75 g excreted by other means. Normal adults have a net zero balance, with ingestion of food by day balancing losses by day and night. During illness such as trauma or sepsis this balance is disturbed and there is a negative nitrogen balance, with loss exceeding input.

CALCULATION OF ENERGY EXPENDITURE

Energy expenditure is best measured using indirect calorimetry. However, the basal metabolic rate can be estimated using Schofield equations, which were produced from healthy volunteers. These use the weight of the patient in kilograms (kg) and are dependent on age and gender (Table 5.6). As the equations were developed using healthy volunteers it must be remembered that they do not necessarily apply to patients with disease (e.g. sepsis, undernutrition, or disturbances in hydration, e.g. oedema). Other factors must be added to account for stress, pyrexia, physical activity, growth and development.

SECTION 3

Basic systems

Section contents

Respiratory system

J. Moore-Gillon

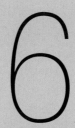

INTRODUCTION

Diseases of the respiratory system account for up to a third of deaths in most countries and for a major proportion of visits to the doctor and time away from work or school. As with every aspect of diagnosis in medicine, the key to success is a clear and carefully recorded history; symptoms may be trivial or extremely distressing, but either may indicate serious and life-threatening disease.

THE HISTORY

Most patients with respiratory disease will present with one or more of the following symptoms.

BREATHLESSNESS

Everyone becomes breathless on strenuous exertion. Breathlessness inappropriate to the level of physical exertion, or even occurring at rest, is called *dyspnoea*. Its mechanisms are complex and not fully understood. It is not due simply to a lowered blood oxygen tension (*hypoxia*) or to a raised blood carbon dioxide tension (*hypercapnia*), although these may play a significant part. People with cardiac disease (see Chapter 7) may become dyspnoeic as well as those with primarily respiratory problems.

Is the dyspnoea related only to exertion? How far can the patient walk at a normal pace on the level? This may take some skill to elicit, as few people note their symptoms in this form, but a brief discussion about what they can do in their daily lives usually gives a good estimate of their mobility.

Is there variability in the symptom? Are there good days and bad days and, very importantly, are there any times of day or night that are usually worse than others? Variable airways obstruction due to asthma is very often worse at night and in the early morning. By contrast, people with predominantly irreversible airways obstruction due to chronic obstructive pulmonary disease (COPD) will often say that as long as they are sitting in bed they feel quite normal; it is exercise that troubles them.

COUGH

A cough may be dry or it may be productive of sputum.

- How long has the cough been present? A cough lasting a few days following a cold has less significance than one lasting several weeks in a middle-aged smoker, which may be the first sign of a malignancy.
- Is the cough worse at any time of day or night? A dry cough at night may be an early symptom of asthma, as may cough that comes in spasms lasting several minutes.
- Is the cough aggravated by anything, for example dust, pollen or cold air? The increased reactivity of the airways seen in asthma, and in some normal people for several weeks after viral respiratory infections, may present in this way. Severe coughing, whatever its cause, may be followed by vomiting.

SPUTUM

- Is sputum produced?
- What does it look like? Children and some adults swallow sputum, but it is always worth asking for a description of its colour and consistency. Yellow or green sputum is usually purulent. People with asthma may produce small amounts of very thick or jelly-like sputum, sometimes in the shape of a cast of the airways. Eosinophils may accumulate in the sputum in asthma, causing a purulent appearance even when no infection is present.
- How much is produced? When severe lung damage in infancy and childhood was common, bronchiectasis was often found in adults. The amount of sputum produced daily often exceeded a cupful. Bronchiectasis is now rare, and chronic bronchitis causes the production of smaller amounts of sputum.

HAEMOPTYSIS

Haemoptysis means the coughing of blood in the sputum. It should *never* be dismissed without very careful evaluation of the patient. The potentially serious significance of blood in the sputum is well known, and fear often leads patients not to mention it: a specific question is always necessary.

- Is there any blood in the sputum? Is it fresh or altered? How often has it been seen, and for how long?

Blood may be coughed up alone, or sputum may be bloodstained. It is sometimes difficult for the patient to describe whether or not the blood has originated from the chest or whether it comes from the gums or nose, or even from the stomach. They should always be asked about associated conditions such as epistaxis (nosebleeds), or the subsequent development of melaena (altered blood in the stool), which occurs in the case of upper gastrointestinal bleeding. Usually, however, it is clear that the blood originates from the chest, and this is an indication for further investigation.

WHEEZING

Always ask whether the patient hears any noises coming from the chest. Even if a wheeze is not present when you examine the patient, it is useful to know that they have noticed it on occasions. Sometimes, wheezing will have been noticed by others (especially by a partner at night, when asthma is worse) but not by the patient.

Sometimes *stridor* (see below) may be mistaken for wheezing by both patient and doctor. This serious finding usually indicates narrowing of the larynx, trachea or main bronchi.

PAIN IN THE CHEST

Apart from musculoskeletal aches and pains consequent upon prolonged bouts of coughing, chest pain caused by lung disease usually arises from the pleura. Pleuritic pain is sharp and stabbing, and is made worse by deep breathing or coughing. It occurs when the pleura is inflamed, most commonly by infection in the underlying lung. More constant pain, unrelated to breathing, may be caused by local invasion of the chest wall by a lung or pleural tumour.

A spontaneous pneumothorax causes pain which is worse on breathing but which may have more of an aching character than the stabbing pain of pleurisy. If a pulmonary embolus causes infarction of the lung, pleurisy – and hence pleuritic pain – may occur, but an acute pulmonary embolus can also cause pain which is not stabbing in nature.

OTHER SYMPTOMS

Quite apart from the common symptoms of respiratory disease, there are some other aspects of the history that are particularly relevant to the respiratory system.

EAR, NOSE AND THROAT

Some questions related to the *ear, nose* and *throat* are often relevant. Recurrent sinusitis and rhinitis may be linked to asthma or, less commonly, bronchiectasis. A change in the voice may indicate involvement of the left recurrent laryngeal nerve by a carcinoma of the lung. Sometimes patients using inhalers for asthma, and especially inhaled steroids, develop hoarseness or weakness of the voice, which improves on changing the treatment. Do not ascribe hoarseness to this cause in older patients, as carcinoma of the vocal cords can also be present with hoarseness or a change in the quality of the voice. Laryngoscopy is always indicated.

THE SMOKING HISTORY

Always take a full smoking history – and do so in a sympathetic and non-condemnatory way, or you are unlikely to get an accurate picture. The time for advice about smoking cessation is after completion of your assessment, not at the outset. Simply asking 'Do you smoke?' is not enough. Novices will be astonished at how often closer probing of the answer 'no' reveals that the patient gave up yesterday, or that they state their intention of doing so from the time of your consultation. Age of starting and stopping if an ex-smoker, and average consumption for both current and ex-smokers, are the bare minimum information needed.

Identification of an individual as a current or ex-smoker will greatly influence the interpretation you place on your findings upon history and examination. Almost all cases of lung cancer and chronic obstructive pulmonary disease (COPD) occur in those who have smoked.

THE FAMILY HISTORY

There is a strong inherited susceptibility to asthma. Associated conditions such as eczema and hay fever may also be present in relatives of those with asthma, particularly in those who develop the condition when young.

THE OCCUPATIONAL HISTORY

No other organ is as susceptible to the working environment as the lungs. Several hundred different substances have now been recognized as causing occupational asthma. Paint sprayers, workers in the electronics, rubber or plastics industries, and woodworkers are relatively commonly affected. Always ask about a relationship between symptoms and work.

Damage from inhalation of asbestos may take decades to become manifest, most seriously as malignant mesothelioma. In industrialized countries this once extremely rare tumour of the pleura has become more common, and will become even more common in the next 20 years. In middle-aged individuals who present with a pleural effusion – often the first sign of a mesothelioma – you will need to ask about possible asbestos exposure in jobs right back to the time of leaving school.

THE EXAMINATION

GENERAL ASSESSMENT

An examination of the respiratory system is incomplete without a simultaneous general assessment (Box 6.1). Watch the patient as they come into the room, during your history taking, and while they are undressing and climbing on to the couch. If this is a hospital inpatient, is there breathlessness just on moving in bed? What is on the bedside table – inhalers, tissues, a sputum pot, an oxygen mask? What is the physique and state of general nourishment of the patient?

For the examination the patient should be resting comfortably on a bed or couch, supported by pillows so that they can lean back comfortably at an angle of 45°.

The hands should be inspected for *clubbing, pallor* or *cyanosis*. The lips and tongue should be inspected for central cyanosis, which almost always indicates poor oxygenation of the blood by the lungs, whereas peripheral cyanosis alone is usually due to poor peripheral perfusion. A breathless patient may be using the accessory muscles of respiration (e.g. sternomastoid), and in the presence of severe COPD many patients find it easier to breathe out through pursed lips (Fig. 6.1).

As well as your general visual assessment, *listen* to the patient. What is the nature of the voice – is it hoarse? Is the patient capable of producing a normal, explosive cough, or is the voice weak or non-existent even when they are asked to cough? Is there *wheezing* audible, usually loudest in expiration, or is there *stridor*, a high-pitched *inspiratory* noise?

In a significant asthma attack the pulse rate is usually raised. The systolic blood pressure also falls during the severe inspiratory effort of acute asthma, and the degree of this fall (the degree of pulsus paradoxus) can be used as a measure of asthma severity.

Box 6.1 Points to note in a general assessment

- Physique
- Voice
- Breathlessness
- Clubbing
- Cyanosis or pallor
- Intercostal recession
- Use of accessory respiratory muscles
- Venous pulses
- Lymph nodes

EXAMINATION OF THE CHEST

RELEVANT ANATOMY

The interpretation of signs in the chest often causes problems for the beginner. A revision of the relevant anatomy may help.

The *bifurcation of the trachea* corresponds on the anterior chest wall with the sternal angle, the transverse bony ridge at the junction of the body of the sternum and the manubrium sterni. Posteriorly, the level is at the disc between the fourth and fifth thoracic vertebrae. The ribs are most easily counted downwards from the second costal cartilage, which articulates with the sternum at the extremity of the sternal angle.

A line from the second thoracic spine to the sixth rib in the mammary line corresponds to the upper border of the lower lobe (major interlobar fissure). On the right side a horizontal line from the sternum at the level of the fourth costal cartilage, drawn to meet the line of the major interlobar fissure, marks the boundary between the upper and middle lobes (the minor interlobar fissure). The greater part of each lung, as seen from behind, is composed of the

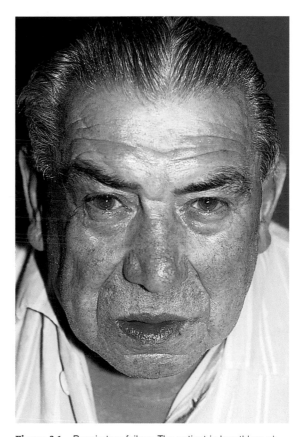

Figure 6.1 Respiratory failure. The patient is breathless at rest and there is central cyanosis with blueness of the lips and face. The lips are pursed during expiration, a characteristic feature of chronic obstructive pulmonary disease (COPD). This facial appearance is often accompanied by heart failure with peripheral oedema (cor pulmonale).

55

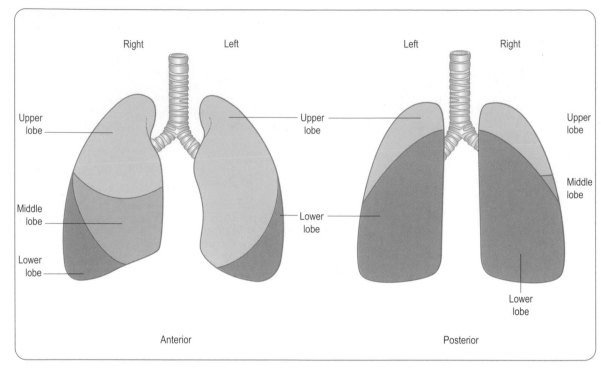

Figure 6.2   Anterior and posterior aspects of the lungs.

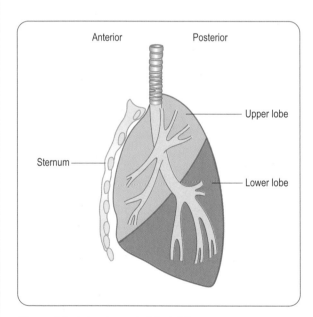

Figure 6.3   Lateral aspect of the left lung.

that listening is only one part of the examination of the chest. Obtaining the maximum possible information from your examination requires you to *look*, then to *feel*, and only then to *listen*.

LOOKING: INSPECTION OF THE CHEST

Appearance of the chest

First, are there any obvious scars from previous surgery? Are there any lumps visible beneath the skin, or any lesions on the skin itself?

The normal chest is bilaterally symmetrical and elliptical in cross-section. The chest may be distorted by disease of the ribs or spinal vertebrae, as well as by underlying lung disease (Box 6.2).

Kyphosis (forward bending) or *scoliosis* (lateral bending) of the vertebral column will lead to asymmetry of the chest, and if severe may significantly restrict lung movement.

A normal chest X-ray is seen in Figure 6.4.

Severe airways obstruction, particularly long term, as in COPD (Figs 6.1, 6.5) may lead to overinflated

lower lobe; only the apex belongs to the upper lobe. The middle and upper lobes on the right side and the upper lobe on the left occupy most of the area in front (Fig. 6.2). This is most easily visualized if the lobes are thought of as two wedges fitting together, not as two cubes piled one on top of the other (Fig. 6.3).

The stethoscope is so much part of the 'image' of a doctor that it is very easy for the student to forget

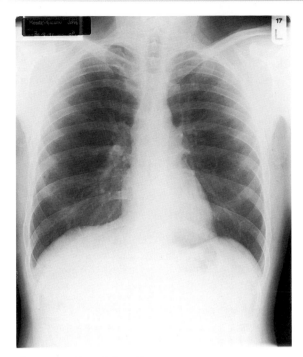

Figure 6.4 Normal chest X-ray.

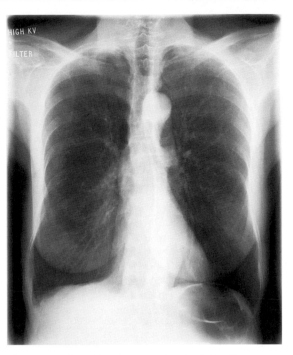

Figure 6.5 Chest X-ray in severe chronic obstructive pulmonary disease.

lungs. On examination the chest may be 'barrel-shaped', most easily appreciated as an increased anteroposterior diameter. On X-ray the hemidiaphragms appear lower than usual, and flattened.

Movement of the chest

Look at the *chest movements*. Are they symmetrical? If they seem to be diminished on one side, that is likely to be the side on which there is an abnormality. Intercostal recession – a drawing-in of the intercostal spaces with inspiration – may indicate severe upper airways obstruction, as in laryngeal disease, or tumours of the trachea. In COPD the lower ribs often move inwards on inspiration instead of the normal outwards movement.

Venous pulses

The *venous pulses* in the neck (see Chapter 7) should be inspected. A raised venous pressure is usually indicative of right heart failure but can be due to obstruction of the superior vena cava, usually because of malignancy in the upper mediastinum.

Respiratory rate and rhythm

The normal rate of respiration in a relaxed adult is about 14–16 breaths per minute (Box 6.3). *Tachypnoea* is an increased respiratory rate observed by the doctor, whereas *dyspnoea* is the symptom of breathlessness experienced by the patient. *Apnoea* means cessation of respiration.

Cheyne–Stokes breathing is the name given to a disturbance of respiratory rhythm in which there is

---

Box 6.3 Observing the chest

- Rate of respiration
- Rhythm of respiration
- Chest expansion
- Symmetry

---

cyclical deepening and quickening of respiration, followed by diminishing respiratory effort and rate, sometimes associated with a short period of complete apnoea, the cycle then being repeated. This is often observed in severely ill patients, and particularly in severe cardiac failure, narcotic drug poisoning and neurological disorders. It is occasionally seen – especially during sleep – in elderly patients without any obvious serious disease.

Some patients may have apnoeic episodes during sleep owing to complete cessation of respiratory effort (*central apnoea*) or, much more commonly, apnoea despite continuation of respiratory effort. This is known as obstructive apnoea and is due to obstruction of the upper airways by soft tissues in the region of the pharynx.

FEELING: PALPATION OF THE CHEST

Lymph nodes

The *lymph nodes* in the supraclavicular fossae, cervical regions and axillary regions should be palpated. If they are enlarged this may be secondary to the spread of malignant disease from the chest, and such findings will influence decisions regarding treatment.

Swellings and tenderness

It is useful to palpate any part of the chest that presents an obvious *swelling*, or where the patient complains of pain (Box 6.4). Feel gently, as pressure may increase the pain. It is often important, particularly in the case of musculoskeletal pain, to identify a site of tenderness (Box 6.5).

Trachea and heart

The *positions* of the cardiac impulse and trachea should then be determined. Feel for the trachea by putting the second and fourth fingers of the examining hand on each edge of the sternal notch and use the third finger to assess whether the trachea is central or deviated to one side. Avoid heavy-handedness in this situation – it is uncomfortable for the patient if the examiner is rough. A slight deviation of the trachea to the right may be found in healthy people.

Displacement of the cardiac impulse without displacement of the trachea may be due to scoliosis, to a congenital funnel depression of the sternum or to enlargement of the left ventricle. In the absence of these conditions a significant displacement of the cardiac impulse or trachea, or of both together, suggests that the position of the mediastinum has been altered by disease of the lungs or pleura. The mediastinum may be *pushed* away from the affected side by a pleural effusion or pneumothorax. Fibrosis or collapse of the lung will *pull* the mediastinum towards the affected side.

Chest expansion

As well as by simple inspection, possible asymmetrical expansion of the chest may be further explored by palpation. Face the patient and place the fingertips of both hands on either side of the lower ribcage, so that the tips of the thumbs meet in the midline in front of – but not touching – the chest. A deep breath by the patient will increase the distance between the thumbs and indicate the degree of expansion. If one thumb remains closer to the midline, this suggests diminished expansion on that side.

Tactile vocal fremitus is detected by palpation, but this is not a commonly used routine examination technique. It is discussed further under Auscultation, below.

FEELING: PERCUSSION OF THE CHEST

The technique of percussion was probably developed as a way of ascertaining how much fluid remained in barrels of wine or other liquids. Auenbrugger applied percussion to the chest having learned this method in his father's wine cellar. Effective percussion is a knack that requires consistent practice; do so upon yourself or on willing colleagues, as percussion can be uncomfortable for patients if performed repeatedly and inexpertly.

The middle finger of the left hand is placed on the part to be percussed and pressed firmly against it. The back of the distal interphalangeal joint is then struck with the tip of the middle finger of the right hand (vice versa if you are left-handed). The movement should be at the *wrist* rather than at the elbow. The percussing finger is bent so that its terminal phalanx is at right-angles and it strikes the other finger perpendicularly. As soon as the blow has been given, the striking finger is raised: the action is a tapping movement.

The two most common mistakes made by the beginner are, first, failing to ensure that the finger of the left hand is applied flatly and firmly to the chest wall and, second, striking the percussion blow from the elbow rather than from the wrist.

The character of the sound produced varies both qualitatively and quantitatively (Box 6.6). When the air in a cavity of sufficient size and appropriate shape is set vibrating a resonant sound is produced, and there is also a characteristic sensation felt by the

---

Box 6.4 Points to note on palpation of the chest

- Swelling
- Pain and tenderness
- Tracheal position
- Cardiac impulse
- Asymmetry
- Tactile vocal fremitus

Box 6.5 Causes of pain and tenderness in the chest

- A recent injury of the chest wall, or inflammatory conditions
- Intercostal muscular pain – as a rule, localized painful spots can be discovered on pressure
- A painful costochondral junction
- Secondary malignant deposits in the rib
- Herpes zoster before the appearance of the rash

Box 6.6 Points to note on percussion of the chest

- Resonance
- Dullness
- Pain and tenderness

finger placed on the chest. Try tapping a hollow cupboard and then a solid wall – the feeling is different, as well as the sound. The sound and feel of resonance over a healthy lung has to be learned by practice, and it is against this standard that possible abnormalities of percussion must be judged.

The normal degree of resonance varies between individuals, and in different parts of the chest in the same individual, being most resonant below the clavicles anteriorly and the scapulae posteriorly where the muscles are relatively thin, and least resonant over the scapulae. On the right side, there is loss of resonance inferiorly as the liver is encountered. On the left side the lower border overlaps the stomach, so there is a transition from lung resonance to tympanitic stomach resonance.

Always systematically compare the percussion note on the two sides of the chest, moving backwards and forwards from one side to the other, not all the way down one side and then down the other. Percuss over the clavicles; traditionally, this is done without an intervening finger on the chest, but there is no reason for this and it is more comfortable for the patient if the finger of the left hand is used in the usual way. Percuss three or four areas on the anterior chest wall, comparing left with right. Percuss the axillae, then three or four areas on the back of the chest.

Reduction of resonance (i.e. the percussion note is said to be *dull*) occurs in two important circumstances:

- When the underlying lung is more solid than usual, usually because of consolidation
- When the pleural cavity contains fluid, i.e. a pleural effusion is present.

Less commonly, a dull percussion note may be due to a thickened pleura. The percussion note is most dull when there is underlying fluid, as in a pleural effusion. Pleural effusion causes the sensation in the percussed finger to be similar to that felt when a solid wall is percussed. This is often called *stony dullness*. By comparing side with side, it is usually easy to detect a unilateral pleural effusion. Pleural effusion usually leads to decreased chest wall movement. Effusions may occur bilaterally in some patients, and this may be more difficult to detect clinically.

An *increase in resonance*, or hyperresonance, is more difficult to detect than dullness. It may be noticeable when the pleural cavity contains air, as in pneumothorax. Sometimes, however, in this situation one is tempted to think that the slightly duller side is the abnormal side. Further examination and chest X-ray will reveal the true situation.

LISTENING: AUSCULTATION OF THE CHEST
Listen to the chest with the diaphragm, not the bell, of the stethoscope (chest sounds are relatively high-pitched, and therefore the diaphragm is more sensitive than the bell). Ask the patient to take deep breaths in and out *through the mouth*. Demonstrate what you would like the patient to do, and then check visually that they are doing it while you listen to the chest.

As with percussion, you should listen in comparable positions to each side alternately, switching back and forth from one side to the other to compare (Box 6.7).

The breath sounds
Breath sounds have *intensity* and *quality*. The intensity (or loudness) of the sounds may be normal, reduced or increased. The quality of normal breath sounds is described as *vesicular*.

Breath sounds will be normal in intensity when the lung is inflating normally, but may be reduced if there is localized airway narrowing, if the lung is extensively damaged by a process such as emphysema, or if there is intervening pleural thickening or pleural fluid. Breath sounds may be of increased intensity in very thin subjects.

Breath sounds probably originate from turbulent airflow in the larger airways. When you place your stethoscope upon the chest, you are listening to how those sounds have been changed on their journey from their site of origin to the position of your stethoscope diaphragm. Normal lung tissue makes the sound quieter, and selectively filters out some of the higher frequencies. The resulting sound that you hear is called a *vesicular* breath sound. There is usually no distinct pause between the end of inspiration and the beginning of expiration.

When the area underlying the stethoscope is airless, as in consolidation, the sounds generated in the large airways are transmitted more efficiently, so they are louder and there is less filtering of the high frequencies. The resulting sounds heard by the stethoscope are termed *bronchial breathing*, classically heard over an area of consolidated lung in cases of pneumonia. The sound resembles that obtained by listening over the trachea, although the

---

Box 6.7   Points to note on auscultation of the chest

- Vesicular breath sounds
- Bronchial breath sounds
- Vocal fremitus and resonance
  - whispering pectoriloquy
  - aegophony
- Added sounds
  - pleural rub
  - wheezes
  - crackles

noise there is much louder. The quality of the sound is rather harsh, the higher frequencies being heard more clearly. The expiratory sound has a more sibilant (hissing) character than the inspiratory one, and lasts for most of the expiratory phase.

The intensity and quality of all breath sounds is so variable from patient to patient and in different situations that it is only by repeated auscultation of the chests of many patients that one becomes familiar with the normal variations and learns to recognize the abnormalities.

Added sounds

Added sounds are abnormal sounds that arise in the lung itself or in the pleura. The added sounds most commonly arising in the lung are best referred to as *wheezes* and *crackles*. Older terms such as *râles* to describe coarse crackles, *crepitations* to describe fine crackles, and *rhonchi* to describe wheezes are poorly defined, have led to confusion and are best avoided.

Wheezes are musical sounds associated with airway narrowing. Widespread *polyphonic wheezes*, particularly heard in expiration, are the most common and are characteristic of diffuse airflow obstruction, especially in asthma and COPD. These wheezes are probably related to dynamic compression of the bronchi, which is accentuated in expiration when airway narrowing is present. A fixed *monophonic* wheeze can be generated by localized narrowing of a single bronchus, as may occur in the presence of a tumour or foreign body. It may be inspiratory or expiratory, or both, and may change its intensity in different positions.

Wheezing generated in smaller airways should not be mistaken for *stridor* associated with laryngeal disease or localized narrowing of the trachea or the large airways. Stridor almost always indicates a serious condition requiring urgent investigation and management. The noise is often both inspiratory and expiratory. It may be heard at the open mouth without the aid of the stethoscope. On auscultation of the chest, stridor is usually loudest over the trachea.

Crackles are short, explosive sounds often described as bubbling or clicking. When the large airways are full of sputum, a coarse rattling sound may be heard even without the stethoscope. However, crackles are not usually produced by moistness in the lungs. It is more likely that they are produced by sudden changes in gas pressure related to the sudden opening of previously closed small airways. Crackles at the beginning of inspiration are common in patients with chronic obstructive pulmonary disease. Localized loud and coarse crackles may indicate an area of bronchiectasis. Crackles are also heard in pulmonary oedema. In diffuse interstitial fibrosis, crackles are characteristically fine in character and late inspiratory in timing.

The *pleural rub* is characteristic of pleural inflammation and usually occurs in association with pleuritic pain. It has a creaking or rubbing character and in some instances can be felt with the palpating hand as well as being audible with the stethoscope.

Take care to exclude false added sounds. Sounds resembling pleural rubs may be produced by movement of the stethoscope on the patient's skin or of clothes against the stethoscope tubing. Sounds arising in the patient's muscles may resemble added sounds: in particular, the shivering of a cold patient makes any attempt at auscultation almost useless. The stethoscope rubbing over hairy skin may produce sounds that resemble fine crackles.

Vocal resonance

You will note from the above that when listening to the breath sounds you are detecting – with your stethoscope – vibrations that have been made in the large airways. Vocal resonance is the resonance in the chest of sounds made by the voice. When testing vocal resonance, you are detecting vibrations transmitted to the chest from the vocal cords as the patient repeats a phrase, usually the words 'ninety-nine'. The ear perceives not the distinct syllables but a resonant sound, the intensity of which depends on the loudness and depth of the patient's voice and the conductivity of the lungs. As always in examining the chest, each point examined on one side should be compared at once with the corresponding point on the other side.

Not surprisingly, conditions that increase or reduce conduction of the breath sounds to the stethoscope have similar effects on the vocal resonance. Consolidated lung conducts sounds better than air-containing lung, so in consolidation the vocal resonance is increased and the sounds are louder and often clearer. In such circumstances, even when the patient whispers a phrase (e.g. 'one, two, three') the sounds may be heard clearly; this is known as *whispering pectoriloquy*. Above the level of a pleural effusion, or in some cases over an area of consolidation, the voice may sound nasal or bleating; this is known as *aegophony*, but is an unusual physical finding.

Vocal fremitus

Vocal fremitus is detected with the hand on the chest wall. It should therefore perhaps be regarded as part of palpation, but it is usually carried out after auscultation (see below). As with vocal resonance, the patient is asked to repeat a phrase such as 'ninety-nine'. The examining hand feels distinct vibrations when this is done. Some examiners use the ulnar border of the hand, but there is no good reason for this: the flat of the hand, including the fingertips, is far more sensitive.

From the above, it should be clear that listening to the breath sounds, listening to the vocal resonance and eliciting vocal fremitus are all doing essentially the same thing: they are investigating how vibrations generated in the larynx or large airways are transmitted to the examining instrument – the stethoscope in the first two cases and the fingers in the third. It follows that in the various pathological situations, all three physical signs should behave in similar ways. Where there is consolidation, the breath sounds are better transmitted to the stethoscope, so they are louder and there is less attenuation of the higher frequencies – 'bronchial breathing' is heard. Similarly, the vocal resonance and the vocal fremitus are increased. Where there is a pleural effusion, the breath sounds are quieter or absent and the vocal resonance and vocal fremitus are reduced.

The intelligent student should now ask: 'Why try and elicit all three signs?'. The experienced physician will answer: 'Because it is often difficult to interpret the signs that have been elicited'.

PUTTING IT TOGETHER: AN EXAMINATION OF THE CHEST

There is no single perfect way of examining the chest, and most doctors develop their own minor variations of order and procedure. The following is one scheme that combines efficiency with thoroughness:

- Observe the patient generally, and the surroundings.
- Ask the patient's permission for the examination, and ensure they are lying back comfortably at 45°.
- Examine the hands.
- Check the face for anaemia or cyanosis.
- Observe the respiratory rate.
- Inspect the chest movements and the anterior chest wall.
- Feel the position of the trachea, and check for lymphadenopathy.
- Feel the position of the apex beat.
- Check the symmetry of the chest movements by palpation.
- Percuss the anterior chest and axillae.

Sit the patient forward:

- Inspect the posterior chest wall.
- Percuss the back of the chest.
- Listen to the breath sounds.
- Check the vocal resonance.
- Check the tactile vocal fremitus.

If you are examining a hospital inpatient, *always* take the opportunity to turn the pillow over before lying the patient back again: a cool, fresh pillow is a great comfort to an ill person.

- Listen to the breath sounds on the front of the chest.

- Check the vocal resonance.
- Check the tactile vocal fremitus.

Stand back for a moment and reflect upon whether you have omitted anything:

- Thank the patient and ensure they are dressed or appropriately covered.

PUTTING IT TOGETHER: INTERPRETING THE SIGNS

Developing an appropriate differential diagnosis on the basis of the signs you have elicited requires thought and practice. Keeping the following in mind will help:

- If movements are diminished on one side, there is likely to be an abnormality on that side.
- The percussion note is dull over a pleural effusion and over an area of consolidation – the duller the note, the more likely it is to be a pleural effusion.
- The breath sounds, the vocal resonance and the tactile vocal fremitus are quieter or less obvious over a pleural effusion, and louder or more obvious over an area of consolidation.
- Over a pneumothorax, the percussion note is more resonant than normal but the breath sounds, vocal resonance and tactile vocal fremitus are quieter or reduced. Pneumothorax is easily missed.

OTHER INVESTIGATIONS

SPUTUM EXAMINATION

AT THE BEDSIDE
Hospital inpatients should have a sputum pot and this must be inspected (Box 6.8). *Mucoid sputum* is characteristic in patients with chronic bronchitis when there is no active infection. It is clear and sticky and not necessarily produced in a large volume. Sputum may become *mucopurulent* or *purulent* when bacterial infection is present in patients with bronchitis, pneumonia, bronchiectasis or a lung abscess. In these last two conditions the quantities may be large and the sputum is often foul-smelling.

Box 6.8   Characteristics to note when assessing sputum

- Mucoid
- Purulent
- Frothy
- Bloodstained
- Rusty

Occasionally asthmatics have a yellow tinge to the sputum, owing to the presence of many eosinophils. A particularly tenacious form of mucoid sputum may also be produced by people with asthma, and sometimes they cough up casts of the bronchial tree, particularly after an attack. Patients with bronchopulmonary aspergillosis may bring up black sputum or sputum with black parts in it: this is the fungal element of the *Aspergillus*.

When sputum is particularly foul-smelling the presence of anaerobic organisms should be suspected. Pink or white frothy sputum may be brought up by very ill patients with pulmonary oedema, for example in acute left ventricular failure. Rusty-coloured sputum is characteristic of pneumococcal lobar pneumonia. Blood may be coughed up alone, or bloodstained sputum produced, with bronchogenic carcinoma, pulmonary tuberculosis, pulmonary embolism, bronchiectasis or pulmonary hypertension (e.g. with mitral stenosis).

IN THE LABORATORY

Sputum may be examined under the microsope in the laboratory for the presence of pus cells and organisms, and may be cultured in an attempt to identify the causative agent of an infection. It is seldom practical to wait for the results of such examinations, and most clinical decisions have to be based on the clinical probability of a particular infection being present.

Tuberculosis, a disease that is becoming more common in all parts of the world, requires specialized techniques of laboratory microscopy and culture to identify the responsible organisms, and if the diagnosis is suspected these tests must be specifically requested. The examination of sputum for malignant cells is useful in helping establishing a diagnosis of lung cancer.

LUNG FUNCTION TESTS

Measurements of respiratory function may provide valuable information. First, in conjunction with the clinical assessment and other investigations they may help establish a diagnosis. Second, they will help indicate the severity of the condition. Third, serial measurements over time will show changes indicating disease progression or, alternatively, a favourable response to treatment. Finally, regular monitoring of lung function in chronic diseases such as idiopathic pulmonary fibrosis, cystic fibrosis or obstructive airways disease may warn of deterioration.

Simple respiratory function tests fall into three main groups:

- Measuring the size of the lungs
- Measuring how easily air flows into and out of the airways
- Measuring how efficient the lungs are in the process of gas exchange.

A *spirometer* will measure how much air can be exhaled after a maximal inspiration: the patient breathes in as far as he or she can, then blows out into the spirometer until no more air at all can be breathed out. This volume is called the *vital capacity* (VC). The amount of air in the lungs at full inspiration is a measure of the *total lung capacity*, and that still remaining after a full expiration is called the *residual volume*.

The actual value of total lung capacity cannot be measured with a spirometer. The simplest way of determining it is to get the patient to inspire a known volume of air containing a known concentration of helium. Measuring the new concentration of helium that exists after mixing with the air already in the lungs enables the total lung capacity to be calculated. Subtraction of the vital capacity from this value gives the residual volume.

Usually, vital capacity is measured after the patient has blown as hard and fast as possible into the spirometer, when the measurement is known as the *forced vital capacity* or FVC. In normal lungs VC and FVC are almost identical, but in COPD compression of the airways during a forced expiration leads to closure of the airways earlier than usual, and FVC may be less than VC.

Figure 6.6(a) shows the trace produced by a spirometer. Time in seconds is on the *x*-axis and volume in litres is on the *y*-axis. Thus, the trace moves *up* during expiration assessing FVC, and *along* the *x*-axis as time passes during expiration.

The volume of air breathed out in the first second of a forced expiration is known as the *forced expiratory volume in the first second* – almost always abbreviated to FEV_1. In normal lungs the FEV_1 is >70% of FVC. When there is obstruction to airflow, as in COPD, the time taken to expire fully is prolonged and the ratio of FEV_1 to FVC is reduced. An example is shown in Figure 6.6(b). A trace like this is described as showing an obstructive ventilatory defect. As noted above, the FVC may be reduced in severe airways obstruction, but in such cases the FEV_1 is reduced even more and the FEV_1/FVC ratio remains low.

Some lung conditions restrict expansion of the lungs but do not interfere with the airways. In such individuals both FEV_1 and FVC are reduced in proportion to each other, so the ratio remains normal even though the absolute values are reduced. Figure 6.6(c) shows a trace of this kind, a restrictive ventilatory defect in a patient with diffuse pulmonary fibrosis.

Look again at the normal expiratory spirogram (Fig. 6.6(a)). The slope of the trace is steepest at the onset of expiration. The trace thus shows that the rate of change of volume with time is greatest in early expiration: in other words, the rate of airflow is greatest then. This measurement, the *peak expiratory flow rate* (PEFR), is readily measured with a

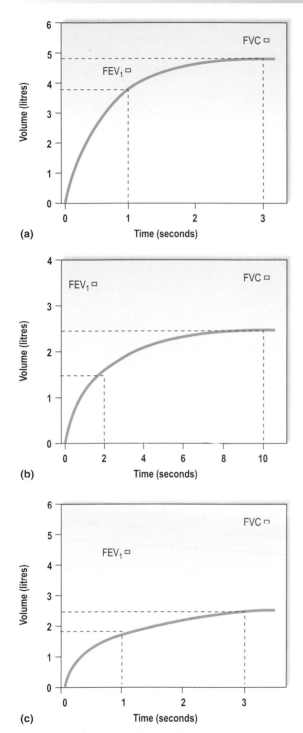

(a)

(b)

(c)

Figure 6.6 **(a)** Normal expiratory spirometer trace.
(b) Spirometer trace showing an obstructive defect. Note the
very prolonged (10 second) expiration. **(c)** Spirometer trace
showing a restrictive defect.

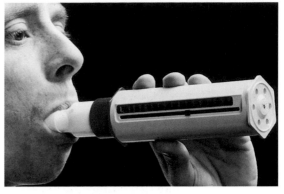

Figure 6.7 A mini-peak flow meter.

peak flow meter. A simplified version of this device
is shown in Figure 6.7. This mini-peak flow meter is
light and inexpensive, and people with asthma can
use it to monitor themselves and alter their medication, as suggested by their doctor, at the first signs of
any fall in peak flow measurement which indicates
a deterioration in their condition.

Normal gas exchange consists of the uptake of
oxygen into the pulmonary capillary blood and the
release of carbon dioxide into the alveoli. For this to
be achieved, the ventilation of the lungs by air and
their perfusion by blood need to be anatomically
matched. An approximation of the efficiency of
the process of gas exchange may be obtained by
measuring the pulmonary transfer factor for carbon
monoxide. This is assessed with apparatus similar
to that used for the helium-dilution technique for
measuring lung volumes. Instead of using helium,
which does not easily enter the blood, a known and
very low concentration of carbon monoxide is used.
This gas is very readily bound by the haemoglobin
in the pulmonary capillaries. The patient inspires to
total lung capacity (TLC), holds the breath for 10
seconds, then expires fully. The difference between
the inspired carbon monoxide concentration and
the expired concentration is a measure of the effi
ciency of gas exchange, and can be expressed per
unit lung volume if TLC is simultaneously measured
by the helium-dilution technique.

ARTERIAL BLOOD SAMPLING

In a sample of arterial blood the partial pressures of
oxygen (PaO_2) and of carbon dioxide ($PaCO_2$), and
the pH, can be measured. The arterial $PaCO_2$ will
reflect the effective ventilation of alveoli that are
adequately perfused with blood so that efficient gas
exchange can take place. Provided the rate of production of carbon dioxide by the body remains
constant, the $PaCO_2$ will be directly related to the
level of alveolar ventilation. The normal range is
4.7–6.0 kPa (36–45 mmHg). When alveolar ventilation is reduced, the $PaCO_2$ will rise. A number of
different conditions may reduce alveolar ventilation.

Alveolar ventilation rises, and $PaCO_2$ may fall, in
response to a metabolic acidosis, in very anxious
individuals, and in many lung conditions that tend
to reduce the oxygenation of the blood.

The PaO_2 is normally in the range 11.3–14.0 kPa (80–100 mmHg). Any lung disease that interferes with gas exchange may reduce arterial PaO_2.

IMAGING THE LUNG AND CHEST

ANATOMY
See page 56.

THE CHEST X-RAY
The chest X-ray is an important extension of the clinical examination (Box 6.9). This is particularly so in patients with respiratory symptoms, and a normal X-ray taken some time before the development of symptoms should therefore not be accepted as a reason for not taking an up-to-date film. In many instances it is of great value to have previous X-rays for comparison, but if these are lacking then careful follow-up with subsequent films may provide the necessary information.

The standard chest X-ray is a posteroanterior (PA) view taken with the film against the front of the patient's chest and the X-ray source 2 m behind the patient (see Fig. 6.4). The X-ray is examined systematically on a viewing box according to the following plan:

The position of the patient
Is the patient straight or rotated? If straight, the inner ends of the clavicles will be disposed symmetrically with reference to the vertebral column. Any rotation will tend particularly to alter the appearance of the mediastinum and the hilar shadows.

The outline of the heart and the mediastinum
Is this normal in size, shape and position?

The position of the trachea
This is seen as a dark column representing the air within the trachea. Is the trachea centrally placed or deviated to either side?

The diaphragm
Can the diaphragm be seen on each side? Is it normal in shape and position? Normally, the anterior end of the sixth or seventh rib crosses the mid-part of the diaphragm on each side, although the diaphragm on the right is usually a little higher than on the left.

Are the cardiophrenic angles clearly seen?

The lung fields
For radiological purposes, the lung fields are divided into three zones:

- The *upper zone* extends from the apex to a line drawn through the lower borders of the anterior ends of the second costal cartilages.
- The *mid-zone* extends from this line to one drawn through the lower borders of the fourth costal cartilages.
- The *lower zone* extends from this line to the bases of the lungs.

Each zone is systematically examined on both sides, and any area that appears abnormal is carefully compared with the corresponding area on the opposite side. The minor interlobar fissure, which separates the right, upper and middle lobes, may sometimes be seen running horizontally in the third and fourth interspace on the right side.

The bony skeleton
- Is the chest symmetrical?
- Is scoliosis present?
- Are the ribs unduly crowded or widely spaced in any area?
- Are cervical ribs present?
- Are any ribs eroded or absent?

As well as the standard AP view, lateral views are sometimes carried out to help localize any lesion that is seen. In examining a lateral view, as in Figure 6.8, follow this plan:

- Identify the sternum anteriorly and the vertebral bodies posteriorly. The cardiac shadow lies anteriorly and inferiorly.
- There should be a lucent (dark) area retrosternally which has approximately the same density as the area posterior to the heart and anterior to the vertebral bodies. Check for any difference between the two, or for any discrete lesion in either area.
- Check for any collapsed vertebrae.
- The lowest vertebrae should appear darkest, becoming whiter as they progress superiorly. Interruption of this smooth gradation suggests an abnormality overlying the vertebral bodies involved.

THE CT SCAN
The routine chest X-ray consists of shadows at all depths in the chest superimposed on one another. In computed tomography (CT) scanning, X-rays are passed through the body at different angles and the resulting information is processed by computer to

---

Box 6.9   Points to note when assessing the chest X-ray

- Bony skeleton
- Position of the patient
- Position of the trachea
- Outline of heart
- Outline of mediastinum
- Diaphragm
- Lung fields

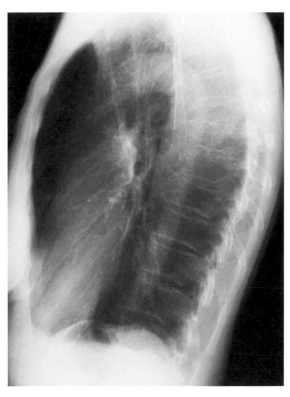

Figure 6.8 A lateral chest X-ray.

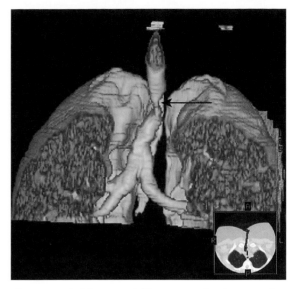

Figure 6.9 A CT-generated 3D reconstruction demonstrating that the patient has a tracheal stenosis (arrowed). (Courtesy of Professor R. H. Reznek.)

generate a series of cross-sectional images. A thoracic CT scan thus comprises a series of cross-sectional 'slices' through the thorax at various levels.

The CT scan is a vital part of the staging of lung cancer, and inoperability may be demonstrated by evidence on CT of mediastinal involvement. CT scanning will demonstrate the presence of dilated and distorted bronchi, as in bronchiectasis. Diffuse pulmonary fibrosis will be shown by a modified high-resolution/thin-section scan technique. Emboli in the pulmonary arteries can be demonstrated by a rapid data acquisition spiral CT technique, and has advantages over isotope lung scanning (see below) in diagnosing pulmonary embolism in patients with pre-existing lung disease. Many scanners can now generate three-dimensional representations of the thoracic structures (Fig. 6.9).

RADIOISOTOPE IMAGING
In the lungs the most widely used radioisotope technique is combined *ventilation and perfusion scanning*, used to aid the diagnosis of pulmonary embolism.

The perfusion scan is performed by injecting intravenously a small dose of macroaggregated human albumin particles labelled with technetium-99m (^{99m}Tc). A gamma-camera image is then built up of the radioactive particles impacted in the pulmonary vasculature; the distribution of perfusion in the lung can then be seen. The ventilation scan is obtained by inhalation of a radioactive gas such as krypton-81m (^{81m}Kr), again using scanning to identify the distribution of the radioactivity.

Blood is usually diverted away from areas of the lung that are unventilated, so a *matched* defect on both the ventilation and perfusion scans usually indicates parenchymal lung disease. If there are areas of ventilated lung which are not perfused (i.e. an *unmatched* defect), this is evidence in support of an embolism to the unperfused area. Figure 6.10 shows a ventilation–perfusion isotope scan. The unmatched defects (areas ventilated by the inspired air but not perfused by blood) suggest a high probability of pulmonary embolism.

MAGNETIC RESONANCE IMAGING
Magnetic resonance imaging (MRI) is useful in demonstrating mediastinal abnormalities and can help evaluate invasion of the mediastinum and chest wall by tumour. Apart from the fact that it does not use ionizing radiation, currently it has few other advantages over CT in imaging the thorax. MRI is particularly degraded by movement artefact in imaging the chest, because of the relatively long data acquisition time, but faster scanners may in the future overcome this drawback.

ULTRASOUND
Ultrasound reveals much less detail than CT scanning but has the advantages that it does not involve radiation and that it gives 'real-time' images – the operator can visualize what is happening as it happens.

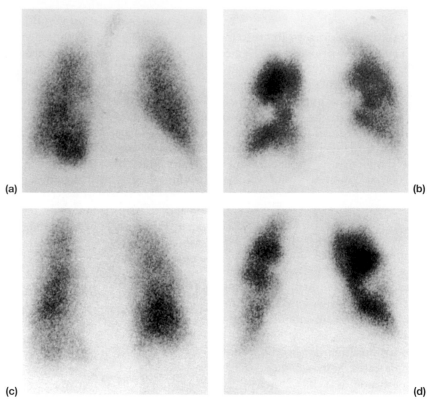

Figure 6.10   Ventilation/perfusion isotope scan of the lungs. Segmental and subsegmental loss of perfusion (b & d) can be seen with relatively normal ventilation (a & c). The clear punched-out areas in the perfusion (b & d) scans indicate areas of reduced isotope concentration during the perfusion scan. Thus these are areas of reduced blood flow. The ventilation scans show normal aeration of the lungs as depicted by the isotope distribution in the pulmonary airways. These sequences of scans are suggestive of pulmonary embolism because they show impaired perfusion with normal ventilation.

Ultrasound is used for examining diaphragmatic movement. A paralysed hemidiaphragm – usually a result of damage to the phrenic nerve by a mediastinal tumour – does not move downward during inspiration. If the patient is asked to make a sudden inspiratory effort, as in sniffing, the non-paralysed side of the diaphragm moves down, so intrathoracic pressure drops, and the paralysed side moves *up*.

Ultrasound is also valuable in distinguishing pleural thickening from pleural fluid – with real-time imaging the latter can be seen to move with changes in posture. When such fluid is present, ultrasound may be used to aid placement of a catheter to drain the collection, and also to steer a draining catheter accurately into an intrapulmonary abscess.

FLEXIBLE BRONCHOSCOPY

Bronchoscopy is an essential tool in the investigation of many forms of respiratory disease. For discrete abnormalities, such as a mass seen on chest X-ray and suspected to be a lung cancer, bronchoscopy is usually indicated to investigate its nature. Under local anaesthesia, the flexible bronchoscope is passed through the nose, pharynx and larynx, down the trachea, and the bronchial tree is then inspected. Figure 6.11 shows a lung cancer seen down the bronchoscope. Flexible biopsy forceps are passed down a channel inside the bronchoscope, and are used to obtain tissue samples for histological examination. Similarly, aspirated bronchial secretions and brushings of any endobronchial abnormality can be sent to the laboratory for cytological examination.

At bronchoscopy, specimens are also taken for microbiological examination in order to determine the nature of any infecting organisms. In diffuse interstitial lung disease, such as sarcoidosis or pulmonary fibrosis, the technique of transbronchial biopsy can be used to obtain small specimens of lung parenchyma for histological examination to help confirm the diagnosis.

PLEURAL ASPIRATION AND BIOPSY

A pleural effusion can give rise to diagnostic problems and, sometimes, management problems

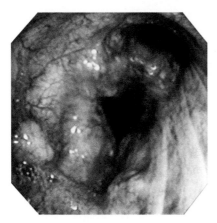

Figure 6.11 A lung cancer, seen down the bronchoscope.

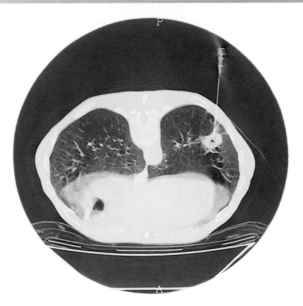

Figure 6.12 A CT-guided percutaneous biopsy in progress. The radio-dense (white) structure penetrating the chest wall is the biopsy needle.

when the amount of fluid causes respiratory embarrassment. When a pleural effusion is seen as a presenting feature in a middle-aged or older patient, the most likely cause is a malignancy. Less commonly, particularly in younger patients, it may be due to tuberculosis. In either case the diagnosis is best obtained by both aspiration of the fluid and pleural biopsy. Aspiration alone has a lower diagnostic yield.

After anaesthetizing the skin, subcutaneous tissues and pleura, pleural fluid may be aspirated by syringe and needle for microbiological and cytological examination. Large pleural effusions may need to be drained by an indwelling catheter, left in situ until the fluid has been fully removed. As noted above, ultrasound guidance can be helpful, particularly if the fluid is *loculated* in various pockets.

Cytological examination of pleural fluid may demonstrate the presence of malignant cells. Many polymorphs may be seen if the effusion is secondary to an underlying pneumonic infection. With tuberculosis the fluid usually contains many lymphocytes, although tubercle bacilli are rarely seen. Therefore almost all pleural fluid samples should be cultured for possible tuberculosis, because this infection can coexist with other pathologies and it is so important not to miss it. In empyema, pus is present in the pleural cavity; this has a characteristic appearance and will be full of white cells and organisms.

The pleural fluid should also be examined for protein content. A transudate resulting from cardiac or renal failure can be distinguished from an exudate – which usually results from pleural inflammation – by its lower protein content (<30 g/L).

Biopsies of the pleura can be obtained percutaneously and under local anaesthesia using an *Abram's pleural biopsy needle*. This technique can be used when there is pleural fluid present to obtain pleural tissue for histological examination and, whenever tuberculosis is a possibility, for microbiological culture. If ultrasound examination shows the pleura to be thickened, biopsies may be obtained with the aid of ultrasound screening by Abram's needle, a Tru-cut needle and similar techniques.

THORACOSCOPY

This technique enables the pleural cavity to be examined directly and biopsies taken under direct vision. The procedure is commonly performed under a general anaesthetic by a surgeon who uses a rigid thoracoscope after the lung has been deflated. More recently, flexible thoracoscopes have been developed that can sometimes be used under local anaesthetic.

LUNG BIOPSY

As noted above, the technique of transbronchial biopsy can be used to obtain samples of lung parenchyma. Such specimens are often too small for diagnosis, however. In this circumstance, biopsies of the lung taken at thoracoscopy may be of value. Occasionally, a formal open lung biopsy obtained at thoracotomy may be necessary.

When there is a discrete, localized lesion it may be possible to obtain a biopsy percutaneously with the aid of CT scanning to direct the insertion of the biopsy needle (Fig. 6.12).

IMMUNOLOGICAL TESTS

Sometimes asthma is related to the development of type I hypersensitivity to certain allergens. Part of the assessment of such patients might include skin sensitivity tests, in which minute quantities of the suspected allergen are introduced intradermally. Delayed (type IV, cell-mediated) hypersensitivity is shown by the Mantoux and Heaf tests, used to detect the presence of sensitivity to tubercular protein.

Precipitating antibodies in the circulating blood are present in patients with some fungal diseases, such as bronchopulmonary aspergillosis or aspergilloma. In patients suspected of having an allergic alveolitis antibodies may be demonstrated to the relevant antigens. Immunoglobulin E (IgE) levels are often raised in patients with asthma.

CLINICAL IMAGES

Figures 6.13–6.18 illustrate some of the clinical points of this chapter.

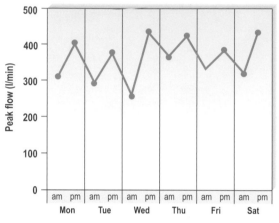

Figure 6.13 A peak-flow chart. Typical diurnal variation of peak flow, worse in the mornings, seen in a young asthmatic during an exacerbation.

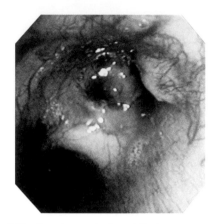

Figure 6.15 Bronchoscopic view of the tumour seen radiologically in Figure 6.14 – histology showed a squamous carcinoma.

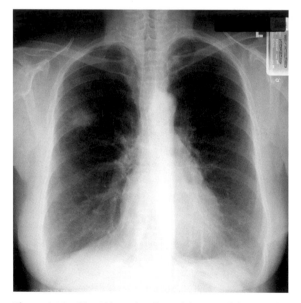

Figure 6.14 Chest X-ray showing a right upper lobe mass in a 70-year-old smoker presenting with haemoptysis.

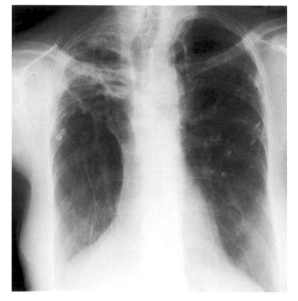

Figure 6.16 Chest X-ray showing right apical scarring and tracheal deviation (detectable clinically) from previous tuberculosis, and hyperinflation of the lungs due to chronic obstructive pulmonary disease in a 66-year-old long-term smoker with 5 years of increasing breathlessness.

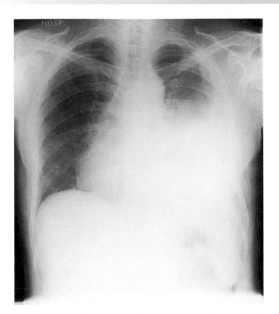

Figure 6.17 Chest X-ray showing a large left pleural effusion in a young man with a 4-month history of malaise, fever, night sweats and weight loss. The diagnosis of tuberculosis was confirmed on histology of a pleural biopsy and culture of the pleural fluid.

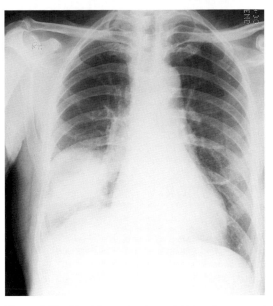

Figure 6.18 Chest X-ray showing a right basal pmeumonia in a previously fit 40-year-old man with fever, breathlessness, central cyanosis and pleuritic pain. Chest signs included bronchial breathing and a pleural rub in the right lower zone. The cyanosis was due to the shunting of deoxygenated blood through the consolidated lung, the increased respiratory rate leading to a low $Pa\text{CO}_2$ because of increased clearance of carbon dioxide by the unaffected alveoli. *Streptococcus pneumoniae* was grown on blood cultures.

7 Cardiovascular system

A. Timmis

INTRODUCTION

The 20th century saw major changes in patterns of cardiovascular disease. In the developed world syphilitic and tuberculous involvement of the cardiovascular system became rare, and the incidence of rheumatic disease declined considerably. Myocardial and conducting tissue disease, on the other hand, were diagnosed with increasing frequency and the importance of arterial hypertension became well recognized. Coronary artery disease emerged as the major cardiovascular disorder of the era, becoming the most common cause of premature death throughout Europe, North America and Australasia. At the beginning of the new millennium coronary artery disease shows signs of loosening its grip on the developed world. Elsewhere, however, its prevalence is greatly increasing, and in the underdeveloped world it now threatens to overtake malnutrition and infectious disease as the major cause of death.

As patterns of cardiovascular disease changed, so did the cardiologist's diagnostic tools. A century that started with the stethoscope, the sphygmomanometer, the chest X-ray and a very rudimentary electrocardiogram saw the development of a variety of new imaging modalities, using ultrasound, radioisotopes, X-rays and magnetic resonance. This non-invasive capability was complemented by introduction of the catheterization laboratory, permitting angiographic imaging, electrophysiological recording and tissue biopsy of the heart. Add to this the resources of the chemical pathology, bacteriology and molecular biology laboratories, and the array of diagnostic technology available to the modern cardiologist becomes almost overwhelming. Nevertheless, most of the common cardiac disorders encountered in clinical practice can still be diagnosed at the bedside on the basis of a careful history and physical examination. Indeed, this simple fact defines the true art of cardiology and remains as relevant now as it was before recent technological advances.

THE CARDIAC HISTORY

The history should record details of presenting symptoms, of which the most common are chest pain, fatigue and dyspnoea, palpitations, and presyncope or syncope (see below). Previous illness should also be recorded, as it may provide important clues about the cardiac diagnosis – thyroid, connective tissue and neoplastic disorders, for example, can all affect the heart. Rheumatic fever in childhood is important because of its association with valvular heart disease and hypertension; and diabetes and dyslipidaemias because of their association with coronary artery disease. Smoking is a major risk factor for coronary artery disease. Alcohol abuse may predispose to cardiac arrhythmias and cardiomyopathy. The cardiac history should quantify both habits in terms of pack-years smoked and units of alcohol consumed. The family history should always be documented because coronary artery disease and hypertension often run in families, as do some of the less common cardiovascular disorders, such as hypertrophic cardiomyopathy. Indeed, in patients with hypertrophic cardiomyopathy a family history of sudden death is probably the single most important indicator of risk. Finally, the drug history should be recorded, as many commonly prescribed drugs are potentially cardiotoxic. β-Blockers and some calcium channel blockers (diltiazem, verapamil), for example, can cause symptomatic bradycardias, and tricyclic antidepressants and β-agonists can cause tachyarrhythmias. Vasodilators cause variable reductions in blood pressure which can lead to syncopal attacks, particularly in patients with aortic stenosis. The myocardial toxicity of certain cytotoxic drugs (notably doxorubicin and related compounds) is an important cause of cardiomyopathy.

CHEST PAIN

Myocardial ischaemia, pericarditis and aortic dissection are common cardiovascular causes of chest pain.

MYOCARDIAL ISCHAEMIA

Ischaemia of the heart results from an imbalance between myocardial oxygen supply and demand, producing pain called *angina* (Boxes 7.1, 7.2). Angina is usually a symptom of atherosclerotic coronary artery disease, which impedes myocardial

Box 7.1 Angina

Typical patient
- Middle-aged or elderly man or woman often with a family history of coronary heart disease and one or more of the major reversible risk factors (smoking, hypertension, hypercholesterolaemia)

Major symptoms
- Exertional chest pain and shortness of breath. Pain often described as 'heaviness' or 'tightness', and may radiate into arms, neck or jaw

Major signs
- None, although hypertension and signs of hyperlipidaemia (xanthelasmata, xanthomas) may be present
- Peripheral vascular disease, evidenced by absent pulses or arterial bruits, is commonly associated with coronary heart disease

Diagnosis
- Typical history is most important diagnostic tool
- ECG: often normal; may show Q waves in patients with previous myocardial infarction
- Stress test: exertional ST depression
- Isotope perfusion scan: exertional perfusion defects
- Coronary arteriogram: confirms coronary artery disease

Additional investigations
- Blood sugar and lipids to rule out diabetes and dyslipidaemia

Comments
- A careful history is the single most important means of diagnosing angina

Box 7.2 Causes of angina

Impaired myocardial oxygen supply
- Coronary artery disease
  - atherosclerosis
  - arteritis in connective tissue disorders
  - diabetes mellitus
- Coronary artery spasm
- Congenital coronary artery disease
  - arteriovenous fistula
  - anomalous origin from pulmonary artery
- Severe anaemia

Increased myocardial oxygen demand
- Left ventricular hypertrophy
  - hypertension
  - aortic valve disease
  - hypertrophic cardiomyopathy
- Tachyarrhythmias

Box 7.3 Causes of coronary artery disease

- Atherosclerosis
- Arteritis
  - systemic lupus erythematosus
  - polyarteritis nodosa
  - rheumatoid arthritis
  - ankylosing spondylitis
  - syphilis
  - Takayasu's disease
- Embolism
  - infective endocarditis
    left atrial/ventricular thrombus
  - left atrial/ventricular tumour
  - prosthetic valve thrombus
  - complication of cardiac catheterization
- Coronary mural thickening
  - amyloidosis
  - radiation therapy
  - Hurler's disease
  - pseudoxanthoma elasticum
- Other causes of coronary luminal narrowing
  - aortic dissection
  - coronary spasm
- Congenital coronary artery disease
  - anomalous origin from pulmonary artery
  - arteriovenous fistula

oxygen supply. Other causes of coronary artery disease (Box 7.3) are rare. The history is diagnostic if the location of the pain, its character, its relation to exertion and its duration are typical. The patient describes retrosternal pain which may radiate into the arms, the throat or the jaw. It has a constricting character, is provoked by exertion and relieved rapidly by rest.

MYOCARDIAL INFARCTION, UNSTABLE ANGINA (Box 7.4)
In these life-threatening cardiac emergencies the pain is similar in location and character to angina but is usually more severe, more prolonged, and unrelieved by rest.

PERICARDITIS
This also causes central chest pain, which is sharp in character and aggravated by deep inspiration, cough or postural changes. It is usually idiopathic or caused by Coxsackie B infection. It may also occur

as a complication of myocardial infarction, but other causes are seen less commonly (Box 7.5).

AORTIC DISSECTION (Box 7.6)
This produces severe tearing pain in either the front or the back of the chest. The onset is abrupt, unlike the crescendo quality of ischaemic cardiac pain.

Box 7.4   Acute myocardial infarction

Typical patient
- Middle-aged (male) or elderly (either sex), often with a family history of coronary heart disease and one or more of the major reversible risk factors (smoking, hypertension, hypercholesterolaemia)
- In many patients there is no preceding history of angina

Major symptoms
- Chest pain and shortness of breath. Pain usually prolonged and often described as 'heaviness' or 'tightness', with radiation into arms, neck or jaw. Alternative descriptions include 'congestion' or 'burning', which may be confused with indigestion

Major signs
- Ischaemic myocardial damage, fourth heart sound, dyskinetic precordial impulse
- Autonomic disturbance, tachycardia (anterior MI), bradycardia (inferior MI), sweating, vomiting, syncope

Diagnosis
- Markers of injury: raised CKMB and troponins
- ECG: may be normal or show ST depression or T-wave change (non-ST elevation myocardial infarction). ST elevation myocardial infarction denotes higher risk

Additional investigations
- Biochemistry: blood sugar and lipids to rule out diabetes and dyslipidaemia
- Risk stratification: echocardiogram (LV function) and stress testing (reversible ischaemia)

Comments
- History and troponin testing most useful diagnostic tools

Box 7.5   Causes of acute pericarditis

- Idiopathic
- Infective
  - viral (Coxsackie B, influenza, herpes simplex)
  - bacterial (*Staphylococcus aureus, Mycobacterium tuberculosis*)
- Connective tissue disease
  - systemic lupus erythematosus
  - rheumatoid arthritis
  - polyarteritis nodosa
- Uraemia
- Malignancy (e.g. breast, lung, lymphoma, leukaemia)
- Radiation therapy
- Acute myocardial infarction
- Post myocardial infarction/cardiotomy (Dressler's syndrome)

Box 7.6   Aortic dissection

Typical patient
- Middle-aged or elderly patient with a history of hypertension or arteriosclerotic disease
- Occasionally younger patient with aortic root disease (e.g. Marfan's syndrome)

Major symptoms
- Chest pain

Major signs
- Often none
- Sometimes regional arterial insufficiency (e.g. occlusions of coronary artery causing myocardial infarction, carotid or verterbral artery causing stroke, spinal artery causing hemi- or quadriplegia); subclavian artery occlusion may cause differential blood pressure in either arm; aortic regurgitation; cardiac tamponade; sudden death

Diagnosis
- CXR: widened mediastinum, occasionally with left pleural effusion
- Transoesophageal echocardiogram: confirms dissection
- CT scan: confirms dissection
- MRI scan: confirms dissection

Additional investigations
- None

Comments
- Having established the diagnosis, emergency surgery is usually necessary, particularly if the dissection involves the ascending thoracic aorta

Rare cardiovascular causes of chest pain include mitral valve disease associated with massive left atrial dilatation. This causes discomfort in the back, sometimes associated with dysphagia due to oesophageal compression. Aortic aneurysms can also cause pain in the chest owing to local compression.

DYSPNOEA

Dyspnoea is an abnormal awareness of breathing occurring either at rest or at an unexpectedly low level of exertion. It is a major symptom of many cardiac disorders, particularly left heart failure (Table 7.1), but its mechanisms are complex. In acute pulmonary oedema and orthopnoea, dyspnoea is due mainly to the elevated left atrial pressure that characterizes left heart failure (Box 7.7). This produces

Table 7.1 Causes of heart failure

Ventricular pathophysiology	Clinical examples
Restricted filling	Mitral stenosis
	Hypertrophic cardiomyopathy
Pressure loading	Hypertension
	Aortic stenosis
	Coarctation of the aorta
Volume loading	Mitral regurgitation
	Aortic regurgitation
Contractile impairment	Coronary artery disease
	Dilated cardiomyopathy
	Myocarditis
Arrhythmia	Severe bradycardia
	Severe tachycardia

Box 7.7   Acute LVF

Typical patient
- Patient with acute myocardial infarction or known left ventricular disease

Major symptoms
- Severe dyspnoea and variable circulatory collapse

Major signs
- Low-output state (hypotension, oliguria, cold periphery); tachycardia; S3; sweating; crackles at lung bases

Diagnosis
- CXR: bilateral air space consolidation with typical perihilar distribution
- Echocardiogram: usually confirms left ventricular disease

Additional investigations
- ECG: may show evidence of acute or previous myocardial infarction
- Blood gas analysis: shows variable hypoxaemia

Comments
- Although most cases are caused by acute myocardial infarction or advanced left ventricular disease, it is vital to exclude valvular disease or myxoma, which are potentially correctable by surgery

Box 7.8   Congestive heart failure

Typical patient
- Middle-aged (male) or elderly (either sex) patient with a history of myocardial infarction or long-standing hypertension
- In cases where there is no clear cause, always inquire about alcohol consumption

Major symptoms
- Exertional fatigue and shortness of breath, with orthopnoea in advanced cases

Major signs
- Fluid retention: basal crackles, raised jugular venous pressure (JVP), peripheral oedema
- Reduced cardiac output: cool skin, peripheral cyanosis
- Other findings: third heart sound

Diagnosis
- ECG: usually abnormal; often shows Q waves (previous myocardial infarction) or left ventricular hypertrophy (hypertension)
- CXR: cardiac enlargement, congested lung fields
- Echocardiogram: LV dilatation with regional (coronary heart disease) or global (cardiomyopathy) contractile impairment

Additional investigations
- Renal function as prelude to diuretic and ACE inhibitor therapy
- Blood count to rule out anaemia

Comments
- The echocardiogram is the single most important diagnostic test in the patient with heart failure

EXERTIONAL DYSPNOEA

This is the most troublesome symptom in heart failure (Box 7.8). Exercise causes a sharp increase in left atrial pressure and this contributes to the pathogenesis of dyspnoea by causing pulmonary congestion (see above). However, the severity of dyspnoea does not correlate closely with exertional left atrial pressure, and other factors must therefore be important. These include respiratory muscle fatigue and the effects of exertional acidosis on peripheral chemoreceptors. As left heart failure worsens, exercise tolerance deteriorates. In advanced disease the patient is dyspnoeic at rest.

ORTHOPNOEA

In patients with heart failure lying flat causes a steep rise in left atrial pressure, resulting in pulmonary congestion and severe dyspnoea. To obtain uninterrupted sleep extra pillows are required, and in

a corresponding elevation of the pulmonary capillary pressure and increases transudation into the lungs, which become oedematous and stiff. The extra effort required to ventilate the stiff lungs causes dyspnoea. In exertional dyspnoea, however, other mechanisms apart from changes in left atrial pressure are also important.

advanced disease the patient may choose to sleep sitting in a chair.

PAROXYSMAL NOCTURNAL DYSPNOEA

Frank pulmonary oedema on lying flat wakes the patient from sleep with distressing dyspnoea and fear of imminent death. The symptoms are corrected by standing upright, which allows gravitational pooling of blood to lower the left atrial pressure, the patient often feeling the need to obtain air at an open window.

FATIGUE

Exertional fatigue is an important symptom of heart failure and is particularly troublesome towards the end of the day. It is caused partly by deconditioning and muscular atrophy but also by inadequate oxygen delivery to exercising muscle, reflecting impaired cardiac output.

PALPITATION

Awareness of the heartbeat is common during exertion or heightened emotion. Under other circumstances it may be indicative of an abnormal cardiac rhythm. A description of the rate and rhythm of the palpitation is essential. Extrasystoles are common but rarely signify important heart disease. They are usually experienced as 'missed' or 'dropped' beats; the forceful beats that follow may also be noticed. Rapid irregular palpitation is typical of atrial fibrillation. Rapid regular palpitation of abrupt onset occurs in atrial, junctional and ventricular tachyarrhythmias.

DIZZINESS AND SYNCOPE

Cardiovascular disorders produce dizziness and syncope by transient hypotension, resulting in abrupt cerebral hypoperfusion. Recovery is usually rapid, unlike with other common causes of syncope (e.g. stroke, epilepsy, overdose).

POSTURAL HYPOTENSION

Syncope on standing upright reflects inadequate baroreceptor-mediated vasoconstriction. It is common in the elderly. Abrupt reductions in blood pressure and cerebral perfusion cause the patient to fall to the ground, whereupon the condition corrects itself.

VASOVAGAL SYNCOPE

This is caused by autonomic overactivity, usually provoked by emotional or painful stimuli, less commonly by coughing or micturition. Only rarely are syncopal attacks so frequent as to be significantly disabling ('malignant' vasovagal syndrome). Vasodilatation and inappropriate slowing of the pulse combine to reduce blood pressure and cerebral perfusion. Recovery is rapid if the patient lies down.

CAROTID SINUS SYNCOPE

Exaggerated vagal discharge following external stimulation of the carotid sinus (e.g. from shaving, or a tight shirt collar) causes reflex vasodilatation and slowing of the pulse. These may combine to reduce blood pressure and cerebral perfusion in some elderly patients, causing loss of consciousness.

VALVULAR OBSTRUCTION

Fixed valvular obstruction in aortic stenosis may prevent a normal rise in cardiac output during exertion, such that the physiological vasodilatation that occurs in exercising muscle produces an abrupt reduction in blood pressure and cerebral perfusion, resulting in syncope. Vasodilator therapy may cause syncope by a similar mechanism. Intermittent obstruction of the mitral valve by left atrial tumours (usually myxoma) may also cause syncopal episodes (Fig. 7.1).

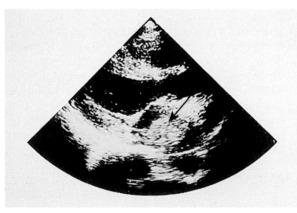 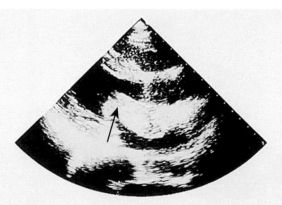

Figure 7.1   Left atrial myxoma: 2D echocardiogram (long axis view). During diastole, the tumour (arrowed) prolapses through the mitral valve and obstructs left ventricular filling.

STOKES–ADAMS ATTACKS

These are caused by self-limiting episodes of asystole (Fig. 7.2) or rapid tachyarrhythmias (including ventricular fibrillation). The loss of cardiac output causes syncope and striking pallor. Following restoration of normal rhythm recovery is rapid and associated with flushing of the skin as flow through the dilated cutaneous bed is re-established.

THE CARDIAC EXAMINATION

A methodical approach is recommended, starting with inspection of the patient and proceeding to examination of the radial pulse, measurement of heart rate and blood pressure, examination of the neck (carotid pulse, jugular venous pulse), palpation of the anterior chest wall, auscultation of the heart, percussion and auscultation of the lung bases, and, finally, examination of the peripheral pulses and auscultation for carotid and femoral arterial bruits.

INSPECTION OF THE PATIENT

Chest wall deformities such as pectus excavatum should be noted, as these may compress the heart and displace the apex, giving a spurious impression of cardiac enlargement. Large ventricular or aortic aneurysms may cause visible pulsations. Superior vena caval obstruction is associated with prominent venous collaterals on the chest wall. Prominent venous collaterals around the shoulder occur in axillary or subclavian vein obstruction.

ANAEMIA

This may exacerbate angina and heart failure. Pallor of the mucous membranes is a useful but sometimes misleading physical sign, and diagnosis requires laboratory measurement of the haemoglobin concentration.

CYANOSIS

This is a blue discoloration of the skin and mucous membranes caused by increased concentration of reduced haemoglobin in the superficial blood vessels.

Peripheral cyanosis may result when cutaneous vasoconstriction slows the blood flow and increases oxygen extraction in the skin and the lips. It is physiological during cold exposure. It also occurs in heart failure, when reduced cardiac output produces reflex cutaneous vasoconstriction. In mitral stenosis, cyanosis over the malar area produces the characteristic mitral facies.

Central cyanosis may result from the reduced arterial oxygen saturation caused by cardiac or pulmonary disease. It affects not only the skin and the lips but also the mucous membranes of the mouth. Cardiac causes include pulmonary oedema (which prevents adequate oxygenation of the blood) and congenital heart disease. Congenital defects associated with central cyanosis include those in which desaturated venous blood bypasses the lungs by ('reversed') shunting through septal defects or a patent ductus arteriosus (e.g. Eisenmenger's syndrome, Fallot's tetralogy).

CLUBBING OF THE FINGERS AND TOES

In congenital cyanotic heart disease clubbing is not present at birth but develops during infancy and may become very marked. Infective endocarditis is the only other cardiac cause of clubbing.

OTHER CUTANEOUS AND OCULAR SIGNS OF INFECTIVE ENDOCARDITIS

These are caused by immune complex deposition in the capillary circulation. A vasculitic rash is common, as are splinter haemorrhages in the nailbed, although these are a very non-specific finding. Other 'classic' manifestations of endocarditis, including Osler's nodes (tender erythematous nodules in the pulps of the fingers), Janeway lesions (painless erythematous lesions on the palms) and Roth's spots (erythematous lesions in the optic fundi) are now rarely seen.

COLDNESS OF THE EXTREMITIES

In patients hospitalized with severe heart failure this is an important sign of reduced cardiac output. It is caused by reflex vasoconstriction of the cutaneous bed. Measurement of skin temperature provides a useful indirect means of monitoring cardiac output in the intensive care unit.

PYREXIA

Infective endocarditis is invariably associated with pyrexia, which may be low grade or 'swinging' in nature if paravalvular abscess develops. Pyrexia also occurs for the first 3 days after myocardial infarction.

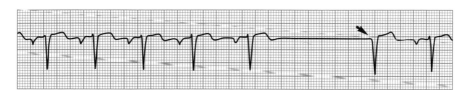

Figure 7.2 Prolonged sinus arrest. After the fifth sinus beat there is a pause of about 1.8 seconds terminated by a nodal escape beat (arrowed) before sinus rhythm resumes.

OEDEMA

Subcutaneous oedema that pits on digital pressure is a cardinal feature of congestive heart failure. Pressure should be applied over a bony prominence (tibia, lateral malleoli, sacrum) to provide effective compression. Oedema is caused by salt and water retention by the kidney. Two mechanisms are responsible:

- *Reduced sodium delivery to the nephron.* This is caused by reduced glomerular filtration caused by constriction of the preglomerular arterioles in response to sympathetic activation and angiotensin II production.
- *Increased sodium reabsorption from the nephron.* This is the more important mechanism. It occurs particularly in the proximal tubule early in heart failure but, as failure worsens, renin–angiotensin activation stimulates aldosterone release, which increases sodium reabsorption in the distal nephron.

Salt and water retention expands plasma volume and increases the capillary hydrostatic pressure. Hydrostatic forces driving fluid out of the capillary exceed the osmotic forces reabsorbing it, so that oedema fluid accumulates in the interstitial space. The effect of gravity on capillary hydrostatic pressure ensures that oedema is most prominent around the ankles in the ambulant patient and over the sacrum in the bedridden patient. In advanced heart failure oedema may involve the legs, genitalia and trunk. Transudation into the peritoneal cavity (ascites), the pleural and pericardial spaces may also occur.

ARTERIAL PULSE

The arterial pulses should be palpated for evaluation of rate, rhythm, character and symmetry.

RATE AND RHYTHM

By convention, both are assessed by palpating the right radial pulse. Rate, expressed in beats per minute (bpm), is measured by counting over a timed period of 15 seconds. Normal sinus rhythm is regular, but in young patients may show phasic variation in rate during respiration (*sinus arrhythmia*). An irregular rhythm usually indicates atrial fibrillation, but may also be caused by frequent ectopic beats or self-limiting paroxysmal arrhythmias. In patients with atrial fibrillation the rate should be measured by auscultation at the cardiac apex, because beats that follow very short diastolic intervals may create a 'pulse deficit' by not generating sufficient pressure to be palpable at the radial artery.

CHARACTER

This is defined by the volume and waveform of the pulse and should be evaluated at the right carotid artery (i.e. the pulse closest to the heart and least subject to damping and distortion in the arterial tree). Pulse volume provides a crude indication of stroke volume, being small in heart failure and large in aortic regurgitation. The waveform of the pulse is of greater diagnostic importance (Fig. 7.3). Aortic stenosis produces a slowly rising carotid pulse; in aortic regurgitation, on the other hand, the large stroke volume vigorously ejected produces a rapidly rising carotid pulse, which collapses in early diastole owing to backflow through the aortic valve. In mixed aortic valve disease a *biphasic pulse* with two systolic peaks is occasionally found. *Alternating pulse* – alternating high and low systolic peaks – occurs in severe left ventricular failure but the mechanism for this is unknown. *Paradoxical pulse* – an inspiratory decline in systolic pressure greater than 10 mmHg – occurs in cardiac tamponade and, less frequently, in constrictive pericarditis and obstructive pulmonary disease (Fig. 7.4). It represents an exaggeration of the normal inspiratory decline in systolic pressure and is not, therefore, truly paradoxical.

SYMMETRY

Symmetry of the radial, brachial, carotid, femoral, popliteal and pedal pulses should be confirmed. A

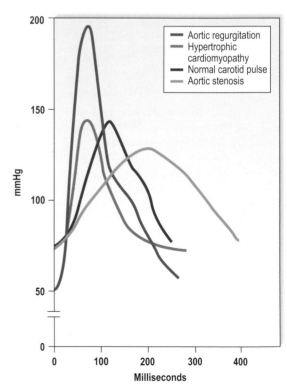

Figure 7.3 The waveform of the pulse is characterized by the rate of rise of the carotid upstroke. Note that in aortic regurgitation the upstroke is rapid and followed by abrupt diastolic 'collapse'. In hypertrophic cardiomyopathy the upstroke is also rapid and the pulse has a jerky character. In aortic stenosis the upstroke is slow with a plateau.

reduced or absent pulse indicates an obstruction more proximally in the arterial tree, caused usually by atherosclerosis or thromboembolism, less commonly by aortic dissection. Coarctation of the aorta causes symmetrical reduction and delay of the femoral pulses compared with the radial pulses.

MEASUREMENT OF BLOOD PRESSURE

Blood pressure is measured indirectly by sphygmomanometry. Supine and erect measurements should be obtained to provide an assessment of baroreceptor function. A cuff of at least 40% the arm circumference in width is attached to a mercury or aneroid manometer and inflated around the extended arm. Auscultation over the brachial artery reveals five phases of *Korotkoff sounds* as the cuff is deflated:

- *Phase 1*: the first appearance of the sounds marking systolic pressure
- *Phase 2 and 3*: increasingly loud sounds
- *Phase 4*: abrupt muffling of the sounds
- *Phase 5*: disappearance of the sounds.

Phase 5 provides a better measure of diastolic blood pressure than phase 4, not only because it corresponds more closely with directly measured diastolic pressure, but also because its identification is less subjective. Nevertheless, in those conditions where Korotkoff sounds remain audible despite complete deflation of the cuff (aortic regurgitation, arteriovenous fistula, pregnancy) phase 4 must be used for the diastolic measurement.

JUGULAR VENOUS PULSE

Fluctuations in right atrial pressure during the cardiac cycle generate a pulse that is transmitted backwards into the jugular veins. It is best examined while the patient reclines at 45°. If the right atrial pressure is very low, however, visualization of the jugular venous pulse may require a smaller reclining angle. Alternatively, manual pressure over the upper abdomen may be used to produce a transient

increase in venous return to the heart which elevates the jugular venous pulse (hepatojugular reflux).

JUGULAR VENOUS PRESSURE

The normal upper limit is 4 cm vertically above the sternal angle. This is about 9 cm above the right atrium and corresponds to a pressure of 6 mmHg. Elevation of the jugular venous pressure indicates elevation of the right atrial pressure unless the superior vena cava is obstructed, producing engorgement of the neck veins (Box 7.9). During inspiration the pressure within the chest falls and there is a fall in the jugular venous pressure. In constrictive pericarditis, and less commonly in tamponade, inspiration produces a paradoxical rise (*Kussmaul's sign*) in the jugular venous pressure (JVP) because the increased venous return cannot be accommodated within the constricted right side of the heart (Fig. 7.5).

WAVEFORM OF JUGULAR VENOUS PULSES

The jugular venous pulse has a flickering character caused by 'a' and 'v' waves separated by 'x' and 'y'

Box 7.9   Causes of elevated jugular venous pressure

- Congestive heart failure
- Cor pulmonale
- Pulmonary embolism
- Right ventricular infarction
- Tricuspid valve disease
- Tamponade
- Constrictive pericarditis
- Hypertrophic/restrictive cardiomyopathy
- Superior vena cava obstruction
- Iatrogenic fluid overload, particularly in surgical and renal patients

---

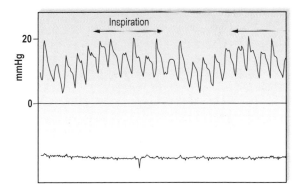

Figure 7.5 Kussmaul's sign. Jugular venous pressure recording in a patient with tamponade. The venous pressure is raised and there is a particularly prominent systolic 'x' descent, giving the waveform of the JVP an unusually dynamic appearance. Note the inspiratory rise in atrial pressure (Kussmaul's sign) reflecting the inability of the tamponaded right heart to accommodate the inspiratory increase in venous return.

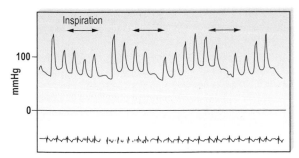

Figure 7.4 Paradoxical pulse (radial artery pressure signal). The patient had severe tamponade. Note the exaggerated (>10 mmHg) decline in arterial pressure during inspiration.

descents. The 'a' wave produced by atrial systole precedes tricuspid valve closure. It is followed by the 'x' descent (marking descent of the tricuspid valve ring), which is interrupted by the diminutive 'c' wave as the tricuspid valve closes. Atrial pressure then rises again, producing the 'v' wave as the atrium fills passively during ventricular systole. The decline in atrial pressure as the tricuspid valve opens to allow ventricular filling produces the 'y' descent. Important abnormalities of the pattern of deflections are shown in Figure 7.6.

PALPATION OF THE CHEST WALL

The apex beat is defined as the lowest and most lateral point at which the cardiac impulse can be

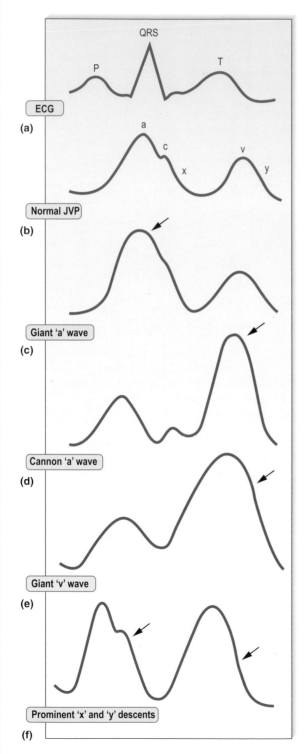

Figure 7.6 Waveform of the jugular venous pulse. **(a)** The ECG is portrayed at the top of the illustration. Note how electrical events precede mechanical events in the cardiac cycle. Thus the P wave (atrial depolarization) and the QRS complex (ventricular depolarization) precede the 'a' and 'v' waves, respectively, of the JVP. **(b)** Normal JVP. The 'a' wave produced by atrial systole is the most prominent deflection. It is followed by the 'x' descent, interrupted by the small 'c' wave marking tricuspid valve closure. Atrial pressure then rises again ('v' wave) as the atrium fills passively during ventricular systole. The decline in atrial pressure as the tricuspid valve opens produces the 'y' descent. **(c)** Giant 'a' wave. Forceful atrial contraction against a stenosed tricuspid valve or a non-compliant hypertrophied right ventricle produces an unusually prominent 'a' wave. **(d)** Cannon 'a' wave. This is caused by atrial systole against a closed tricuspid valve. It occurs when atrial and ventricular rhythms are dissociated (complete heart block, ventricular tachycardia) and marks coincident atrial and ventricular systole. **(e)** Giant 'v' wave. This is an important sign of tricuspid regurgitation. The regurgitant jet produces pulsatile systolic waves in the JVP. **(f)** Prominent 'x' and 'y' descents. These occur in constrictive pericarditis and give the JVP an unusually dynamic appearance. In tamponade only the 'x' descent is usually exaggerated.

palpated. Its location inferior or lateral to the fifth intercostal space or the midclavicular line, respectively, usually indicates cardiac enlargement. Palpable third and fourth heart sounds give the apical impulse a double thrust. In the past considerable importance was attached to the character of the apical impulse ('thrusting' in aortic valve disease, 'tapping' in mitral stenosis), but this is of very limited practical value in the modern era.

Left ventricular aneurysms can sometimes be palpated medial to the cardiac apex. Right ventricular enlargement produces a systolic thrust in the left parasternal area. The turbulent flow responsible for heart murmurs may produce palpable vibrations (*thrills*) on the chest wall, particularly in aortic stenosis, ventricular septal defect and patent ductus arteriosus.

AUSCULTATION OF THE HEART

The diaphragm and bell of the stethoscope permit appreciation of high- and low-pitched auscultatory events, respectively. The apex, lower left sternal edge, upper left sternal edge and upper right sternal edge should be auscultated in turn. These locations correspond respectively to the mitral, tricuspid, pulmonary and aortic areas, and loosely identify sites at which sounds and murmurs arising from the four valves are best heard.

FIRST SOUND (S1)

This corresponds to mitral and tricuspid valve closure at the onset of systole. It is accentuated in mitral stenosis because prolonged diastolic filling through the narrowed valve ensures that the thickened leaflets are widely separated at the onset of systole. Thus valve closure generates unusually vigorous vibrations. In advanced mitral stenosis the valve is rigid and immobile and S1 becomes soft again.

SECOND SOUND (S2)

This corresponds to aortic and pulmonary valve closure following ventricular ejection. S2 is single during expiration. Inspiration, however, causes physiological splitting into aortic followed by pulmonary components because increased venous return to the right side of the heart delays pulmonary valve closure. Important abnormalities of S2 are illustrated in Figure 7.7.

THIRD AND FOURTH SOUNDS (S3, S4)

These low-frequency sounds occur early and late in diastole, respectively. When present they give a characteristic 'gallop' to the cardiac rhythm. Both sounds are best heard with the bell of the stethoscope at the cardiac apex. They are caused by abrupt tensing of the ventricular walls following rapid diastolic filling. Rapid filling occurs early

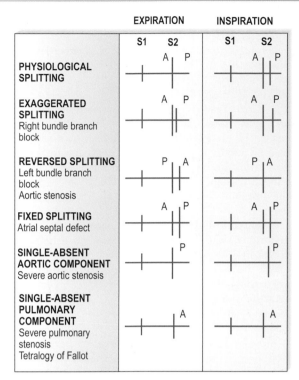

Figure 7.7 Splitting of the second heart sound. The first sound, representing mitral and tricuspid closure, is usually single, but the aortic and pulmonary components of the second sound normally split during inspiration as increased venous return delays right ventricular emptying. Abnormal splitting of the second heart sound is an important sign of heart disease.

in diastole (S3) following atrioventricular valve opening, and again late in diastole (S4) due to atrial contraction. S3 is physiological in children and young adults but usually disappears after the age of 40. It also occurs in high-output states caused by anaemia, fever, pregnancy and thyrotoxicosis. After the age of 40 S3 is nearly always pathological, usually indicating left ventricular failure or, less commonly, mitral regurgitation or constrictive pericarditis. In the elderly S4 is sometimes physiological. More commonly, however, it is pathological, and occurs when vigorous atrial contraction late in diastole is required to augment filling of a hypertrophied, non-compliant ventricle (e.g. hypertension, aortic stenosis, hypertrophic cardiomyopathy).

SYSTOLIC CLICKS AND OPENING SNAPS

Valve opening, unlike valve closure, is normally silent. In aortic stenosis, however, valve opening produces a click in early systole which precedes the ejection murmur. The click is only audible if the valve cusps are pliant and non-calcified, and is particularly prominent in the congenitally bicuspid valve. A click later in systole suggests mitral valve prolapse, particularly when followed by a murmur.

In mitral stenosis, elevated left atrial pressure causes forceful opening of the thickened valve leaflets. This generates a snap early in diastole that precedes the mid-diastolic murmur.

HEART MURMURS   (Fig. 7.8)

These are caused by turbulent flow within the heart and great vessels. Occasionally the turbulence is caused by increased flow through a normal valve – usually aortic or pulmonary – producing an 'innocent' murmur. However, murmurs may also indicate valve disease or abnormal communications between the left and right sides of the heart (e.g. septal defects).

Rheumatic heart disease has become much less common in the western world, although it remains common elsewhere, and is the cause of many of the classic heart murmurs (Box 7.10). Heart murmurs are defined by four characteristics: *loudness, quality, location* and *timing*.

The *loudness* of a murmur reflects the degree of turbulence. This relates to the volume and velocity of flow and not the severity of the cardiac lesion. Loudness is graded on a scale of 1 (barely audible) to 6 (audible even without application of the stethoscope to the chest wall). The *quality* of a murmur relates to its frequency and is best described as low-, medium- or high-pitched. The *location* of a murmur on the chest wall depends on its site of origin and has led to the description of four valve areas (see above). Some murmurs radiate, depending on the velocity and direction of blood flow. The sound of the high-velocity systolic flow in aortic stenosis and mitral regurgitation, for example, is directed towards the neck and the axilla, respectively; that of the high-velocity diastolic flow in aortic regurgitation is directed towards the left sternal edge. Murmurs are *timed* according to the phase of systole or diastole during which they are audible. It is inadequate to describe the timing of a murmur as systolic or diastolic without more specific reference to the length of the murmur and the phase of systole or diastole during which it is heard: *systolic* murmurs are either midsystolic, pansystolic or late systolic; *diastolic* murmurs are either early diastolic, mid-diastolic or presystolic in timing. Continuous murmurs are audible in both phases of the cardiac cycle.

A *midsystolic* ('*ejection*') murmur is caused by turbulence in the left or right ventricular outflow tracts during ejection. It starts following opening of the aortic or pulmonary valve, reaches a crescendo in midsystole and disappears before the second heart sound. The murmur is loudest in the aortic

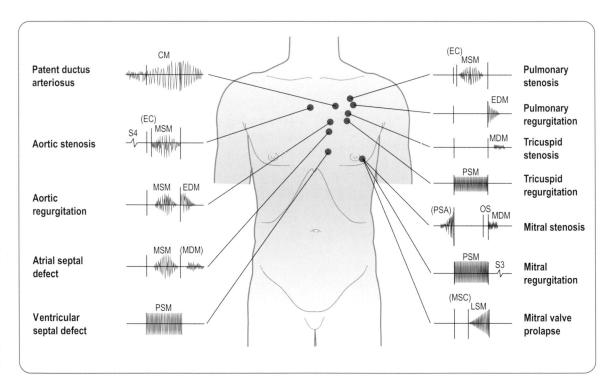

Figure 7.8 Heart murmurs. These are caused by turbulent flow within the heart and great vessels, and may indicate valve disease. Heart murmurs (defined by loudness, quality, location, radiation and timing) may be depicted graphically as shown in this illustration. CM, continuous murmur; MSM, midsystolic murmur; PSM, pansystolic murmur; LSM, late systolic murmur; EDM, early diastolic murmur; MDM, mid-diastolic murmur; PSA, presystolic accentuation of murmur; EC, ejection click; MSC, midsystolic click; OS, opening snap; S3, third heart sound; S4, fourth heart sound. Parentheses indicate those auscultatory findings that are not constant.

Box 7.10   Rheumatic heart disease

Typical patient
- Middle-aged woman, less commonly man, with a history of childhood rheumatic fever (often not recognized or dismissed as trivial feverish illness). The mitral valve is almost invariably affected, commonly with associated aortic valve involvement. Right-sided valves less commonly affected. Presentation is usually with exertional dyspnoea, less commonly with unexplained atrial fibrillation or unheralded stroke
- Pregnant woman presenting abruptly with atrial fibrillation and pulmonary oedema

Major symptoms
- Mitral valve disease: dyspnoea or symptoms of frank congestive failure
- Aortic valve disease: dyspnoea, sometimes angina or syncope

Major signs
- Mitral stenosis: AF, signs of fluid retention (raised JVP ± peripheral oedema and basal crackles in lung fields), loud S1, opening snap in early diastole followed by low-pitched mid-diastolic murmur best heard at cardiac apex. With increasing calcification the valve gets more rigid and the loud S1 and opening snap disappear
- Mitral regurgitation: AF, signs of fluid retention, pansystolic murmur best heard at cardiac apex, often with third heart sound
- Aortic stenosis: slow rising carotid pulse, ejection systolic murmur best heard at base of heart
- Aortic regurgitation: fast rising carotid pulse, ejection systolic murmur with early diastolic murmur best heard at left sternal edge

Diagnosis
- Echocardiogram: diagnostic of rheumatic heart disease, Doppler studies providing additional information about the severity of valvular stenosis or regurgitation

Treatment
- Diuretics for fluid retention and vasodilators to increase forward flow through regurgitant left-sided valves. Digoxin or β-blockers for rate control in AF plus warfarin to protect against embolism. Symptomatic mitral valve disease that fails to respond to treatment requires valve surgery (repair or replacement) or, in selected cases of mitral stenosis, percutaneous valvuloplasty. Symptomatic aortic valve disease always requires consideration for valve replacement

area (with radiation to the neck) when it arises from the left ventricular outflow tract, and in the pulmonary area when it arises from the right ventricular outflow tract. It is best heard with the diaphragm of the stethoscope while the patient sits forward. Important causes of *aortic ejection murmurs* are aortic stenosis and hypertrophic cardiomyopathy. Aortic regurgitation also produces an ejection murmur due to increased stroke volume and velocity of ejection. *Pulmonary ejection murmurs* may be caused by pulmonary stenosis or infundibular stenosis (Fallot's tetralogy). In atrial septal defect the pulmonary ejection murmur results from right ventricular volume loading and does not indicate organic valvular disease. 'Innocent' murmurs unrelated to heart disease are always midsystolic in timing and are caused by turbulent flow in the left (sometimes right) ventricular outflow tract. In most cases there is no clear cause, but they may reflect a hyperkinetic circulation in conditions such as anaemia, pregnancy, thyrotoxicosis or fever. They are rarely louder than grade 3, often vary with posture, may disappear on exertion, and are not associated with other signs of heart disease.

Pansystolic murmurs are audible throughout systole from the first to the second heart sounds. They are caused by regurgitation through incompetent atrioventricular valves and by ventricular septal defects. The pansystolic murmur of *mitral regurgitation* is loudest at the cardiac apex and radiates into the left axilla. It is best heard using the diaphragm of the stethoscope with the patient lying on the left side. The murmurs of *tricuspid regurgitation* and *ventricular septal defect* are loudest at the lower left sternal edge. Inspiration accentuates the murmur of tricuspid regurgitation because the increased venous return to the right side of the heart increases the regurgitant volume. *Mitral valve prolapse* may also produce a pansystolic murmur but, more commonly, prolapse occurs in midsystole, producing a click followed by a late-systolic murmur.

Early diastolic murmurs are high pitched and start immediately after the second heart sound, fading away in mid-diastole. They are caused by regurgitation through incompetent aortic and pulmonary valves and are best heard using the diaphragm of the stethoscope while the patient leans forward. The early diastolic murmur of *aortic regurgitation* radiates from the aortic area to the left sternal edge, where it is usually easier to hear, in maintained expiration with the patient leaning forward. *Pulmonary regurgitation* is loudest at the pulmonary area.

Mid-diastolic murmurs are caused by turbulent flow through the atrioventricular valves. They start after valve opening, relatively late after the second sound, and continue for a variable period during mid-diastole. *Mitral stenosis* is the principal cause of a mid-diastolic murmur which is best heard at the cardiac apex using the bell of the stethoscope while the patient lies on the left side. Increased flow across a non-stenotic mitral valve occurs in *ventricular septal defect* and *mitral regurgitation* and may produce a mid-diastolic murmur. In severe *aortic regurgitation*, preclosure of the anterior leaflet of the mitral valve by the regurgitant jet may produce mitral turbulence associated with a mid-diastolic murmur (Austin Flint murmur). A mid-diastolic murmur at the lower left sternal edge, accentuated by inspiration, is caused by *tricuspid stenosis* and also by conditions that increase tricuspid flow (e.g. atrial septal defect, tricuspid regurgitation).

In *mitral or tricuspid stenosis*, atrial systole produces a presystolic murmur immediately before the first heart sound. The murmur is perceived as an accentuation of the mid-diastolic murmur associated with these conditions. Because presystolic murmurs are generated by atrial systole they do not occur in patients with atrial fibrillation.

Continuous murmurs are heard during systole and diastole, and are uninterrupted by valve closure. The commonest cardiac cause is *patent ductus arteriosus*, in which flow from the high-pressure aorta to the low-pressure pulmonary artery continues throughout the cardiac cycle, producing a murmur over the base of the heart which, though continuously audible, is loudest at end systole and diminishes during diastole. Ruptured sinus of Valsalva aneurysm also produces a continuous murmur.

FRICTION RUBS AND VENOUS HUMS

A friction rub occurs in pericarditis. It is best heard in maintained expiration with the patient leaning forward as a high-pitched scratching noise audible during any part of the cardiac cycle and over any part of the left precordium. A continuous venous hum at the base of the heart reflects hyperkinetic jugular venous flow. It is particularly common in infants and usually disappears on lying flat.

THE ELECTROCARDIOGRAM

The electrocardiogram (ECG) records the electrical activity of the heart at the skin surface. A good-quality 12-lead ECG is essential for the evaluation of almost all cardiac patients.

ELECTROPHYSIOLOGY

GENERATION OF ELECTRICAL ACTIVITY

The wave of depolarization that spreads through the heart during each cardiac cycle has vector properties defined by its direction and magnitude. The net direction of the wave changes continuously during each cardiac cycle and the ECG deflections change accordingly, being positive as the wave approaches the recording electrode and negative as it moves away. Electrodes orientated along the axis

of the wave record larger deflections than those orientated at right-angles. Nevertheless, the size of the deflections is determined principally by the magnitude of the wave, which is a function of muscle mass. Thus the ECG deflection produced by depolarization of the atria (P wave) is smaller than that produced by the depolarization of the more muscular ventricles (QRS complex). Ventricular repolarization produces the T wave.

INSCRIPTION OF THE QRS COMPLEX

The ventricular depolarization vector can be resolved into two components:

- Septal depolarization – spreads from left to right across the septum
- Ventricular free wall depolarization – spreads from endocardium to epicardium.

Left ventricular depolarization dominates the second vector component, the resultant direction of which is from right to left. Thus electrodes orientated to the left ventricle record a small negative deflection (Q wave) as the septal depolarization vector moves away, followed by a large positive deflection (R wave) as the ventricular depolarization vector approaches. The sequence of deflections for electrodes orientated towards the right ventricle is in the opposite direction (Fig. 7.9).

Any positive deflection is termed an R wave. A negative deflection before the R wave is termed a Q wave (this must be the first deflection of the complex), whereas a negative deflection following the R wave is termed an S wave.

ELECTRICAL AXIS

Because the mean direction of the ventricular depolarization vector (the electrical axis) shows a wide range of normality, there is corresponding variation in QRS patterns consistent with a normal ECG. Thus correct interpretation of the ECG must take

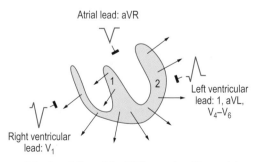

Figure 7.9 Inscription of the QRS complex. The septal depolarization vector (1) produces the initial deflection of the QRS complex. The ventricular free-wall depolarization vector (2) produces the second deflection, which is usually more pronounced. Lead aVR is oriented towards the cavity of the left ventricle and records an entirely negative deflection.

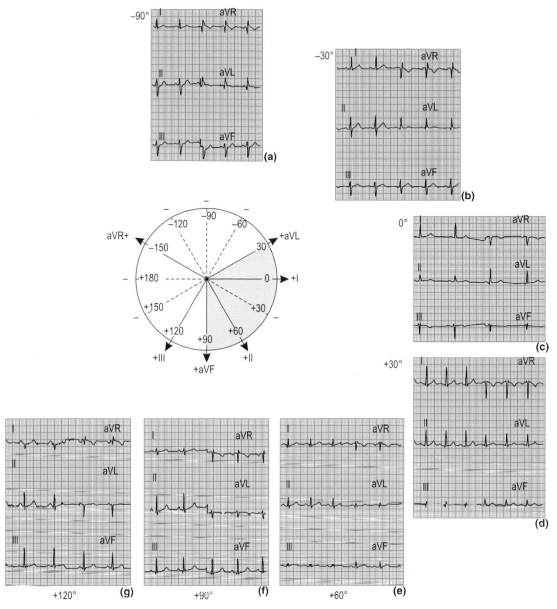

Figure 7.10 Mean frontal QRS axis. This is the mean direction of the LV depolarization vector in those leads (I–aVF) that lie in the frontal plane of the heart. It lies at right-angles to the lead in which the net QRS deflexion is least pronounced. It is quantified using a hexaxial reference system. The QRS axis shows a wide range of normality from –30° to 90°. Thus despite the different ECG patterns in this illustration, only recordings **(a)** and **(g)** are abnormal, owing to left and right axis deviation, respectively.

account of the electrical axis. The frontal plane axis is determined by identifying the limb lead in which the net QRS deflection (positive and negative) is least pronounced. This lead must be at right-angles to the frontal plane electrical axis, which is defined using an arbitrary hexaxial reference system (Fig. 7.10).

NORMAL 12-LEAD ECG

This is illustrated in Figure 7.11. Leads I–III are the standard bipolar leads, which each measure the potential difference between two limbs:

- *Lead I*: left arm to right arm
- *Lead II*: left leg to right arm
- *Lead III*: left leg to left arm.

The remaining leads are unipolar, connected to a limb (aVR to aVF) or to the chest wall (V_1–V_6). Because the orientation of each lead to the wave of depolarization is different, the direction and magnitude of ECG deflections is also different in each lead. Nevertheless, the sequence of deflections (P wave, QRS complex, T wave) is identical. In some patients a small U wave can be seen following

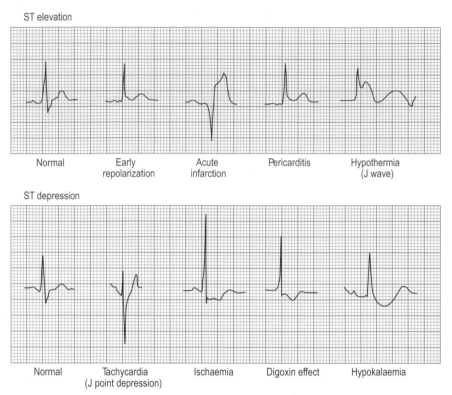

ST elevation

| Normal | Early repolarization | Acute infarction | Pericarditis | Hypothermia (J wave) |

ST depression

| Normal | Tachycardia (J point depression) | Ischaemia | Digoxin effect | Hypokalaemia |

Figure 7.14 ST segment morphology: common causes of ST segment elevation and depression. Note that depression of the J point (junction between the QRS complex and ST segment) is physiological during exertion and does not signify myocardial ischaemia. Planar depression of the ST segment, on the other hand, is strongly suggestive of myocardial ischaemia.

causes of ST depression are digitalis therapy and hypokalaemia.

T-WAVE MORPHOLOGY

The orientation of the T wave should be directionally similar to the QRS complex. Thus T-wave inversion is normal in leads with dominantly negative QRS complexes (aVR, V_1, and sometimes lead III). Pathological T-wave inversion occurs as a non-specific response to various stimuli (e.g. viral infection, hypothermia). More important causes of T-wave inversion are ventricular hypertrophy, myocardial ischaemia and myocardial infarction. Exaggerated peaking of the T wave is the earliest ECG change in ST elevation myocardial infarction. It also occurs in hyperkalaemia.

CLINICAL APPLICATIONS OF ECG

DIAGNOSIS OF CORONARY HEART DISEASE

The territories supplied by the three major coronary arteries, although variable, are highly circumscribed, the left anterior descending artery supplying the anterior wall, the circumflex artery the lateral wall, and the right coronary artery the inferior wall of the left ventricle. The regional distribution of coronary flow has important implications for electrocardiography (and diagnostic imaging), patients with coronary heart disease showing *regional* electrocardiographic (or wall motion) abnormalities whereas patients with diffuse myocardial disease (e.g. cardiomyopathy) show more widespread changes.

STABLE ANGINA

The ECG is often normal in patients with stable angina unless there is a history of myocardial infarction, when pathological Q waves or T-wave inversion may be present.

EXERCISE STRESS TESTING

This is one of the most widely used tests for evaluating the patient with chest pain. The patient is usually exercised on a treadmill, the speed and slope of which can be adjusted to increase the workload gradually. The exercise ECG provides important *diagnostic* information. Thus, in patients with coronary artery disease, exercise-induced increases in myocardial oxygen demand may outstrip oxygen delivery through the atheromatous arteries, resulting in regional ischaemia. This causes planar or downsloping ST segment depression, with

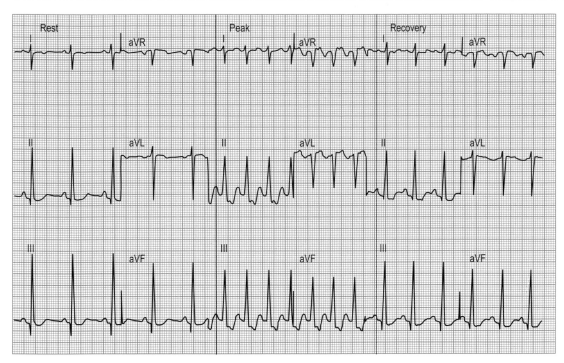

Figure 7.15 Exercise ECG: ischaemic changes in inferior standard leads (II, III and aVF). At rest the ST segments are isoelectric. Exercise causes tachycardia and provokes 3 mm of downsloping ST depression in leads II, III and aVF. The changes reverse during recovery. The findings suggest exertional ischaemia affecting the inferior wall of the heart. The probability of coronary artery disease is high.

reversal during recovery (Fig. 7.15). The diagnostic accuracy of stress testing is not 100%, and Bayes' theorem predicts that false positive and false negative results will be common when the probability of coronary disease is very low (as in young women) or very high (as in elderly patients with typical symptoms), respectively. The exercise ECG also provides important *prognostic* information: an increased risk of myocardial infarction or sudden death is indicated by ST depression very early during exercise, by an exertional fall in blood pressure, or by exercise-induced ventricular arrhythmias. In these cases, urgent coronary arteriography is required.

ACUTE CORONARY SYNDROMES

Acute myocardial infarction and less severe acute coronary syndromes present similarly with unprovoked – often severe – ischaemic cardiac pain, and a reliable differential diagnosis cannot be made using clinical criteria. However, measurement of cardiac biomarkers 12 hours after the onset of symptoms, in particular troponin I or T (see below), and observation of the 12-lead ECG resolves this important question. The combination of typical symptoms plus raised troponins (troponin positive) is diagnostic of myocardial infarction, which is categorized as ST elevation myocardial infarction (STEMI) or

non-ST elevation myocardial infarction (non-STEMI), depending on the ECG findings. Typical symptoms unassociated with either troponin release or ST elevation are diagnosed as troponin-negative acute coronary syndrome or unstable angina. It therefore follows that acute myocardial infarction and unstable angina may be associated with a completely normal ECG or with ST depression (Fig. 7.16) or T-wave changes, the differential diagnosis depending on the presence or absence of raised troponins. In STEMI the evolution of ECG changes is characteristic, although it may be aborted by timely reperfusion therapy (thrombolysis or primary stenting). Peaking of the T wave followed by ST segment elevation occur during the first hour of pain (Fig. 7.17). The changes are regional, and reciprocal ST depression may be seen in the opposite ECG leads. Usually a pathological Q wave occurs during the following 24 hours and thereafter persists indefinitely. The ST segment returns to the isoelectric line within 2–3 days, and T-wave inversion may occur. The ECG is a useful indicator of infarct location. Changes in leads II, III and aVF indicate inferior infarction (Fig. 7.18), whereas changes in leads V_1–V_6 indicate anteroseptal (V_1–V_3) or anterolateral (V_1–V_6) infarction (Fig. 7.19). When the infarct is located posteriorly ECG changes may be difficult to detect, but dominant R waves in leads V_1 and V_2 often develop (Fig. 7.18).

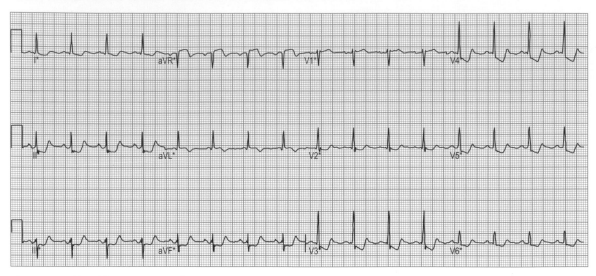

Figure 7.16 Unstable angina or non-ST elevation myocardial infarction (depending on troponin release): 12-lead ECG showing planar/downsloping ST depression in the inferolateral territory.

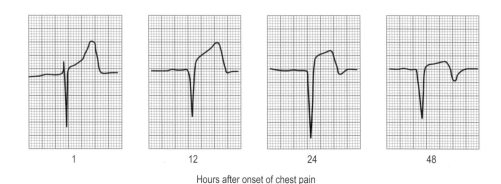

| 1 | 12 | 24 | 48 |

Hours after onset of chest pain

Figure 7.17 AMI: evolution of ECG changes. Elevation of the ST segment occurs during the first hour of chest pain. The Q wave develops during the subsequent 24 hours and usually persists indefinitely. Within a day of the attack the ST segment usually returns to the isoelectric line and T-wave inversion may occur.

DETECTION OF CARDIAC ARRHYTHMIAS

Electrocardiographic documentation of the arrhythmia should be obtained prior to instituting treatment. In patients with sustained arrhythmias a 12-lead recording at rest is usually diagnostic, but a long continuous recording of the lead showing the clearest P wave (if present) should also be obtained. In patients with paroxysmal arrhythmias special techniques may be required for electrocardiographic documentation.

IN-HOSPITAL ECG MONITORING

Patients who have had out-of-hospital cardiac arrest or severe, arrhythmia-induced heart failure should undergo ECG monitoring in hospital under the continuous surveillance of trained staff.

AMBULATORY (HOLTER) ECG MONITORING

Patients with intermittent palpitation or dizzy attacks should have a continuous 24-hour ECG recording while engaging in normal activities. Portable cassette recorders are available for this purpose. Analysis of the tape often identifies the cardiac arrhythmias, particularly if symptoms were experienced during the recording (Fig. 7.20).

PATIENT-ACTIVATED ECG RECORDING

For patients with very infrequent symptoms the detection rate with 24-hour ambulatory monitoring is low and patient-activated recorders are therefore more useful. When symptoms occur the patient applies the recorder to the chest wall. The recorder may then transmit the ECG by telephone to the hospital for scrutiny by the physician. Alternatively, miniaturized recording devices can be implanted

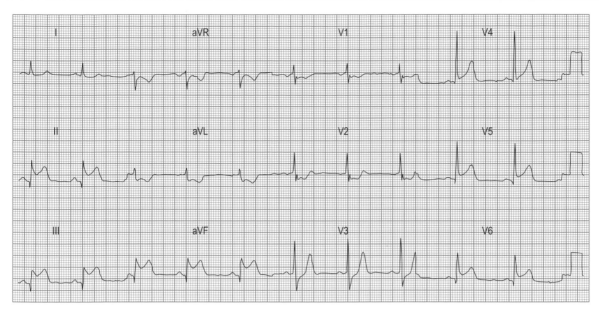

Figure 7.18 Acute inferoposterior infarction. ECG 2 hours after the onset of chest pain. Typical ST elevation in leads II, III and aVF with reciprocal ST depression in aVL is diagnostic of inferior myocardial infarction. Prominent R waves in leads V_1 and V_2 associated with ST depression indicate posterior extension of the infarct. This pattern may reflect occlusion of the right coronary artery or a dominant circumflex coronary artery.

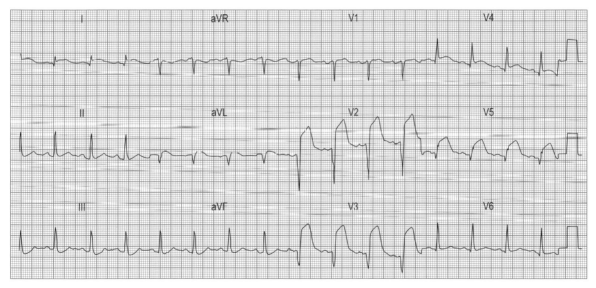

Figure 7.19 Acute anterior infarction. ECG 1 hour after the onset of chest pain. Typical ST elevation in leads V_1–V_5 is diagnostic of anterior myocardial infarction. Additional ST elevation in standard leads I and aVL indicates lateral extension of the infarct. This pattern usually reflects proximal occlusion of the left anterior descending coronary artery.

subcutaneously using local anaesthetic and interrogated electronically in the event of symptoms.

EXERCISE TESTING
The ECG recorded during exercise may be helpful when there is a history of exertional palpitation. Arrhythmias provoked by ischaemia or increased sympathetic activity are more likely to be detected during exercise.

TILT TESTING
When malignant vasovagal syndrome is suspected, ECG and blood pressure recordings during tilting from supine to erect posture can be helpful. Abnormal bradycardia and hypotension sufficient to produce presyncope or syncope are strongly suggestive of the diagnosis.

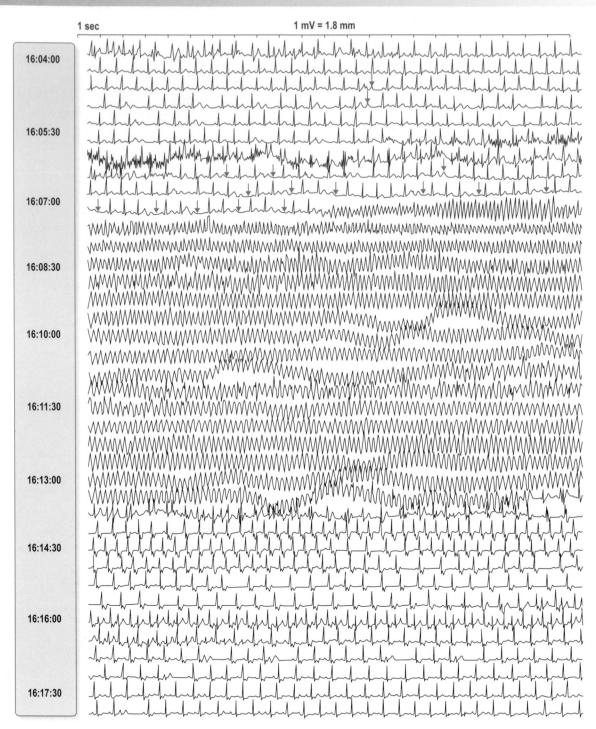

Figure 7.20 Ventricular tachycardia: Holter recording. When tachycardias are paroxysmal in nature, continuous ECG monitoring is often necessary to document the arrhythmia. Here a Holter recording illustrates a long burst of rapid VT lasting a total of 6 minutes. Preceding the VT there is second-degree heart block (arrows).

PROGRAMMED CARDIAC STIMULATION

This technique requires cardiac catheterization with catheter-mounted electrodes. Premature stimuli are introduced into the atria or ventricles with a view to stimulating re-entry arrhythmias. In the normal heart sustained arrhythmias are rarely provoked by premature stimuli. Thus arrhythmia provocation during programmed stimulation is usually diagnostic, particularly when the arrhythmia reproduces symptoms. To test the efficacy of treatment the test can be repeated after the administration of anti-arrhythmic drugs.

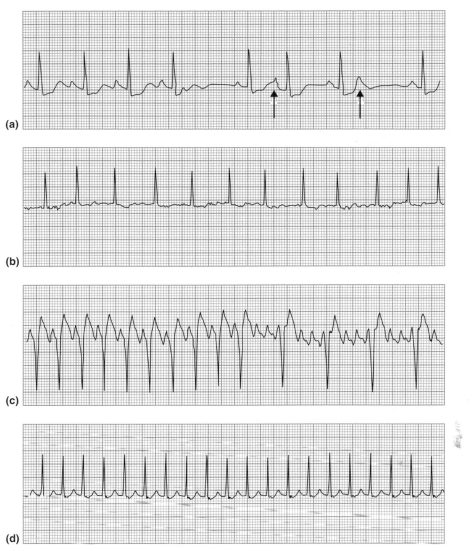

Figure 7.21 Atrial arrhythmias: **(a)** Ectopic beats. After the fourth sinus beat there is a very early P wave which, finding the AV node refractory, is not conducted to the ventricle. This produces a pause before the next sinus beat, which itself is followed by a somewhat later atrial ectopic beat (arrowed), which is conducted normally. This is followed by a sinus beat, following which the T wave is distorted by another early atrial ectopic (arrowed), which is also blocked. **(b)** Atrial fibrillation. Note the irregular fibrillatory waves and the irregular ventricular response. The ventricular rate is fairly slow because the patient was treated with a β-blocker. **(c)** A flutter. AV conduction is first with 2:1 block, giving a ventricular rate of about 150/min and then gives way to 4:1 block. Sawtooth flutter waves at a rate of 300/min are clearly visible. **(d)** AV junctional re-entrant tachycardia (AVJRT). Often called supraventricular tachycardia (SVT), this arrhythmia causes a regular tachycardia, rate 180/min.

DIAGNOSIS OF ATRIAL ARRHYTHMIAS (Fig. 7.21)

The ECG in atrial arrhythmias shows a narrow and morphologically normal QRS complex when ventricular depolarization occurs by normal His–Purkinje pathways. Rate-related or pre-existing bundle branch block, however, results in broad ventricular complexes that are difficult to distinguish from ventricular tachycardia.

ATRIAL ECTOPIC BEATS

These rarely indicate heart disease. They often occur spontaneously, but may be provoked by toxic stimuli such as caffeine, alcohol and cigarette smoking. They are caused by the premature discharge of an atrial ectopic focus; an early and often bizarre P wave is essential for the diagnosis. The premature impulse enters and depolarizes the sinus node such that a partially compensatory pause occurs before the next sinus beat during resetting of the sinus node.

ATRIAL FIBRILLATION

This is often idiopathic. It is common in hypertensive heart disease, mitral valve disease, thyrotoxicosis and left ventricular failure. It also occurs after major surgery and in response to various toxic stimuli, particularly alcohol. Atrial activity is chaotic and mechanically ineffective. P waves are therefore absent and are replaced by irregular fibrillatory waves (rate 400–600/min). The long refractory period of the atrioventricular node ensures that only some of the atrial impulses are conducted, to produce an irregular ventricular rate of 130–200 bpm. If the atrioventricular node is diseased the ventricular rate is slower, but in the presence of a rapidly conducting accessory pathway in Wolff–Parkinson–White syndrome dangerous ventricular rates above 300 bpm may occur.

ATRIAL FLUTTER

This is less common than atrial fibrillation but occurs under identical circumstances. Re-entry mechanisms produce an atrial rate close to 300 bpm. The normal atrioventricular node conducts with 2:1 block, giving a ventricular rate of 150 bpm. Higher degrees of block may reflect intrinsic disease of the atrioventricular node or the effects of nodal blocking drugs. The ECG characteristically shows sawtooth flutter waves, which are most clearly seen when the block is increased by carotid sinus pressure.

DIAGNOSIS OF JUNCTIONAL ARRHYTHMIAS

These are often called supraventricular tachycardias (SVTs) and are usually paroxysmal without obvious cardiac or extrinsic causes. They are re-entry arrhythmias caused either by an abnormal pathway between the atrium and the atrioventricular node (atrionodal pathway) or by an accessory atrioventricular pathway (bundle of Kent), as seen in Wolff–Parkinson–White syndrome. Like atrial arrhythmias, ventricular depolarization usually occurs by normal His–Purkinje pathways, producing a narrow QRS complex which confirms the supraventricular origin of the arrhythmia. Rate-related or pre-existing bundle branch block, on the other hand, produces broad ventricular complexes difficult to distinguish from ventricular tachycardia.

ATRIOVENTRICULAR JUNCTIONAL RE-ENTRY TACHYCARDIA (AVJRT)

The abnormal atrionodal pathway provides the basis for a small re-entry circuit. In sinus rhythm the electrocardiogram is usually normal, although occasionally the PR interval is short (Lown–Ganong–Levine syndrome). During tachycardia the rate is

150–250 bpm (Fig. 7.21). The arrhythmia is usually self-limiting but will sometimes respond to carotid sinus pressure. If this fails, intravenous verapamil or adenosine are usually effective by blocking the re-entry circuit within the atrioventricular node. Anti-tachycardia pacing or DC cardioversion may also be used. Many patients are now being treated by catheter ablation to destroy the abnormal atrionodal pathway and avoid the need for long-term drug therapy (see below).

WOLFF–PARKINSON–WHITE SYNDROME (WPW)

This congenital disorder, which affects 0.12% of the population, is caused by an accessory pathway (bundle of Kent) between the atria and the ventricles. During sinus rhythm, atrial impulses conduct more rapidly through the accessory pathway than the atrioventricular node, such that the initial phase of ventricular depolarization occurs early (pre-excitation) and spreads slowly through the ventricles by abnormal pathways. This produces a short PR interval and slurring of the initial QRS deflection (δ wave). The remainder of ventricular depolarization, however, is rapid because the delayed arrival of the impulse conducted through the atrioventricular node rapidly completes ventricular depolarization by normal His–Purkinje pathways (Fig. 7.22). Cardiac arrhythmias affect about 60% of patients with WPW syndrome and are usually re-entrant (rate 150–250 bpm) triggered by an atrial premature beat (Fig. 7.23). In most patients the re-entry arrhythmia is 'orthodromic', with anterograde conduction through the atrioventricular node and retrograde conduction through the accessory pathway. This results in a narrow complex tachycardia (without pre-excitation) that is indistinguishable from AVJRT. Occasionally, the re-entry circuit is in the opposite direction ('antidromic'), producing a very broad, pre-excited tachycardia.

Patients with WPW syndrome are more prone than the general population to atrial fibrillation. If the accessory pathway is able to conduct the fibrillatory impulses rapidly to the ventricles, it may result in ventricular fibrillation and sudden death. Digoxin (and to a lesser extent verapamil) should be avoided because it shortens the refractory period of the accessory pathway and can heighten the risk. Patients with dangerous accessory pathways of this type require ablation of the pathway, either surgically or, preferably, by catheter techniques. Ablation therapy also cures AVJRT and is treatment of choice in patients with frequent attacks.

DIAGNOSIS OF VENTRICULAR ARRHYTHMIAS

VENTRICULAR PREMATURE BEATS

These may occur in normal individuals, either spontaneously or in response to toxic stimuli such as caffeine or sympathomimetic drugs. They are caused

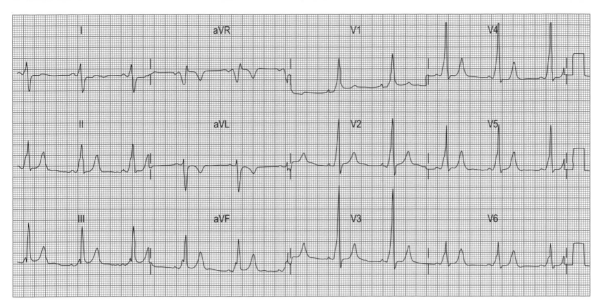

Figure 7.22 WPW syndrome: 12-lead ECG. Ventricular pre-excitation is reflected on the surface ECG by a short PR interval and a slurred upstroke to the QRS complex (δ wave). The remainder of the QRS complex is normal because delayed arrival of the impulse conducted through the AV node rapidly completes ventricular depolarization through normal His–Purkinje pathways.

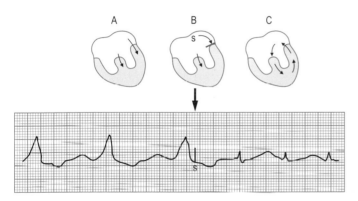

Figure 7.23 Wolff–Parkinson–White syndrome: re-entry tachycardia recorded at fast paper speed. Just after the third pre-excited (broad) complex a premature atrial pacing stimulus (S) initiates an impulse that is blocked in the bundle of Kent but conducted normally through the AV node, producing ventricular depolarization without pre-excitation. Thus the QRS complex is narrow and lacks a δ wave. The impulse is conducted retrogradely through the bundle of Kent, re-enters the proximal conducting system and completes the re-entry circuit, initiating a self-sustaining orthodromic re-entry tachycardia (last three complexes).

by the premature discharge of a ventricular ectopic focus that produces an early and broad QRS complex (Fig. 7.24). The premature impulse may be conducted backwards into the atria, producing a retrograde P wave, but penetration of the sinus node is rare. Thus, resetting of the sinus node does not usually occur and there is a fully compensatory pause before the next sinus beat.

VENTRICULAR TACHYCARDIA
This is always pathological. It is defined as three or more consecutive ventricular beats at a rate above 120 per minute. Ventricular depolarization inevitably occurs slowly by abnormal pathways, producing a broad QRS complex. This distinguishes it from most atrial and junctional tachycardias which have a narrow QRS complex, although differential diagnosis may be more difficult for atrial or junctional tachycardias with a broad QRS

complex caused by rate-related or pre-existing bundle branch block (Fig. 7.25). Nevertheless, ventricular tachycardia can usually be identified by careful scrutiny of the 12-lead ECG (Fig. 7.26). *Support* for the diagnosis is provided by a very broad QRS complex (>140 ms), extreme left or right axis deviation, concordance of the QRS deflections in V_1–V_6 (either all positive or all negative), and configurational features of the QRS complex, including an 'rSR' complex in V_1 and a QS complex in V_6. *Confirmation* of the diagnosis is provided by any evidence of AV dissociation: either P waves, at a slower rate than the QRS complexes, 'marching through' the tachycardia (Fig. 7.27(a)), or ventricular capture and/or fusion beats, in which the dissociated atrial rhythm penetrates the ventricle by conduction through the AV node and interrupts the tachycardia, producing sometimes a normal ventricular complex (capture, Fig. 7.27(a)) or, more

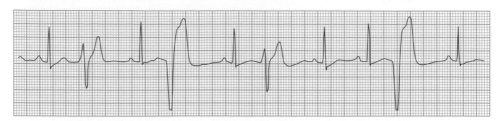

Figure 7.24 Multifocal, ventricular ectopic beats. Frequent broad complex ectopic beats are seen early after the sinus beats. Note, however, that the ectopic beats have two different morphologies, indicating that they arise from different foci. Note also that the coupling interval (interval between QRS complex and ectopic beat) is identical for beats arising from any particular focus.

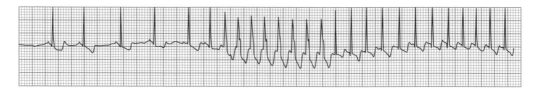

Figure 7.25 Paroxysmal AV nodal re-entrant tachycardia. This Holter recording shows sinus rhythm giving way to a broad complex tachycardia. However, this is clearly the result of temporary bundle branch block because it converts spontaneously to a narrow complex tachycardia, confirming that the arrhythmia is junctional not ventricular in origin.

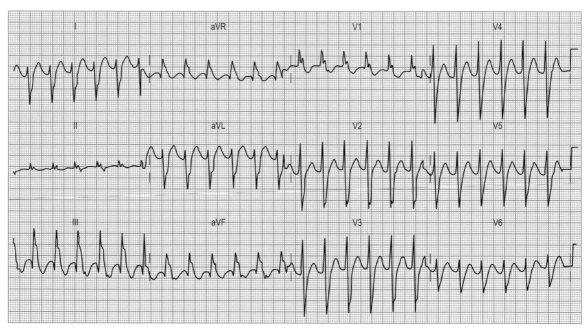

Figure 7.26 Ventricular tachycardia: 12-lead ECG. The recording shows a broad complex tachycardia. The following features suggest or confirm the ventricular origin of the tachycardia: very broad QRS complex (>140 ms); extreme right axis deviation; atrioventricular dissociation – note the dissociated P waves seen clearly in leads II and V_1; the 'rSR' complex in V_1.

commonly, a broad hybrid complex (fusion) that is part sinus and part ventricular in origin (Fig. 7.27(b)). *Torsades de pointes*, a broad complex tachycardia with changing wavefronts, also provides unequivocal evidence of ventricular tachycardia and is particularly characteristic of the arrhythmia that complicates long QT syndrome, often resulting in sudden death. The syndrome may be inherited as an autosomal dominant (Romano–Ward syndrome) or as an autosomal recessive (Lange–Nielsen syndrome) trait, when it is associated with congenital deafness.

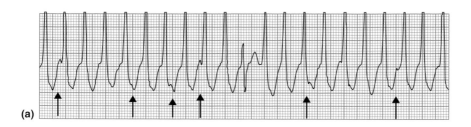

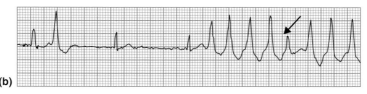

Figure 7.27 **(a)** Ventricular tachycardia: AV dissociation. P waves (arrowed) can be seen 'marching through' the tachycardia, confirming its ventricular origin. The tachycardia is interrupted by a narrow capture beat. **(b)** Ventricular tachycardia: fusion. In this example VT is initiated by a very early ventricular ectopic beat (morphologically similar to the previous isolated ectopic beat) and is interrupted by a fusion beat (arrowed), confirming the ventricular origin of the tachycardia.

VENTRICULAR FIBRILLATION

This occurs most commonly in severe myocardial ischaemia, either with or without frank infarction. It is a completely disorganized arrhythmia characterized by irregular fibrillatory waves with no discernible QRS complexes. There is no effective cardiac output and death is inevitable unless resuscitation with direct current cardioversion is instituted rapidly.

DIAGNOSIS OF SINOATRIAL DISEASE (Fig. 7.28 and Box 7.11)

Sinus node discharge is not itself visible on the surface ECG, but the atrial depolarization it triggers produces the P wave. The spontaneous discharge of the normal sinus node is influenced by a variety of neurohumoral factors, particularly vagal and sympathetic activity, which respectively slow and quicken the heart rate. In *sinoatrial disease* sinus node discharge may be abnormally slow, blocked (with failure to activate atrial depolarization), or absent altogether. Under these circumstances the sinus rate may be very slow, the atrium may fibrillate, or pacemaker function may be assumed by foci lower in the atrium, the atrioventricular node or the His–Purkinje conducting tissue in the ventricles. The intrinsic rate of these 'escape' pacemaker foci is slower than the normal sinus rate.

SINUS BRADYCARDIA (<50 BPM)

This is physiological during sleep and in trained athletes, but in other circumstances often reflects sinoatrial disease, particularly when the heart rate fails to increase normally with exercise.

SINOATRIAL BLOCK

If the sinus impulse is blocked and fails to trigger atrial depolarization, a pause occurs in the ECG. No P wave is seen during the pause owing to the absence of atrial depolarization. The electrically 'silent' sinus discharge, however, continues uninterrupted. Thus the pause is always a precise multiple of preceding P–P intervals. Sinoatrial block that cannot be abolished by atropine-induced vagal inhibition usually indicates sinoatrial disease, particularly with pauses longer than 2 seconds.

SINUS ARREST

Failure of sinus node discharge produces a pause on the ECG that bears no relation to the preceding P–P interval. Pauses longer than 2 seconds are usually pathological. Prolonged pauses are often terminated by an escape beat from a 'junctional' focus in the bundle of His.

BRADYCARDIA–TACHYCARDIA SYNDROME

In this syndrome atrial bradycardias are interspersed by paroxysmal tachyarrhythmias, usually atrial fibrillation. Nevertheless, it is the bradycardia that usually causes symptoms, particularly dizzy attacks and blackouts.

DIAGNOSIS OF ATRIOVENTRICULAR BLOCK

In *atrioventricular block* (Fig. 7.29) conduction is delayed or completely interrupted, either in the atrioventricular node or in the bundle branches (Box 7.12). When conduction is merely delayed (e.g. first-degree atrioventricular block, bundle branch block),

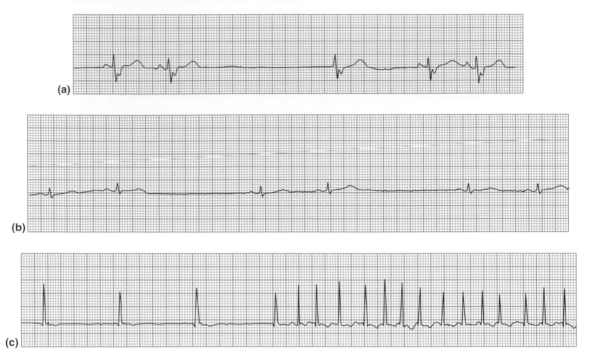

Figure 7.28 Sinoatrial disease. **(a)** Sinus arrest with late junctional escape. After the second sinus beat there is a long pause, interrupted by a single junctional escape beat, before sinus rhythm is re-established. **(b)** Sinoatrial block. Pauses after the second and fourth complexes are the result of sinoatrial block, which has prevented sinus impulses from depolarizing the atrium. No P waves are seen but, because the sinus discharge continues uninterrupted, the pauses are each a precise multiple of the preceding PP interval. Sinoatrial block is probably rare. **(c)** Bradycardia–tachycardia syndrome. A slow junctional rhythm gives way to rapid atrial fibrillation.

the heart rate is unaffected. When conduction is completely interrupted, however, the heart rate may slow sufficiently to produce symptoms. In second-degree atrioventricular block, failure of conduction is, by definition, intermittent, and if sufficient sinus impulses are conducted to maintain an adequate ventricular rate symptoms may be avoided. In third-degree atrioventricular block there is complete failure of conduction and continuing ventricular activity depends on the emergence of an escape rhythm. If the block is within the atrioventricular node the escape rhythm usually arises from a focus just below the node in the bundle of His (junctional escape), and is often fast enough to prevent symptoms. If both bundle branches are blocked, however, the escape rhythm must arise from a focus lower in the ventricles. Ventricular escape rhythms of this type are nearly always associated with symptoms because they are not only very slow but also unreliable, and may stop altogether, producing prolonged asystole.

FIRST-DEGREE ATRIOVENTRICULAR BLOCK
Delayed atrioventricular conduction causes prolongation of the PR interval (>0.20 s). Ventricular depolarization occurs rapidly by normal His–Purkinje pathways and the QRS complex is usually narrow.

SECOND-DEGREE ATRIOVENTRICULAR BLOCK: MOBITZ TYPE I (WENCKEBACH)
This commonly occurs in inferior myocardial infarction. Successive sinus beats find the atrioventricular node increasingly refractory until failure of conduction occurs. The delay permits recovery of nodal function, and the process may then repeat itself. The ECG shows progressive prolongation of the PR interval, culminating in a dropped beat. Block is within the atrioventricular node itself and ventricular depolarization occurs rapidly by normal pathways. Thus the QRS complex is usually narrow.

SECOND-DEGREE ATRIOVENTRICULAR BLOCK: MOBITZ TYPE II
This always indicates advanced conducting tissue disease affecting the bundle branches. The ECG typically shows a normal PR interval with bundle branch block in conducted beats, and intermittent block in the other bundle branch resulting in complete failure of atrioventricular conduction and dropped beats.

THIRD-DEGREE (COMPLETE) ATRIOVENTRICULAR BLOCK
The atrial and ventricular rhythms are 'dissociated' because none of the atrial impulses are conducted. Thus the ECG shows regular P waves (unless the

Box 7.11   Sinoatrial disease

Typical patient
- Elderly, often with no previous cardiac history

Causes
- Acute: myocardial infarction, coronary artery disease, drugs (e.g. β-blockers, digitalis), hypothermia, atrial surgery
- Chronic: idiopathic fibrotic disease, congenital heart disease, ischaemic heart disease, amyloid

Major symptoms
- Intermittent syncopal or presyncopal attacks
- Patients may also complain of exertional fatigue (chronotropic incompetence) or palpitations (tachycardia–bradycardia syndrome)

Major signs
- Often none
- Sometimes sinus bradycardia or slow atrial fibrillation

Diagnosis
- ECG: often normal. May show sinus bradycardia or slow atrial fibrillation
- Ambulatory ECG: 24-hour Holter recording may show pauses diagnostic of sinoatrial disease

Additional investigations
- None

Comments
- Documentation of the sinus pauses (or very slow AF) during an attack of symptoms provides the most robust diagnostic information

Box 7.12   Causes of atrioventricular heart block

Acute
- Myocardial infarction
- Drugs (e.g. β-blockers, verapamil, digitalis, adenosine)
- Surgical or catheter ablation of bundle of His

Chronic
- Idiopathic fibrosis of both bundle branches
- Ischaemic heart disease
- Congenital heart disease
- Calcific aortic valve disease
- Chagas' disease
- Infiltrative disease (amyloid haemochromatosis)
- Granulomatous disease (sarcoid, tuberculosis)

atrium is fibrillating) and regular but slower QRS complexes occurring independently of each other. When block is within the atrioventricular node (e.g. inferior myocardial infarction, congenital atrioventricular block), a junctional escape rhythm with a reliable rate (40–60 bpm) takes over (see Fig. 7.29). Ventricular depolarization occurs rapidly by normal pathways, producing a narrow QRS complex. However, when block is within the bundle branches (e.g. idiopathic fibrosis) there is always extensive conducting tissue disease. The ventricular escape rhythm is slow and unreliable, with a broad QRS complex (Fig. 7.29).

RIGHT BUNDLE BRANCH BLOCK
This may be a congenital defect but is more commonly the result of organic conducting tissue disease. Right ventricular depolarization is delayed, resulting in a broad QRS complex with an 'rSR' pattern in lead V_1 and prominent S waves in leads I and V_6.

LEFT BUNDLE BRANCH BLOCK
This always indicates organic conducting tissue disease. The entire sequence of ventricular depolarization is abnormal, resulting in a broad QRS complex with large slurred or notched R waves in leads I and V_6.

THE CHEST X-RAY

Good-quality posteroanterior (PA) and lateral chest X-rays are always helpful in the assessment of the cardiac patient (Fig. 7.30).

CARDIAC SILHOUETTE

Although the PA chest X-ray exhibits a wide range of normality, the maximum diameter of the heart should not be more than 50% of the widest diameter of the thorax. Cardiac enlargement is caused either by dilatation of the cardiac chambers or by pericardial effusion (Fig. 7.31). Myocardial hypertrophy only affects heart size if very severe.

VENTRICULAR DILATATION
The PA chest X-ray does not reliably distinguish left from right ventricular dilatation. For this, the lateral chest X-ray is more helpful. Dilatation of the posteriorly located left ventricle encroaches on the retrocardiac space, whereas dilatation of the anteriorly located right ventricle encroaches on the retrosternal space.

ATRIAL DILATATION
Right atrial dilatation is usually due to right ventricular failure, but occurs as an isolated finding in tricuspid stenosis and Ebstein's anomaly. It produces cardiac enlargement without specific radiographic signs.

Left atrial dilatation occurs in left ventricular failure and mitral valve disease (Fig. 7.32). Radiographic signs are:

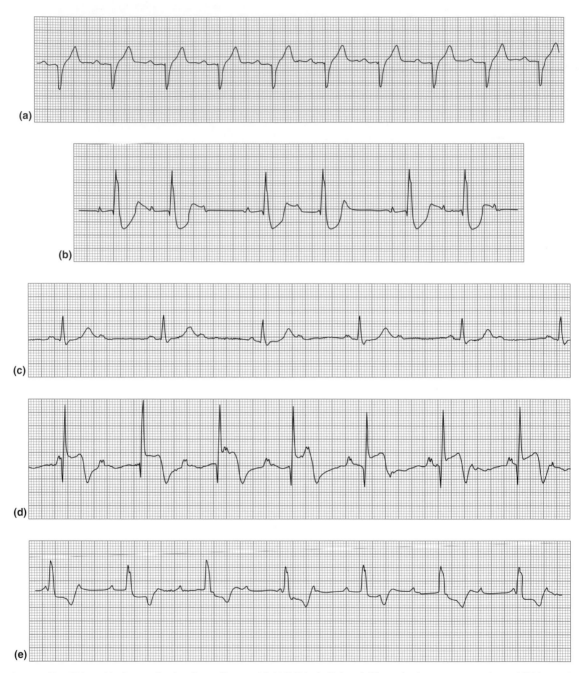

Figure 7.29 Atrioventricular conducting tissue disease. **(a)** 1° AV block. Delayed AV conduction causes a prolonged PR interval (>0.20 s). **(b)** 2° AV block, Wenckebach type. This is also called Mobitz type I block and occurs within the AV node. Three Wenckebach cycles are shown. Successive sinus beats find the AV node increasingly refractory until failure of conduction occurs. This delay permits recovery of nodal function and the process repeats itself. **(c)** 2° AV block at bundle branch level (Mobitz type II). This is standard lead I. Note that the PR interval of conducted beats is normal but the QRS complex shows right bundle branch block. Intermittent block in the left bundle results in failure of conduction of alternate P waves. **(d)** 3° (complete) AV block at level of AV node. In this patient with acute inferior myocardial infarction there is complete failure of AV conduction, as reflected by the dissociated atrial and ventricular rhythms. Note the regular P waves and the regular slower QRS complexes occurring independently of one another. Because block is at the level of the AV node a junctional escape rhythm has taken over with a narrow QRS complex. **(e)** 3° (complete) AV block at bundle branch level. The atrial and ventricular rhythms are dissociated because none of the atrial impulses are conducted. The ECG shows regular P waves and regular but slower QRS complexes. Because the escape rhythm is ventricular in origin the QRS complexes are broad and the rate is slow.

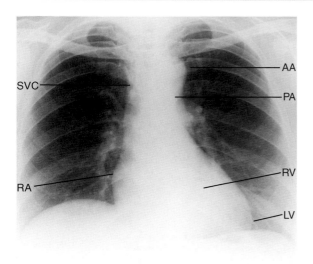

Figure 7.30 Normal chest X-ray: posteroanterior projection. Note the heart is not enlarged (cardiothoracic ratio <50%) and the lung fields are clear. SVC, superior vena cava; RA, right atrium; AA, aortic arch; LV, left ventricle; PA, pulmonary artery; RV, right ventricle.

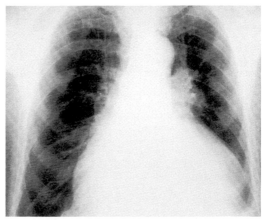

Figure 7.32 Left atrial dilatation. This is a penetrated PA chest X-ray in a patient with mitral stenosis. The dilated, posteriorly located left atrium is clearly visible. Note flattening of the left heart border, the widening of the carina and the double-density sign at the right heart border.

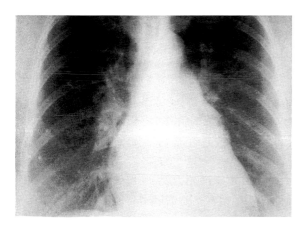

Figure 7.31 Pericardial effusion with tamponade: chest X-ray. There is a left hilar mass caused by carcinoma. Pericardial infiltration has produced effusion and tamponade, evidenced by the severe cardiac enlargement. Malignant disease is now the most common cause of tamponade in most developed countries.

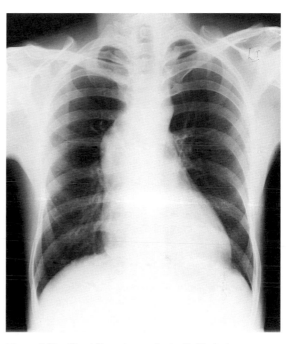

Figure 7.33 Chest X-ray in a patient with Marfan's syndrome. Note the dilatation of the ascending aorta.

- Flattening and later bulging of the left heart border below the main pulmonary artery
- Elevation of the left main bronchus, with widening of the carina
- Appearance of the medial border of the left atrium behind the right side of the heart (double-density sign).

VASCULAR DILATATION

Aortic dilatation caused by aneurysm or dissection may produce widening of the entire upper medi-astinum. Localized dilatation of the proximal aorta occurs in aortic valve disease and produces a prominence in the right upper mediastinum (Fig. 7.33). Dilatation of the main pulmonary artery occurs in pulmonary hypertension and pulmonary stenosis and produces a prominence below the aortic knuckle (Fig. 7.34).

INTRACARDIAC CALCIFICATION

Because the radiodensity of cardiac tissue is similar to that of blood, intracardiac structures can rarely

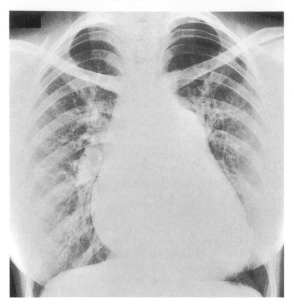

Figure 7.34 Pulmonary arterial hypertension illustrating cardiomegaly and enlargement of the main pulmonary artery and hilar arteries. Vessels beyond the hilum are normal or small, notably in the lower zones. The patient, a 19-year-old woman, had severe primary pulmonary hypertension.

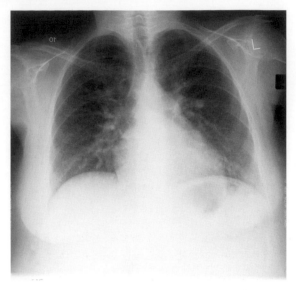

Figure 7.35 Atrial septal defect: chest X-ray. Note the prominent proximal pulmonary arteries and the pulmonary plethora reflecting increased pulmonary flow.

be identified unless they are calcified. Valvular, pericardial or myocardial calcification may occur, and usually indicates important disease of these structures. Calcification is best appreciated on the deeply penetrated lateral chest X-ray.

LUNG FIELDS

Common lung field abnormalities in cardiovascular disease are caused either by altered pulmonary flow or by increased left atrial pressure.

ALTERED PULMONARY FLOW

Increments in pulmonary flow sufficient to cause radiographic abnormalities are caused by left-to-right intracardiac shunts (e.g. atrial septal defect, Fig. 7.35), ventricular septal defect, patent ductus arteriosus). Prominence of the vascular markings gives the lung fields a plethoric appearance. Reductions in pulmonary flow, on the other hand, cause reduced vascular markings. This may be regional (e.g. pulmonary embolism) or global (e.g. severe pulmonary hypertension, see Fig. 7.34).

INCREASED LEFT ATRIAL PRESSURE

This occurs in mitral stenosis and left ventricular failure and produces corresponding rises in pulmonary venous and pulmonary capillary pressures. Prominence of the upper lobe veins is an early radiographic finding. As the left atrial and pulmonary capillary pressures rise above 18 mmHg transudation into the lung produces interstitial pulmonary oedema, characterized by prominence of the inter-

lobular septa, particularly at the lung bases (Kerley B lines). Further elevation of pressure leads to alveolar pulmonary oedema, characterized by perihilar 'bat's wing' shadowing (Fig. 7.36).

OTHER LUNG FIELD ABNORMALITIES

Pulmonary infarction

Localized and typically wedge-shaped areas of consolidation are occasionally seen in pulmonary embolic disease, although more often the bronchial circulation protects against ischaemic damage.

Pneumonic consolidation and abscess

In patients with right-sided endocarditis infected pulmonary emboli commonly cause septic foci within the lung fields.

INTERSTITIAL LUNG DISEASE

In long-standing pulmonary hypertension complicating rheumatic mitral valve disease, haemosiderosis (stippled shadowing throughout the lung fields) was once a common X-ray finding. It is now rarely seen.

BONY ABNORMALITIES

Bony abnormalities are unusual in cardiovascular disease, apart from coarctation of the aorta and thoracic outlet syndromes. In coarctation, dilated bronchial collateral vessels erode the inferior aspect of the ribs to produce notches, although they are rarely present before adolescence. Cervical ribs may compress the neurovascular bundle in the thoracic outlet, and special thoracic outlet views are necessary for radiographic diagnosis.

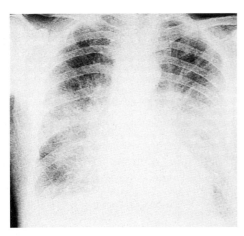

Figure 7.36 Chest X-ray in acute left ventricular failure: the patient had severe pulmonary oedema caused by acute myocardial infarction. The heart is not yet enlarged, but there is prominent alveolar pulmonary oedema in a perihilar ('bat's-wing') distribution. Note the bilateral pleural effusions.

ECHOCARDIOGRAPHY

Echocardiography is one of the most versatile non-invasive imaging techniques in clinical cardiology. Because it does not use ionizing radiation it is free of known risk and can be employed safely throughout pregnancy. Transthoracic imaging with the transducer applied to the chest wall is usually satisfactory, but better-quality information is obtained via the transoesophageal approach, in which the transducer is mounted on a probe and positioned in the oesophagus, directly behind the heart. This provides better-quality images because there are no intervening ribs or lung tissue and the probe is closely applied to the posterior aspect of the heart. It is particularly useful for imaging the left atrium, the aorta and prosthetic heart valves.

PRINCIPLES

PHYSICS
A transducer containing a piezoelectric element converts electrical energy into an ultrasound beam that can be directed towards the heart. The beam is reflected when it strikes an interface between tissues of different densities. The reflected ultrasound, or *echo*, is converted back to electrical energy by the piezoelectric element, which permits the construction of an image using two basic units of information:

- The *intensity* of the echoes, which defines the density difference at tissue interfaces within the heart
- The *time* taken for echoes to arrive back at the transducer, which defines the distance of the cardiac structures from the transducer.

Density differences within the heart are greatest between the blood-filled chambers and the myocardial and valvular tissues, all of which are clearly visible on the echocardiogram. Because the depth of the myocardial and valvular tissues with respect to the transducer changes constantly throughout the cardiac cycle, the time taken for echo reflection changes accordingly. Thus, real-time imaging throughout the cardiac cycle provides a dynamic record of cardiac function.

M-MODE ECHOCARDIOGRAM (Fig. 7.37(a))
This provides a unidimensional 'ice-pick' view through the heart. Continuous recording on photographic paper provides an additional time dimension, thereby permitting appreciation of the dynamic component of the cardiac image. By convention, cardiac structures closest to the transducer are displayed at the top of the record and more distant structures are displayed below. Thus, on the transthoracic M-mode echocardiogram, anteriorly located ('right-sided') structures lie above the posteriorly located ('left-sided') structures, but on the transoesophageal echocardiogram the display is reversed.

**TWO-DIMENSIONAL
ECHOCARDIOGRAM** (Fig. 7.37(b))
This provides more detailed information about morphology than the M-mode recording. By projecting a fan of echoes in an arc of up to 80° a two-dimensional 'slice' through the heart can be obtained, the precise view depending on the location and angulation of the transducer.

CLINICAL APPLICATIONS

CONGENITAL HEART DISEASE
Echocardiography, particularly the two-dimensional technique, has revolutionized the diagnosis of congenital heart disease, in the majority of cases obviating the need for invasive investigation by cardiac catheterization (Fig. 7.38). The relationships of the cardiac chambers and their connections with the great vessels are readily determined. Valvular abnormalities and septal defects can also be recognized. Recent technology has permitted in utero fetal imaging for the antenatal diagnosis of cardiac defects.

MYOCARDIAL DISEASE
Echocardiography permits accurate assessment of cardiac dilatation, hypertrophy and contractile function. Congestive cardiomyopathy produces ventricular dilatation with *global* contractile impairment (Fig. 7.39). This must be distinguished from the *regional* contractile impairment that follows myocardial infarction in patients with coronary artery disease (Fig. 7.40). Hypertrophic cardiomyopathy is characterized by thickening (hypertrophy)

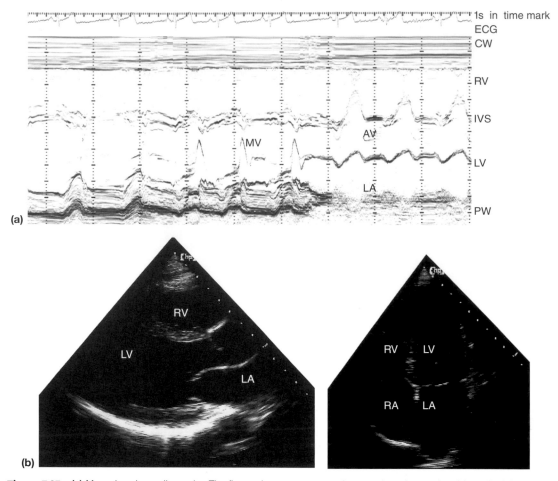

Figure 7.37 **(a)** M-mode echocardiography. The figure shows a sweep as the transducer is angulated from the left ventricle to the aortic root. **(b)** Transthoracic 2D echocardiography. Parasternal long axis and apical four-chamber views are shown. The dots are a 1 cm scale. CW, chest wall; RV, right ventricle; IVS, interventricular septum; LV, left ventricle; PW, posterior LV wall; MV, mitral valve; AV, aortic valve; LA, left atrium.

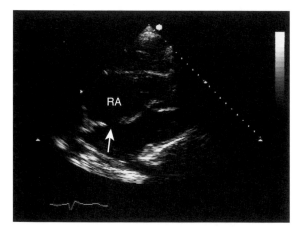

Figure 7.38 Atrial septal defect: 2D echocardiogram (subcostal view). In this view, good views of the interatrial septum can usually be obtained without resorting to transoesophageal echocardiography. Note the ASD (arrowed) and the dilatation of the right atrium (RA).

of the left ventricular myocardium, usually with disproportionate involvement of the interventricular septum (asymmetric septal hypertrophy). In aortic and hypertensive heart disease, on the other hand, left ventricular hypertrophy is usually symmetrical (Fig. 7.41).

VALVULAR DISEASE   (Boxes 7.13–7.16)
Echocardiography is of particular value for identifying both structural and dynamic valvular abnormalities and any associated chamber dilatation or hypertrophy. The severity of valvular involvement in congenital, rheumatic, degenerative and infective disease may thus be defined; the technique is diagnostic of bicuspid aortic valve and mitral valve prolapse, and readily identifies valve thickening and calcification in rheumatic and calcific disease (Figs 7.41, 7.42). Vegetations in infective endocarditis can usually be visualized if they are large enough (>3 mm, Fig. 7.43). The transoesophageal approach

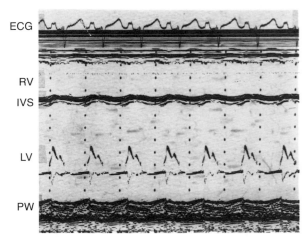

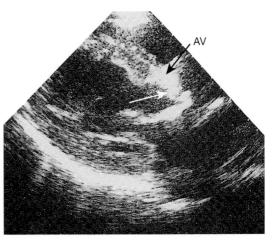

Figure 7.39 Dilated cardiomyopathy: echocardiogram. This M-mode study shows severe dilatation of the left ventricular cavity and severe global contractile impairment. The patient later underwent successful heart transplantation.

Figure 7.41 Aortic stenosis and left ventricular hypertrophy: 2D echocardiogram (long axis view). The aortic valve (AV) is grossly thickened and highly echogenic. Concentric LV hypertrophy is present.

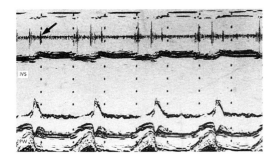

Figure 7.40 Heart failure: echocardiogram. This M-mode study shows considerable dilatation of the left ventricle. Note that the interventricular septum (IVS) is almost akinetic, but the posterior wall (PW) is contracting normally. Regional contractile impairment of this type indicates coronary heart disease. The phonocardiogram recorded simultaneously shows normal first and second heart sounds and also a third heart sound (arrowed).

oesophageal technique is also helpful for diagnosing aortic disease, such as aneurysm and dissection, as it provides better views of the thoracic aorta than are possible with conventional 2D echocardiography (Fig. 7.46).

STRESS ECHOCARDIOGRAPHY

This is increasingly being used for the diagnosis of myocardial ischaemia in suspected coronary disease. Left ventricular imaging during increasing dobutamine infusion permits assessment of regional wall motion in response to adrenergic stress. Decreasing systolic wall motion or wall thickening indicates ischaemia and the need for further investigation. Stress echocardiography is also used to identify myocardial 'viability' in the patient with heart failure, and improvement in regional hypokinesis in response to dobutamine infusion, indicating 'hibernating' (and hence potentially salvageable) myocardium likely to respond favourably to revascularization by angioplasty or bypass surgery.

DOPPLER ECHOCARDIOGRAPHY

Doppler echocardiography permits evaluation of the direction and velocity of blood flow within the heart and great vessels. It is widely used for measuring the severity of valvular stenosis and identifying valvular regurgitation and intracardiac shunts through septal defects.

PRINCIPLES

PHYSICS
According to the Doppler principle, when an ultrasound beam is directed towards the bloodstream

is usually necessary for endocarditis involving prosthetic heart valves.

PERICARDIAL DISEASE
Although the echocardiogram is of little value in constrictive pericarditis, it is the most sensitive technique available for the diagnosis of pericardial effusion (Fig. 7.44). The effusion appears as an echo-free space distributed around the ventricles but usually avoiding the potential space behind the left atrium.

OTHER CLINICAL APPLICATIONS
Intracardiac tumours, particularly myxomas and thrombi, are readily visualized by echocardiography (see Fig. 7.1), and the oesophageal instrument has found important application for identifying thrombus in the left atrial appendage (Fig. 7.45). The

---

Box 7.13   Aortic stenosis

Typical patient
- Middle-aged (congenitally bicuspid valve) or elderly (degenerative calcific disease) man or woman

Major symptoms
- Exertional shortness of breath is usual presenting symptom
- Angina may also occur and, in advanced cases, syncopal attacks or sudden death

Major signs
- Carotid pulse: slow upstroke with plateau
- Auscultation: fourth heart sound at cardiac apex; ejection systolic murmur at base of heart, radiating to neck. The murmur may be preceded by an ejection click if the valve is mobile and not heavily calcified

Diagnosis
- ECG: left ventricular hypertrophy
- CXR: dilatation of ascending aorta
- Echocardiogram: calcified immobile aortic valve with left ventricular hypertrophy. Doppler studies permit quantification of the severity of stenosis

Additional investigations
- Cardiac catheterization is necessary to evaluate coronary arteries in patients being considered for aortic valve replacement surgery

Comments
- Aortic stenosis is now the commonest acquired valve lesion in developed countries

---

Box 7.14   Aortic regurgitation

Typical patient
- Young men (Marfan's syndrome etc.) or older patients (long-standing hypertension) with dilating disease of the aortic root

Major symptoms
- Exertional shortness of breath is usual presenting symptom
- Angina may also occur

Major signs
- Carotid pulse: sharp upstroke with early diastolic collapse
- Blood pressure: systolic hypertension with wide pulse pressure
- Auscultation: early diastolic murmur at left sternal edge. Third heart sound at cardiac apex in severe cases. Mid-diastolic murmur (Austin Flint) may be heard at apex owing to preclosure of mitral valve by regurgitant jet

Diagnosis
- ECG: left ventricular hypertrophy
- CXR: cardiac enlargement with dilatation of ascending aorta
- Echocardiogram: often normal valve with dilated aortic root. Doppler studies confirm regurgitant jet

Additional investigations
- Cardiac catheterization is necessary to evaluate coronary arteries in older patients (age >50) being considered for aortic valve replacement surgery

Comments
- The timing of valve replacement surgery is difficult but should anticipate irreversible left ventricular contractile failure

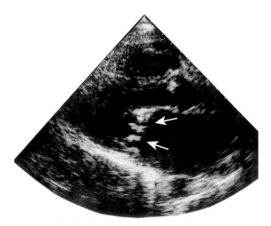

Figure 7.42   Mitral stenosis: 2D echocardiogram (parasternal long axis view). The mitral valve leaflets are densely thickened (arrowed) and the left atrium is severely dilated.

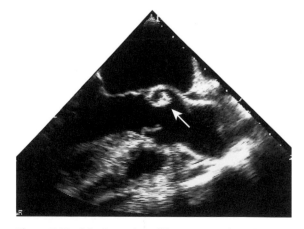

Figure 7.43   Infective endocarditis: transoesophageal echocardiogram. A vegetation (arrowed) is adherent to the aortic valve leaflet.

Box 7.15 Mitral stenosis

Typical patient
- Young to middle-aged woman with a history of rheumatic fever in childhood

Major symptoms
- Exertional shortness of breath with orthopnoea in advanced cases
- Palpitations commonly signal the development of atrial fibrillation, which puts the patient at serious risk of peripheral embolism and stroke

Major signs
- Pulse: atrial fibrillation in many cases
- Auscultation: loud S1 with early diastolic opening snap, followed by low-pitched mid-diastolic murmur best heard at cardiac apex. If the patient is in sinus rhythm there is presystolic accentuation of the murmur

Diagnosis
- ECG: atrial fibrillation usually
- CXR: signs of left atrial enlargement (flat left heart border, widening of carinal angle, and double-density sign at right heart border). Pulmonary congestion
- Echocardiogram: rheumatic mitral valve and left atrial dilatation. Doppler studies confirm diastolic jet

Additional investigations
- Cardiac catheterization is necessary to evaluate coronary arteries in patients aged >50 being considered for mitral valve replacement surgery

Comments
- In patients with atrial fibrillation, anticoagulation with warfarin is mandatory to protect against stroke

Box 7.16 Mitral regurgitation

Typical patient
- Mitral valve prolapse (floppy mitral valve) causes regurgitation of variable severity, and more commonly affects women at almost any age
- Patients with subvalvular disease (papillary muscle dysfunction or chordal rupture) are usually elderly men or women

Major symptoms
- Exertional shortness of breath with orthopnoea in advanced cases
- Palpitations commonly signal the development of atrial fibrillation, which puts the patient at serious risk of peripheral embolism and stroke

Major signs
- Pulse: often sinus rhythm, but may be atrial fibrillation
- Auscultation: pansystolic murmur at cardiac apex, radiating to axilla. Often associated with third heart sound

Diagnosis
- ECG: atrial fibrillation, but may be normal
- CXR: cardiac enlargement with variable signs of left atrial enlargement, though these are usually less marked than in mitral stenosis. Pulmonary congestion in severe cases
- Echocardiogram: prolapsing (floppy) mitral valve may be seen; in subvalvular disease the valve often appears normal. Left ventricular and left atrial dilatation. Doppler studies confirm regurgitant jet

Additional investigations
- Cardiac catheterization is necessary to evaluate coronary arteries in patients aged >50 being considered for mitral valve replacement surgery

Comments
- In patients with atrial fibrillation, anticoagulation with warfarin is mandatory to protect against stroke

the frequency of the sound waves reflected from the blood cells is altered. The frequency shift or Doppler effect is related to the direction and velocity of flow. If continuous-wave Doppler is used, blood flow at any point along the path of the ultrasound beam is detected, such that a 'clean' Doppler signal from the area of interest may be difficult to obtain. Pulsed Doppler, however, has a range-gating facility that permits frequency sampling from any specific point within the heart, preselected on the echocardiogram. This lends greater precision to the technique. Nevertheless, pulsed Doppler is less able than continuous-wave Doppler to quantify very high-velocity jets, such as those that occur in aortic stenosis.

COLOUR-FLOW MAPPING
This has been a major technological advance. Instead of the unidirectional ultrasound beam used

in continuous-wave and pulsed Doppler imaging, the beam is rotated through an arc. Frequency sampling throughout the arc permits the construction of a colour-coded map, red indicating flow towards and blue away from the transducer. Colour flow data can be superimposed on the standard 2D echocardiogram to identify precisely the patterns of flow within the four chambers of the heart. This simplifies the interpretation of Doppler imaging and provides more useful qualitative data, although it is less useful for quantitative assessment of valve

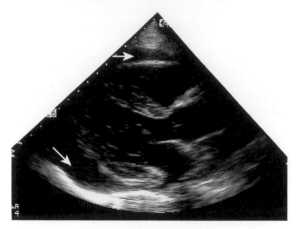

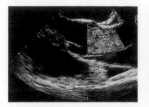
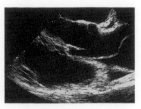

Figure 7.46 Aortic dissection: transoesophageal echocardiogram. Right panel: this longitudinal axis transoesophageal echocardiogram reveals the dilated aortic root and an S-shaped flap traversing the lumen. Left panel: same patient with colour Doppler superimposed to show flow in the true lumen.

Figure 7.44 Pericardial effusion: 2D echocardiogram (parasternal long axis view). Note the echo-free space (arrowed) around the heart, but not behind the left atrium.

permits quantification of the stenosis by the application of the Bernoulli equation:

$$\text{pressure gradient} = 4 \times \text{velocity}^2.$$

CARDIOVASCULAR RADIONUCLIDE IMAGING

PRINCIPLES

All radionuclide techniques require the internal administration of a radioisotope; the distribution of radioactivity in the area of interest is then imaged with a gamma camera. Ideally, the isotope should be distributed homogeneously in that part of the cardiovascular system under investigation: thus, isotopes that remain in the intravascular space during imaging are used for radionuclide angiography. In myocardial perfusion scintigraphy, however, isotopes taken up by the myocardium are required. Because of their potential toxicity, isotopes with a short half-life are usually used.

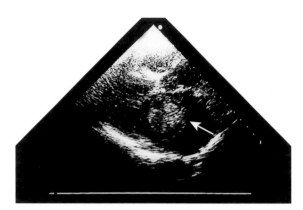

Figure 7.45 Mitral stenosis: 2D echocardiogram (long axis view). The left atrium is severely dilated and a large thrombus (arrowed) is visible, emphasizing the importance of anticoagulation in patients with mitral valve disease and atrial fibrillation.

CLINICAL APPLICATIONS

RADIONUCLIDE VENTRICULOGRAPHY

This method is used for assessment of ventricular function. Red cells labelled with technetium-99m (^{99m}Tc) are allowed to equilibrate in the blood pool and the heart is then imaged under the gamma camera (Fig. 7.48). The waxing and waning of radioactivity within the ventricular chambers during diastole and systole, respectively, permits the construction of a dynamic ventriculogram. Left ventricular contractile function can be evaluated quantitatively, by calculating the ejection fraction, or qualitatively by observing wall movement. Global left ventricular impairment is characteristic of cardiomyopathy, whereas regional defects are seen after myocardial infarction. Stress radionuclide angiography using exercise or peripheral cold stimulation (cold pressor test) is used to detect myocardial ischaemia: provocation of reversible regional wall motion abnormalities is strongly suggestive of coronary artery disease.

gradients, which requires the precision of conventional Doppler technique.

CLINICAL APPLICATIONS

In paediatric cardiology the combination of 2D echocardiography and colour-flow Doppler mapping has made possible the 'non-invasive' diagnosis of a large majority of congenital defects, often without the need for cardiac catheterization. These techniques have also revolutionized the diagnosis of valvular disease in all age groups. In valvular regurgitation, the retrograde flow that occurs after valve closure is readily detected by Doppler echocardiography, although only an approximate estimate of its severity is possible (Fig. 7.47). In valvular stenosis the peak velocity (as opposed to the volume) of flow across the valve is directly related to the degree of stenosis. Thus measurement of Doppler flow velocity (ideally by continuous wave)

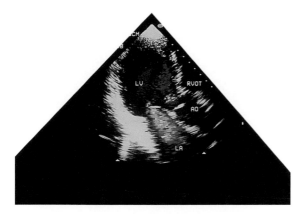

Figure 7.47 Mitral regurgitation: colour-flow Doppler. This is an apical long axis view of the heart showing a large jet of mitral regurgitation (blue) occupying most of the left atrial cavity (LA).

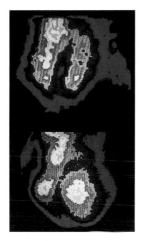

Figure 7.48 Radionuclide ventriculography: colour-coded study showing systolic and diastolic frames in a patient with dilated cardiomyopathy. The left ventricular cavity is severely dilated with contractile failure.

MYOCARDIAL PERFUSION SCINTIGRAPHY

This method is used for the diagnosis of coronary artery disease (Fig. 7.49). The investigation requires a standardized exercise stress test with continuous ECG monitoring in order to provoke myocardial ischaemia in susceptible subjects. Thallium-201 (^{201}Tl) is now giving way to ^{99m}Tc-labelled MIBI which provides better image quality. Isotope is injected intravenously at peak exercise and the heart is imaged under a gamma camera. Isotope is distributed homogeneously in normally perfused myocardium, ischaemic or infarcted areas appearing as scintigraphic defects. If ^{201}Tl is used, repeat imaging after 2–4 hours' rest permits the reassessment of scintigraphic defects – those that disappear (reversible defects) indicate areas of exercise-induced ischaemia, those that persist (fixed defects) indicate infarcted myocardium. If ^{99m}Tc-labelled

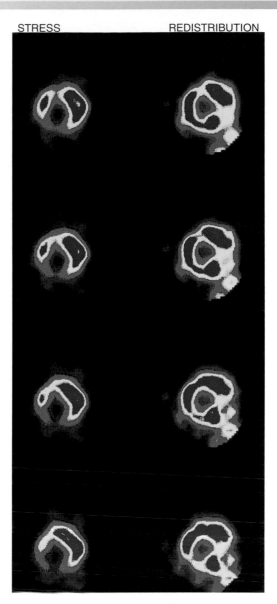

STRESS   REDISTRIBUTION

Figure 7.49 Isotope perfusion scan. These are tomographic slices across the short axis of the left ventricle. An inferior wall defect is seen during stress, but it largely disappears during rest as isotope 'redistributes' into the ischaemic area. A smaller fixed defect is seen in the anterior wall, indicating infarction in that territory.

MIBI is used, resting images for assessment of reversibility require a separate injection of isotope 24 hours after (or before) the exercise images.

POSITRON EMISSION TOMOGRAPHY (PET)

Originally a research tool, PET scanning is now used clinically to determine 'viability' in patients with heart failure (see Stress echocardiography). Simultaneous assessment of myocardial perfusion using ^{13}N ammonia and glucose uptake using a glucose analogue permits the identification of viable but dysfunctional myocardium, in which perfusion

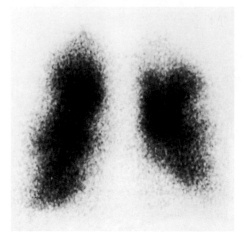
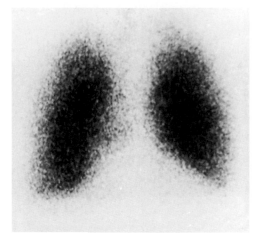

Figure 7.50 Ventilation (right) and perfusion (left) lung scans in pulmonary embolism. Contrast the homogeneous distribution of isotope in the ventilation scan with the regional defects in the perfusion scan.

is impaired but metabolic activity in terms of glucose uptake remains normal. This perfusion–metabolic 'mismatch' indicates viable muscle likely to respond favourably to revascularization by angioplasty or bypass surgery.

PULMONARY SCINTIGRAPHY (RADIOISOTOPE IMAGING)

This method is used for the diagnosis of pulmonary embolism (Fig. 7.50). ^{99m}Tc-labelled microspheres injected intravenously become trapped within the pulmonary capillaries. The normal pulmonary perfusion scintigram shows a homogeneous distribution of radioactivity throughout both lung fields. Pulmonary embolism causes regional impairment of pulmonary flow, which results in a perfusion defect on the scintigram; however, the appearance is nonspecific and occurs in many other pulmonary disorders, particularly chronic obstructive pulmonary disease. Specificity is enhanced by simultaneous ventilation scintigraphy. Inhaled xenon-133 (^{133}Xe) is distributed homogeneously throughout the normal lung and, in pulmonary embolism (unlike other pulmonary disorders), distribution remains homogeneous. Thus a scintigraphic perfusion defect not 'matched' by a ventilation defect is highly specific for pulmonary embolism.

COMPUTED TOMOGRAPHY

PRINCIPLES

Computed tomography (CT) measures the attenuation of X-rays after they have traversed body tissues. Attenuation is greatest for tissues such as bone, which are relatively radio-opaque, and least for tissues such as lung or fat, which are relatively radiolucent. From X-ray attenuation measurements, taken as a sensor rotates around the chest, cross-sectional images are constructed. Image resolution is excellent, and contrast injection into a peripheral vein provides adequate opacification of the blood pool for the identification of intracardiac structures. In the past, the clinical application of CT in cardiology was limited by image acquisition times of up to 5 seconds, during which the constant motion of the heart degraded the image. The current generation of ultrafast CT scanners with image acquisition times of less than 1 second provide high-resolution cardiac images in both static and video mode; measurements of blood flow can also be obtained by the application of indicator dilution principles.

CLINICAL APPLICATIONS

CT (with contrast enhancement) is widely used for the non-invasive diagnosis of aortic dissection, when two contrast columns separated by an intimal flap can be clearly seen (Fig. 7.51). It is also used for accurate assessment of pericardial thickness in constrictive disease (Fig. 7.52) and in the diagnosis of cardiac tumours. Additional applications of ultrafast CT include the evaluation of graft patency following coronary bypass surgery, analysis of ventricular wall motion, and blood flow quantification in congenital heart disease, permitting dynamic assessment of shunts and other defects. With the new generation of multislice scanners image quality is yet further enhanced, and quantification of coronary calcification using a scoring method is finding widespread application as a marker of coronary risk in asymptomatic individuals, scores >100 providing an indication for secondary prevention treatment and ischaemia testing.

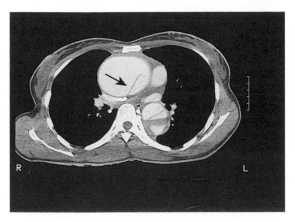

Figure 7.51 Aortic dissection: CT scan (Marfan's syndrome). The ascending aorta is severely dilated and the intimal flap (arrowed) clearly visible. This flap extends around the arch (not seen here) into the descending aorta, where again it is clearly visible.

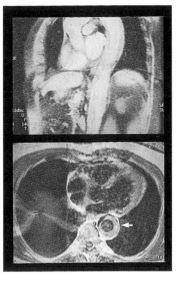

Figure 7.53 Aortic dissection: MRI scan. The upper panel (coronal section) reveals an extensive aortic dissection extending from the aortic root through the arch and into the descending aorta. The lower panel reveals a transverse view through the heart and descending aorta. Note the thrombus in the false lumen surrounding the true lumen in the descending aorta (arrowed).

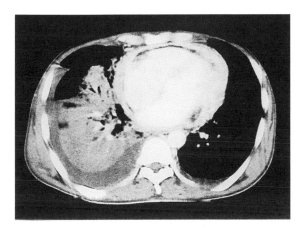

Figure 7.52 Non-calcific pericardial constriction: CT scan. There is consolidation in the right lung and severe pericardial thickening. The patient had pulmonary tuberculosis with pericardial involvement and presented with fever and signs of constriction. Antituberculous therapy caused regression of all symptoms and signs, although the patient is at major risk of developing constriction later as the pericardium becomes fibrotic and calcified.

MAGNETIC RESONANCE IMAGING

PRINCIPLES

Magnetic resonance imaging (MRI) utilizes the fact that certain nuclei with an intrinsic spin generate magnetic fields and behave like tiny bar magnets. Placed in a magnetic field, these nuclei align and adopt a resonant frequency that is unique to that nucleus and the strength of the magnetic field. If the nuclei are exposed to pulsed radiowaves of that frequency, they resonate and release energy, which allows their location to be determined.

For imaging purposes, the patient lies in a strong magnetic field which is artificially graded. The hydrogen protons of fat and water are imaged and, on exposure to pulsed radiowaves, they resonate at different frequencies in different parts of the imaging zone. Analysis of the emitted frequencies permits the construction of tomographic and three-dimensional images of the heart. If data acquisition is gated to a specific part of the cardiac cycle, motion artefact is eliminated and excellent image resolution can be obtained.

CLINICAL APPLICATIONS

MRI is now widely used for the diagnosis of aortic dissection (Fig. 7.53) and for imaging cardiac tumours. Emerging applications include coronary artery imaging without the need for cardiac catheterization, the identification of histological and metabolic disorders of the myocardium, and assessment of myocardial perfusion using paramagnetic contrast agents. These new applications have secured a central role for MRI in clinical cardiology.

CARDIAC CATHETERIZATION

Catheters introduced into an artery or vein may be directed into the left or right sides of the heart, respectively. Vascular access is usually percutaneous, using the femoral vessels, or by surgical cutdown, using the antecubital vessels. Originally developed for diagnostic purposes, catheter techniques are now being used increasingly for the interventional management of cardiovascular disease.

CARDIAC ANGIOGRAPHY

Coronary arteriography uses relatively small volumes of contrast (5–8 mL) injected manually, but other angiographic procedures require much larger amounts (up to 50 mL), introduced by power injection. Digital subtraction techniques permit a reduction in contrast volume but at present have only a limited role in cardiovascular angiographic diagnosis (see below). Until recently, images have been recorded on high-speed cine film or video, to provide a dynamic record of ventricular wall movement, blood flow and intravascular anatomy. The current generation of angiographic laboratories, however, use digital technology and provide better-quality images that can be stored electronically.

AORTIC ROOT ANGIOGRAPHY

Injection of contrast into the aortic root demonstrates the vascular anatomy in suspected aneurysm or dissection, and also permits evaluation of aortic valve function (Fig. 7.54). The normal aortic valve prevents diastolic backflow of contrast, but in aortic regurgitation variable opacification of the left ventricle occurs, depending on the severity of the valve lesion.

LEFT VENTRICULAR ANGIOGRAPHY

Contrast injection into the left ventricle defines ventricular anatomy and wall motion, and also permits evaluation of mitral valve function (Fig. 7.55). Dilatation of the ventricle and contractile dysfunction occurs in left ventricular failure. Exaggerated

contractile function with systolic obliteration of the cavity occurs in hypertrophic cardiomyopathy. Filling defects within the ventricular lumen may indicate thrombus or neoplasm. The normal mitral valve prevents systolic backflow of contrast into the left atrium, but in mitral regurgitation variable atrial opacification occurs, depending on the severity of the valve lesion.

CORONARY ARTERIOGRAPHY

This is the only reliable technique for diagnostic imaging of the coronary arteries. Indications are summarized in Box 7.17. The technique requires selective injection of contrast into the left and right coronary arteries (Fig. 7.56), and multiple views in different projections are necessary for a complete study. Intraluminal filling defects or occlusions indicate coronary artery disease, which is nearly always caused by atherosclerosis.

PULMONARY ARTERIOGRAPHY

Injection of contrast medium into the main pulmonary artery opacifies the arterial branches throughout both lung fields. The normal flow distribution is homogeneous. Vascular occlusions with regional perfusion defects usually indicate pul-

---

Box 7.17   Indications for coronary arteriography

- Severe angina unresponsive to medical treatment
- Unstable angina
- Angina or a positive exercise test following myocardial infarction
- Cardiac arrhythmias when there is clinical suspicion of underlying coronary artery disease
- Preoperatively in patients requiring valve surgery when advanced age (>50) or angina suggest a high probability of coronary artery disease

---

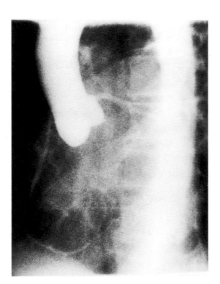

Figure 7.54   Aortic root angiogram: normal study. Contrast injection provides an X-ray image of the ascending aorta. The coronary arteries arising from the sinuses of Valsalva are clearly seen.

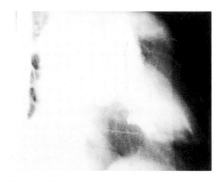

Figure 7.55   Left ventricular angiogram showing mitral regurgitation. Contrast injection into the left ventricle has resulted in prompt opacification of the left atrium owing to backflow across the diseased mitral valve.

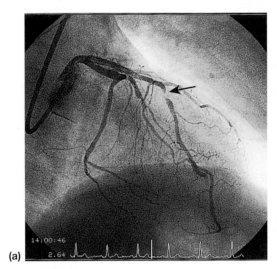
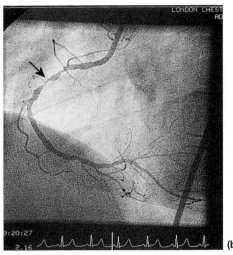

(a) (b)

Figure 7.56 Coronary arteriograms. **(a)** Left anterior descending disease (arrowed). This tight stenosis threatens the coronary supply to the anterior wall of the left ventricle. **(b)** Right coronary artery disease (arrowed). Serial stenoses in this dominant right coronary artery threaten the supply to the inferior wall of the heart.

monary thromboembolism (particularly when intra-luminal filling defects are present), but may also occur in advanced emphysema.

INTRACARDIAC PRESSURE MEASUREMENT

Cardiac catheterization for measurement of blood flow and pressure within the heart and great vessels is widely used both for diagnostic purposes and to guide treatment. The fluid-filled catheter is attached to a pressure transducer, which converts the pressure waves into electrical signals. For measurement of right-sided pressures the catheter is directed by the venous route into the right atrium and then advanced through the right ventricle into the pulmonary artery. For measurement of left-sided pressures, the catheter is directed by the arterial route into the ascending aorta and advanced retrogradely through the aortic valve into the left ventricle. Because access to the left atrium is technically difficult, left atrial pressure is usually measured indirectly using the pulmonary artery wedge pressure.

The pulmonary artery wedge pressure is obtained during right heart catheterization by advancing the catheter distally into the pulmonary arterial tree until the tip wedges in a small branch. Alternatively, a catheter with a preterminal balloon (Swan–Ganz catheter) may be used. Inflation of the balloon in the pulmonary artery causes the catheter tip to be carried with blood flow into a more distal branch, which becomes occluded by the balloon. Regardless of which method is used, the wedge pressure recorded at the catheter tip is a more or less accurate measure of the left atrial pressure transmitted

retrogradely through the pulmonary veins and capillaries.

HAEMODYNAMIC EVALUATION OF VALVULAR STENOSIS

In the normal heart there is no pressure gradient across an open valve. Such a gradient usually indicates valvular stenosis (Fig. 7.57) and, as stenosis worsens, the pressure gradient increases. This therefore provides a useful index of the severity of stenosis. However, it must be recognized that the pressure gradient is itself influenced by the flow through the valve. For example, if output is very low the gradient may be small despite the presence of severe stenosis. This applies particularly to the aortic valve because flow velocity is normally high.

HAEMODYNAMIC EVALUATION OF INTRACARDIAC SHUNTS

Left-to-right intracardiac shunts through atrial or ventricular septal defects introduce 'arterialized' blood into the right side of the heart. This results in an abrupt increase or step-up in the oxygen saturation of venous blood at the level of the shunt, which can be detected by right heart catheterization. Thus, by drawing serial blood samples for oxygen saturation from the pulmonary artery, right ventricle, right atrium and vena cava, the shunt may be localized to the site at which the step-up in oxygen saturation occurs. The magnitude of the step-up is related to the size of the shunt, but precise quantification of the shunt requires measurement of pulmonary and systemic blood flow. The extent to which the pulmonary–systemic flow ratio exceeds 1 is a measure of the size of the shunt.

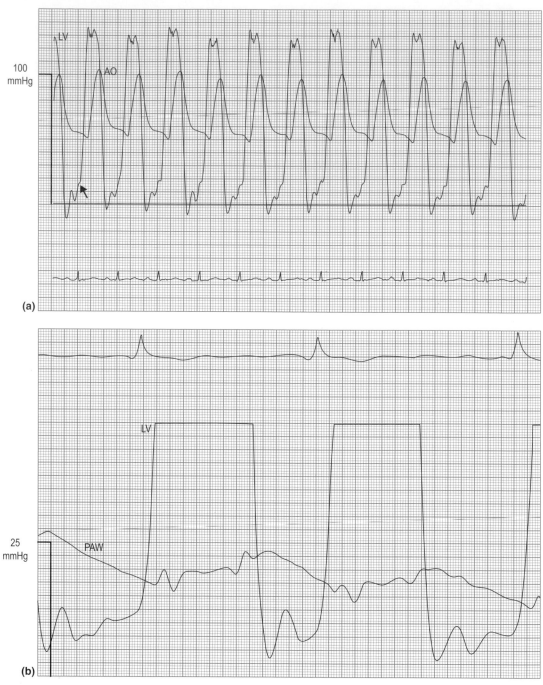

Figure 7.57 Valvular stenosis: pressure signals. **(a)** Aortic stenosis: simultaneous left ventricular (LV) and aortic (AO) pressure signals. In the normal heart the pressure signals should be essentially similar throughout systole. Here there is a peak systolic gradient of about 50 mmHg across the aortic valve. Note the prominent 'a' wave (arrowed), reflecting the major contribution that atrial systole makes to filling of the hypertrophied, non-compliant ventricle. Note also the pulsus alternans indicating left ventricular failure. **(b)** Mitral stenosis: simultaneous recordings of the pulmonary artery wedge (PAW) and left ventricular (LV) pressure signals. In the normal heart the pressure signals should be superimposed throughout diastole. Here there is a pressure gradient >10 mmHg, indicating severe mitral stenosis. Note that the patient is in AF and the pressure gradient varies inversely with the RR interval, tending to increase as the RR interval shortens.

Box 7.18   Constriction

Typical patient
- Middle-aged or elderly patient with a long history of progressive debilitation

Major symptoms
- Dyspnoea and weight loss with abdominal discomfort

Major signs
- Fluid retention with raised JVP (prominent 'x' and 'y' descents), hepatomegaly and peripheral oedema; diastolic filling sound ('pericardial knock'); paradoxical rise in JVP with inspiration (Kussmaul's sign)

Diagnosis
- This is a clinical diagnosis, confirmed by demonstration of increased pericardial thickness (± calcification) on CT or MRI scan

Additional investigations
- CXR: often normal, but occasionally shows pericardial calcification on lateral film

Comments
- Tuberculosis no longer commonest cause in developed countries, where most cases are idiopathic

Box 7.19   Tamponade

Typical patient
- Either middle-aged or elderly patient with malignant disease (usually breast or lung), or patients of any age with tuberculosis

Major symptoms
- Dyspnoea and variable circulatory collapse

Major signs
- Low-output state (hypotension, oliguria, cold periphery); tachycardia; paradoxical pulse; raised JVP with rapid 'x' descent; paradoxical rise in JVP on inspiration (Kussmaul's sign)

Diagnosis
- This is a clinical diagnosis, confirmed by echocardiographic demonstration of pericardial infusion

Additional investigations
- ECG: low-voltage QRS complexes with alternating electrical axis
- Tests for aetiological diagnosis: these might include serological tests for rheumatoid and SLE, and tests for malignant or tuberculous disease

Comments
- Any cause of pericardial effusion may produce tamponade, malignant disease being the commonest cause in developed countries. Pericardiocentesis relieves the tamponade. Pericardial fluid should always be sent for cytological and bacteriological analysis

HAEMODYNAMIC EVALUATION OF CONSTRICTION AND TAMPONADE   (Boxes 7.18, 7.19)

In constrictive pericarditis and tamponade diastolic relaxation of the ventricles is impeded, preventing adequate filling. Compensatory increments in atrial pressures occur to help maintain ventricular filling, and because these disorders usually affect both ventricles equally, the filling pressures also equilibrate. Thus simultaneous left- and right-sided recordings in constrictive pericarditis and tamponade show characteristic elevation and equalization of the filling pressures (atrial or ventricular end-diastolic), with loss of the normal differential (Fig. 7.58). Exactly similar physiology characterizes restrictive cardiomyopathy, in which infiltrative disease (usually amyloid in the UK) impedes relaxation of the ventricles.

MEASUREMENT OF CARDIAC OUTPUT

Cardiac output measurement is increasingly being used in intensive care units to characterize cardiovascular status and monitor responses to treatment. It is usually calculated by application of the Fick principle. A Swan–Ganz catheter with a right atrial portal and a terminal thermistor is positioned in the pulmonary artery. A known volume of cold saline (usually 10 ml) is injected into the right atrium and the temperature reduction in the pulmonary artery is recorded at the thermistor. The contour of the cooling curve is dependent on cardiac output, which is calculated by measuring the area under the curve using a bedside computer.

A relatively simple non-invasive measure of cardiac output can be obtained by Doppler echocardiography using the 'area–length' method. Thus, the length of the column of blood ejected by the left ventricle during a single beat is obtained by multiplying the Doppler aortic flow velocity (cm/s) by the ejection time (s). The length of the column of blood is then multiplied by the echocardiographic cross-sectional area of the aorta to yield stroke volume (ml/beat). Cardiac output is the product of stroke volume and heart rate.

INTRAVASCULAR ULTRASOUND

An ultrasound transducer mounted at the tip of a coronary catheter can now be used to provide cross-sectional images of the artery. The technique permits visualization of coronary plaques and provides information about plaque composition and structure that cannot be obtained from angiographic

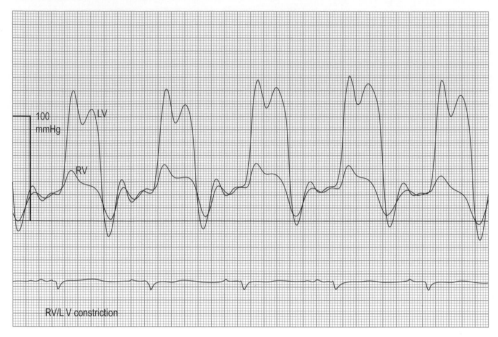

Figure 7.58 Pericardial constriction: left (LV) and right (RV) ventricular pressure signals. Like tamponade and restrictive cardiomyopathy, constriction usually affects both ventricles equally and the diastolic pressures must rise and equilibrate to maintain ventricular filling. Thus in diastole the pressure signals are superimposed with a typical 'dip and plateau' configuration ('square root' sign).

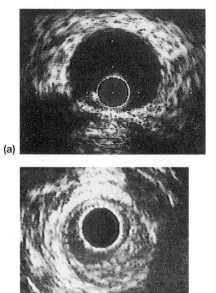

Figure 7.59 Intravascular ultrasound. **(a)** Normal cross-sectional ultrasound scan in a distal segment of the right coronary artery. The ultrasound's transducer is clearly visible at the intersection of the horizontal and vertical centimetre scales. **(b)** Coronary artery disease: a large semilunar coronary plaque extending from the 1 o'clock to the 7 o'clock position is shown severely reducing the coronary arterial lumen.

images (Fig. 7.59). Indeed, it is already apparent from ultrasound studies that coronary arteries that appear angiographically normal may in reality be extensively diseased. Intravascular ultrasound has already found a clinical role in coronary angioplasty and stenting, when 'before and after' images can be used to document satisfactory patency of the vessel and correct deployment of the stent. Potential future developments include the identification of lipid-laden vulnerable coronary plaques which are prone to rupture, putting the patient at risk of acute coronary events.

PATHOLOGY LABORATORY SUPPORT

HAEMATOLOGY LABORATORY

Anaemia is an important diagnosis in the cardiac patient and is confirmed by measurement of the circulating haemoglobin concentration. It exacerbates angina by adversely affecting the myocardial oxygen supply–demand relationship, and also exacerbates heart failure by increasing the cardiac work necessary to meet oxygen demands of metabolizing tissues. Rarely, anaemia is a consequence of, rather than a contributor to, heart disease. Thus, in infective endocarditis a normochromic normocytic anaemia is almost invariable, reflecting the adverse effects of chronic illness on erythropoiesis. Chronic haemolysis occasionally occurs in patients with mechanical prosthetic heart valves and is caused by traumatic erythrocyte damage. Anaemia is usually low grade, but if severe may require removal of the prosthesis and substitution with a xenograft.

BIOCHEMISTRY LABORATORY

CARDIAC ENZYMES AND OTHER MARKERS OF MYOCARDIAL INJURY

Following myocardial infarction, enzymes and structural proteins released into the circulation by the necrosing myocytes provide biochemical markers of injury. Until recently, creatine kinase (CK) was the most widely used marker, the isoenzyme MB being highly specific for myocardial injury. However, newer serum markers of myocardial injury are now replacing enzymatic markers, particularly the highly specific troponins T and I, measured 12 hours after the onset of symptoms. Indeed, these form the basis of the new definition of myocardial infarction, which is now diagnosed in any patient with raised circulating troponins who presents with cardiac chest pain, or who develops regional ST elevation on the 12-lead ECG. Implicit in this new definition is the fact that myocardial infarction may be diagnosed in patients without ST elevation. In non-ST elevation myocardial infarction (non-STEMI) the increase in circulating troponin concentration is a useful measure of risk and is widely used to guide decisions about cardiac catheterization and coronary revascularization.

RENAL FUNCTION

Renal function should always be measured in the cardiac patient. Renal dysfunction is a major cause (and consequence) of hypertension, whereas in heart failure progressive deterioration of renal function is almost inevitable as perfusion of the kidneys becomes threatened. Renal function may also deteriorate in response to treatment with diuretics and ACE (angiotensin-converting enzyme) inhibitors, and careful monitoring is essential as these drugs are introduced. Cardiac drugs that are excreted through the kidneys (e.g. digoxin) should be used cautiously if renal function is impaired. In the patient with established renal failure, accelerated coronary artery disease and heart failure commonly occur, reflecting the combined effects of dyslipidaemia, hypertension, arterial endothelial dysfunction, anaemia and volume loading on the cardiovascular system. Indeed, cardiovascular disease is the major cause of death in patients with renal failure.

ELECTROLYTES

Serum potassium interacts importantly with the cardiac conduction system, patients with hypokalaemia being at risk of lethal cardiac arrhythmias; hyperkalaemia may also cause bradyarrhythmias and heart block. Patients presenting with acute coronary syndromes commonly have hypokalaemia, reflecting the effects of sympathoadrenal activation on membrane-bound sodium-potassium ATPase, and this may require correction because of its association with lethal arrhythmias. In patients on thiazide or loop diuretics, potassium supplements (or potassium-sparing diuretics) are usually necessary to protect against hypokalaemia unless ACE inhibitors are also given. Serum potassium should always be measured in patients with hypertension, not only to provide a baseline before the introduction of diuretic therapy, but also as a simple screening test for primary aldosteronism.

GLUCOSE AND LIPIDS

Blood glucose and lipid profiles should be analysed in all patients with suspected vascular disease. Fasting samples should be obtained for glucose, triglycerides, total cholesterol and high- and low-density lipoprotein cholesterol. In high-risk individuals, particularly those with diabetes, and in all

---

Box 7.20   Infective endocarditis

Typical patient
- Elderly man or woman with mitral or aortic valve disease (often not previously recognized)
- Younger patients with congenital heart defects (usually VSD or PDA)
- Also at risk are patients with prosthetic heart valves or a history of intravenous drug abuse

Major symptoms
- Non-specific feverish ('flu-like') illness

Major signs
- Fever and heart murmur (usually aortic or mitral regurgitation)
- Splinter haemorrhages and vasculitic rash may occur
- Clubbing, Osler's nodes and Roth's spots are rare

Diagnosis
- Blood culture: usually provides bacteriological diagnosis
- Echocardiogram: usually reveals valvular regurgitation ± vegetation

Additional investigations
- Haematology: leukocytosis; normochromic, normocytic anaemia
- Inflammatory markers: raised ESR and CRP
- Urinalysis: haematuria

Comments
- Formerly a disease of young adults, now seen more commonly in the elderly
- Diagnosis should always be considered in patients with fever and a heart murmur

Table 7.2 Organisms implicated in endocarditis

Organism	Typical source of infection	First choice antibiotics (pending sensitivity studies)
Streptococcus viridans	Upper respiratory tract	Benzylpenicillin: gentamicin
Streptococcus faecalis	Bowel and urogenital tract	Ampicillin: gentamicin
Anaerobic streptococcus	Bowel	Ampicillin: gentamicin
Staphylococcus epidermidis	Skin	Flucloxacillin: gentamicin
Fungi: Candida, histoplasmosis	Skin and mucous membranes	Amphotericin B*: 5-fluorocytosine*
Coxiella burnettii	Complication of Q fever	Chloramphenicol*: tetracycline*
Chlamydia psittaci	Contact with infected birds	Tetracycline* and erythromycin
Acute disease		
Staphylococcus aureus	Skin	Flucloxacillin: gentamicin
Streptococcus pneumoniae	Complication of pneumonia	Benzylpenicillin: gentamicin
Neisseria gonorrhoeae	Venereal	Benzylpenicillin: gentamicin

*These drugs are not bactericidal, and valve replacement is nearly always necessary to eradicate infection.

Box 7.21   Jones's criteria for the diagnosis of rheumatic fever

Major criteria
- Carditis
- Polyarthritis
- Erythema marginatum
- Chorea
- Subcutaneous nodules

Minor criteria
- Fever
- Arthralgia
- Previous rheumatic fever
- Elevated ESR
- Prolonged PR intervals

patients with established coronary artery disease, statin therapy is essential regardless of the baseline lipid profile. This lowers LDL ('bad') cholesterol, but if HDL ('good') cholesterol is low, treatment with nicotinic acid or fibrates should be added. Treatment of diabetes protects against microvascular complications, and in hyperglycaemic patients with acute myocardial infarction infusion of insulin and glucose is usually recommended.

BACTERIOLOGY LABORATORY

BLOOD CULTURE   (Box 7.20)
In suspected infective endocarditis, treatment must not be delayed beyond the time necessary to obtain three to four blood samples for culture (Table 7.2). Aerobic, anaerobic and fungal cultures should be performed. Occasionally, bone marrow cultures are helpful for detection of Candida and Brucella endocarditis. Coxiella and Chlamydia can never be cultured from the blood and must be diagnosed by serological tests. Failure to detect bacteraemia may be due to pretreatment with antibiotics, inadequate sampling (up to six blood samples should be taken over 24 hours), or infection with unusual microorganisms.

SEROLOGY
If a recent streptococcal throat infection can be confirmed by demonstrating an elevated serum antistreptolysin O titre, Jones's criteria may be used for the diagnosis of rheumatic fever (Box 7.21). The presence of two major criteria, or one major and two minor criteria, indicates a high probability of rheumatic fever. In suspected viral pericarditis or myocarditis the aetiological diagnosis depends on the demonstration of elevated viral antibody titres in acute serum samples, which decline during convalescence. Virus may sometimes be cultured from throat swabs and stools.

Gastrointestinal system

M. Glynn

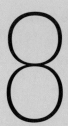

INTRODUCTION

The human gastrointestinal (GI) tract is a complex system of serially connected organs approximately 8 m in length, extending from the mouth to the anus, which, together with its connected secretory glands, controls the passage, processing, absorption and elimination of ingested material. Symptoms of GI disorders are often vague, and signs of abnormality few unless the disease is advanced. The liver, biliary system and pancreas are embryologically part of the GI tract. Symptoms of disease in these organs can also be non-specific, but each can give specific clinical features. Finally, from the standpoint of systematic history taking and examination, the kidneys, groins and genitalia are considered in this chapter.

SYMPTOMS OF GASTROINTESTINAL DISEASE

In normal health there is some awareness of the functioning of the gut, and this can be partly related to body needs. For example, thirst and hunger are common symptoms, and the latter may be associated with epigastric discomfort. A dry mouth can suggest the need to drink. Swallowing is normally perceived, and there is temperature sensation in the upper and mid-oesophagus, as well as in the mouth. Vigorous peristaltic contractions in the gut, the movement of gas and fluid in the gut – called borborygmi – and the experience of a sensation of fullness in the colon and rectum prior to defecation, or during constipation and the call to stool, are all aspects of the normal sensation of gut activity.

It is always sensible to remember that although it may be convenient for doctors to classify symptoms according to their anatomical site of origin, patients present with single symptoms or groups of symptoms that characterize functional or disease processes. Therefore, a history taking that follows these likely processes is more likely to lead to a meaningful diagnosis. This is particularly true in the GI tract and abdomen because many patients present with symptoms that are not easily referable to a clear anatomical site.

The common symptoms of gastrointestinal and abdominal disease are listed in Box 8.1 and are discussed individually below.

DYSPHAGIA (AND ODYNOPHAGIA)

Dysphagia is the awareness of something sticking in the throat or retrosternally during swallowing, and odynophagia is pain as food or drink descends the oesophagus. Dysphagia often has a significant cause, which can be malignant, and almost always needs investigation. An oesophageal or upper gastric carcinoma usually presents with dysphagia for solids, progressing fairly quickly to liquids also, and with accompanying weight loss. A benign stricture (or rarely an oesophageal pouch) may follow the same pattern, but much less rapidly. Neurogenic dysphagia may present with greater difficulty in swallowing liquids than solids, sometimes associated with aspiration or coughing. Odynophagia (pain during swallowing) may indicate infection of the oesophageal mucosa, classically candida oesophagitis associated with HIV infection.

Box 8.1 Common symptoms of gastrointestinal and abdominal disease

- Dysphagia and odynophagia
- Heartburn and reflux
- Indigestion
- Flatulence
- Vomiting
- Anorexia
- Constipation
- Diarrhoea
- Alteration of bowel pattern
- Abdominal pain
- Abdominal distension
- Weight loss
- Haematemesis
- Rectal bleeding
- Melaena
- Jaundice
- Itching
- Urinary symptoms

HEARTBURN

This is due to acid reflux from the stomach into the oesophagus. It causes pain in the epigastrium, retrosternally and in the neck. It is occasionally difficult to distinguish from angina pectoris, and may cause atypical chest pain in various sites. It occurs particularly at night when the patient lies flat in bed, or after bending or stooping when abdominal pressure is increased. Alcohol often induces heartburn.

REFLUX

Reflux is a symptom that occurs when acid or bile regurgitates into the mouth, causing a bitter taste and a disagreeable sensation.

INDIGESTION (DYSPEPSIA)

Dyspepsia is the medical term for indigestion, a symptom that includes epigastric pain, heartburn, distension, nausea or 'an acid feeling' occurring after eating or drinking. The symptom is subjective and frequent. In many patients there is no demonstrable cause, but it may be associated with *Helicobacter* infection, peptic ulceration, acid reflux, and occasionally upper GI malignancy.

FLATULENCE

Flatulence describes excessive wind. It is associated with belching, abdominal distension and the passage of flatus per rectum. It is only infrequently associated with organic disease of the gastrointestinal tract, but usually represents a functional disturbance, some of which is due to excessive swallowed air. In some patients it is clearly related to certain foods, such as vegetables.

VOMITING

Vomiting is a neurogenic response triggered by chemoreceptors in the brainstem or reflexly through irritation of the stomach. Vomiting consists of a phase of nausea followed by hypersalivation, pallor, sweating and hyperventilation. Retching, an involuntary effort to vomit, then occurs, followed by expulsion of gastric contents through the mouth and sometimes through the nose. Most nausea and vomiting of gastrointestinal origin is associated with local discomfort in the abdomen. Non-GI disease, such as raised intracranial pressure or metabolic disturbance, should be suspected if there is painless vomiting not associated with eating.

ANOREXIA

This term refers to loss of appetite, although some patients with GI disease have an appetite for food but feel full after just a few mouthfuls. It often indicates important pathology, particularly in the upper GI tract.

CONSTIPATION

The frequency of bowel action varies greatly from person to person. In a western population the statistical norm is between three bowel actions per day and three per week. Constipation is a subjective complaint. Patients feel constipated when they sense that they have not adequately emptied the bowel by defecation. The term is sometimes used to describe the passage of hard stools, irrespective of frequency. In clinical practice, the passage of formed stool less often than three times per week is usually taken to indicate an abnormality of bowel frequency, and if unresponsive to simple treatment or if there are associated features then investigation may be needed.

DIARRHOEA

Diarrhoea is also subjective, but the regular passage of more than three stools per day or the passage of a large amount of stool (>300 g/day) can certainly be called diarrhoea. It is common as a result of dietary indiscretion or from viral or bacterial infection. Chronic diarrhoea should raise the possibility of inflammatory bowel disease or malabsorption with steatorrhoea. Steatorrhoea is the passage of pale, bulky stools containing excess fats that commonly float in water and are difficult to flush away.

ABDOMINAL PAIN

Abdominal pain is a common symptom that often accompanies serious diagnoses but which frequently has no definable cause. As with any pain it is important to characterize its site, intensity, character, areas of radiation, duration and frequency, together with aggravating and relieving factors and associated features. The particular clinical problem of acute abdominal pain is discussed on page 136. The particular characteristics of pain from certain frequent and important causes are in Box 8.2. When described as colicky, the pain is coming in waves. These waves are more frequent in pain from the gut, but vary over a longer period when pain is from the biliary or renal tract. Abdominal pain may be due to causes that are not specifically in the abdomen, such as metabolic disorders (porphyria or lead poisoning) or depression.

ABDOMINAL DISTENSION

Abdominal distension has many causes, which include flatus, fluid (e.g. ascites or ovarian cyst) and pregnancy. Marked enlargement of the major organs is sometimes noted by the patient, as is the presence of a large mass lesion.

WEIGHT LOSS

Weight loss may be due to lack of food intake (anorexia, dysphagia or vomiting), malabsorption

---

Box 8.2   Particular characteristics of pain from frequent and important causes (the regions of the abdomen are in Figure 8.5 – the loin is lateral and posterior to the lumbar area)

• Peptic ulcer	epigastric, burning or gnawing, radiates through to back, meal related, wakes the patient, relieved by antacid
• Gastric cancer	epigastric, severe, partly meal related, not relieved by antacid
• Pancreatic	high epigastric, severe, felt front-to-back, immediately after eating, relieved by sitting forward
• Midgut	Periumbilical, colicky, some relation to meals
• Lower gut	Periumbilical or suprapubic, colicky, some relief from bowel action
• Biliary	Right upper quadrant, severe, colicky (but over long time period), radiates to right shoulder, accompanied by nausea
• Renal colic	Loin-to-groin, colicky, very severe, accompanied by nausea
• Functional	Anywhere in the abdomen, colicky, accompanied by bloating, relieved by bowel action

---

Box 8.3   Peripheral stigmata (signs) of chronic liver disease

Skin, nails and hands
- Spider naevi – small telangiectatic superficial blood vessels with a central feeding vessel
- Clubbing
- Leukonychia – expansion of the paler half-moon at the base of the nail
- Palmar erythema – seen on the thenar and hypothenar eminences, often with a blotchy appearance
- Bruising
- Dupuytren's contracture – can occur in the absence of liver disease
- Scratch marks – particularly in cholestatic liver disease

Endocrine – due to excess oestrogens
- Gynaecomastia
- Testicular atrophy
- Loss of axillary and pubic hair

Other
- Parotid swelling – particularly in alcohol-related liver disease
- Hepatic fetor – characteristic sweet-smelling breath
- Hepatic flap – a sign of encephalopathy and advanced disease

---

of nutrients, or a systemic effect of important diseases such as cancer (within or outside the GI tract), inflammatory bowel disease or chronic infections such as TB (within or outside the GI tract).

HAEMATEMESIS
Haematemesis results from bleeding in the upper GI tract (above the duodenojejunal flexure), causing the vomiting of blood. Blood that lies in gastric juice for a while turns black, and when vomited may look like ground coffee. Reports of vomiting blood by the patient or a bystander may be unreliable.

MELAENA
Melaena describes altered blood that has passed through a significant length of the GI tract and looks jet-black, tarry, and with a particularly characteristic smell. It should indicate bleeding above the ileocaecal valve, but occasionally may originate in the right colon.

RECTAL BLEEDING
If the blood is bright red, separate from the stool or just on the toilet paper this usually indicates a source in the sigmoid colon, rectum or anal canal, haemorrhoids being the commonest cause. If darker red and mixed with the stool this usually indicates a source above the rectum, of which carcinoma is the most important cause. Large-volume rectal bleeding in an ill patient can have an upper GI source.

JAUNDICE
Jaundice implies disease of the liver or the biliary tract, although it may also occur from excessive haemolysis. It causes yellowness of the skin and conjunctiva, and may be associated with other cutaneous and systemic features of liver disease, often with dark urine (see below).

URINARY SYMPTOMS
These are discussed in Chapter 14.

PHYSICAL EXAMINATION OF THE GI TRACT AND ABDOMEN

GENERAL SIGNS

Assessment of the nutritional state (Chapter 5) is particularly important in patients with suspected GI disease. Systemic features of GI disease may be evident on general examination. Peripheral signs of *chronic liver disease* are listed in Box 8.3. Of these, the most common and useful are *spider naevi* (Fig. 8.1) (the presence of up to five small ones can be normal) and palmar erythema (Fig. 8.2) (the blotchy appearance often being more important

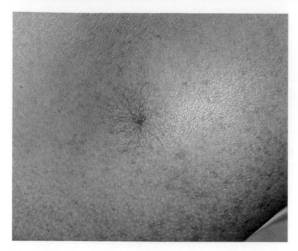

Figure 8.1 A typical spider naevus, with a central arteriole and fine radiating vessels.

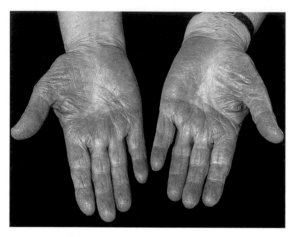

Figure 8.2 Palmar erythema in chronic liver disease (sparing the centre of the palms).

than the overall redness). *Inflammatory bowel disease* may give rise to clubbing, arthritis, uveitis and skin changes, including erythema nodosum (tender raised red lumps on the extensor surface of the limbs) and the much rarer pyoderma gangrenosum. *Anaemia* accompanies many GI diseases, as does oedema, and lymphadenopathy can be secondary to GI malignancy.

It is helpful when examining the patient, recording in notes or communicating information to colleagues to remember the surface anatomy of the structures related to the GI tract and abdomen (Figs 8.3, 8.4) and to think of the abdomen as being divided into regions (Fig. 8.5). The two *lateral vertical* planes pass from the femoral artery below to cross the costal margin close to the tip of the ninth costal cartilage. The two *horizontal* planes, the subcostal and interiliac, pass across the abdomen to connect the lowest points on the costal margin and the tubercles of the iliac crests, respectively.

Remember that the area of each region will depend on the width of the subcostal angle and the proximity of costal margin to iliac crest, in addition to other features of body habitus, which vary greatly from one patient to the next.

INSPECTION

The patient should be lying supine with the arms loosely by his or her sides, on a couch or mattress, the head and neck supported by enough pillows – normally one or two – for comfort (Fig. 8.6). A sagging mattress makes examination, particularly palpation, difficult. Make sure there is good light, that the room is warm and that the hands are warm. A shivering patient cannot relax and vital signs may be missed, especially on palpation.

Stand on the patient's right side and expose the abdomen by turning down all the bedclothes except the upper sheet. The clothing should then be drawn up to just above the xiphisternum and the sheet folded down to the level of the symphysis pubis Fig. 8.6. Traditional teaching was to expose the patient 'from nipples to knees'. In the modern era, however, when patient dignity is of paramount importance, this approach is not acceptable. However, inspection of the groins and genitalia must not be neglected and needs to be carried out with discretion, with full explanations as to the reasons, and leaving these areas exposed for the minimum time. There have been many patients presenting with intestinal obstruction due to a strangulated femoral or inguinal hernia where the diagnosis has been missed initially owing to lack of a proper inspection of the groins in an effort to save embarrassment. Inspection is an important and neglected part of abdominal examination. It is well worth spending 30 seconds observing the abdomen from different positions to note the following features.

SHAPE

Is the abdomen of normal contour and fullness, or distended? Is it scaphoid (sunken)?

- *Generalized fullness* or *distension* may be due to fat, fluid, flatus, faeces or a fetus.
- *Localized distension* may be symmetrical and centred around the umbilicus, as in the case of small bowel obstruction, or asymmetrical as in gross enlargement of the spleen, liver or ovary.
- Make a mental note of the site of any such swelling or distension; think of the anatomical structures in that region and note if there is any movement of the swelling, either with or independent of respiration.
- Remember that chronic urinary retention may cause palpable enlargement in the lower abdomen.

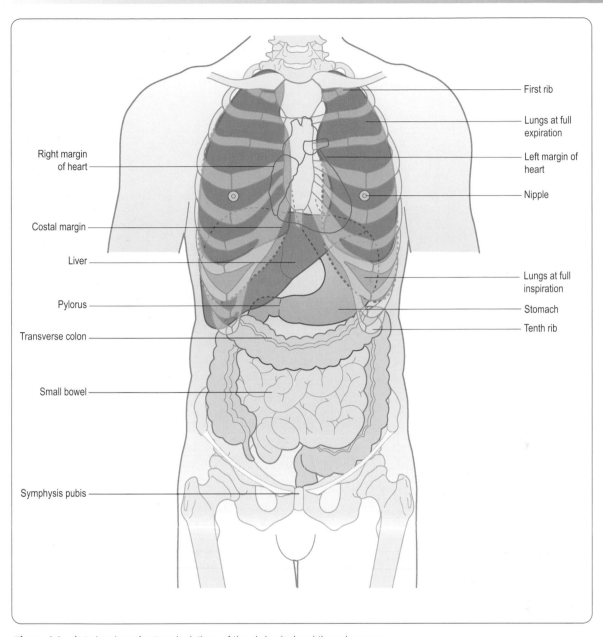

Figure 8.3 Anterior view of external relations of the abdominal and thoracic organs.

A *scaphoid* abdomen is seen in advanced stages of starvation and malignant disease, particularly carcinoma of the oesophagus and stomach.

THE UMBILICUS
Normally the umbilicus is slightly retracted and inverted. If it is everted then an umbilical hernia may be present, and this can be confirmed by feeling an expansile impulse on palpation of the swelling when the patient coughs. The hernial sac may contain omentum, bowel or fluid. A common finding in the umbilicus of elderly obese people is a concentration of inspissated desquamated epithelium and other debris (*omphalolith*).

MOVEMENTS OF THE ABDOMINAL WALL
Normally there is a gentle rise in the abdominal wall during inspiration and a fall during expiration; the movement should be free and equal on both sides. In *generalized peritonitis* this movement is absent or markedly diminished (the 'still, silent abdomen'). To aid the recognition of intra-abdominal movements shine a light across the patient's abdomen. Even small movements of the intestine may then be detected by alterations in the pattern of shadows cast over the abdomen.

Visible pulsation of the abdominal aorta may be noticed in the epigastrium and is a frequent finding in nervous, thin patients. It must be distinguished

Labels on figure:
- First rib
- Lungs at full expiration
- Left margin of heart
- Nipple
- Lungs at full inspiration
- Stomach
- Tenth rib
- Right margin of heart
- Costal margin
- Liver
- Pylorus
- Transverse colon
- Small bowel
- Symphysis pubis

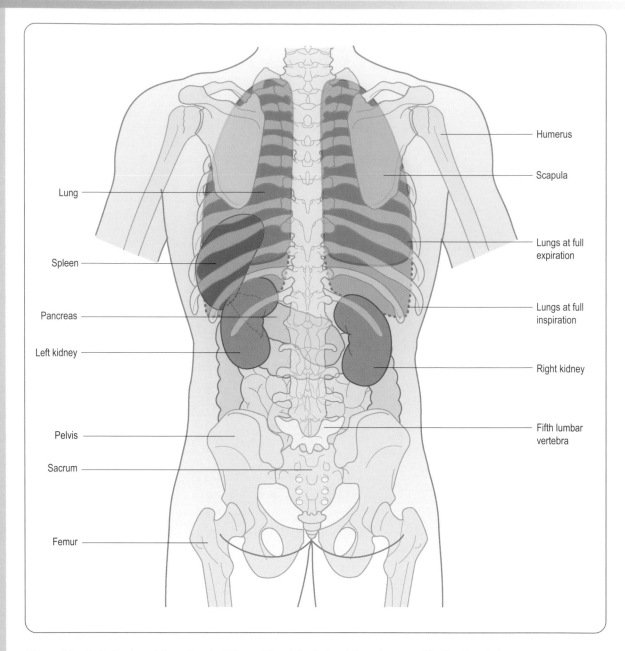

Figure 8.4 Posterior view of the external relations of the abdominal and thoracic organs. The liver is not shown.

from an aneurysm of the abdominal aorta, where pulsation is more obvious and a widened aorta is felt on palpation.

Visible peristalsis of the stomach or small intestine may be observed in three situations:

● *Obstruction at the pylorus.* Visible peristalsis may occur where there is obstruction at the pylorus, produced either by fibrosis following chronic duodenal ulceration or, less commonly, by carcinoma of the stomach in the pyloric antrum. In pyloric obstruction a diffuse swelling may be seen in the left upper abdomen but, where obstruction is long-standing with severe gastric distension,

this swelling may occupy the left mid and lower quadrants. Such a stomach may contain a large amount of fluid and, on shaking the abdomen, a splashing noise is usually heard ('*succussion splash*'). This splash is frequently heard in healthy patients for up to 3 hours after a meal, so enquire when the patient last ate or drank. In *congenital pyloric stenosis of infancy* not only may visible peristalsis be apparent, but also the grossly hypertrophied circular muscle of the antrum and pylorus may be felt as a 'tumour' to the right of the midline in the epigastrium. Both these signs may be elicited more easily after the infant has been fed. Standing behind the mother with the

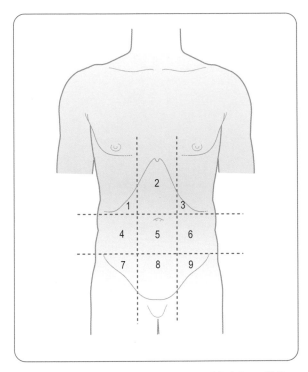

Figure 8.5 Regions of the abdomen. 1 and 3: right and left hypochondrium; 2: epigastrium; 4 and 6: right and left lumbar; 5: umbilical; 7 and 9: right and left iliac; 8: hypogastrium or suprapubic.

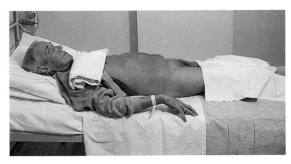

Figure 8.6 Position of the patient and exposure for abdominal examination. Note that the genitalia must be exposed.

child on her lap may allow the child's abdominal musculature to relax sufficiently to feel the walnut-sized swelling.

- *Obstruction in the distal small bowel.* Peristalsis may be seen where there is intestinal obstruction in the distal small bowel or coexisting large and small bowel hold-up produced by distal colonic obstruction, with an incompetent ileocaecal valve allowing reflux of gas and liquid faeces into the ileum. Not only is the abdomen distended and tympanitic (hyperresonant), but the distended coils of small bowel may be visible in a thin patient and tend to stand out in the centre of the abdomen in a 'ladder pattern'.

- *As a normal finding* in very thin, elderly patients with lax abdominal muscles or large, wide-necked incisional herniae seen through an abdominal scar.

SKIN AND SURFACE OF THE ABDOMEN

In marked abdominal distension the skin is smooth and shiny. *Striae atrophica* or *gravidarum* are white or pink wrinkled linear marks on the abdominal skin. They are produced by gross stretching of the skin with rupture of the elastic fibres and indicate a recent change in size of the abdomen, such as is found in pregnancy, ascites, wasting diseases and severe dieting. Wide purple striae are characteristic of Cushing's syndrome and excessive steroid treatment.

Note any *scars*, their site, and whether they are old (white) or recent (red or pink), linear or stretched (and therefore likely to be weak and contain an incisional hernia). Common examples are shown in Figure 8.7.

Look for *prominent superficial veins*, which may be apparent in three situations (Fig. 8.8): thin veins over the costal margin, usually of no significance; occlusion of the inferior vena cava; and venous anastomoses in portal hypertension. *Inferior vena caval obstruction* not only causes oedema of the limbs, buttocks and groins, but in time distended veins on the abdominal wall and chest wall appear. These represent dilated anastomotic channels between the superficial epigastric and circumflex iliac veins below and the lateral thoracic veins above, conveying the diverted blood from long saphenous vein to axillary vein; the direction of flow is therefore upwards. If the veins are prominent enough, try to detect the direction in which the blood is flowing by occluding a vein, emptying it by massage and then looking for the direction of refill. Distended veins around the umbilicus (caput medusae) are uncommon but signify *portal hypertension*, other signs of which may include splenomegaly and ascites. These distended veins represent the opening up of anastomoses between portal and systemic veins and occur in other sites, such as oesophageal and rectal varices.

Pigmentation of the abdominal wall may be seen in the midline below the umbilicus, where it forms the linea nigra and is a sign of pregnancy. *Erythema ab igne* is a brown mottled pigmentation produced by constant application of heat, usually a hot water bottle or heat pad, on the skin of the abdominal wall. It is a sign that the patient is experiencing severe ongoing pain, such as from chronic pancreatitis.

Finally, uncover and inspect both groins, and the penis and scrotum of a male, for any swellings and to ensure that both testes are in their normal position. Then bring the sheet up back up to the level of the symphysis pubis.

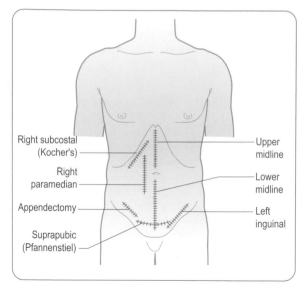

Right subcostal (Kocher's)
Right paramedian
Appendectomy
Suprapubic (Pfannenstiel)
Upper midline
Lower midline
Left inguinal

Figure 8.7 Some commonly used abdominal incisions. The midline and oblique incisions avoid damage to the innervation of the abdominal musculature and the later development of incisional herniae.

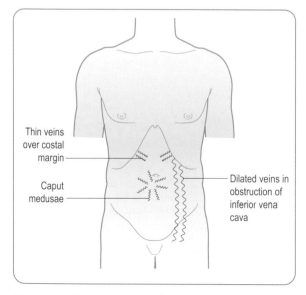

Thin veins over costal margin
Caput medusae
Dilated veins in obstruction of inferior vena cava

Figure 8.8 Prominent veins of the abdominal wall.

PALPATION

Palpation is the most important part of the abdominal examination. Tell the patient to relax as best they can and to breathe quietly, and assure them that you will be as gentle as possible. Enquire about the site of any pain and come to this region last. These points, together with unhurried palpation with a warm hand, will give the patient confidence and allow the maximum amount of information to be obtained.

When palpating, the wrist and forearm should be in the same horizontal plane where possible, even

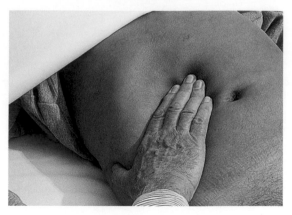

Figure 8.9 Correct method of palpation. The hand is held flat and relaxed, and 'moulded' to the abdominal wall.

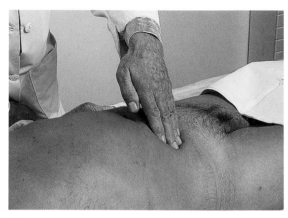

Figure 8.10 Incorrect method of palpation. The hand is held rigid and mostly not in contact with the abdominal wall.

if this means bending down or kneeling by the patient's side (Fig. 8.9). The best palpation technique involves moulding the relaxed right hand to the abdominal wall, not to hold it rigid. The best movement is gentle but with firm pressure, with the fingers held almost straight but with slight flexion at the metacarpophalangeal joints, and certainly avoid sudden poking with the fingertips (Fig. 8.10).

Palpation of intra-abdominal structures is an imperfect process in which the great sensitivity of the sense of touch and pressure is heavily masked by the abdominal wall tissue. It is unusual for structures to be very easily palpable, and so it is necessary to concentrate fully on the task and to try and visualize the normal anatomical structures and what might be palpable beneath the examining hand. It may be necessary to repeat the palpation more slowly and deeply. Putting the left hand on top of the right allows increased pressure to be exerted (Fig. 8.11), such as with an obese or very muscular patient.

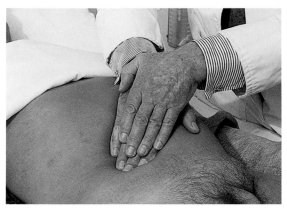

Figure 8.11 Method of deep palpation in an obese, muscular or poorly relaxed patient.

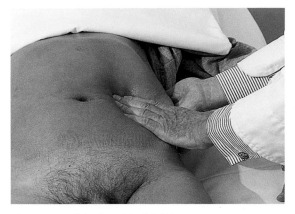

Figure 8.12 Palpation of the left kidney.

A small proportion of patients find it impossible to relax their abdominal muscles when being examined. In such cases it may help to ask them to breathe deeply, to bend their knees up, or to distract their attention in other ways. No matter how experienced the examiner, little will be gained from palpation of a poorly relaxed abdomen.

It is helpful to have a logical sequence to follow and, if this is done as a matter of routine, then no important point will be omitted. The following scheme is suggested, which may need to be varied according to the site of any pain:

- Start in the left lower quadrant of the abdomen, palpating lightly, and repeat for each quadrant.
- Repeat using slightly deeper palpation examining each of the nine areas of the abdomen.
- Feel for the left kidney.
- Feel for the spleen.
- Feel for the right kidney.
- Feel for the liver.
- Feel for the urinary bladder.
- Feel for the aorta and para-aortic glands and common femoral vessels.
- If a swelling is palpable, spend time eliciting its features.
- Palpate both groins.
- Examine the external genitalia.

All the organs in the upper abdomen (liver, spleen, kidneys, stomach, pancreas, gallbladder) move downward with inspiration (with the spleen moving more downwards and medially). Thus asking the patient to take a deep breath while examining makes detection of these organs easier, as something that is moving is easier to detect than something stationary. However, to avoid confusing one's sensation, when the patient breathes the examining hand should be still so that the organ in question 'comes on to the examining hand', or 'slips by underneath it'.

LEFT KIDNEY

The left hand is placed anteriorly in the left lumbar region and the right is placed posteriorly in the left loin (Fig. 8.12). Ask the patient to take a deep breath in, press the right hand forwards and the left hand backwards, upwards and inwards. The left kidney is not usually palpable unless it is either low in position or enlarged. Its lower pole, when palpable, is felt as a rounded firm swelling between both right and left hands (i.e. bimanually palpable) and it can be pushed from one hand to the other, in an action known as 'ballotting'.

SPLEEN

Like the left kidney, the spleen is not normally palpable. It has to be enlarged to two or three times its usual size before it becomes palpable, and then is felt beneath the left subcostal margin. Enlargement takes place in a superior and posterior direction before it becomes palpable subcostally. Once the spleen has become palpable, the direction of further enlargement is downwards and towards the right iliac fossa (Fig. 8.13). Place the flat of the left hand over the lowermost ribcage posterolaterally, thereby restricting the expansion of the left lower ribs on inspiration and concentrating more of the inspiratory movement into moving the spleen downwards. The right hand is placed beneath the costal margin well out to the left. Ask the patient to breathe in deeply, and press in deeply with the fingers of the right hand beneath the costal margin, at the same time exerting considerable pressure medially and downwards with the left hand (Fig. 8.14). Repeat this manoeuvre with the right hand moving more medially beneath the costal margin on each occasion (Fig. 8.15). If enlargement of the spleen is suspected from the history and it is still not palpable, turn the patient half on to the right side, ask them to relax back on to your left hand, which is now supporting the lower ribs, and repeat the examination as above. Alternatively, the spleen may be very large and the

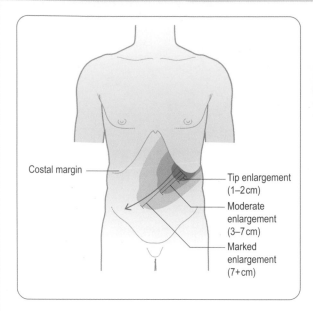

Figure 8.13   The direction of enlargement of the spleen. The spleen has a characteristic notched shape and the organ moves downwards during full inspiration.

Costal margin

Tip enlargement (1–2 cm)

Moderate enlargement (3–7 cm)

Marked enlargement (7+ cm)

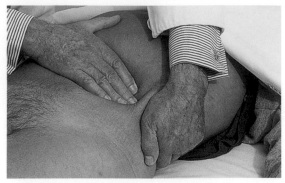

Figure 8.14   Palpation of the spleen. Start well out to the left.

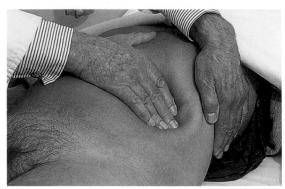

Figure 8.15   Palpation of the spleen more medially than in Figure 8.14.

lower edge much lower than at first suspected. It may help to ask the patient to place their left hand on your right shoulder while you are palpating for the spleen.

In minor degrees of enlargement the spleen will be felt as a firm swelling with smooth, rounded borders. Where considerable splenomegaly is present, its typical characteristics include a firm swelling appearing beneath the left subcostal margin in the left upper quadrant of the abdomen, which is dull to percussion, moves downwards on inspiration, is not bimanually palpable, whose upper border cannot be felt (i.e. one cannot 'get above it'), and in which a notch can often – though not invariably – be felt in the lower medial border. The last three features distinguish the enlarged spleen from an enlarged kidney; in addition, there is usually a band of colonic resonance anterior to an enlarged kidney.

RIGHT KIDNEY

Feel for the right kidney in much the same way as for the left. Place the right hand horizontally in the right lumbar region anteriorly with the left hand placed posteriorly in the right loin. Push forwards with the left hand, ask the patient to take a deep breath in, and press the right hand inwards and upwards (Fig. 8.16). The lower pole of the right kidney, unlike the left, is commonly palpable in thin patients, and is felt as a smooth, rounded swelling which descends on inspiration and is bimanually palpable and may be 'ballotted'.

LIVER

Sit on the couch beside the patient. Place both hands side by side flat on the abdomen in the right sub-costal region lateral to the rectus, with the fingers pointing towards the ribs. If resistance is encountered, move the hands further down until this resistance disappears. Exert gentle pressure and ask the patient to breathe in deeply. Concentrate on whether the edge of the liver can be felt moving downwards and under the examining hand (Fig. 8.17).

Repeat this manoeuvre working from lateral to medial regions to trace the liver edge as it passes upwards to cross from right hypochondrium to epigastrium. Another commonly employed though less accurate method of feeling for an enlarged liver is to place the right hand below and parallel to the right subcostal margin. The liver edge will then be felt against the radial border of the index finger (Fig. 8.18). The liver is often palpable in normal patients without being enlarged. The lower edge of the liver can be clarified by percussion (see below), as can the upper border in order to determine overall size: a palpable liver edge can be due to enlargement or to displacement downwards by lung pathology. Hepatomegaly is conventionally measured in centimetres palpable below the right costal margin, which should be determined with a ruler if possible.

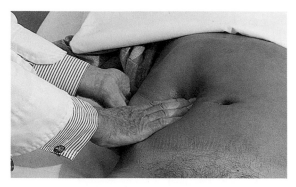

Figure 8.16 Palpation of the right kidney.

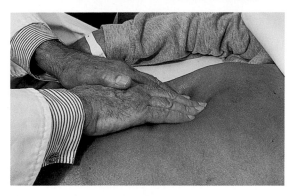

Figure 8.17 Palpation of the liver: preferred method.

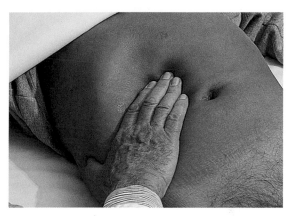

Figure 8.18 Palpation of the liver: alternative method.

Try and make out the character of the liver's surface (i.e. whether it is soft, smooth and tender as in heart failure, very firm and regular as in obstructive jaundice and cirrhosis, or hard, irregular, painless and sometimes nodular, as in advanced secondary carcinoma). In tricuspid regurgitation the liver may be felt to pulsate. Occasionally a congenital variant of the right lobe projects down lateral to the gallbladder as a tongue-shaped process, called Riedel's lobe. Though uncommon, it is important to be aware of this because it may be mistaken either for the gallbladder itself or for the right kidney.

GALLBLADDER

The gallbladder is palpated in the same way as the liver. The normal gallbladder cannot be felt. When it is distended, however, it forms an important sign and may be palpated as a firm, smooth, or globular swelling with distinct borders, just lateral to the edge of the rectus abdominis near the tip of the ninth costal cartilage. It moves with respiration. Its upper border merges with the lower border of the right lobe of the liver, or disappears beneath the costal margin and therefore can never be felt (Fig. 8.19). When the liver is enlarged or the gallbladder grossly distended, the latter may be felt not in the hypochondrium but in the right lumbar or even as low down as the right iliac region.

The ease of definition of the rounded borders of the gallbladder, its comparative mobility on respiration, the fact that it is not normally bimanually palpable, and that it seems to lie just beneath the abdominal wall helps to identify such a swelling as gallbladder rather than a palpable right kidney. A painless gallbladder can usually be palpated in the following clinical situations:

- In a jaundiced patient with *carcinoma of the head of the pancreas* or other malignant causes of obstruction of the common bile duct (below the entry of the cystic duct), the ducts above the obstruction become dilated, as does the gallbladder (see Courvoisier's Law, below).
- In *mucocele of the gallbladder* a gallstone becomes impacted in the neck of a collapsed,

empty, uninfected gallbladder and mucus continues to be secreted into its lumen (Fig. 8.20). Eventually, the uninfected gallbladder is so distended that it becomes palpable. In this case the bile ducts are normal and the patient is not jaundiced.

- In *carcinoma of the gallbladder* the gallbladder may be felt as a stony, hard, irregular swelling, unlike the firm, regular swelling of the two above-mentioned conditions.

Murphy's sign

In acute inflammation of the gallbladder (*acute cholecystitis*) severe pain is present. Often an exquisitely tender but indefinite mass can be palpated; this represents the underlying acutely inflamed gallbladder walled off by greater omentum. Ask the patient to breathe in deeply, and palpate for the gallbladder in the normal way; at the height of inspiration the breathing stops with a gasp as the mass is felt. This represents Murphy's sign. The sign is *not* found in chronic cholecystitis or uncomplicated cases of gallstones.

Courvoisier's Law

This states that in the presence of jaundice a palpable gallbladder makes gallstone obstruction of the

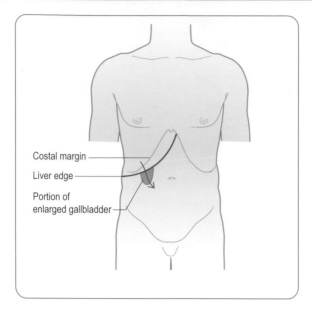

Figure 8.19   Palpation of an enlarged gallbladder, showing how it merges with the inferior border of the liver so that only the fundus of the gallbladder and part of its body can be palpated.

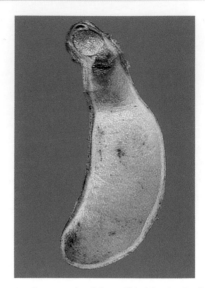

Figure 8.20   A mucocele of the gallbladder that is distended and thin walled.

common bile duct an unlikely cause (because it is likely that the patient will have had gallstones for some time, and these will have rendered the wall of the gallbladder relatively fibrotic and therefore non-distensible). However, the converse is not true, because the gallbladder is not palpable in many patients who do prove to have malignant bile duct obstruction.

THE URINARY BLADDER

Normally the urinary bladder is not palpable. When it is full and the patient cannot empty it (retention of urine), a smooth firm regular oval-shaped swelling will be palpated in the suprapubic region and its dome (upper border) may reach as far as the umbilicus. The lateral and upper borders can be readily made out, but it is not possible to feel its lower border (i.e. the swelling is 'arising out of the pelvis'). The fact that this swelling is symmetrically placed in the suprapubic region beneath the umbilicus, that it is dull to percussion, and that pressure on it gives the patient a desire to micturate, together with the signs above, confirms such a swelling as the bladder (Fig. 8.21).

In women, however, a mass that is thought to be a palpable bladder must be differentiated from a gravid uterus (firmer, mobile side to side, and vaginal signs different), a fibroid uterus (may be bosselated, firmer, and vaginal signs different) and an ovarian cyst (usually eccentrically placed to left or right side).

THE AORTA AND COMMON FEMORAL VESSELS

In most adults the aorta is not readily felt, but with practice it can usually be detected by deep palpation

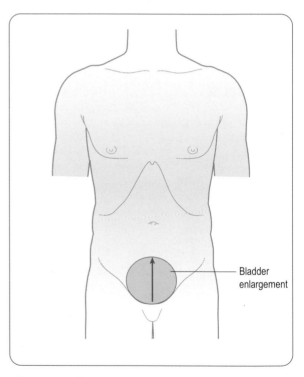

Figure 8.21   Physical signs in retention of urine; a smooth, firm and regular swelling arising out of the pelvis which one cannot 'get below' and which is dull to percussion.

a little above and to the left of the umbilicus. In thin patients, particularly women with a marked lumbar lordosis, the aorta is more easily palpable. Palpation of the aorta is one of the few occasions when the fingertips are used as a means of palpation. Press the extended fingers of both hands, held side by side, deeply into the abdominal wall in the position

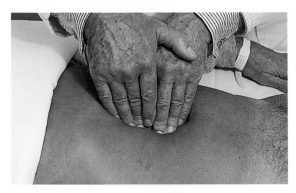

Figure 8.22 Palpation of the abdominal aorta.

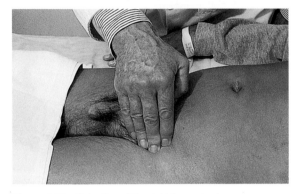

Figure 8.23 Palpation of the right femoral artery.

shown in Figure 8.22; make out the left wall of the aorta and note its pulsation. Remove both hands and repeat the manoeuvre a few centimetres to the right. In this way the pulsation and width of the aorta can be estimated. It is difficult to detect small aortic aneurysms; where an aneurysm is large, its presence and width may be assessed by placing the extended fingertips on either side of it with the palms flat on the abdominal wall and the fingers pointing towards each other. When the fingertips are either side of an aneurysm it should be clear that they are being separated by each pulsation, and not just moved up and down (this latter manoeuvre can involve very deep palpation, and the patient should be warned).

The common femoral vessels are found just below the inguinal ligament at the midpoint between the anterior superior iliac spine and the symphysis pubis. Place the pulps of the right index, middle and ring fingers over this site in the right groin and palpate the wall of the vessel. Note the strength and character of its pulsation and then compare it with the opposite femoral pulse (Fig. 8.23).

Lymph nodes lying along the aorta (para-aortic nodes) are palpable only when considerably enlarged. They are felt as rounded, firm, often confluent fixed masses in the umbilical region and epigastrium along the left border of the aorta.

CAUSES OF DIAGNOSTIC DIFFICULTY ON PALPATION

In many patients, especially those with a thin or lax abdominal wall, faeces in the colon may simulate an abdominal mass. The sigmoid colon is frequently palpable, particularly when loaded with hard faeces. It is felt as a firm, tubular structure about 12 cm in length, situated low down in the left iliac fossa parallel to the inguinal ligament. The caecum is often palpable in the right iliac fossa as a soft, rounded swelling with indistinct borders. The transverse colon is sometimes palpable in the epigastrium. It feels somewhat like the pelvic colon but rather larger and softer, with distinct upper and lower borders and a convex anterior surface. A faecal 'mass' will usually have disappeared or moved on repeat examination, and may retain an indentation with pressure (not the case with a colonic malignancy).

In the epigastrium, the muscular bellies of the rectus abdominis lying between its tendinous intersections can mimic an underlying mass and give rise to confusion. This can usually be resolved by asking the patient to tense the abdominal wall (by lifting the head off the pillow), when the 'mass' may be felt to contract.

WHAT TO DO WHEN AN ABDOMINAL MASS IS PALPABLE

When a swelling in the abdomen is palpable first make sure that it is not a normal structure, as described above. Consider whether it could be due to enlargement of the liver, spleen, right or left kidney, gallbladder, urinary bladder, aorta or para-aortic nodes. The aim of examination of a mass is to decide the organ of origin and the pathological nature. In doing this it is helpful to bear in the mind the following points.

Site

Feeling the swelling while the patient lifts their head and shoulders off the pillow to tense the anterior abdominal wall, will differentiate between a mass in the abdominal wall and one within the abdominal cavity.

Note the region occupied by the swelling. Think of the organs that normally lie in or near this region, and consider whether the swelling could arise from one of them. For instance, a swelling in the right upper quadrant most probably arises from the liver, right kidney, hepatic flexure of colon or gallbladder.

Now, if the swelling is in the upper abdomen, try and determine whether it is possible to 'get above it' – that is, to feel the upper border of the swelling as it disappears above the costal margin, and similarly, if it is in the lower abdomen, whether one can 'get below it'. If one cannot 'get above' an upper abdominal swelling, a hepatic, splenic, renal or gastric origin should be suspected. If one cannot 'get below' a lower abdominal mass the swelling probably arises in the bladder, uterus, ovary, or occasionally the upper rectum.

Size and shape

As a general rule, gross enlargement of the liver, spleen, uterus, bladder or ovary presents no undue difficulty in diagnosis. On the other hand, swellings arising from the stomach, small or large bowel, retroperitoneal structures such as the pancreas, or the peritoneum (see Mobility and attachments, below), may be difficult to diagnose. The larger a swelling arising from one of these structures, the more it tends to distort the outline of the organ of origin (e.g. a large renal mass can feel as if it is arising from intraperitoneal organs).

Surface, edge and consistency

The pathological nature of a mass is suggested by a number of features. A swelling that is hard, irregular in outline and nodular is likely to be *malignant*, whereas a regular, round, smooth, tense swelling is likely to be *cystic*. A solid, ill-defined and tender mass suggests an inflammatory lesion, as in Crohn's disease of the ileocaecal region.

Mobility and attachments

Swellings arising in the liver, spleen, kidneys, gallbladder and distal stomach all show downward movement during inspiration, owing to the normal downward diaphragmatic movement, and such structures cannot be moved with the examining hand. Tumours of the small bowel and transverse colon, cysts in the mesentery, and large secondary deposits in the greater omentum, are not usually influenced by respiratory movements, but may move easily on palpation.

When the swelling is completely fixed it usually signifies one of three things:

- A mass of retroperitoneal origin (e.g. pancreas)
- Part of an advanced tumour with extensive spread to the anterior or posterior abdominal walls or abdominal organs
- A swelling resulting from severe chronic inflammation involving other organs (e.g. diverticulitis of the sigmoid colon or a tuberculous ileocaecal mass).

In the lower abdomen, the side-to-side mobility of a fibroid or pregnant uterus rapidly establishes such a swelling as uterine in origin and as not arising from the urinary bladder.

Is it bimanually palpable or pulsatile?

Bimanually palpable swellings in the lumbar region are usually renal in origin. Just occasionally, however, a posteriorly situated gallbladder or a mass in the posteroinferior part of the right lobe of the liver may give the impression of being bimanually palpable. Carefully note whether a swelling exhibits pulsation, and decide whether any pulsation comes from the mass or is transmitted.

PERCUSSION

Details of how to percuss correctly are given in Chapter 6. The normal percussion note over most of the abdomen is resonant (tympanic) except over the liver, where the note is dull. A normal spleen is not large enough to render the percussion note dull. A resonant percussion note over suspected enlargement of liver or spleen weighs against there being true enlargement.

In obese patients tympanic areas of the abdomen may not give a truly resonant percussion note, and palpation of such things as a large liver is more difficult. If hepatomegaly is suspected, rhythmic percussion just above the suspected lower border of the liver as the patient breathes in and out deeply can elicit a note that changes cyclically between dull and hollow, and eliciting this change may be more certain than the character of the fixed and unchanging note.

DEFINING THE BOUNDARIES OF ABDOMINAL ORGANS AND MASSES

Liver

The upper and lower borders of the right lobe of the liver can be mapped out accurately by percussion. Start anteriorly, at the fourth intercostal space, where the note will be resonant over the lungs, and work vertically downwards.

Over a normal liver, percussion will detect the upper border at about the fifth intercostal space (just below the right nipple in men). The dullness extends down to the lower border at or just below the right subcostal margin, giving a normal liver vertical height of 12–15 cm. The normal dullness over the upper part of the liver is reduced in severe emphysema, in the presence of a large right pneumothorax, and after laparotomy or laparoscopy.

Spleen

Percussion over a substantially enlarged spleen provides rapid confirmation of the findings detected on palpation (see Fig. 8.14). Dullness extends from the left lower ribs into the left hypochondrium and left lumbar region.

Urinary bladder

The findings in a patient with urinary retention are usually unmistakable on palpation (see Fig. 8.21). The dullness on percussion, and clear difference from the adjacent bowel, provides reassurance that the swelling is cystic or solid and not gaseous.

Other masses

The boundaries of any localized swelling in the abdominal cavity, or in the walls of the abdomen, can sometimes be defined more accurately by percussion than palpation, as for the urinary bladder.

DETECTION OF ASCITES AND ITS DIFFERENTIATION FROM OVARIAN CYST AND INTESTINAL OBSTRUCTION

Three common causes of diffuse enlargement of the abdomen are:

- The presence of free fluid in the peritoneum (*ascites*)
- A massive ovarian cyst
- Obstruction of the large bowel, distal small bowel, or both.

Percussion rapidly distinguishes between these three, as can be seen in Figure 8.24. Other helpful symptoms or signs that are usually present are listed in Box 8.4.

The use of ultrasound to detect ascites has shown that quite a lot needs to be present to detect clinically – probably more than 2 L. It is unwise and unreliable to diagnose ascites unless there is sufficient free fluid present to give generalized enlargement of the abdomen. The cardinal sign created by ascites is shifting dullness. A fluid thrill may also be present, but it would be unwise to diagnose ascites based on this sign alone.

To demonstrate *shifting dullness*, lie the patient supine. Place your fingers in the longitudinal axis on the midline near the umbilicus and begin percussion moving your fingers laterally towards the right flank. When dullness is first detected (in normal individuals dullness is only over the lateral abdominal musculature) keep your fingers in that position and ask the patient to roll on their left side. Wait a few seconds for any peritoneal fluid to redistribute, and if ascites is present the percussion note should have become resonant. This shift in the area of dull-ness can be confirmed by finding the left border of dullness with the patient still on their left side and seeing whether it shifts when the patient returns to the supine position, or by repeating the original manoeuvre but towards the other side of the abdomen.

To elicit a *fluid thrill* the patient is again laid supine. Place one hand flat over the lumbar region of one side and ask an assistant to put the side of their hand longitudinally and firmly in the midline of the abdomen. Then flick or tap the opposite lumbar region (Fig. 8.25). A fluid thrill or wave is felt as a definite and unmistakable impulse by the detecting hand held flat in the lumbar region. (The purpose of the assistant's hand is to damp any impulse that may be transmitted through the fat of the abdominal wall.) As a rule a fluid thrill is felt only when there is a large amount of ascites present which is under tension, and it is not a very reliable sign.

Box 8.4   Clinical features of marked abdominal swelling

Gross ascites
- Dull in flanks
- Umbilicus everted and/or hernia present
- Shifting dullness positive
- Fluid thrill positive

Large ovarian cyst
- Resonant in flank
- Umbilicus vertical and drawn up
- Large swelling felt arising out of pelvis which one cannot 'get below'

Intestinal obstruction
- Resonant throughout
- Colicky pain
- Vomiting
- Recent cessation of passage of stool and flatus
- Increased and/or 'noisy' bowel sounds

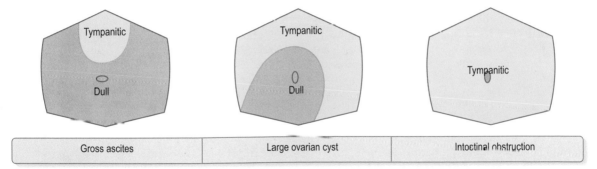

Figure 8.24   Three types of diffuse enlargement of the abdomen.

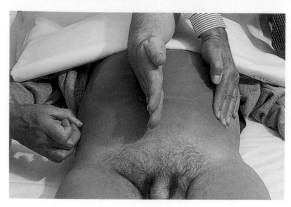

Figure 8.25 Eliciting a fluid thrill.

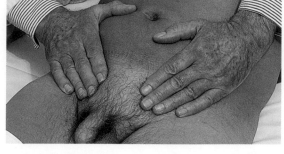

Figure 8.26 Palpating the groins to detect an expansile impulse on coughing.

AUSCULTATION

Auscultation of the abdomen is for detecting bowel sounds and vascular bruits.

BOWEL SOUNDS

The stethoscope should be placed on one site on the abdominal wall (just to the right of the umbilicus is best) and kept there until sounds are heard. It should not be moved from site to site. Normal bowel sounds are heard as intermittent low- or medium-pitched gurgles interspersed with an occasional high-pitched noise or tinkle.

In *simple acute mechanical obstruction of the small bowel* the bowel sounds are excessive and exaggerated. Frequent loud low-pitched gurgles (*borborygmi*) are heard, often rising to a crescendo of high-pitched tinkles and occurring in a rhythmic pattern with peristaltic activity. The presence of such sounds occurring at the same time as the patient experiences bouts of colicky abdominal pain is highly suggestive of small bowel obstruction. In between the bouts of peristaltic activity and colicky pain, the bowel is quiet and no sounds are heard on auscultation.

If obstruction progresses, leading to bowel necrosis, peristalsis ceases and sounds lessen in volume and frequency. In *generalized peritonitis* bowel activity rapidly disappears and a state of *paralytic ileus* ensues, with gradually increasing abdominal distension. The abdomen is 'silent', but one must listen for several minutes before being certain that there are no sounds. Frequently towards the end of this period a short run of faint, very high-pitched tinkling sounds is heard. This represents fluid spilling over from one distended loop to another and is characteristic of ileus.

A *succussion splash* may be heard without a stethoscope and also on auscultation in pyloric stenosis, in advanced intestinal obstruction with grossly distended loops of bowel, and in paralytic ileus. Lie the patient supine and place the stethoscope over the epigastrium. Roll the patient briskly from side to side, and if the stomach is distended with fluid a splashing sound will be heard.

VASCULAR BRUITS

Listen for bruits by applying the stethoscope lightly above and to the left of the umbilicus (aorta), the iliac fossae (iliac arteries), the epigastrium (coeliac or superior mesenteric arteries), laterally in the mid-abdomen (renal arteries), or over the liver (increased blood flow in liver tumours – classically primary liver cancer). If an arterial bruit is heard it is a significant finding, which indicates turbulent flow in the underlying vessel, due either to stenosis or to aneurysm.

THE GROINS

Once the groins have been inspected, ask the patient to turn the head to one side and cough. Look at both inguinal canals for any expansile impulse. If none is apparent, place the left hand in the left groin so that the fingers lie over and in line with the inguinal canal; place the right hand similarly in the right groin (Fig. 8.26). Now ask the patient to give a loud cough and feel for any expansile impulse with each hand. When a person coughs, the muscles of the abdominal wall contract violently and this imparts a definite – though not expansile – impulse to the palpating hands, which is a source of confusion to the inexperienced. Trying to differentiate this normal contraction from a small, fully reducible inguinal hernia is difficult, and the matter can usually be resolved only when the patient is standing up.

The femoral vessels have already been felt (Fig. 8.23) and auscultated. Now palpate along the femoral artery for enlarged inguinal nodes, feeling with the fingers of the right hand, and carry this palpation medially beneath the inguinal ligament towards the perineum. Then repeat this on the left side. A patient who complains of a lump in the groin should be examined *both lying down and standing up.*

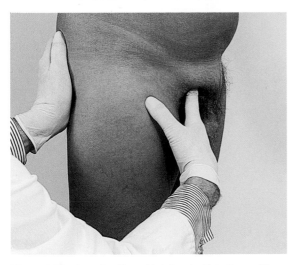

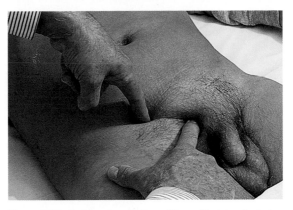

Figure 8.28 Left hand: palpation of the pubic tubercle; index finger occluding the deep inguinal ring. Right hand: index finger on the pubic tubercle.

Figure 8.27 Locating the pubic tubercle. Note the position of the examiner, at the side of the patient, with one hand supporting the buttock.

WHAT TO DO IF A PATIENT COMPLAINS OF A LUMP IN THE GROIN

A lump in the groin or scrotum is a common clinical problem in all age groups. Most are due either to herniae or to enlarged inguinal nodes; inguinal herniae are considerably more common than femoral, with an incidence ratio of 4:1. In the scrotum, *hydrocele* of the tunica vaginalis or a cyst of the epididymis are common causes of painless swelling; *acute epididymo-orchitis* is the most frequent cause of a painful swelling. Generalized diseases such as *lymphoma* may present as a lump in the groin. Usually the diagnosis of a lump in the groin or scrotum can be made simply and accurately. Remember that the patient should be examined not only lying down, but also standing up.

Ask the patient to stand in front of you, get him to point to the side and site of the swelling, and note whether it extends into the scrotum. Get him to turn his head to one side and give a loud cough; look for an expansile impulse and try to decide whether it is above or below the crease of the inguinal ligament. If an expansile impulse is present on inspection, it is likely to be a hernia, so move to whichever side of the patient the lump is on. Stand beside and slightly behind the patient. If the right groin is being examined, place the left hand over the right buttock to support the patient, the fingers of the right hand being placed obliquely over the inguinal canal. Now ask the patient to cough again. If an expansile impulse is felt then the lump must be a hernia.

Next, decide whether the hernia is *inguinal* or *femoral*. The best way to do this is to determine the relationship of the sac to the pubic tubercle. To locate this structure push gently upwards from beneath the neck of the scrotum with the index finger (Fig. 8.27), but do not invaginate the neck of

the scrotum as this is painful. The tubercle will be felt as a small bony prominence 2 cm from the midline on the pubic crest. In thin patients the tubercle is easily felt, but this is not so in the obese. If there is any difficulty, follow upwards the tendon of adductor longus, which arises just below the tubercle.

If the hernial sac passes *medial to and above* the index finger placed on the pubic tubercle, then the hernia must be inguinal; if it is *lateral to and below*, then the hernia must be femoral in site.

If it has been decided that the hernia is inguinal, then one needs to know these further points:

- *What are the contents of the sac?* Bowel tends to gurgle, is soft and compressible, whereas *omentum* feels firmer and is doughy in consistency.
- *Is the hernia fully reducible or not?* It is best to lie the patient down to decide this. Ask the patient whether the hernia is reducible, and if so get them to reduce it and confirm it yourself. (It is more painful if the examiner reduces it.)
- *Is the hernia direct or indirect?* Again, it is best to lie the patient down to decide this. Inspection of the direction of the impulse is often diagnostic, especially in thin patients. A direct hernia tends to bulge straight out through the posterior wall of the inguinal canal, whereas with an indirect hernia the impulse can often be seen to travel obliquely down the inguinal canal. Another helpful point is to place one finger just above the midinguinal point over the deep inguinal ring (Fig. 8.28). If the hernia is fully controlled by this finger then it must be an indirect inguinal hernia.

Apart from a femoral hernia, the differential diagnosis of an inguinal hernia includes a large *hydrocele of the tunica vaginalis*, a large *cyst of the epididymis* (one should be able to 'get above' and feel the upper border of both of these in the scrotum), an *undescended or ectopic testis* (there will be an empty scrotum on the affected side), a *lipoma* of the cord, and a *hydrocele of the cord*.

In considering the *differential diagnosis of a femoral hernia*, one must think not only of an inguinal hernia but of a *lipoma* in the femoral triangle, an *aneurysm* of the femoral artery (expansile pulsation will be present), a *sapheno-varix* (the swelling disappears on lying down, has a bluish tinge to it, there are often varicose veins present and there may be a venous hum), a *psoas abscess* (the mass is fluctuant, and may be compressible beneath the inguinal ligament to appear above it in the iliac fossa), and an *enlarged inguinal lymph node*. Whenever the latter is found the feet, legs, thighs, scrotum, perineum and the pudendal and perianal areas must be carefully scrutinized for a source of infection or primary tumour.

The examination is completed by following the same scheme in the opposite groin.

THE MALE GENITALIA

It is important to examine the genitalia in men presenting with abnormalities in the groin, and in many acute or subacute abdominal syndromes; thus disease of the genitalia may lead to abdominal symptoms, such as pain or swelling. It is vital to give a careful and ongoing explanation of what is involved and why, throughout this part of the examination. A more detailed description of the examination of the male genitalia is given in Chapter 27.

THE FEMALE GENITALIA

These are described in Chapters 15 and 27. As in men, examination of the genitalia is an important part of overall examination and it is vital to give a careful and ongoing explanation of what is involved and why, throughout this part of the examination.

THE ANUS AND RECTUM

The left lateral position is best for routine examination of the rectum (Fig. 8.29). Make sure that the buttocks project over the side of the couch and that the knees are drawn well up, and that a good light is available. Put on disposable gloves and stand behind the patient's back, facing their feet. Explain what you are about to do, that you will be as gentle as possible, and that you will stop the examination if requested at any point.

INSPECTION

Separate the buttocks carefully and inspect the perianal area and anus. Note the presence of any abnormality of the perianal skin, such as inflammation, which may vary in appearance from mild erythema to a raw, red, moist, weeping dermatitis, or in chronic cases thickened white skin with exag-

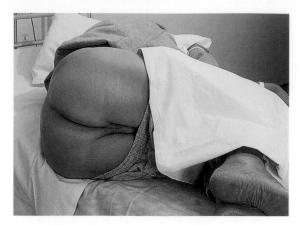

Figure 8.29   Left lateral position for rectal examination.

geration of the anal skin folds. The latter form *anal skin tags*, which may follow not only *severe pruritus* but also occur when prolapsing piles have been present over a period of time. Tags should not be confused with *anal warts* (condylomata acuminata), which are sessile or pedunculated papillomata with a red base and a white surface. Anal warts may be so numerous as to surround the anal verge, and even extend into the anal canal. Note any 'hole' or dimple near the anus with a telltale bead of pus or granulation tissue surrounding it, which represents the external opening of a *fistula in ano*. It is usually easy to distinguish a fistula in ano from a *pilonidal sinus*, where the opening lies in the midline of the natal cleft but well posterior to the anus.

There are a number of painful anorectal conditions that can usually be diagnosed readily on inspection. An *anal fissure* usually lies directly posterior in the midline. The outward pathognomonic sign of a chronic fissure is a tag of skin at the base (sentinel pile). If pain allows, the fissure can easily be demonstrated by gently drawing apart the anus to reveal the tear in the lining of the anal canal.

A *perianal haematoma* (thrombosed external pile) occurs as a result of rupture of a vein of the external haemorrhoidal plexus. It is seen as a small (1 cm), tense, bluish swelling on one aspect of the anal margin and is exquisitely tender to the touch. In *prolapsed strangulated piles* there is gross swelling of the anal and perianal skin, which looks like oedematous lips, with a deep red or purple strangulated pile appearing in between – and sometimes partly concealed by – the oedema of the swollen anus. In a *perianal abscess* an acutely tender, red, fluctuant swelling is visible which deforms the outline of the anus. It is usually easy to distinguish this from an *ischiorectal abscess*, where the anal verge is not deformed, the signs of acute inflammation are often lacking, and the point of maximum tenderness is located midway between the anus and the ischial tuberosity.

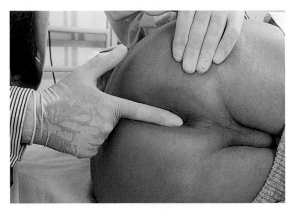

Figure 8.30 Correct method for insertion of the index finger in rectal examination. The pulp of the finger is placed flat against the anus.

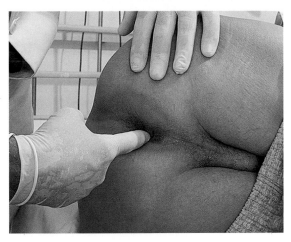

Figure 8.31 Incorrect method of introduction of finger into the anal canal.

Note the presence of any ulceration. Finally, if rectal *prolapse* is suspected, ask the patient to bear down (as if trying to pass stool) and note whether any pink rectal mucosa or bowel appears through the anus, or whether the perineum itself bulges downwards. Downward bulging of the perineum during straining on bending down, or in response to a sudden cough, indicates weakness of the pelvic floor support musculature, usually because of denervation of these muscles. This sign is often found in women after childbirth, in women with faecal or urinary incontinence, and in patients with severe chronic constipation.

DIGITAL EXAMINATION (PALPATION)

Put a generous amount of lubricant on the gloved index finger of the right hand, place the *pulp* of the finger (not the tip) flat on the anus (Figs 8.30, 8.31) and press firmly and slowly (flexing the finger) in a slightly backwards direction. After initial resistance the anal sphincter relaxes and the finger can be passed into the anal canal. If severe pain is elicited on attempting this manoeuvre then further examination should be abandoned, as it is likely the patient has a fissure and the rest of the examination will be very painful and unhelpful.

Feel for any thickening or irregularity of the wall of the canal, making sure that the finger is turned through a full circle (180° each way). Assess the tone of the anal musculature: it should normally grip the finger firmly. If there is any doubt, ask the patient to contract the anus on the examining finger. A cough will induce a brisk contraction of the external anal sphincter, which should be readily appreciated. In the old and infirm with anal incontinence or prolapse almost no appreciable contraction will be felt. With experience it is usually possible to feel a shallow groove just inside the anal canal which marks the dividing line between the external and the internal sphincter. The anorectal ring may be felt as a stout band of muscle surrounding the junction between the anal canal and rectum.

Now pass the finger into the rectum. The examiner's left hand should be placed on the patient's right hip, and later it can be placed in the suprapubic position to exert downward pressure on the sigmoid colon. Try to visualize the anatomy of the rectum, particularly in relation to its anterior wall. The rectal wall should be assessed with sweeping movements of the finger through 360°, 2, 5 and 8 cm inwards or until the finger cannot be pushed any higher. Repeat these movements as the finger is being withdrawn. In this way it is possible to detect *malignant ulcers, proliferative and stenosing carcinomas, polyps* and *villous adenomas*. The hollow of the sacrum and coccyx can be felt posteriorly. Laterally, on either side, it is usually possible to reach the side walls of the pelvis. In men one should feel anteriorly for the *rectovesical pouch, seminal vesicles* (normally not palpable) and the *prostate*. In a patient with a pelvic abscess, however, pus gravitates to this pouch, which is then palpable as a boggy, tender swelling lying above the prostate. Malignant deposits will feel hard and irregular. In infection of the seminal vesicles these structures become palpable as firm, almost tubular swellings deviating slightly from the midline just above the level of the prostate.

Assessment of the *prostate gland* is important. It forms a rubbery, firm swelling about the size of a large nut. Run the finger over each lateral lobe, which should be smooth and regular. Between the two lobes lies the median sulcus, which is palpable as a faint depression running vertically between each lateral lobe. Although it is possible to say on rectal examination that a prostate is enlarged, accurate assessment of its true size is not possible. In carcinoma of the prostate the gland loses its rubbery consistency and becomes hard, the lateral lobes tend to be irregular and nodular, and there is distortion or loss of the median sulcus.

The *cervix* is felt as a firm, rounded mass projecting back into the anterior wall of the rectum. This is often a disconcerting finding for the inexperienced. The body of a *retroverted uterus, fibroid mass, ovarian cyst, malignant nodule* or *pelvic abscess* may all be palpated in the pouch of Douglas (rectouterine pouch), which lies above the cervix. This aspect of rectal examination forms an essential part of pelvic assessment in female patients.

On withdrawing the finger after rectal examination look at it for evidence of mucus, pus and blood. If in doubt wipe the finger on a white swab. Finally, be sure to wipe the patient clean before telling them that the examination is complete, and also tell them to be careful as they roll to the supine position as they will be very near the edge of the couch or bed.

THE ACUTE ABDOMEN

HISTORY

The patient usually presents with *acute abdominal pain*. As with any pain, its site, severity, radiation, character, time and circumstances of onset, and any aggravating or relieving features are all important.

SITE

When the visceral peritoneum is predominantly involved in an acute process pain is often referred in a developmental distribution, and so when assessing acute abdominal pain it is often helpful to think of the embryological development of the gut. Foregut structures are proximal to the duodenojejunal flexure, and pain from here will often be felt in the upper abdomen. The small bowel and the colon around to the mid-transverse originate from the midgut and may produce pain in the periumbilical region, such as in the early phases of acute appendicitis. Pain from structures developing from the hindgut will be felt in the lower abdomen. As any disease process advances and the parietal peritoneum is irritated, pain is felt at the site of the affected organ, such as in the right iliac fossa in the later stages of acute appendicitis.

Ask the patient to point to the site of maximal pain with one finger. If pain is experienced mostly in the *upper abdomen* think of perforation of a gastric or duodenal ulcer, cholecystitis or pancreatitis. If pain is located in the *mid-abdomen*, disease of the small bowel is likely. Pain in the *right iliac fossa* is commonly due to appendicitis and pain in the *left iliac fossa* to diverticulitis. In women the menstrual history is important, as *low abdominal pain* of acute onset is often due to salpingitis, but rupture of an ectopic pregnancy should also be considered. The coexistence of *severe back and abdominal pain* may

indicate a ruptured abdominal aneurysm or a dissecting aneurysm.

SEVERITY

Try to assess the severity of the pain. Ask whether it keeps the patient awake. In women who have had children, compare the severity with labour pains. Sometimes comparison to the pain of a fractured bone is useful.

RADIATION

If pain radiates from the right subcostal region to the shoulder or to the interscapular region, inflammation of the gallbladder (cholecystitis) is a likely diagnosis. If pain begins in the loin but then is felt in the lumbar region a renal stone or renal infection should be considered. Pain beginning in the loin and radiating to the groin is likely to be due to a ureteric calculus, and umbilical pain radiating to the right iliac fossa is usually due to appendicitis. Central upper abdominal pain, later radiating through to the back, is common in pancreatitis.

CHARACTER AND CONSTANCY

Constant severe pain felt over many hours is likely to be due to infection. For example, diverticulitis or pyelonephritis can present in this manner. *Colicky pain*, on the other hand (i.e. pain lasting a few seconds or minutes and then passing off, leaving the patient free of pain for a further few minutes), is typical of small bowel obstruction. If such pain is suddenly relieved after several hours of severe pain, perforation of a viscus should be considered. Large bowel obstruction produces a more constant pain than small bowel obstruction, but colic is usually prominent. Biliary and renal colic are also variable in severity, but with a longer period of variation than small bowel colic, and also with a much more sudden onset than relief.

MODE OF ONSET

In obstruction from mechanical disorders, such as that due to biliary or ureteric stone, or obstruction of the bowel from adhesions or volvulus, the onset of colicky pain is usually sudden. It is often related to activity or movement in the previous few hours. In infective and inflammatory disorders the pain usually has a slower onset, sometimes over several days, and there is no relation to activity. Recent ingestion of a rich, heavy meal sometimes precedes pancreatitis. Alcohol excess or the ingestion of aspirin or non-steroidal anti-inflammatory drugs are sometimes precipitating features in patients presenting with perforated peptic ulcer or with haematemesis.

RELIEVING FEATURES

Abdominal pain relieved by rest suggests an infective or inflammatory disorder. Pancreatic pain is classically relieved by sitting forward.

VOMITING

A history of vomiting is not in itself very helpful because vomiting occurs as a response to pain of any type. However, effortless projectile vomiting often denotes pyloric stenosis or high small bowel obstruction. In peritonitis the vomitus is usually small in amount but vomiting is persistent. There may be a faeculent smell to the vomitus when there is low small bowel obstruction. Persistent vomiting with associated diarrhoea strongly suggests gastro-enteritis. Patients with a perforated ulcer do not usually vomit.

MICTURITION

Increased frequency of micturition occurs both in urinary tract infections and in other pelvic inflammatory disorders, as well as in patients with renal infections or ureteric stones. In the latter, haematuria commonly occurs.

APPETITE AND WEIGHT

In patients with a chronic underlying disorder, such as abdominal cancer, there may be a history of anorexia and weight loss, although weight loss also occurs in a variety of other disorders. Sudden loss of appetite clearly indicates a disorder of sudden onset.

OTHER FEATURES

It is important to note whether there have been previous episodes of abdominal pain and whether or not they have been severe. The patient may have noticed swellings at the site of a hernial orifice, indicating the likelihood of an obstructed hernia, or there may be a history of blunt or penetrating abdominal trauma. Sometimes the patient may be aware of increasing abdominal distension, a phenomenon indicating intestinal obstruction or paralytic ileus, probably associated with an inflammatory or infective underlying bowel disorder. Food poisoning may be suggested by a history of ingestion of unusual foods or a meal in unfamiliar surroundings. The menstrual history should never be forgotten, particularly in relation to the possibility of an ectopic pregnancy. Enquiry should always be made as to a purulent vaginal discharge, indicating salpingitis, or of discharge of mucus, pus or blood from the rectum, suggesting ulcerative colitis.

EXAMINATION

Certain features are important in all patients presenting with an acute abdominal crisis. An assessment of the vital signs and of the patient in general is essential. The physical signs found on inspection and on auscultation of the abdomen have already been discussed.

GUARDING

Guarding is an involuntary reflex contraction of the muscles of the abdominal wall overlying an inflamed viscus and peritoneum, producing localized rigidity. It indicates localized peritonitis. What is felt on examination is spasm of the muscle, which prevents palpation of the underlying viscus. Guarding is seen classically in uncomplicated acute appendicitis. It is very important to distinguish this sign from voluntary contraction of muscle.

RIGIDITY

Generalized or 'board-like' rigidity is an indication of diffuse peritonitis. It can be seen as an extension of guarding, with involuntary reflex rigidity of the muscles of the anterior abdominal wall. It is quite unmistakable on palpation, as the whole abdominal wall feels hard and 'board-like', precluding palpation of any underlying viscus. The least downward pressure with a palpating hand in a patient with generalized rigidity produces severe pain. It may be differentiated from voluntary spasm by asking the patient to breathe: in voluntary spasm the abdominal wall will be felt to relax during expiration.

REBOUND TENDERNESS

Rebound tenderness is present if, when palpating slowly and deeply over a viscus and then releasing the palpating hand, the patient experiences sudden pain. Rebound tenderness is not always a reliable sign and should be interpreted with caution, particularly in patients with a low pain threshold, but is often a useful adjunct to detecting peritoneal inflammation.

PERCUSSION

The absence of dullness over the liver can indicate free intraperitoneal gas and hence a perforated viscus.

RADIOLOGY

A plain X-ray of the abdomen is an important immediate investigation in the diagnosis of the acute abdomen, especially in suspected perforation or obstruction (Fig. 8.32).

EXAMINATION OF ABDOMINAL FLUIDS

EXAMINATION OF VOMIT

The character of the vomit varies with the nature of the food ingested and the absence or presence of bile, blood or intestinal obstruction. In pyloric stenosis the vomit is usually copious and sour smelling, containing recognizable food eaten many hours previously and exhibiting froth on the surface after standing. The presence of much mucus gives

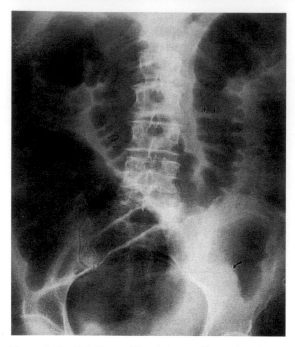

Figure 8.32 Plain X-ray of the abdomen. Obstruction of the large bowel due to carcinoma of the sigmoid colon. Most of the colon is dilated with gas, indicating obstruction, but there appears to be no gas below the sigmoid region.

vomit a viscid consistency. Brisk haematemesis, such as from a large vessel in an ulcer, will cause the patient to vomit essentially pure blood. Bright red blood that is 'vomited' nearly always originates from the naso- or oropharynx and not from the stomach. Slower upper GI bleeding leads to the blood mixing with gastric juice and becoming darker and an appearance likened to that of ground coffee.

Vomit that contains dark green bile may resemble vomit containing blood, but usually red and green parts can be distinguished. Faeculent vomit, characteristic of advanced intestinal obstruction, is brown in colour, rather like vomited tea, and has a faecal odour. Vomit containing formed faeces is rare but indicates a communication between the stomach and the transverse colon, usually from a colonic carcinoma or gastric ulcer.

EXAMINATION OF FAECES

Examination of the faeces is an investigation of great importance that is all too easily omitted. No patient with bowel disturbance has been properly examined until the stools have been inspected.

FAECAL AMOUNT
Note whether the stools are copious or scanty, and whether they are hard, formed, semiformed or liquid.

FAECAL COLOUR
Black stools may be produced by altered blood or the ingestion of iron or bismuth. In haemorrhage occurring high up in the intestine the altered blood makes the stools dark, tarry-looking and with a characteristic and offensive smell. *Pallor* of the stools may be due to lack of entry of bile into the intestine, as in obstructive jaundice; to dilution and rapid passage of the stool through the intestine, as in diarrhoea; or to an abnormally high fat content, as in malabsorption.

FAECAL ODOUR
In jaundice the stools are often very offensive. Cholera stools, on the other hand, contain very little organic matter and are almost free from odour. The stools of acute bacillary dysentery are almost odourless, whereas those of amoebic dysentery have a characteristic odour, something like that of semen. Melaena stools have a characteristic smell.

ABNORMAL STOOLS
Watery stools are found in all cases of profuse diarrhoea and after the administration of purgatives. In cholera the stools – known as *rice-water* stools – are colourless, almost devoid of odour, alkaline in reaction, and contain a number of small flocculi consisting of shreds of epithelium and particles of mucus. Purulent or pus-containing stools are found in severe dysentery or ulcerative colitis. Slimy stools are due to the presence of an excess of mucus, and point to a disorder of the large bowel. The mucus may envelop the faecal masses or may be intimately mixed with them.

Bloody stools vary in appearance according to the site of the haemorrhage. If the bleeding takes place high up, the stools look like tar. In an intussusception they may look like redcurrant jelly. Large bowel bleeding above the rectum may produce darker red visible blood, whereas bleeding from the rectum or anus may streak the faeces bright red, and haemorrhoidal bleeding may just be found on the toilet paper. A brisk upper GI bleed can lead to bright red rectal bleeding.

The stools of bacillary dysentery consist at first of faecal material mixed with blood and pus, and later of blood and pus without faecal material. Those of amoebic dysentery characteristically consist of fluid faecal material, mucus and small amounts of blood. The stools of steatorrhoea are very large, pale and putty- or porridge-like, sometimes frothy with a visible oily film, and often float. They are apt to stick to the sides of the toilet and are difficult to flush away.

TESTS FOR FAECAL OCCULT BLOOD
Several methods are available. For ease of use and safety the guaiac test (Haemoccult) is the most widely used. A filter paper impregnated with guaiac

turns blue in the presence of haemoglobin when hydrogen peroxide is added. The test depends on the oxidation of guaiac in the presence of haemoglobin. Other substances with peroxidase activity, including dietary substances such as bananas, pineapple, broccoli and radishes, can produce a false positive reaction, and ascorbic acid may cause false negative results. Therefore, dietary preparation is necessary for accurate screening testing, for example when screening a population in the early detection of colonic cancer. In ordinary clinical use the test is sensitive to faecal blood losses of about 20 mL/day. This test can be used on patients on a normal diet, but it may not detect small amounts of gastrointestinal bleeding. The test may be negative in the presence of lesions that bleed intermittently or slightly, particularly those situated in the upper GI tract. Spectroscopic methods and isotopic methods using radiolabelled red cells that can localize the source of bleeding in the gut are also available.

TESTS FOR FAECAL FAT

Fat is present in food as neutral fat or triglyceride. It is split to a greater or lesser degree by lipases, mainly of the pancreas, into glycerol and fatty acids. Some of the fatty acids, if unabsorbed, combine with bases to form soaps. Fat may therefore be found in the faeces as neutral fat, fatty acids and soaps.

Estimation of the proportion of split and unsplit fats present has been found unreliable as a method of distinguishing pancreatic from non-pancreatic steatorrhoea because of the effects of bacterial activity on neutral fats.

For estimation of the fat in the stools, the patient may be placed on a diet containing 50 g of fat per day. The fat present in the stools collected over at least 3 days is then estimated, and should not exceed 6 g (11–18 mmol) per day. It has been found that equally reliable results are obtained if the patient eats a normal diet, provided a 3–5-day collection is made.

Faecal fat testing has largely been replaced by the measurement of faecal elastase.

STOOL MICROBIOLOGY   (see also Appendix 2)

Reliable microbiological examination of the stool is vital for accurate diagnosis of acute and chronic diarrhoea. All stool samples for microbiological examination should reach the laboratory as fresh as possible, and if amoebic or similar infection is suspected then microscopy should be performed with the stool still as close to body temperature as possible.

Any microbiological finding must be correlated with the history, as many patients are healthy carriers of organisms that can be pathogenic in other situations. If *Clostridium difficile* infection is suspected in a patient with diarrhoea following use of antibiotics, the laboratory must be asked to look for the clostridium toxin as well as the organism.

ASPIRATION OF PERITONEAL FLUID

Aspiration of peritoneal fluid (*paracentesis abdominis*) is undertaken for diagnostic and therapeutic purposes. Most patients with significant ascites should have an initial diagnostic aspiration to help differentiate the causes. In cirrhotic patients with ascites whose condition deteriorates the complication of spontaneous bacterial peritonitis must be excluded because it has no specific signs, has a significant mortality, and substantially affects prognosis. Therapeutic paracentesis may be needed in cirrhotic patients for whom diuretics are contraindicated or have not worked, and in patients with ascites due to malignancy.

First make sure that the bladder is empty (pass a catheter if there is any doubt). The patient should be lying flat, or propped up at a slight angle. The aspiration is usually performed in the flanks, a little outside the midpoint of a line drawn from the umbilicus to the anterior superior iliac spine. With suitable sterile precautions, the skin at the chosen point should be infiltrated with local anaesthetic and the anaesthetic then injected down to the parietal peritoneum. For a simple diagnostic puncture, a 30 mL syringe and an 18 G needle can be used. If it is intended to drain a significant quantity of fluid, a trocar and flanged cannula (which can be fixed to the skin with adhesive tape) should be employed (a peritoneal dialysis catheter is often suitable). A diagnostic tap should be performed before inserting the trocar and cannula to ensure that fluid can be obtained at the chosen site. A tiny incision should be made in the anaesthetized area of the skin before the trocar and cannula are inserted. The cannula is attached to a drainage bag and the drainage rate should be limited to 1 L/hour. Because of the risk of infection the drainage catheter should not be left in situ for more than 6 hours. In general, diuretics are preferable to therapeutic drainage.

The fluid withdrawn is sent for bacteriological and cytological examination and chemical analysis. Transudates, such as occur in heart failure, cirrhosis and the nephrotic syndrome, normally have a protein content less than 25 g/L (i.e. less than two-thirds the concentration of albumin in the plasma). Exudates occurring in tuberculous peritonitis or in the presence of secondary malignancy usually contain more than 25 g/L protein. This method of distinction, however, is somewhat unreliable. Lymphocytes in the fluid are characteristic features of tuberculous peritonitis, but acid-fast bacilli are often not seen on staining. Bloodstained fluid strongly suggests a malignant cause, and malignant cells may also be demonstrated (Fig. 8.33).

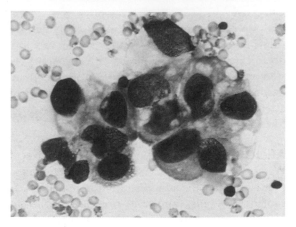

Figure 8.33   Ascites cytology. A group of tumour cells showing random orientation and large abnormal nucleoli indicating malignancy. Ascitic fluid from a patient with ovarian carcinoma. May–Grünwald–Giemsa stain. ×160.

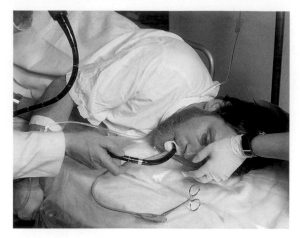

Figure 8.34   A patient undergoing endoscopy of the upper gastrointestinal tract. The plastic guard between the teeth prevents the instrument being bitten. The patient may have received a pharyngeal local anaesthetic spray or light sedation with midazolam.

In ascites due to cirrhosis some of the sample should also be inoculated into blood culture bottles. However, in spontaneous bacterial peritonitis the cultures are often negative and the diagnosis is based primarily on the finding of 500 or more neutrophils per mm^3 fluid and an unexpectedly high protein content, results that should lead to the use of appropriate broad-spectrum antibiotics.

SPECIAL TECHNIQUES IN THE EXAMINATION OF THE GI TRACT

There are a number of common and important methods of examining the oesophagus, stomach and duodenum, the small and large intestine, the liver, gallbladder, biliary tree and pancreas.

UPPER GASTROINTESTINAL ENDOSCOPY

In the last 30 years the developments of the fibreoptic endoscope, and more recently of videoendoscopy, have revolutionized the inspection of the upper gastrointestinal tract (Fig. 8.34). With these instruments it is possible to inspect directly as far as the duodenal loop, with or without light sedation and local pharyngeal anaesthesia. Because of the ability to photograph and biopsy any suspicious lesions, this technique is the investigation of choice for demonstrating structural abnormalities in the upper gut. Therapeutic endoscopy is replacing surgery in many cases of bleeding oesophageal varices, bleeding peptic ulcer (Fig. 8.35) and oesophageal stricture. In inoperable cancer of the oesophagus, palliative prostheses (stents) can be inserted endoscopically.

OESOPHAGEAL FUNCTION STUDIES

The oesophageal phase of swallowing can be assessed by barium swallow and may show slowing

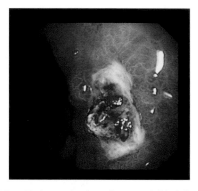

Figure 8.35   Endoscopic view of a recently bled duodenal ulcer with a visible blood vessel on its surface.

or arrest of transit of the food bolus in the oesophagus. In special clinical applications manometric studies of pressure changes during swallowing are used to localize functional abnormalities in the coordination of oesophageal peristalsis, for example achalasia and oesophageal spasm.

In patients with epigastric and retrosternal discomfort (*heartburn*) related to eating or to lying supine, reflux of acid from the stomach into the lower oesophagus should be suspected. Acid reflux can best be detected by monitoring the pH in the lower oesophagus over a 24-hour period. The pH measuring probe, attached to an oesophageal line, is placed in the lower oesophagus, 5 cm above the oesophagogastric junction, for 24 hours and the pH recorded continuously. The patient indicates when pain is experienced by pressing an electronic marker on the recorder to see if there is a close correlation with the degree of acidity. This investigation has found a major clinical application in the differential diagnosis of acid reflux pain from cardiac pain.

GASTRIC SECRETORY STUDIES AND SERUM GASTRIN LEVELS

Measurement of stomach acid secretion was formerly much used for the assessment of patients with peptic ulcer disease, and for the diagnosis of hyperacidity caused by the rare gastrin-secreting tumours (Zollinger–Ellison syndrome), but serum gastrin estimation is now the investigation of choice.

In normal subjects the *basal acid output* is no more than a few millilitres per hour, containing up to 10 mmol/L of hydrogen ion. The *maximal acid output*, measured during 1 hour after the administration of pentagastrin (6.0 mg/kg body weight), a synthetic analogue of the naturally occurring human hormone gastrin, may reach 27 mmol/L/h in males and 25 mmol/L/h in females. In most patients with Zollinger–Ellison syndrome the ratio of basal to maximum acid secretion is raised as much as sixfold.

Measurement of serum gastrin must be made fasting, after quite a long period without acid-suppression therapy, and collected into special preservative. In Zollinger–Ellison patients the level of gastrin in the serum is increased above 100 ng/L. Serum gastrin levels are also increased in renal failure, pernicious anaemia, after vagotomy, and during acid-suppression therapy.

TESTS FOR *HELICOBACTER PYLORI*

In recent years the role of infection by *Helicobacter pylori* in the pathogenesis of gastric and duodenal ulceration has become increasingly well documented, although the exact causative link is not fully understood. *H. pylori* is a Gram-negative spiral bacillus found in the gastric antrum in about 60% of patients with gastritis or gastric ulceration, and in almost all patients with duodenal ulceration. There are many asymptomatic carriers in the general population. Patients carrying *H. pylori* in the stomach will have IgG antibodies in the serum and these will remain present for a long period after successful treatment. *H. pylori* can be detected by microscopy or culture of gastric mucosal biopsies obtained during endoscopy, and can be detected in the stool, but the most convenient test depends on the ability of the organism to break down urea to ammonia.

H. pylori is rich in urease. In a simple clinical test a gastric biopsy is placed in contact with a pellet or solution containing urea and a coloured pH indicator. The colour of the substrate changes when the pH is greater than 6, indicating the conversion of urea to ammonia by urease in *H. pylori*. A variant of this method uses ^{13}C-labelled urea, given to the patient by mouth. The patient's breath is monitored for labelled carbon dioxide, indicating breakdown of the ingested urea by urease-containing organisms in the upper GI tract.

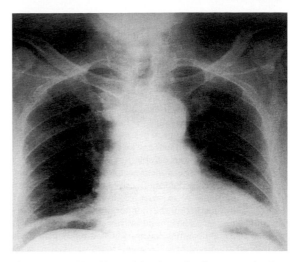

Figure 8.36 Plain X-ray of the chest showing gas under the right and left diaphragms after perforation of the duodenal ulcer. The patient was admitted in shock with abdominal pain and abdominal rigidity.

H. pylori can be rendered undetectable but not eradicated by acid-suppression therapy, which for reliable results should be stopped 2 weeks before any testing.

RADIOLOGY OF THE UPPER GASTROINTESTINAL TRACT

PLAIN RADIOGRAPHS

Plain radiographs of the chest and abdomen with the patient both supine and in the erect position are of great value in cases of suspected peritonitis due to a perforated viscus, when gas may be seen under the diaphragm, usually on the right side (Fig. 8.36). A plain abdominal X-ray is useful in suspected intestinal obstruction or ileus, when dilated bowel loops may be seen with fluid levels appearing on the erect X-ray.

BARIUM SWALLOW

Direct observation of the passage of a radio-opaque barium solution through the pharynx and oesophagus into the stomach remains an important investigation of dysphagia. In addition to structural abnormalities such as neoplasia or stricture, disorders of motor function can be detected that might otherwise escape diagnosis. Lack of progress of barium through an apparently normal lower oesophageal sphincter on swallowing in a patient with dysphagia indicates the presence of *achalasia*, a disorder of neuromuscular coordination of the oesophageal body and failure of the lower sphincter to relax.

A careful radiological assessment of the stomach and duodenum which have been coated with swallowed barium and then inflated with a gas-forming tablet has the ability to demonstrate benign ulcers and tumours, as well as assessing gastric outflow, but the ability to take endoscopic biopsies has meant that barium radiology is now a secondary investigation to upper GI endoscopy.

SMALL INTESTINE

BARIUM FOLLOW-THROUGH X-RAYS

The small intestine may be studied by taking films of the abdomen at intervals after swallowing barium contrast. Abnormalities in the transit time to the colon and in small bowel pattern (e.g. dilatation, narrowing, increase in transverse barring or flocculation) may be demonstrated in malabsorption. Areas of narrowing with proximal dilatation, fistulae and mucosal abnormalities may be produced by Crohn's disease. Small bowel diverticula or neoplasms may also be demonstrated. The amount and type of barium used for examination of the stomach/duodenum and of the small bowel are different, and so a barium follow-through should be requested as a specific examination and not as an add-on to a barium meal.

SMALL BOWEL ENEMA

This is an alternative to the barium follow-through examination and involves intubating the duodenum and passing small quantities of a non-flocculating barium suspension down the tube. This method is particularly valuable for detecting isolated focal lesions and strictures.

RADIOISOTOPE STUDIES

In inflammatory bowel disease the location of the disease, and a measure of its activity, can be obtained by radioisotope studies using the patient's own white blood cells that have been radiolabelled.

SMALL INTESTINAL ENDOSCOPY AND BIOPSY

Samples of small intestinal mucosa are valuable for histological diagnosis in various types of malabsorption. Direct biopsy of the lower duodenum at conventional upper gastrointestinal endoscopy is usually sufficient for diagnosis of coeliac disease, but jejunal tissue can also be obtained using a push-type flexible enteroscope. Endoscopic biopsy techniques have now largely replaced remote biopsy by Crosby capsule. If necessary full-thickness jejunal biopsies, useful for diagnosing neuromuscular gut disorders, can be obtained by laparoscopy. Excellent endoscopic images of the whole of the small bowel can now be obtained by wireless capsule endoscopy, but as yet biopsies are not possible by this method.

If coeliac disease is suspected serum antibodies to gliadin, reticulin and endomysial antigens are a useful screening test (provided there is no IgA deficiency), but a biopsy is essential to fully complete or fully exclude the diagnosis. The low-power view of the villi is as important as the detailed histology. Other malabsorption problems, such as Whipple's disease and chronic giardiasis, may also be seen on duodenal biopsy.

COLON, RECTUM AND ANUS

PROCTOSCOPY

The anal canal and lower rectum can be readily visualized with a rigid proctoscope. Place the patient in the position described for rectal examination and gently pass the lubricated instrument to its full depth. Remove the obturator and inspect the mucosa as the instrument is slowly withdrawn. Haemorrhoids are seen as reddish/blue swellings that bulge into the lumen of the instrument. Asking the patient to strain down as the proctoscope is withdrawn exaggerates the haemorrhoids. The internal opening of an anal fistula, an anal or low rectal polyp and a chronic anal fissure are other abnormalities that may be seen.

RIGID SIGMOIDOSCOPY AND OTHER TESTS IN CHRONIC DIARRHOEA

It is often necessary to examine the rectum and colon more fully than is possible by proctoscopy, and in such cases the rigid sigmoidoscope is employed. Sigmoidoscopy requires skill and experience. In accomplished hands the instrument can be passed for 30 cm. The procedure causes relatively little discomfort and anaesthesia is unnecessary.

Proctitis, polyps and carcinomas may be seen and biopsies taken. Sigmoidoscopy is particularly useful in the differential diagnosis of diarrhoea of colonic origin. Granularity, loss of vascular pattern and ulceration with bleeding may indicate the presence of ulcerative colitis, aphthous ulceration may suggest Crohn's disease, and multiple rounded white macules may be diagnostic of pseudomembranous colitis due to *Clostridium difficile* toxin, usually following antibiotic treatment. In suspected amoebic dysentery the mucous membrane should be inspected and portions of mucus and scrapings from the ulcerated mucosa may be removed and examined microscopically for amoebic cysts.

Urine tests for purgative abuse are useful in the investigation of persistent unexplained diarrhoea.

BARIUM ENEMA

Prior to barium enema the patient must have their bowel prepared with a vigorous laxative, as residual stool or fluid can be mistaken for polyps and other lesions. Impending obstruction is a contraindication to this laxative preparation. A plain X-ray of the abdomen should always be taken in patients with suspected perforation or obstruction before considering a contrast study (see Fig. 8.32). The barium suspension is introduced via a tube into the rectum as an enema and manipulated

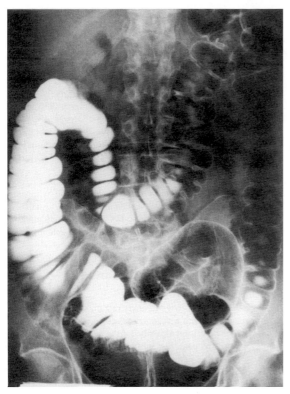

Figure 8.37 Barium enema with air contrast. The right colon is outlined by barium sulphate, and the rectum, left colon and part of the transverse colon are outlined by air with a thin mucosal layer of barium sulphate. Note the normal haustral pattern in the colon and the smooth appearance of the rectum. The anal canal can also be seen.

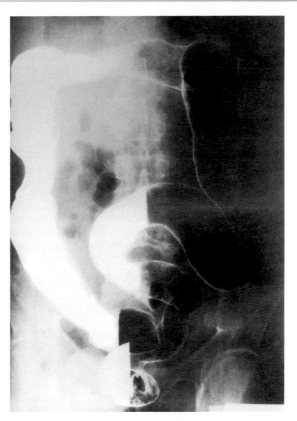

Figure 8.38 Barium enema with air contrast. In this patient with ulcerative colitis the normal mucosal pattern and the haustra themselves have been obliterated. The patient is lying on his right side so that there are clear fluid levels in the barium sulphate suspension in the bowel.

around the rest of the colon to fill it. Screening is performed by a radiologist and films are taken. The barium is then evacuated and further films taken. By this means, obstruction to the colon, tumours, diverticular disease, fistulae and other abnormalities can be recognized.

Following evacuation, air is introduced into the colon. This improves visualization of the mucosa and is especially valuable for detecting small lesions such as polyps and early tumours (Figs 8.37, 8.38).

Patients often find the preparation and procedure uncomfortable and there is a very small risk of perforating the colon.

COLONOSCOPY AND FLEXIBLE SIGMOIDOSCOPY

As in the upper gut, the use of flexible fibreoptic and video instruments has revolutionized the investigation of the colon. Both sigmoidoscopes and colonoscopes are available. The former may be employed in an outpatient setting after a simple enema preparation; the latter require more extensive colon preparation (similar to barium enema X-ray) and sedation, but can also be used in an outpatient procedure. These techniques are invaluable for

obtaining tissue for the diagnosis of inflammatory and neoplastic disease and for removal of neoplastic polyps (Figs 8.39, 8.40). Dilatation of strictures, stenting, laser or other thermal treatments of obstructing tumours can also be applied during endoscopy.

A skilled colonoscopist can reach the caecum in 95% of examinations attempted. There is a very small risk of colonic perforation associated with colonoscopy, and of respiratory arrest with the sedatives.

THE LIVER

BIOCHEMICAL TESTS IN LIVER DISORDERS

These are used in the differential diagnosis of jaundice, to detect liver cell damage in other disorders, and to monitor the results of medical and surgical treatments of the liver, pancreas and biliary systems. These include plasma bilirubin, alkaline phosphatase, serum aminotransferases, plasma proteins and prothrombin time. Serum γ-glutamyl transferase levels are especially sensitive to liver dysfunction as, for example, in alcohol-related liver disease.

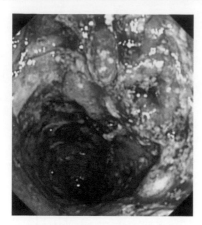

Figure 8.39 View of colonic epithelium at colonoscopy, showing severe ulcerative colitis with extensive ulceration and bleeding.

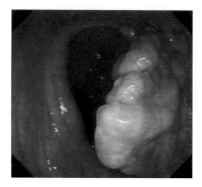

Figure 8.40 Colonoscopic view of a tubulovillous adenoma.

Smooth muscle antibodies are commonly present in the blood in chronic active hepatitis, and other autoantibody studies are used in the investigation of chronic inflammatory liver disease. Antimitochondrial antibodies are found in the blood in over 90% of cases of primary biliary cirrhosis.

Liver disease due to excess iron or copper accumulation can be detected by measurements of these metals and their carrier proteins in blood or urine (for copper). In primary haemochromatosis, genetic studies are very useful in diagnosis. Serum α-fetoprotein is often raised in primary liver cell cancer, which can complicate any cause of cirrhosis, or the carriage of hepatitis B or C.

VIRAL HEPATITIS
Ongoing carriage of viral hepatitis is initially detected by antigen testing (for hepatitis B) and by antibody testing for hepatitis C, D and E. Active infection is detected by the presence of IgM antibody (for hepatitis A, D and E), and by PCR testing for the viral RNA (hepatitis C). At least two antigens and antibodies of hepatitis B can be detected (surface and e), which give information about activity and ongoing disease, and in the latter detection of the viral DNA is helpful.

NEEDLE BIOPSY OF LIVER
Percutaneous needle biopsy is the standard technique for obtaining liver tissue for histological examination. Although needle biopsy can be conducted under mild sedation and local anaesthesia, it should be carried out only in hospital under supervision, and blood should be available for transfusion, if necessary. Generally the method is safe and reliable, but there is a tiny but definite mortality from the procedure owing to leakage of bile and/or blood into the peritoneal cavity from the puncture site. The procedure should therefore always be regarded as a potentially dangerous investigation for which there should be a clear beneficial indication for the patient, and should be performed by an appropriately trained operator. Liver biopsy under ultrasound control can allow the targeting of specific abnormalities and give confidence that the procedure will be safer. Contraindications to biopsy include patients with abnormal clotting times or platelet numbers, obstructive jaundice or ascites.

ULTRASOUND SCANNING

A probe emitting ultrasonic pulses is passed across the abdomen. Echoes detected from within the patient are received by a transducer, amplified and suitably displayed. This technique is the most commonly used method for non-invasive investigation of the liver. It can suggest the presence of cirrhosis and small metastases, and is helpful in the diagnosis of fluid-filled lesions such as cysts and abscesses. Fine needles can be inserted into a suspicious lesion under direct ultrasound guidance for cytology and for drainage of fluid or bile.

The gallbladder is most easily investigated by ultrasound, appearing as an echo-free structure. If stones are present they are usually easily seen as mobile and echo dense, with a characteristic 'acoustic shadow' behind them. Ultrasound detects 95% of gallbladder stones, but only about 50% of stones in the bile ducts themselves. Ultrasound is particularly valuable in detecting dilatation of the bile duct, which may be due to partial or complete obstruction by tumour or gallstones. Ultrasound has largely replaced oral cholecystography for imaging the gallbladder.

Ultrasound is the usual initial technique for investigating the pancreas, is particularly useful in the diagnosis of true and pseudopancreatic cysts, and is essential for percutaneous needle biopsy. It is used extensively for examining other intra-abdominal, pelvic and retroperitoneal organs, and increasingly for imaging the bowel, for example in Crohn's disease.

ISOTOPE SCANNING

A radioisotope of technetium or colloidal gold is injected intravenously and taken up by the reticulo-endothelial system. A gamma camera is used to show the size and shape of the liver. Abnormal areas such as primary or secondary hepatic tumours, abscesses and cysts take up more or less isotope than normal. Technetium-labelled red blood cells can be used to detect the location of sources of bleeding in the GI tract. Isotopes taken up in the bile (HIDA) can give images of the gallbladder and biliary tree.

COMPUTED TOMOGRAPHY (CT) SCANNING

CT can be used to produce cross-sectional images of the liver and other intra-abdominal and retroperitoneal organs. It is particularly helpful in assessing patients with cancer of the oesophagus, stomach, pancreas and colon (Fig. 8.41). Because it can be combined with the injection of vascular contrast it can be helpful in assessing intra-abdominal vascular abnormalities. It can facilitate guided biopsy of abnormalities, and drainage of fluid and other collections. It is also increasingly being used to image the bowel, particularly if there is suspected obstruction.

ENDOSCOPIC ULTRASOUND

Endoscopic ultrasound is more sensitive than CT in staging the mucosal depth of penetration of cancers in the oesophagus and stomach, and is frequently better at lymph node detection, but is less good at detecting distant metastases. It is also valuable in assessing biliary and pancreatic abnormalities and can be used to guide biopsy.

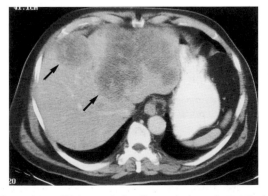

Figure 8.41   CT demonstrating liver metastases from colonic carcinoma. Large, lobulated, non-homogeneous masses (arrowed) replace most of the left lobe of the liver.

MAGNETIC RESONANCE IMAGING (MRI)

Magnetic resonance cholangiopancreatography (MRCP) can give high-quality images of the bile and pancreatic ducts. The safety of this non-invasive technique has reduced the need for more hazardous examinations such as endoscopic retrograde cholangiopancreatography (ERCP), which is reserved for patients requiring therapeutic intervention.

SELECTIVE ANGIOGRAPHY OF GASTROINTESTINAL ARTERIES

Angiography is occasionally used in the investigation of haematemesis or melaena when gastroscopy, colonoscopy and enteroscopy fail to identify the bleeding source. It is most useful if performed when the patient is actively bleeding, but may be of value if an aneurysm or abnormal tumour vasculature is present, and can occasionally detect angiomas. It is an invasive technique that demands a great deal of skill on the part of the radiologist. It is sometimes possible to use therapeutic embolization to treat haemorrhage.

ENDOSCOPIC RETROGRADE CHOLANGIOPANCREATOGRAPHY (ERCP)

Using a special side-viewing duodenoscope, the duodenal papilla is identified and a cannula passed through it into the common bile duct. Radio-opaque contrast is then injected down the cannula and the whole of the biliary system is visualized. The technique is useful in the rapid diagnosis and localization of the different causes of jaundice due to obstruction of the main bile ducts. Needle or forceps biopsy and brush cytology may give a specific diagnosis of strictures of the biliary tree. ERCP has an important therapeutic role in the treatment of jaundice because it allows the removal of bile duct stones, or the placement of stents, which are tubes that facilitate the passage of bile into the duodenum past obstructing lesions such as tumours of the pancreas or bile duct. Such therapies often involve performing a sphincterotomy during ERCP using a cutting diathermy wire within a plastic catheter and passed into the bile duct via the ampulla. The sphincterotomy opens the ampulla and may allow the delivery of stones in the bile duct.

The ERCP procedure can display the entire pancreatic duct system. It is therefore valuable not only in the diagnosis of chronic pancreatitis, but also in defining those cases that could benefit from surgery. In patients with pancreatic carcinoma needle biopsy can be performed at ERCP, and brush cytology of the pancreatic duct may also provide histological proof of the diagnosis. ERCP carries a small mortality rate and may be complicated by pancreatitis, bleeding, perforation or infection.

PERCUTANEOUS TRANSHEPATIC CHOLANGIOGRAPHY

Percutaneous transhepatic cholangiography complements the use of ERCP in patients with jaundice due to obstruction of the main bile ducts, but is usually only possible if the intrahepatic bile ducts are seen to be dilated on ultrasound. The site of obstruction caused by tumours of the head of the pancreas, or benign and malignant bile duct strictures, can be accurately localized and differentiated. This technique is usually used only if ERCP fails. It also has a therapeutic function. Transhepatic drains can be placed to treat cholangitis and sepsis, stents can be placed to relieve obstruction, gallstones can be removed, and wires can be passed into the duodenum to allow stenting at ERCP.

PANCREATIC FUNCTION TESTS

Pancreatic function tests are now rarely used in diagnosis. In suspected pancreatic malabsorption, a therapeutic trial of pancreatic supplementation may be the easiest confirmatory test. If a definitive test is wanted the pancreolauryl test can be used, which relies on the collection in the urine of a substance that can only be absorbed after GI breakdown by pancreatic enzymes. In chronic pancreatitis faecal elastase may be reduced. Measurement of the blood amylase level is still valuable in the diagnosis of acute pancreatitis.

Locomotor system

D. D'Cruz

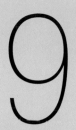

INTRODUCTION

Musculoskeletal symptoms are a major cause of pain and disability, accounting for a quarter of all general practitioner consultations and having important economic consequences. In later life, musculoskeletal diseases are the single most important cause of disability, requiring considerable health and social service resources. The autoimmune connective tissue diseases, although much less common, cause significant morbidity and may be fatal if not recognized and treated early.

The objectives of performing a musculoskeletal assessment are:

- to make an accurate diagnosis
- to assess the severity and consequences of the condition
- to construct a clear management plan.

The clinical methods involved are largely those practised at the bedside, i.e. a careful, structured history and a thorough examination. Although modern musculoskeletal medicine uses complex imaging and immunological investigations, in most patients with locomotor disorders diagnosis can be achieved at the bedside without complex investigations.

GENERAL ASSESSMENT: THE *GALS* LOCOMOTOR SCREEN

A full assessment of the musculoskeletal system can be time-consuming. The gait, arms, legs and spine (GALS) screen is a rapid and sensitive screening method for detecting musculoskeletal disorders that can easily be incorporated into the general physical examination.

SCREENING HISTORY

If answers to the following three questions are negative, a musculoskeletal disorder is unlikely:

- Do you have any pain or stiffness in your muscles, joints or back?
- Can you dress yourself completely without difficulty?
- Can you walk up and down stairs without difficulty?

Positive answers imply the need for a more detailed assessment, as described in this chapter.

SCREENING EXAMINATION

- **Gait**: Watch the patient *walking* and *turning* back towards you
- **Spine**: inspect the *standing* patient
  - from behind – look for abnormal spinal and paraspinal anatomy and look at the legs
  - from the side – look for abnormal spinal posture (Fig. 9.1), then ask the patient to bend down and try to touch their toes
  - from the front – ask the patient to 'try and put your ear on your left then right shoulder' and watch the neck movements (Fig. 9.2)
  - gently press the midpoint of each supraspinatus muscle to elicit tenderness (Fig. 9.3)
- **Arms**: ask the patient to:
  - 'put your hands behind your head, with your elbows back'; observe shoulder and elbow function (Fig. 9.4)
  - 'put your arms straight out in front of you'; observe elbow extension
  - 'put your hands and fingers out straight and turn them over'; observe pronation and supination and palmar and finger anatomy (Fig. 9.5)
  - 'make a fist with both hands' and observe power grip (Fig. 9.6)
  - gently squeeze the hand across the metacarpals to elicit tenderness and check for swelling (Fig. 9.7)
  - 'touch each fingertip with your thumb' and observe precision movements
- **Legs**: with the patient *still standing*:
  - examine the lower limbs for swelling, deformities or limb shortening
  - then, with the patient *lying* on a couch:
    - flex each hip and knee with a hand on the knee to feel for crepitus
    - passively rotate each hip internally and look for pain or limitation of movement (Fig. 9.8)
    - palpate each knee for warmth and swelling, and press on the patella feeling for an effusion

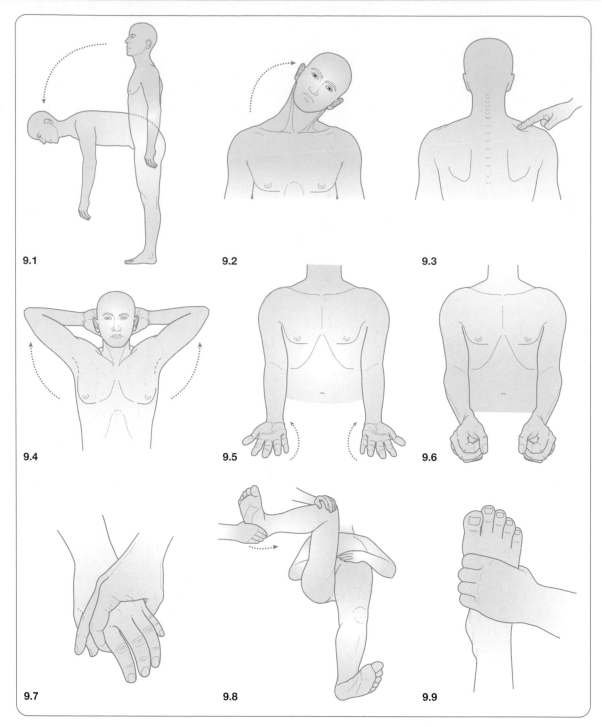

Figure 9.1 Inspect patient from behind and side, observing for normal spinal curves, then ask the patient to 'bend forwards to try and touch your toes'.
Figure 9.2 From the front, ask the patient to 'place your ear on your right then your left shoulder'.
Figure 9.3 Gently press the midpoint of each supraspinatus to elicit the hyperalgesia of fibromyalgia.
Figure 9.4 'Put your hands behind your head, elbows back.' Observe for pain or restricted movement.
Figure 9.5 'Put your hands out palms down and then turn your hands over.'
Figure 9.6 'Make a fist with both hands.'
Figure 9.7 Look for swelling between the heads of the metacarpals and gently squeeze across the MCP joints to elicit tenderness.
Figure 9.8 Gently flex the hips and knees, feeling for crepitus at the knee during movement, and look for pain and restriction of movement. Look for knee effusion.
Figure 9.9 Squeeze across MTP joints and inspect the soles of the feet.

- squeeze gently across the metatarsals for tenderness (Fig. 9.9)
- finally, inspect the soles of the feet for callosities, ulcers.

This examination can be conducted in approximately 2 minutes, especially if the clinician performs the movements and asks the patient to follow them. The precise order of the examination is not important and clinicians usually develop their own pattern of examination.

RECORDING THE RESULTS

The findings of this locomotor screen should be noted routinely in the medical record. For example, a normal screen might be recorded as follows:

Screening questions:	pain	0
	dressing	✓
	walking	✓

with positive answers being elaborated.
Examination:

A (Appearance)		M (Movement)
G	✓	
A	✓	✓
L	✓	✓
S	✓	✓

with abnormal findings indicated, e.g. in rheumatoid arthritis:

A (Appearance)		M (Movement)
G	X	
A	X	X
L	X	X
S	✓	✓

Slow painful gait.
Synovitis of MCP, MTP, wrists and knee joints.

The incorporation of this brief musculoskeletal examination into the routine examination is not a substitute for more detailed assessment as outlined below.

SPECIFIC LOCOMOTOR HISTORY

General demographic details such as age, sex and occupation should be recorded. Start the full musculoskeletal history with the presenting complaint and ask the patient to describe the sequence of symptoms, related features and events since the onset. Characteristic diagnostic points may emerge. For example, the pain from an osteoporotic vertebral fracture which is acute and self-limiting is very different from the severe, constant and gnawing pain of a spinal metastatic deposit that prevents sleep and may be associated with weight loss. Similarly, the acute, severe, usually continuous throbbing pain of joint infection is different from the mechanical pain of osteoarthritis.

Pain may be referred or radiate from an affected joint:

- Neck pain may radiate through the occiput to the vertex or to the shoulder and down the arm, with paraesthesiae if there is nerve root impingement.
- Shoulder joint pain may radiate to the elbow and below.
- Cervical root pain shoots toward the elbow or hand.
- Thoracic spine nerve root pain may radiate around the chest and mimic cardiac pain.
- Lumbar spinal root pain may radiate through the buttock and leg to the knee and below, with paraesthesiae in the foot with a large disc prolapse – this is called 'sciatica'.
- Hip joint pain may radiate to the knee and below.
- Knee pain may radiate above and below the joint.

With these patterns in mind it is prudent to examine the joints above and below the apparently affected area.

JOINT DISEASE

A combination of *pain* and *stiffness*, leading to loss of function, is a classic feature of joint disease. Usually one component predominates, as with stiffness in inflammation, and pain in mechanical joint problems. Therefore, specific questions will establish whether symptoms are *mechanical* (e.g. degenerative joint disease or meniscal tear) or *inflammatory* (e.g. rheumatoid arthritis or gout).

FEATURES OF MECHANICAL JOINT DISEASE

In degenerative joint disease there may be a feeling of stiffness in the affected joint after resting which rapidly disappears with activity. This *inactivity stiffness* typically lasts only a few minutes and nearly always less than 30 minutes. Pain in the affected joint on activity, usually improving with rest, is typical. A clicking sensation in a joint, particularly in the knee, is a common complaint but is usually a normal phenomenon (compare with *crepitus*, p. 156). *Locking* of a joint may occur. In the knee, this means that the knee becomes locked in such a way that it will not extend fully, although it may flex. In other joints locking is less well defined and simply means that at some point through its range of motion the joint becomes stuck, usually associated with pain and often followed by swelling. Locking is due to material within the joint interfering with movement at the articular surfaces. In the knee, this is usually part of one of the menisci, or a cartilaginous loose body.

FEATURES OF INFLAMMATORY JOINT DISEASE

Early morning stiffness
Early morning joint stiffness that persists for more than 30 minutes is an important symptom of active

inflammatory joint disease. Ask about *redness* (rubor), *warmth* (calor), *tenderness/pain* (dolor) and *swelling* (tumour), the classic features of inflammation.

If the history suggests inflammation, and if only one joint is involved (monoarticular disease), always consider infection. Ask if there has been any fever or sweating, and if the joint is inflamed, consider aspirating it to look for infection.

Distribution of joint disease

The pattern of involvement of joints is important in diagnosis. Symmetry is useful in distinguishing various inflammatory arthropathies. There are only a few causes of an exactly symmetrical arthropathy (Box 9.1). Other conditions have such a classic history that this is diagnostic. For example, acute inflammation in the first metatarsophalangeal joint (*hallux*) suggests a diagnosis of gout (Box 9.2). Another typical pattern is the pain and stiffness of the shoulder and hip girdles in polymyalgia rheumatica (Box 9.3).

Recurrent attacks of joint pain

Ask if the same joint is always involved. If not, define the patterns of involvement, the severity and duration of the episodes, and any associated clinical symptoms.

Episodic joint pain

Ask if attacks of joint pain are associated with para-articular redness, with the attacks lasting about 48 hours (occasionally up to 1 week). This is typical of *palindromic rheumatism*, which may progress to rheumatoid arthritis.

Flitting or migratory joint pains

This term is used to describe inflammation beginning in one joint and then involving others, usually one at a time for about 3 days each. Gonococcal arthritis should be considered; this is characterized by typical fleeting skin lesions and urethritis, in addition to joint pain. In rheumatic fever there is associated cardiac involvement, and erythema marginatum and subcutaneous nodules may occur.

The other features in the history that should be brought out are best considered under the differential diagnosis of polyarthritis (Box 9.4). Many arthropathies may have a monoarticular presentation.

Box 9.1   Importance of distribution of joint involvement in differential diagnosis of oligo- or polyarthritis

Typically symmetrical
- Upper and lower limbs
  - rheumatoid arthritis, SLE
- Especially upper limbs
  - haemochromatosis (hand: index, middle MCP joints)

Typically asymmetrical
- psoriatic arthritis

Typically lower limb and asymmetrical
- spondyloarthritis (e.g. ankylosing spondylitis, Reiter's syndrome)
- Document any associated features

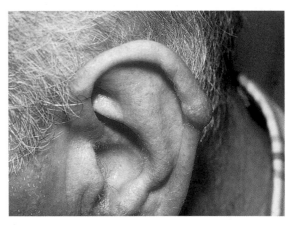

Figure 9.10 Gouty tophus on the ear. Other sites include the elbows, fingers and toes.

Box 9.2   Acute gout

A 48-year-old publican presented with sudden severe pain and swelling of his left big toe. He was unable to weightbear or wear a shoe, and said that he could not even bear the weight of his bedclothes on the toe at night. His past history included hypertension, for which he was taking a thiazide diuretic and his alcohol intake was excessive. On examination he had tophi in the ears (Fig. 9.10) and the left first metatarsophalangeal joint was red, hot, swollen and exquisitely painful to touch. Aspiration of the joint revealed urate crystals.

Box 9.3   Polymyalgia rheumatica

A 74-year-old woman presented with a 2-month history of pain around her hips and shoulders. The key points in the history were that these regions were extremely stiff for 4 hours each morning, and that there was no joint swelling. Clinically there was pain and some limitation of movement at the shoulders and hips, but no synovitis. Her erythrocyte sedimentation rate was 96 mm/1st hour, and she had a dramatic response within 2 days to a moderate dose of prednisolone.

First attack
- Exclude infection by aspiration for culture and crystals
- If negative culture but high-risk group, biopsy: for example tuberculosis in Asian immigrants or immunosuppressed patients

Recurrent attacks
- Flitting (gonococcal arthritis; rheumatic fever)
- Episodic (crystal arthritis; palindromic rheumatism)

Persistent synovitis with none of the above features
- Look for systemic features and check serology (e.g. rheumatoid factor or antinuclear antibody)

INFLAMMATORY CONNECTIVE TISSUE DISEASES

The connective tissue diseases, such as systemic lupus erythematosus (SLE), systemic sclerosis and vasculitides, are multisystem disorders. A careful systems enquiry (see Chapter 1) is essential if this diagnosis is suspected. Associated features of these conditions include systemic symptoms such as weight loss, malaise or fevers, and skin rash, especially if the latter is photosensitive or vasculitic (Fig. 9.11). Oral and genital ulceration, Raynaud's phenomenon and symptoms of neuropathic, cardiac, pulmonary and gastrointestinal involvement may occur. Dry eyes and dry mouth (sicca symptoms) are common in these conditions and can be documented with Schirmer's test (Fig. 9.12). Renal disease is an important complication of the connective tissue diseases, especially in SLE and the systemic vasculitides. Clinical assessment should always include measuring blood pressure and dipstick-testing the urine for blood and protein, and microscopy of the urine sediment for casts or dysmorphic red cells if this is positive (Chapter 14). Ear, nose and throat involvement with sinusitis, facial pain and deafness (Chapter 19) is common in Wegener's granulomatosis and Churg–Strauss syndrome. A history of arterial and venous thromboses or miscarriages, especially in the context of livedo reticularis, should raise the suspicion of the antiphospholipid syndrome.

SOFT TISSUE SYMPTOMS

Soft tissue problems are common and usually consist of pain, a dull ache, tenderness or swelling. In the elderly these symptoms often appear spontaneously, but in younger people there is usually a history of injury or overuse, through either occupation

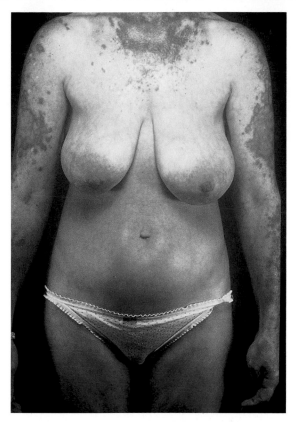

Figure 9.11 Extensive rash in sun-exposed areas in a woman with systemic lupus erythematosus and anti-Ro antibodies.

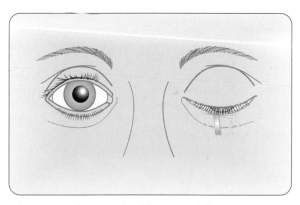

Figure 9.12 A sterile strip of filter paper is hooked over the lower eyelid. Less than 5 mm of wetness after 5 minutes is abnormal and is associated with connective tissue disease.

(e.g. tenosynovitis of the long flexor tendons of the hand) or sport (e.g. Achilles tendinitis). It is important to define the exact site of the symptoms, and the factors that either make them worse or induce relief. The localization of symptoms to specific soft tissue structures can be confirmed by careful examination (Box 9.5). The possible soft tissues involved are *joint*, *tendon*, *ligament*, *bursa* and *muscle*.

Box 9.5   Localization of the site of articular and extra-articular features

Joint
- Diffuse pain and tenderness
- Generalized joint swelling
- Restriction of movement, usually in all directions of movement (specific to each joint)

Tendon
- Localized pain/tenderness at attachment (enthesis) or in the tendon substance
- Swelling, tendon sheath or paratenon
- Pain on resisted movement
- Sometimes pain on stretch (e.g. Achilles)

Ligament
- Localized pain/tenderness at attachment or in ligament substance
- Pain on stretch
- Instability, if major tear

Bursa
- Localized tenderness
- Pain on stretching adjacent structures

Muscle
- Localized or diffuse pain and tenderness
- Pain on resisted action
- Pain on stretch (e.g. hamstring)

Box 9.6   Examination of the musculoskeletal system

General observations
- Gait
- Posture
- Mobility
- Deformity
- Independence: use of wheelchair or walking aids
- Muscle wasting
- Long bones

Fractures
- Joints
- Tendons
- Skin

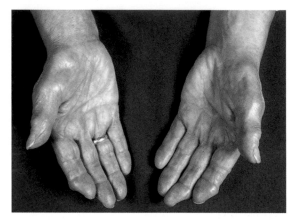

Figure 9.13   Thenar wasting due to carpal tunnel syndrome. This is often associated with osteoarthritis: note nodal change on the terminal interphalangeal joints of the index fingers.

THE BONES

Bone pain is characteristically deep-seated and localized, but referred pain may confuse the clinical picture. In the case of fractures, unless pathological, there will almost always be a history of injury. In athletes, however, a fracture may be due to chronic overuse, as in stress fracture of the tibia or metatarsals in runners. The spontaneous onset of pain may suggest Paget's disease (with bony enlargement, e.g. skull or tibia) or metastatic deposits. Infection must also be considered, particularly in younger patients or in immunodeficiency states. Consider also congenital or familial disorders as predisposing factors, for example multiple osteochondromata or brittle bone disease (*osteogenesis imperfecta*).

EXAMINATION: GENERAL PRINCIPLES

Observe the patient entering the room (Box 9.6). Abnormalities of *gait* and *posture* may provide clues that can be pursued in history-taking. Observation of any difficulty in undressing and getting on to the examination couch will further help in assessment. The patient must always be asked to stand and walk, even when it is obvious that this may be difficult. Note how much help the patient requires from others or from sticks, crutches etc. The musculoskeletal system includes the muscles, bones, joints, and soft tissue structures such as tendons and ligaments. Remember that although muscle wasting may be due to *primary muscle disease* (e.g. polymyositis), it is more commonly secondary to *disuse*, perhaps because of a painful joint, or to *neuropathy* due to nerve root compression or peripheral neuropathy (Fig. 9.13). Examination of the muscles is discussed further in Chapter 10.

THE BONES

The examination of the bones should always be directed by information obtained from the history.

Inspection

Look for any alterations in shape or outline and measure any shortening. In *Paget's disease* (osteitis deformans) bowing of the long bones, particularly the tibia (Fig. 9.14(a) and (b)) and femur, is

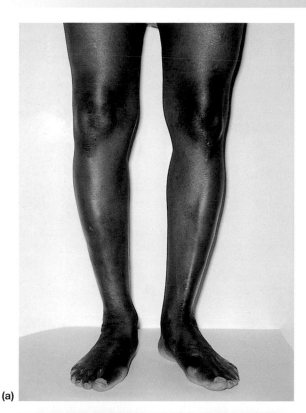

(a)

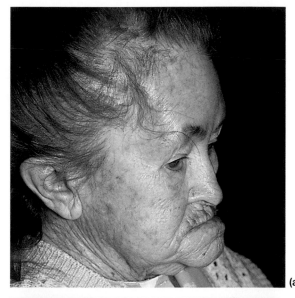

(a)

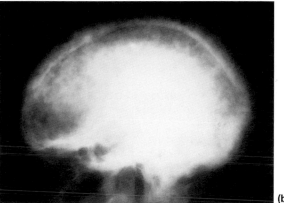

(b)

Figure 9.15 Paget's disease, causing deformity of the skull **(a)**. Note the thickened skull vault with remodelled bone **(b)**.

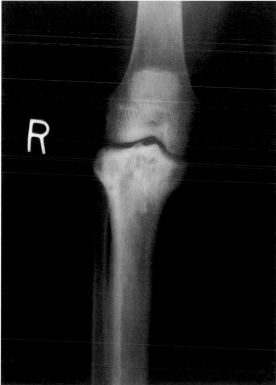

(b)

Figure 9.14 Paget's disease of the right tibia. Note tibial bowing and bony enlargement **(a)** and bony enlargement sclerosis with some patchy porosis in the X-ray of the upper tibia **(b)**.

associated with bony enlargement and, usually, increased local temperature. The skull is also commonly involved, but this may not be apparent until the disease is advanced. Early involvement of the skull bones can be detected on X-rays (Fig. 9.15(a) and (b)). Alterations in the shape of bones also occur in rickets as a result of epiphyseal enlargement. Deformity of the chest in rickets is due to osteochondral enlargement (*rickety rosary*).

Localized swellings of long bones may be caused by infections, cysts or tumours. Spontaneous fractures may occasionally be the presenting symptom in the diagnosis of secondary carcinoma, multiple myeloma, generalized osteitis fibrosa cystica (*hyperparathyroidism*) or osteogenesis imperfecta.

Palpation
On palpation bone tenderness occurs in local lesions when there is destruction, elevation or irritation of the periosteum, as in generalized osteitis fibrosa cystica, myelomatosis, bone infections, occasionally in

carcinomatosis of bones and, rarely, in leukaemia. Injury is the commonest cause.

FRACTURES

Fractures are common and may involve any bone. They are painful, distressing for the patient and expensive for the community (Box 9.7). Fractures in healthy bones commonly involve the long bones and are usually due to trauma. Fractures of the wrists, hips and vertebrae are more frequently complications of bone disease, such as osteoporosis. Multiple rib fractures, caused by falls, may be found in alcoholics, but may only be seen as healed lesions on chest X-ray. Fractures occur without apparent trauma when a bone is weakened by disease, especially with metastatic malignant deposits in bone (*pathological fractures*). Traumatic fractures invariably present with local pain, swelling and loss of function, but pathological fractures may be relatively silent. The history will reveal the circumstances of the trauma, whether accidental or due to physical abuse, and should be carefully documented, if necessary with diagrams or digital photographs of the clinical findings. If clinical photographs are taken prior written consent is needed.

Examination of suspected fracture

It is essential to establish whether the fracture is open (*compound*) or closed. In *closed fractures* the surrounding soft tissues are intact. In *open fractures* the bone communicates with the surface of the skin, either because the primary injury has broken the overlying skin or because deformation at the fracture site has caused the bone ends to penetrate the skin. There is a major risk of infection when the fracture site communicates with the open air.

Deformity is an obvious feature in the majority of fractures. It may be clinically characteristic, as in

Colles' fracture, in which there is a fracture of the distal end of the radius characterized by dorsal displacement and angulation, shortening of the wrist and rotation of the fragment, well summarized in the description 'dinner-fork deformity'. Certain fractures may show little deformity: for example, a fracture of the femoral shaft may be accompanied by only slight deformity, as there is often little separation of the bones at the fracture site and other features are disguised by the thick overlying muscle. A fracture of the neck of the femur causes deformity through external rotation of the foot and shortening of the leg.

Most fractures are characterized by local tenderness and swelling, unless the overlying muscle mass is large. Bony crepitus, due to abnormal motion at the fracture site, is a feature of fractures, but this should not be elicited unless absolutely necessary for diagnosis because it is very painful. However, if it is perceived or has been recognized by the patient, it is diagnostic.

A fracture of the bone may damage the neighbouring soft tissues directly or, alternatively, a fracture may be a marker of severe injury in which direct damage to the soft tissues, such as the nerves and vessels, may have taken place. It is therefore essential to evaluate the nerve and blood supply to a limb distal to the site of the fracture. Impairment of blood supply distal to a fracture is a surgical emergency.

The presence or absence of *pulses* and *cutaneous sensation* and the colour and perfusion of the limb must always be recorded and any changes over time reported. Voluntary movement at joints distal to a fractured long bone, such as ankle movement in a fractured femur, should be noted. If this is absent, nerve injury must be suspected.

THE JOINTS

Examination of the joints can be summarized simply as 'look, feel and move', i.e. *inspection, palpation,* and *range of movement*. With practice the clinician can develop a systematic review of the joints – for example the jaw, cervical spine, shoulder girdle and upper limb, thoracic and lumbar spine, pelvis and lower limb – so that inconspicuous but important joints, such as the temporomandibular, sternoclavicular and sacroiliac, will not be overlooked. Compare the corresponding joints on the two sides of the body and always take care to avoid causing undue discomfort.

Inspection

The detection of joint inflammation is a crucial clinical skill. Inflammation is often associated with *redness* of the joint, and with *tenderness* and *warmth*. Look also for swelling or deformity of the joint. The *overall pattern* of joint involvement should be recorded. Note whether the distribution is symmetrical, as is usual in rheumatoid arthritis

---

Box 9.7   Fractures: clinical features

Type
- Closed
- Compound (open)

Complications
- Accompanying soft tissue injury (indirect)

Features
- Haemorrhage
- Deformity
- Pain
- Crepitus
- Restricted movement

Cause
- Traumatic
- Spontaneous (osteoporosis or metabolic)
- Pathological

(Fig. 9.16), or asymmetrical, as in psoriatic arthropathy or gout (Fig. 9.17). The seronegative spondyloarthropathies (Fig. 9.18) tend to involve predominantly the joints of the lower limb.

Palpation

On palpation of a joint swelling, check first for tenderness. Then determine whether the swelling is due to bony enlargement or osteophytes (e.g.

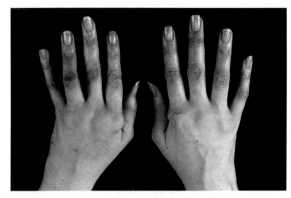

Figure 9.16 Symmetrical joint involvement due to rheumatoid arthritis.

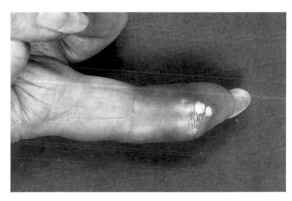

Figure 9.17 Gouty tophi of the index finger.

Heberden's nodes, Fig. 9.19), thickening of synovial tissues such as occurs in inflammatory arthritis, or effusion into the joint space. *Joint effusions* usually have a characteristic smooth outline and *fluctuation* is usually easily demonstrable. Tenderness and enlargement of the ends of long bones, particularly the radius, ulna and tibia, can occur in hypertrophic pulmonary osteoarthropathy: a chest X-ray is essential. Gross disorganization of a joint – nearly always the foot and ankle joints – associated with an absence of deep pain and position sense, occurs in neuropathic (*Charcot*) joints. Charcot joints probably arise from recurrent painless injury and overstretching, and are a feature of severe chronic sensorimotor neuropathy.

Joint tenderness may be graded depending on the patient's reaction to firm pressure of the joint between finger and thumb (Box 9.8). Grade 4 tenderness occurs only in septic arthritis, crystal arthritis and rheumatic fever. In gout, the skin overlying the affected joint is dry, whereas in septic arthritis or rheumatic fever it is usually moist.

If tenderness is present, localize it as accurately as possible and determine whether it arises in the joint or in neighbouring structures, for example in the supraspinatus or bicipital tendon rather than the shoulder joint. Other rheumatic conditions give different types of pain. For example, in conditions such as *complex regional pain syndrome* (CRPS) type I (previously known as reflex sympathetic dystrophy), hyperpathia (abnormal and excessive pain to mildly

Box 9.8   Assessment of joint tenderness
• Grade 1: The patient says the joint is tender
• Grade 2: The patient winces
• Grade 3: The patient winces and withdraws the affected part
• Grade 4: The patient will not allow the joint to be touched

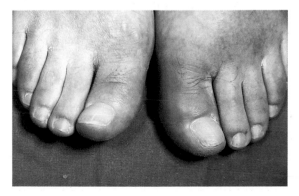

Figure 9.18 Acute synovitis of the interphalangeal joint in reactive arthritis of the left hallux. Differential diagnosis includes gout.

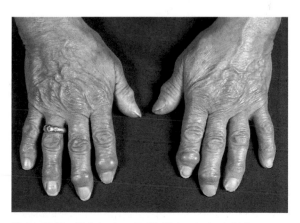

Figure 9.19 Nodal osteoarthritis (Heberden's nodes).

painful stimuli) and allodynia (a sensation of pain to stimuli not normally painful, such as light touch) may often be seen, together with altered sweating and discoloration. In *fibromyalgia* there is widespread diffuse muscle and joint tenderness but no inflammation. A number of characteristic trigger points may be tender around the neck, trunk, upper and lower limbs.

TENDON SHEATH CREPITUS
This is a grating or creaking sensation defined by palpating the tendon while the patient is asked to contract the muscle tendon complex involved. It is particularly common in the hand and is seen in rheumatoid arthritis and systemic sclerosis. In tenosynovitis of the long flexor tendons in the palm, tendon sheath crepitus may be associated with the trigger phenomenon, when the finger becomes caught in flexion and has to be pulled back into extension. Tendon sheath *effusions* can be distinguished from joint swelling by their anatomical location in association with tendons.

JOINT CREPITUS
This can be detected by feeling the joint with one hand while moving it passively with the other. This may indicate osteoarthritis, or loose bodies (cartilaginous fragments) in the joint space, but should be differentiated from non-specific clicking of joints.

RANGE OF MOVEMENT
When examining joints for range of movement it is usually sufficient to estimate the degree of limitation based on comparison with the normal side, or on the examiner's previous experience. For accurate description the actual range of movement should be measured with a protractor (*goniometer*). Both *active* and *passive* movement should be assessed. Active movement, however, may give a poor estimation of true range of movement because of muscle spasm due to pain. If pain is very severe on attempting active movement, and other findings suggest a fracture, take an X-ray before attempting any further examination. In testing the range of passive movement always be gentle, particularly when the joints are painful.

Limitation of movement in a joint may be due to pain, muscle spasm, contracture, inflammation, increased thickness of the capsular or periarticular structures, effusion into the joint space, bony overgrowths, bony ankylosis, mechanical factors such as a torn meniscus, or to painful conditions quite unconnected with the joint.

EXTRA-ARTICULAR FEATURES OF JOINT DISEASE

Some of the extra-articular features of joint disease are listed in Box 9.9.

Box 9.9   Extra-articular features of joint disease

- Cutaneous nodules
- Cutaneous vasculitic lesions
- Lymphadenopathy
- Oedema
- Tendon sheath effusions
- Enlarged bursae
- Ocular inflammation
- Diarrhoea
- Urethritis
- Orogenital ulceration

Box 9.10   Types of subcutaneous nodule

- Gouty tophi caused by urate deposition
- Rheumatoid nodules
- Vasculitic nodules in SLE and systemic vasculitis
- Xanthomatous deposits (hypercholesterolaemia)

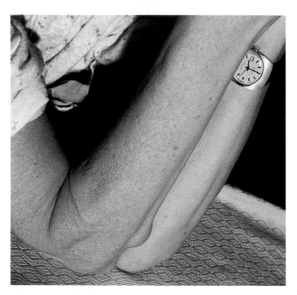

Figure 9.20   Rheumatoid nodule overlying the olecranon of the right arm.

SUBCUTANEOUS NODULES
Subcutaneous nodules are associated with several conditions (Box 9.10). If gout is suspected, inspect the helix of the ear for tophi caused by the subcutaneous deposition of urate, which may also be found overlying joints or in the finger pulps (see Figs 9.10, 9.17). Subcutaneous nodules in rheumatoid arthritis are firm and non-tender; they may be detected by running the examining thumb from the point of the elbow down the proximal portion of the ulna (Fig. 9.20). They can also be found at other pressure and frictional sites, such as bony prominences, including the sacrum. If an olecranon bursa swelling is found, feel also in its wall, as rheumatoid nodules, tophi, or occasionally xanthomata may be found within the swelling. Subcutaneous nodules are not specific to rheumatoid arthritis and may

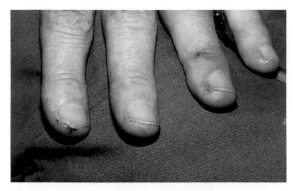

Figure 9.21 Nailfold vasculitis in rheumatoid arthritis. This also occurs in SLE and polyarteritis nodosa.

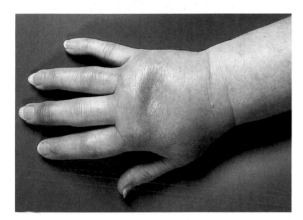

Figure 9.22 Pitting oedema, right hand.

occur in patients with SLE, systemic sclerosis and rheumatic fever.

CUTANEOUS VASCULITIC LESIONS
These may be seen in rheumatoid arthritis, SLE and the systemic vasculitides, including polyarteritis nodosa. They may be small, punched-out necrotic lesions, palpable purpura or vasculitic ulcers, especially on the lower limbs. Small vessel involvement is typically seen at the nail fold (cutaneous infarct, Fig. 9.21), but also occurs at pressure sites. Splinter haemorrhages, the classic feature of bacterial endocarditis (p. 115), may also be a feature of vasculitis and the antiphospholipid syndrome.

LYMPHADENOPATHY
Lymphadenopathy may be found proximal to an inflamed joint, not only in septic arthritis but also in rheumatoid arthritis. Generalized lymphadenopathy, sometimes with splenomegaly, is common in active SLE.

LOCAL OEDEMA
Local oedema is sometimes seen over inflamed joints (Fig. 9.22), but other causes of oedema must be

excluded. Pitting leg oedema may indicate cardiac failure, pericardial effusion or nephrotic syndrome, which can complicate rheumatoid arthritis and SLE.

OTHER SOFT TISSUE SWELLINGS
Tendon sheath effusions are distinguished from joint swellings by their location in association with tendons. Enlarged subcutaneous bursae may be found over pressure areas, particularly at the olecranon surface of the elbow, owing to inflammatory joint disease or secondary to friction. Deeper bursae may be defined only by finding local tenderness or by stressing adjacent tissues (e.g. greater trochanter bursitis).

EXAMINATION OF INDIVIDUAL JOINTS

The range of movement of joints is described in the following pages. All motion should be measured in degrees from a neutral or zero position, which must be defined whenever possible, and compared with the opposite side. Some special features seen at individual joints are set out in each section.

THE SPINE

GENERAL EXAMINATION OF THE VERTEBRAL COLUMN

Inspection
Examine the patient both in standing and in sitting in the erect posture. The normal thoracolumbar spine has an S-shaped curve. If there is an abnormality, note which vertebrae are involved and at what level any vertebral projection is most prominent. Note the presence of any local projections or angular deformity of the spine.

Palpation
The major landmarks are the spinous processes of C7 (the vertebra prominens) and the last rib, which articulates with the twelfth thoracic vertebra. In many patients, however, the last rib cannot be felt distinctly, and this is therefore rather untrustworthy as a guide to this level.

The neutral position of the spine is an upright stance with head erect and chin drawn in. Note any curvature of the spinal column, whether as a whole or of part of it. Abnormal curvature may be in an anterior, posterior or lateral direction (Fig. 9.23). Anterior curvature is termed *lordosis*. There are natural lordotic curves in the cervical and lumbar regions. Posterior curvature is termed *kyphosis*. The thoracic spine usually exhibits a slight smooth kyphosis, which increases in the elderly and especially in osteoporosis. It must be distinguished from a localized angular deformity (*gibbus*, Fig. 9.24) caused by a fracture, by Pott's disease (spinal

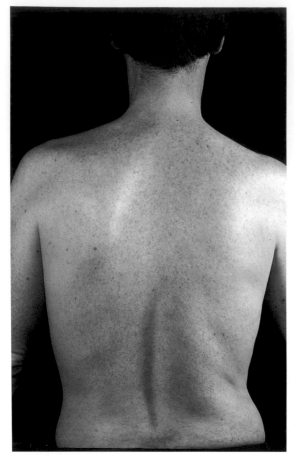

Figure 9.23   Scoliosis of the lumbar spine, due to prolapsed intervertebral disc.

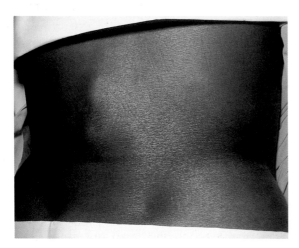

Figure 9.24   Gibbus of the lumbar spine due to tuberculosis.

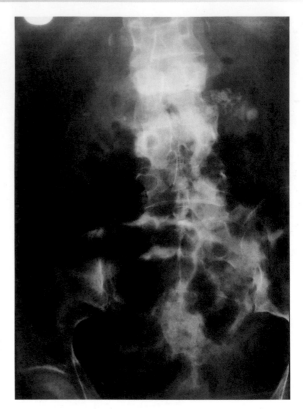

Figure 9.25   X-ray tuberculous discitis. This shows the underlying deformity shown in Figure 9.24. There is tuberculous infection of the intervertebral disc, causing the spinal deformity.

come to point towards the concavity of the curve. The curvature is always greater than appears from inspection of the posterior spinous processes. In scoliosis due to muscle spasm (e.g. with lumbosacral disc protrusion syndromes), the spinal curvature and rotational deformity decrease in flexion. When scoliosis is caused by inequality of leg length it disappears on sitting, because the buttocks then become level. Scoliosis secondary to skeletal anomalies shows in spinal flexion as a 'rib hump' due to the rotation. Kyphosis and scoliosis are often combined, particularly when the cause is an idiopathic spinal curvature, beginning in adolescence.

THE CERVICAL SPINE
The following movements should be tested (Fig. 9.26):

- Rotation (ask the patient to look over one, then the other shoulder)
- Flexion (ask the patient to touch chin to chest)
- Extension (ask the patient to look up to the ceiling)
- Lateral bending (ask the patient to bend the neck sideways and to try to touch the shoulder with the ear without raising the shoulder).

Note any pain or paraesthesiae in the arm reproduced by neck movement, especially on gentle sus-

tuberculosis, Fig. 9.25), or by a metastatic malignant deposit.

Lateral curvature is termed *scoliosis* (Fig. 9.23) and may be towards either side. It is always accompanied by rotation of the bodies of the vertebrae in such a way that the posterior spinous processes

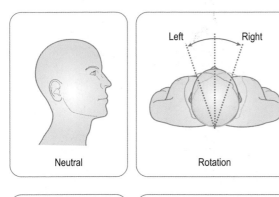

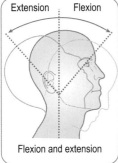

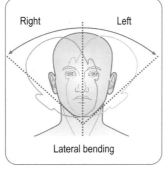

Figure 9.26 Movements of the neck.

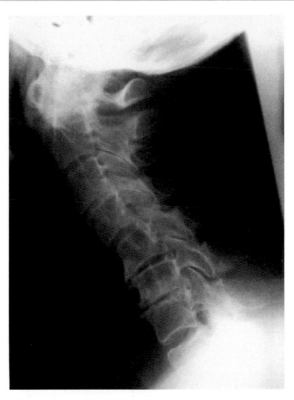

Figure 9.27 Lateral X-ray of cervical spine showing degenerative spondylosis with narrowing of the disc spaces and reversed cervical lordosis between C4 and C6.

tained extension or lateral flexion, suggesting nerve root involvement. If indicated, check for any associated neurological deficit, particularly of radicular or spinal cord type.

In rheumatoid arthritis particular care is necessary in examining the neck, as atlantoaxial instability may lead to damage to the spinal cord when the neck is flexed or extended. If there is any doubt about neck stability in a patient with rheumatoid arthritis arrange for lateral X-rays of the cervical spine in flexion and extension, together with a view of the odontoid peg through the mouth, and defer clinical examination.

In patients with cervical injury *never* try to elicit range of motion of the neck (see Chapter 22). Instead, splint the neck, take a history, look for abnormality of posture (usually in rotation) and check neurological function in the limbs, including both arms and both legs. Take X-rays of the neck in the lateral (Fig. 9.27) and anteroposterior planes, *without* moving the neck. Only if the X-rays are normal should neck movements be examined.

THE THORACIC AND LUMBAR SPINE

The main movement at the thoracic spine is rotation, whereas the lumbar spine can flex, extend, and bend laterally. The following movements should be tested (Fig. 9.28):

- Flexion (ask the patient to try to touch their toes, without bending at the knees)
- Extension (ask the patient to bend backwards)
- Lateral bending (ask the patient to run the hand down the side of the thigh as far as possible
- Thoracic rotation (ask the seated patient, with arms crossed, to twist round to the left and right as far as possible).

In flexion the normal lumbar lordosis should be abolished. The extent of lumbar flexion can be assessed more accurately by marking a vertical 10 cm line on the skin overlying the lumbar spinous processes and the sacral dimples and measuring the increase in the line length on flexion (*modified Schober's test*): this should normally be 5 cm or more. Painful restriction of spinal movement is an important sign of cervical and lumbar spondylosis, but may also be found in vertebral disc disease or other mechanical disorders of the back or neck. A useful clinical aphorism is that a rigid lumbar spine should *always* be investigated for serious pathology, such as infection (e.g. staphylococcal or tuberculous discitis), malignancy or inflammation (e.g. ankylosing spondylitis). Spinal movements may be virtually absent in ankylosing spondylitis (Fig. 9.29), but in the early stages of this condition lateral flexion of the lumbar spine is typically affected first. In mechanical or osteoarthritic back problems flexion and extension are reduced more than lateral movements. In prolapsed intervertebral disc lesions,

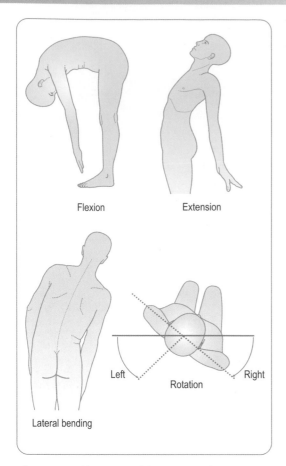

Flexion   Extension

Left   Right

Rotation

Lateral bending

Figure 9.28   Movements of the lumbar and dorsal spine.

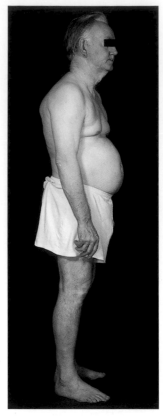

Figure 9.29   Ankylosing spondylitis. Note dorsal kyphosis and protuberant abdomen due to poor chest expansion with abdominal breathing.

sustained gentle lumbar extension may reproduce the low back pain and sciatic radiation.

Chest expansion is a measure of costovertebral movement and should be recorded using a tape measure with the patient's hands behind their head to reduce the possibility of muscular action in the shoulder girdle giving a false reading. Reduced chest expansion is a characteristic early feature in ankylosing spondylitis. Obviously, this may also be a feature of primary pulmonary disease, such as emphysema (see Chapter 6).

Examination of the back is completed by assessing straight leg raising and strength, sensation and reflex activity in the legs. Pain and limitation on *straight leg raising* (SLR) is a feature of prolapsed intervertebral disc, when there is irritation or compression of one of the roots of the sciatic nerve. Tight hamstring muscles may cause a similar picture, but if there is severe pain it is more considerate to lower the leg to just below the limit of SLR and then to see whether gentle passive dorsiflexion of the foot brings back the same pain. If in doubt, dorsiflex the foot once the limit of SLR has been reached. This further stretches the sciatic nerve (the pain increases) but does not affect the hamstrings

(*Lasègue's sign*). The femoral stretch test is a useful confirmatory test and is performed with the patient lying prone: if there is a prolapsed disc at that level flexion at the knee will produce pain in the lower lumbar spine. Sacral sensory loss must always be carefully assessed, because if there is a central lumbosacral disc protrusion, bilateral limitation of straight leg raising may be associated with bladder dysfunction and sacral anaesthesia. This combination requires immediate investigation and treatment and is a surgical emergency.

THE SACROILIAC JOINTS

The surface markings of these joints are two dimples low in the lumbar region. Test for *irritability* in four ways:

- Direct pressure over each sacroiliac joint
- Firm pressure with the side of the hand over the sacrum
- Inward pressure over both iliac bones in an attempt to distort the pelvis
- Flex the hip to 90° and exert firm pressure at the knee through the femoral shaft (this should only be done if the hip and knee are not painful).

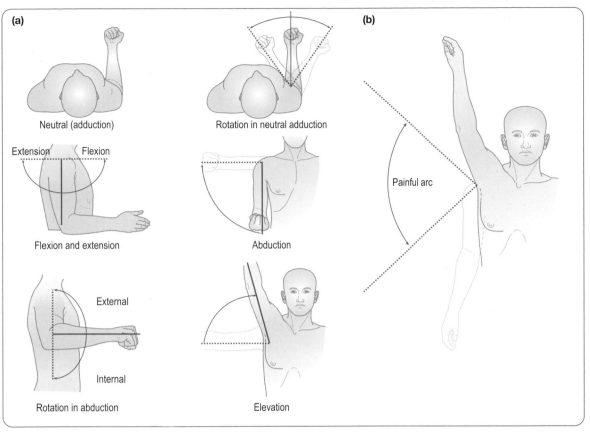

Figure 9.30 **(a)** Movements of the shoulder. **(b)** Painful arc of supraspinatus tendinitis.

In the last three a positive test is only indicated by the patient localizing discomfort to the sacroiliac joint.

THE SHOULDER

The neutral position is with the arm to the side, elbow flexed to 90° and forearm pointing forwards. Because the scapula is mobile, true shoulder (*glenohumeral*) movement can be assessed only when the examiner anchors the scapula between finger and thumb on the posterior chest wall. The following movements should be tested (Fig. 9.30(a) and (b)):

- Flexion
- Extension
- Abduction
- Rotation in abduction
- Rotation in neutral position
- Elevation (also involving scapular movement).

In practice, *internal rotation* can best be compared by recording the height reached by each thumb up the back, representing combined glenohumeral and scapular movement. Similarly, *external rotation* can be assessed by the ability to get the hand to the back of the neck. Limitation of external rotation is a good sign of true glenohumeral disease, which may

occur in adhesive capsulitis (frozen shoulder) or erosive damage from inflammatory arthritis.

Note any pain during the range of movement. In *supraspinatus tendinitis* a full passive range of movement is found but there is a painful arc on abduction, with pain exacerbated on resisted abduction (Fig. 9.30). *Other tendon involvement* should also be defined by pain on resisted action.

Subacromial impingement due to a bursitis or rotator cuff abnormality may produce severe pain at the end of abduction, blocking full elevation. Acute bursitis, however, may be so painful that no abduction is allowed (grade 4 discomfort).

Acromioclavicular joint pain is always very localized and is typically felt in the last 10° of elevation (170–180° arc).

THE ELBOW

The neutral position is with the forearm in extension. The following movements should be tested (Fig. 9.31):

- Flexion
- Hyperextension.

Medial (golfer's elbow) and lateral (tennis elbow) epicondylitis are the most common causes of elbow

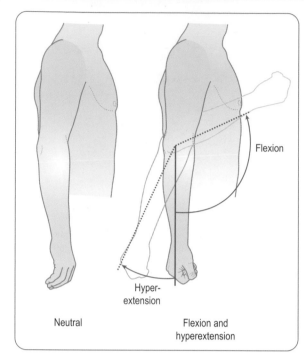

Figure 9.31   Movements of the elbow.

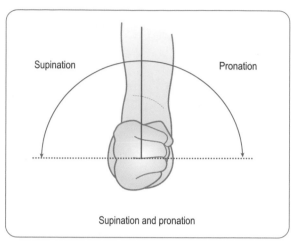

Figure 9.32   Movements of the forearm.

pain. They are characterized by pain on active use, but if severe may be associated with night pain.

Examination must define localized epicondylar tenderness with pain on resisted movement. Wrist extension exacerbates lateral epicondylar tenderness and wrist flexion exacerbates medial epicondylar tenderness. An elbow effusion may be palpated in the posterior triangle formed by the epicondyles and the olecranon.

THE FOREARM

The neutral position is with the arm by the side, elbow flexed to 90° and thumb uppermost. The following movements should be tested (Fig. 9.32):

- Supination
- Pronation.

THE WRIST

The neutral position is with the hand in line with the forearm, and palm down. The following movements should be tested (Fig. 9.33):

- Dorsiflexion (extension)
- Palmar flexion
- Ulnar deviation
- Radial deviation.

Even minor limitation of wrist flexion or extension can be detected by comparing movement in both wrists (Fig. 9.34). Arthritis of the wrist joints is usually due to inflammatory arthritis. Primary osteoarthritis of the wrist is rare, but secondary degenerative change is common.

THE FINGERS

When identifying fingers, use the names *thumb, index, middle, ring* and *little*. Numbering tends to lead to confusion. The neutral position is with the fingers in extension. Test flexion at the metacarpophalangeal (MCP), proximal interphalangeal (PIP) and distal interphalangeal (DIP) joints (Fig. 9.35).

In fractures of the fingers the commonest deformity is rotational. If the finger will flex, make sure it points to the scaphoid tubercle (all the fingers will point individually in this direction). If it will not flex, look end-on at the nail and make sure it is parallel with its fellows.

THE THUMB (CARPOMETACARPAL JOINT)

The neutral position is with the thumb alongside the forefinger, and extended. The following movements should be tested (Fig. 9.36):

- Extension
- Flexion (measured as for the fingers)
- Opposition
- Abduction (not illustrated; movement at right-angles to plane of palm).

THE HAND

DEFORMITIES IN JOINT DISEASE
Examination of the individual joints of the hand may be less informative than inspection of the hand as a whole (Fig. 9.37). The combination of Heberden's nodes and thumb carpometacarpal arthritis occurs in osteoarthritis (see Fig. 9.19). A variety of patterns of deformity are characteristic of long-standing rheumatoid arthritis, for example

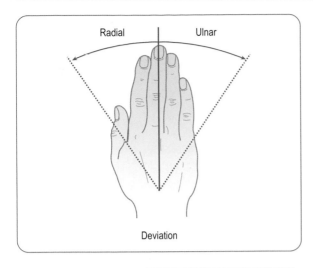

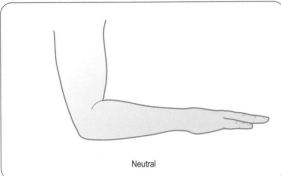

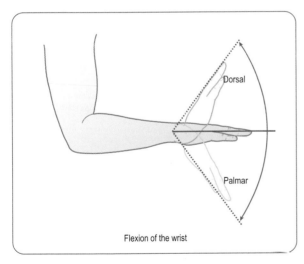

Figure 9.33 Movements of the wrist.

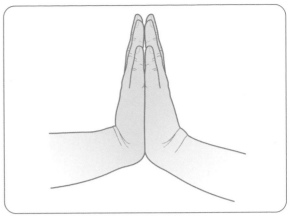

Figure 9.34 Minor limitation of left wrist extension compared with the right. Note the slightly different angulation of the left forearm.

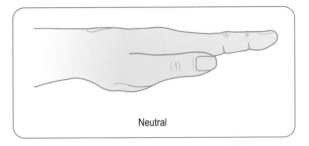

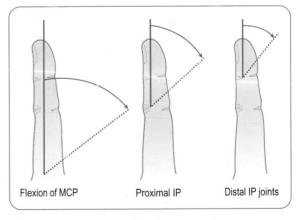

Figure 9.35 Movements of the fingers.

metacarpophalangeal joint subluxation, ulnar deviation of the fingers at the metacarpophalangeal joints, 'swan neck' deformities of the fingers (Fig. 9.38), and 'boutonnière' deformities (flexed proximal and hyperextended distal interphalangeal joints). This is due to the head of the phalanx sliding dorsally between the lateral slips of the extensor tendon, the middle slip having been damaged. In psoriatic arthritis terminal interphalangeal joint swelling may occur, with psoriatic pitting and ridging of the nail (onychopathy) on that digit.

DEFORMITIES DUE TO NEUROPATHY
The hand may adopt a posture typical of a nerve lesion (see Chapter 10). Slight hyperextension of the medial metacarpophalangeal joints with slight flexion of the interphalangeal joints is the 'ulnar claw hand' of an ulnar nerve lesion. There is wasting of the small muscles of the hypothenar eminence, with loss of sensation of the palmar and

163

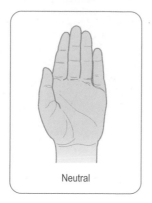

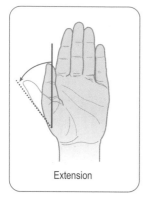

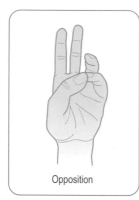

Neutral

Extension

Opposition

Figure 9.36 Movements of the thumb.

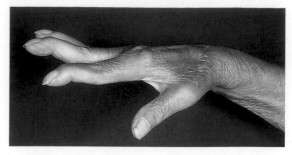

Figure 9.38 Swan-neck deformity of the right hand. Note also wasting of the small muscles of the hand owing to disuse in this patient with rheumatoid arthritis.

ASSESSMENT OF HAND FUNCTION

Assessment of hand function (Fig. 9.37) should include testing hand grip and pinch grip (between index and thumb). The latter may be decreased in lesions in the line of action of the thumb metacarpal, particularly scaphoid fractures.

THE HIP

The neutral position is with the hip in extension and the patella pointing forwards. Ensure the pelvis does not tilt by placing one hand over it while examining the hip with the other. Look for scars and wasting of the gluteal and the thigh muscles. The hip joint is too deeply placed to be accessible to palpation. The following movements should be tested (Fig. 9.39):

- Flexion: measured with knee bent. Opposite thigh must remain in neutral position. Flex the knee as the hip flexes
- Abduction: measured from a line that forms an angle of 90° with a line joining the anterior superior iliac spines
- Adduction (measured in the same manner)
- Rotation in flexion
- Rotation in extension
- Extension: attempt to extend the hip with the patient lying in the lateral or prone position.

ADDITIONAL EXAMINATION OF THE HIP JOINT

- Test for *flexion deformity*. With one hand flat between the lumbar spine and the couch, flex the normal hip fully to the point of abolishing the lumbar lordosis. The spine will come down on to the hand, pressing it on to the couch. If there is a flexion deformity on the opposite side, the leg on that side will move into a flexed position (Thomas's test).
- *Trendelenburg test*. Observe the patient from behind and ask him or her to stand on one leg. In health, the pelvis tilts upwards on the side with the leg raised. When the weightbearing hip is abnormal, owing to pain or subluxation, the pelvis sags downwards due to weakness of the hip abductors on the affected side.

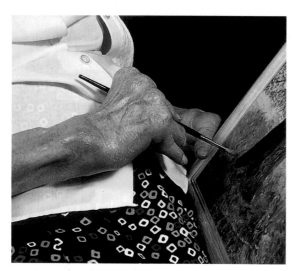

Figure 9.37 Functional ability. Severe joint deformity due to psoriatic arthropathy, but retention of function and artistic ability.

dorsal aspects of the little finger and of the ulnar half of the ring finger. In a median nerve lesion the thenar eminence (abductor pollicis brevis) will be flattened (see Fig. 9.13) and sensory impairment will be found on the palmar surfaces of the thumb, index, middle and radial half of the ring fingers. Remember that carpal tunnel syndrome may be a presenting feature of wrist inflammation.

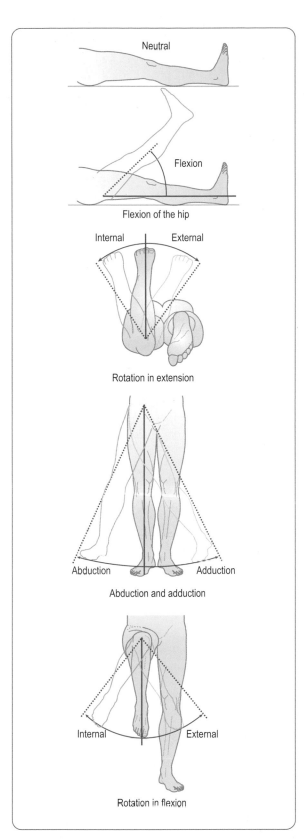

Figure 9.39 Movements of the hip.

- *Measurement of 'true' and 'apparent' shortening.* The length of the legs is measured from the anterior superior iliac spine to the medial malleolus on the same side. Any difference is termed '*true*' shortening and may result from disease of either the hip joint or the neck of the femur on the shorter side. '*Apparent*' shortening is due to tilting of the pelvis and can be measured by comparing the lengths of the two legs, measured from the umbilicus, provided there is no true shortening of one leg. Apparent shortening is usually due to an abduction deformity of the hip.

THE KNEE

A magnetic resonance image (MRI) scan of the normal knee is illustrated in Figure 9.40. The neutral position is complete extension. Observe any valgus (lateral angulation of the tibia) or varus (medial angulation) deformity on the couch and on standing. Look for muscle wasting. The quadriceps, especially its medial part near the knee, wastes rapidly in knee joint disease. Swelling may be obvious, particularly if it distends the suprapatellar pouch. Check the apparent height of the patella and watch to see if it deviates to one side in flexion or extension of the knee. Feel for tenderness at the joint margins, not forgetting the patellofemoral joint. Palpate the ligaments, remembering that the medial collateral ligament is attached 8 cm below the joint line. Measure the girth of the thigh muscles 10 cm above the upper pole of the patella.

JOINT SWELLING
The presence of swelling in the knee joint may be confirmed by the patellar tap test or, for small effusions, by the bulge test, in which the medial parapatellar fossa is emptied by pressure of the flat of the hand sweeping proximally. The bulge is seen to refill as the suprapatellar area is emptied by pressure from the flat hand. Posterior knee joint (Baker's) cysts, particularly in rheumatoid arthritis, may be palpable in the popliteal fossa. They sometimes rupture, producing calf pain, and may then mimic a deep vein thrombosis. When intact, large posterior knee cysts can sometimes cause venous obstruction.

The movements of the knee are flexion and extension (Fig. 9.41). Loss of flexion can be documented by loss of the angle of flexion or loss of heel-to-buttock distance, either in the crouching position or on the couch. Loss of extension is detected by inability to get the back of the knee on to the flat examining couch. Hyperextension must be sought by lifting the foot with the knee extended and comparing with the normal side. Lack of full extension by comparison with the normal constitutes fixed flexion deformity. Loose bodies in the joint cause crepitus, interruption of movement (locking) and pain and effusion (Fig. 9.42).

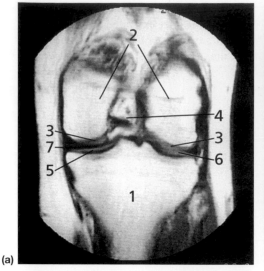

(a)

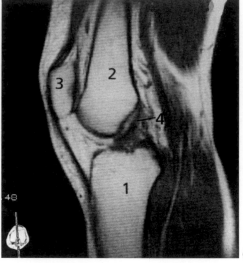

(b)

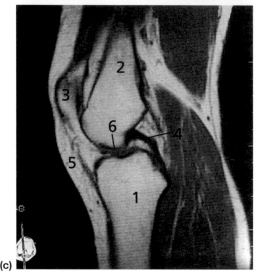

(c)

Figure 9.40 MRI scans of the normal knee (MR image, T$_1$-weighted). **(a)** Scan to show the medial (5) and lateral (6) menisci, origin of the anterior cruciate ligament (4) and the articular cartilages (3) and synovial fluid (7). Other structures: (1) tibia, (2) articular surfaces of femur. **(b)** The anterior cruciate ligament (4). Other structures: (1) tibia, (2) femur, (3) patella. **(c)** The posterior cruciate ligament (4). Other structures: (1) tibia, (2) femur, (3) patella, (5) patellar tendon, (6) joint space.

TESTING FOR STABILITY

Test the stability of the joint by stressing the medial and lateral ligaments, first with the knee in full extension (abnormal motion is due to lax posterior structures) and then in 20° of flexion. Abnormal motion in flexion is due to laxity of the collateral ligaments. With the knee flexed and the foot fixed on the couch by seating your buttock lightly against the patient's toes, check that the hamstrings are relaxed and then try to pull the tibia forward towards you. Abnormal anterior translation implies damage to the anterior cruciate ligament, provided it can be shown that the tibia has not already fallen backwards because of a torn posterior cruciate ligament. Look across both knees similarly flexed to exclude this.

THE ANKLE

The neutral position is with the outer border of the foot at an angle of 90° with the leg, and midway between inversion and eversion. Observe the patient from behind in the standing position. With any long-standing ankle disorder there will be a loss of calf muscle bulk.

Look at the position of the foot with the patient standing. The heel may tilt outwards (*valgus deformity*) in subtalar joint damage. Inward (*varus deformity*) is much less common and usually not so painful. Flattening of the longitudinal arch of the foot also produces valgus at the heel, but the foot curves laterally as well because the change is in the midtarsal joints in addition to the subtalar joint.

The following movements should be tested (Fig. 9.43).

- Dorsiflexion: test with the knee in flexion and extension to exclude tight calf muscles
- Plantar flexion: place a finger on the head of the talus to be sure that it is moving. A hypermobile subtalar joint can mimic movement in an arthrodesed ankle.

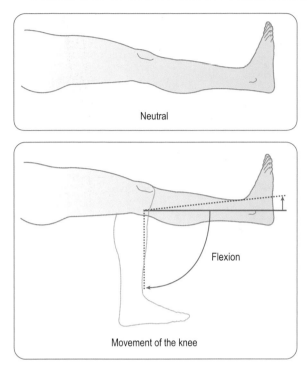

Neutral

Flexion

Movement of the knee

Figure 9.41 Movements of the knee.

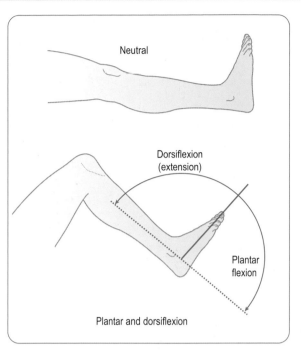

Neutral

Dorsiflexion (extension)

Plantar flexion

Plantar and dorsiflexion

Figure 9.43 Movements of the ankle.

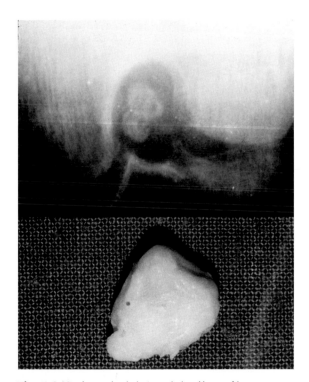

Figure 9.42 Loose body in tunnel view X-ray of knee, showing the loose body in the intercondylar space.

THE FOOT

Remember that complaints apparently relating to the foot may be features of systemic disease, such as gout, or of referred vertebral problems such as a

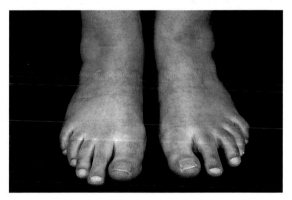

Figure 9.44 Daylight sign, due to metatarsophalangeal joint synovitis in rheumatoid arthritis.

prolapsed intervertebral disc. Look for abnormalities of posture.

Callosities are areas of hard skin under points of abnormal pressure. The most common site is beneath the metatarsal heads because loss of the normal soft tissue pad allows abnormal loading. There may be abnormal spread of two adjacent toes (daylight sign, Fig. 9.44) on weightbearing if there is a bursa between the metatarsal heads. Check for lateral deviation of the big toe (*hallux valgus*), usually associated with abnormal swelling at its base (*a bunion*). There may be deformities affecting any or all toes, with abnormal curvature (*claw toes*), fixed flexion of the terminal joint (*hammer toes*) or overriding.

The following movements should be tested (Fig. 9.45):

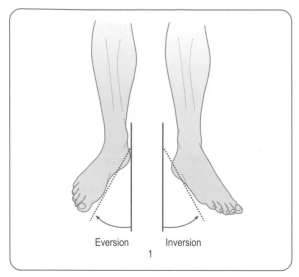

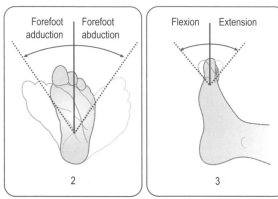

Figure 9.45 Movements of the foot.

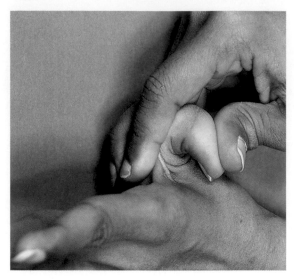

Figure 9.46 Hyperextensibility of the digits in Ehlers–Danlos syndrome.

- Subtalar inversion and eversion: cup the heel in the hands and move it in relation to the tibia without any up and down movement; this eliminates movement at the ankle or midtarsal joints
- Midtarsal inversion/eversion and adduction/abduction: hold the os calcis in the neutral position in one hand and grasp the forefoot in the other
- Metatarsophalangeal and interphalangeal flexion/extension.

Also look for tenderness at the Achilles tendon insertion on the back of the calcaneum and for plantar tenderness at the site of the plantar fascial insertion. Inflammation of these attachments (*enthesopathy*) is common in ankylosing spondylitis and Reiter's syndrome.

THE GAIT

It is best to study gait with the patient's legs and feet fully exposed and *without* shoes or slippers. Ask the patient to walk away from you, to turn around at a given point, and then to walk towards you.

Abnormalities of gait are usually due either to joint problems in the legs or to neurological disorder, although alcohol intoxication or malingering may occasionally cause difficulty. A full examination of the legs and feet should reveal any local cause, which may range from a painful corn to osteoarthritis of the hip. Abnormalities due to neurological disorders are described in Chapter 10.

HYPERMOBILITY

There is a wide variation in the range of normal joint movement, associated with age, sex and race. Excessive laxity or hypermobility of the joints (Fig. 9.46) can be defined in about 10% of healthy subjects and is frequently familial. It is also a feature of two inherited connective tissue disorders: Marfan's syndrome and Ehlers–Danlos syndrome. Repeated trauma, haemarthrosis or dislocation may produce permanent joint damage.

WORK-RELATED MUSCULOSKELETAL DISORDERS

Musculoskeletal pain arising as a result of the patient's occupation is an increasingly recognized cause of disability and economic loss. For example, spinal pain may commonly be ascribed to poor seating in sedentary occupations. Likewise, an occupational history of repetitive movements may be relevant to upper limb pain (*repetitive strain injury*). Assessment by an occupational health physician and an occupational therapist may be needed to consider workplace alterations.

INVESTIGATIONS IN THE RHEUMATIC DISEASES

When a full history and examination have been completed, investigations should be considered to support the working diagnosis or to distinguish between different possible diagnoses. They can broadly be defined as:

- Tests in support of inflammatory disease
- Diagnostic tests including biopsies and radiological investigations.

TESTS IN SUPPORT OF INFLAMMATORY DISEASE

The following acute-phase reactant tests are used in the assessment of inflammatory disease activity and in the subsequent monitoring of the patient.

- *Erythrocyte sedimentation rate (ESR)*. This is a useful screening test, although it has poor specificity, being affected by the levels of haemoglobin, globulins and fibrinogen. Higher mean values are also seen in elderly patients. Automation makes this a relatively cheap test.
- *C-reactive protein (CRP)*. This is a more specific indicator of inflammation and is a good marker of the acute-phase response. A high ESR with a normal CRP is a useful pointer towards connective tissue diseases, especially SLE.
- *Plasma viscosity*. This is a more specific measure of the acute phase response than ESR, but may not be as widely available.
- *Anaemia and thrombocytosis*. Anaemia of chronic disease and a high platelet count often occur in inflammatory disease but are non-specific. Other abnormalities on blood count, such as neutropenia, thrombocytopenia and lymphopenia, are common in SLE.
- *Serum complement*. Low levels of serum complement reflect activation due to immune complex deposition; this may be a marker of disease activity in autoimmune diseases such as SLE. Hereditary complement deficiencies are also associated with SLE.

DIAGNOSTIC TESTS

Diagnostic tests differentiate between specific diseases and are relatively specific investigations.

TESTS FOR RHEUMATOID FACTOR
Rheumatoid factors are autoantibodies in the form of immunoglobulin (Ig) directed against other immunoglobulin G (IgG) molecules. IgM rheumatoid factor can be detected by its ability to clump particles coated with human IgG (*latex test*). This test is positive in about 80% of patients with rheumatoid arthritis. Results are reported as a titre, 1 in 80 or higher being a positive result. The *Rose–Waaler haemagglutination* test used sheep erythrocytes coated with rabbit IgG to detect IgM (titres of 1 in 32 or more are positive); it has now been replaced by other tests. ELISA (enzyme-linked immunosorbent serum assay) techniques are much more sensitive, but produce positive results in many other conditions. Antibodies to cyclic citrullinated peptide (anti-CCP) have emerged as a specific marker for rheumatoid arthritis.

These rheumatoid factor screening tests are useful where a diagnosis of rheumatoid arthritis is suspected, but they are not specific. Rheumatoid factor is frequently found in patients with other connective tissue diseases, for example systemic lupus erythematosus and Sjögren's syndrome, or other inflammatory disorders such as subacute bacterial endocarditis and some viral infections.

ANTINUCLEAR ANTIBODY TESTS
Antinuclear antibody (ANA), often referred to as antinuclear factor (ANF), is a very useful screening test for SLE as it is positive in up to 95% of patients. It is, however, non-specific, being positive in many other connective tissue disorders, including about 20% of patients with rheumatoid arthritis. A positive test in children with arthritis may be associated with chronic iridocyclitis, which is frequently asymptomatic. Slit-lamp examination of the eye is mandatory to confirm the diagnosis.

The ANA test is carried out by incubating the patient's serum with frozen sections of normal tissue (usually rat liver). After washing, a fluorescent antiserum to human IgG is used to detect human antibody adhering to the nuclear antigens. A titre of 1 in 80 or more is significant; adequate standardization is important.

DNA-BINDING TEST
Different immunochemical techniques (Farr assay or ELISA) may be used to detect antibodies to native, double-stranded DNA. Another method is indirect immunofluorescence using the protozoon *Crithidia luciliae*, where the kinetoplast at the tail containing DNA fluoresces. The test is usually reserved for patients with a positive ANA test and is specific for SLE but not as sensitive as ANA. Occasionally it is positive in patients in whom the clinical suspicion of SLE is very high but the ANA test is negative.

ANTIBODY TESTS TO EXTRACTABLE NUCLEAR ANTIGENS (ENA)
These tests may be suggested by a particular type of pattern of staining (*speckled*) in the routine ANA test. They can be summarized in terms of their clinical association as follows:

- *Anti-Ro (SSA)* and *anti-La (SSB)*, typically in Sjögren's syndrome. Also seen in SLE, where they are associated with photosensitivity, and the neonatal lupus syndrome, which may result in congenital heart block and neonatal rashes.
- *Anti-Sm* in 5–10% of patients with SLE: a very specific marker if present.
- *Anti-RNP* (ribonucleoprotein) in some cases of SLE. Also picks out a group of patients who often have a mixed picture of connective tissue disorder and who are therefore often diagnosed as MCTD (*mixed connective tissue disease*). The test can be considered a marker for the combination of clinical features, but the major clinical component of the condition will define management.
- *Anticentromere antibody* is found in 'CREST syndrome' (calcinosis, Raynaud's phenomenon, oesophageal symptoms, sclerodactyly and telangiectasis) and some patients with scleroderma. Often a good prognostic marker.
- *Anti-Scl 70 (DNA topoisomerase I) and anti-RNA polymerase* are found in scleroderma and often associated with severe disease.

Other antibodies used in diagnostic tests include the following:

- *Antineutrophil cytoplasmic antibodies* are a marker for vasculitic conditions. Two immunofluorescence staining patterns occur:
  - cytoplasmic or c-ANCA, with specificity for proteinase 3 (a neutrophil enzyme), is very specific for Wegener's granulomatosis (Fig. 9.47)
  - perinuclear or p-ANCA, with specificity for myeloperoxidase (and some other neutrophil enzymes), occurs in other vasculitic diseases (and inflammatory bowel disease)

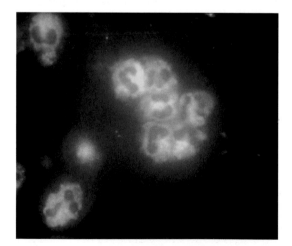

Figure 9.47 Antineutrophil cytoplasmic autoantibodies with cytoplasmic staining (cANCA). This pattern has a high predictive value for a diagnosis of Wegener's granulomatosis.

- *Antiphospholipid antibodies* in high titre may be associated with a syndrome characterized by arterial and venous thromboses (including cerebral infarction), thrombocytopenia and, in women, recurrent pregnancy loss and pregnancy morbidity (*antiphospholipid syndrome*). This antibody may be associated with SLE and called *anticardiolipin antibody* or *lupus anticoagulant*, despite the association with thromboses. A false positive VDRL may also be found in these patients.
- *Anti-Jo 1 (histidyl t-RNA synthetase)* is a marker for the idiopathic inflammatory myopathies such as dermatomyositis and polymyositis, especially when complicated by interstitial lung disease.
- *Human leukocyte antigen (HLA) typing*: The association of tissue antigen HLA-B27 with ankylosing spondylitis remains the strongest association in medicine. Although about 95% of ankylosing spondylitis patients in the UK possess the B27 antigen, it is also found in 8% of the normal population. Ankylosing spondylitis therefore remains a clinical diagnosis, supported by typical radiographic findings. However, in early disease, in children with peripheral arthritis or where the clinical findings are atypical HLA-B27, typing may provide supportive diagnostic value.
- *Antistreptolysin-O (ASO) test*: the presence in the serum of this antibody in a titre greater than 1/200, rising on repeat testing after about 2 weeks, indicates a recent haemolytic streptococcal infection.
- *Viral titres.* Certain viruses, notably parvovirus and Coxsackie virus, may cause transient musculoskeletal symptoms which may be mistaken for systemic diseases. Rising viral titres may be useful in the differential diagnosis.

URIC ACID

A consistently normal plasma uric acid level (<375 mmol/L in women, <425 mmol/L in men) usually excludes the diagnosis of untreated gout. Raised levels occur in many circumstances and do not in themselves establish the diagnosis of gout (see below). On a low-purine diet the 24-hour urinary urate excretion should not exceed 600 mg. Higher levels indicate 'overproduction' of urate and a risk of renal stone formation.

SYNOVIAL FLUID EXAMINATION

Synovial fluid may be obtained for examination from any joint in which it is clinically detectable. The knee is the most convenient source: after infiltration with a local anaesthetic a 21-gauge needle is inserted into the joint on its medial aspect between the patella and the femoral condyle. The aspirated fluid should be placed in a plain sterile container; if a cell count is required, some of the fluid should be mixed with ethylenediaminetetra-acetic acid (EDTA) anticoagulant.

An injured joint can also be aspirated (Box 9.11). The joint swollen after injury may reveal clear pink fluid suggesting a *meniscal lesion*, or show frank blood. The latter is usually indicative of a *torn anterior cruciate ligament*. If blood is aspirated, look at its surface for fat globules. This is derived from the marrow and confirms an intra-articular fracture. Synovial fluid examination is diagnostic in two conditions, *bacterial infections* and *crystal synovitis*, and every effort should be made to obtain fluid when either of these is suspected. Polarized light microscopy can differentiate between the crystals of urate in gout and those of calcium pyrophosphate dihydrate in pseudogout. Outside these conditions, synovial fluid examination is unlikely to be diagnostic. Frank blood may point to trauma, haemophilia or villonodular synovitis, whereas inflammatory (as opposed to degenerative) arthritis is suggested by opaque fluid of low viscosity, with a total white cell count >1000/mL, neutrophils >50%, protein content >35 g/L, and the presence of a firm clot. Culture of this fluid may produce a bacterial growth, usually of staphylococci, but occasionally *Mycobacterium tuberculosis* or other organisms.

BIOPSIES USEFUL IN DIFFERENTIAL DIAGNOSIS

The following biopsies may be useful in the differential diagnosis of rheumatic diseases:

- *Synovial biopsy* is of little value in the differential diagnosis of inflammatory polyarthritis, but should be considered in any unusual monoarthritis to exclude infection, particularly tuberculous, or rare conditions such as sarcoid or amyloid arthropathy, or villonodular synovitis.
- *Rectal biopsy* can be useful in the diagnosis of amyloidosis secondary to chronic inflammatory disease, but renal biopsy may still be necessary if the cause of renal impairment is not clear.
- *Renal biopsy* is essential in the vasculitides or SLE where active glomerulonephritis is suspected. Vasculitis may also be confirmed on

renal biopsy, but in general tissues found to be abnormal on clinical examination or by further investigation (e.g. skin, muscle, sural nerve or liver) should be considered first for diagnostic biopsy in undifferentiated systemic vasculitis.
- *Biopsy of a lip minor salivary gland* may be useful to confirm Sjögren's syndrome.
- *Temporal artery biopsy* is often diagnostic in patients with clinical features of temporal (giant cell) arteritis. This is the investigation of choice.

RADIOLOGICAL EXAMINATION

Certain general principles are important, particularly as all doctors are likely to be asked to give an opinion on X-rays of bones and limbs after traumatic injury, whether minor or more serious (Box 9.12). Common problems are shown in Figures 9.48–9.51. A systematic approach is essential (Box 9.13).

Bone density (Table 9.1) may be normal, reduced (osteopenia) or increased (osteosclerosis). These changes are easy to detect if focal, but difficult if diffuse. When a focal bone lesion (Box 9.14) is noted, look at its position in the bone and at its margins, and note whether there is any focal matrix calcification, whether the cortex of the bone is intact, and whether there is any periosteal reaction around it. Most solitary bone lesions in young people are benign and show no periosteal reaction or swelling around them, and no associated soft tissue swelling. Aggressive (malignant) bone lesions are more common in the elderly. Certain bone metastases have a characteristic appearance (Box 9.15). Isotope imaging is useful in detecting multiple sites of bony involvement in generalized disease and in metastatic cancer. CT imaging is also sensitive in detecting and analysing bony lesions, as it provides good images of the bony margins of the lesions and of the associated soft tissues. MRI is used to assess the extent of the lesion and any local soft tissue invasion.

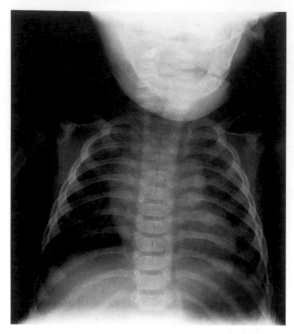

Figure 9.48 Healed fracture of posterior left and right ribs in a 6-month-old infant, classic non-accidental injury (NAI).

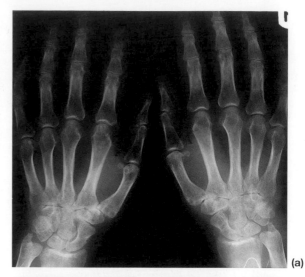

(a)

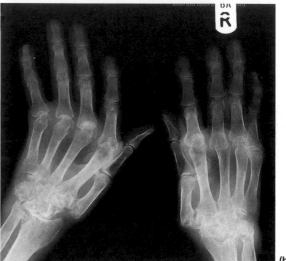

(b)

Figure 9.50 **(a)** Early rheumatoid arthritis: local osteopenia, loss of joint spaces, soft tissue swelling. **(b)** Late rheumatoid arthritis: erosion of periarticular surfaces and ulnar subluxation.

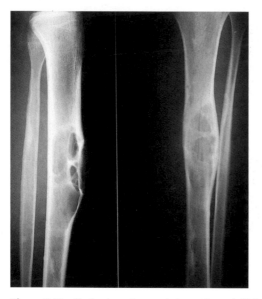

Figure 9.49 Benign bone tumour (adamantinoma). Note the solitary well-defined lucent lesion with a sclerotic margin, and the absence of matrix calcification.

FRACTURES

X-rays are often the first investigation in suspected fractures and in joint disease. In traumatic fractures X-rays are diagnostic and are used to check alignment of the fracture and healing. X-rays of a fracture are also important in excluding pathological fracture associated with metabolic bone disease, a focal benign bone lesion, or neoplastic invasion by metastases. When there is clinical doubt after a non-diagnostic X-ray, an MR scan often reveals the underlying fracture and is the investigation of choice. Radiographs taken to confirm or exclude a fracture must be taken in two planes. It is essential that either the whole limb is turned or the imaging equipment rotated. The limb must not be twisted at the fracture site. When looking for a fracture, run a pen tip or its equivalent around the cortex of the bone as seen on the film (without leaving marks). Any break in continuity will reveal itself; do not confuse an epiphysis with a fracture. Note soft tissue swelling and distension of joints. Always seek a radiology opinion if in doubt.

Table 9.1 Abnormal bone density

Generalized osteopenia	Generalized osteosclerosis	Benign focal lucent lesions	Benign focal sclerotic lesions
Ageing osteoporosis	Osteopetrosis (marble bone disease)	Simple bone cyst, aneurysmal bone cyst	Bone island
	Metastatic bone disease, e.g. prostate and breast cancer	Fibrous cortical defect	Callus after fracture
Disuse, e.g. trauma and neurogenic paralysis Osteogenesis imperfecta	Dietary causes, e.g. hypervitaminosis A, fluorosis	Non-ossifying fibroma	Paget's disease of bone
Acquired metabolic bone disease, e.g. rickets, osteomalacia, hyperparathyroidism	Acquired metabolic bone disease, e.g. renal osteodystrophy	Enchondroma	Bone infarction Osteoid osteoma
Myeloma	Myelofibrosis, sickle cell disease	Fibrous dysplasia, giant cell tumour of bone	Fibrous dysplasia

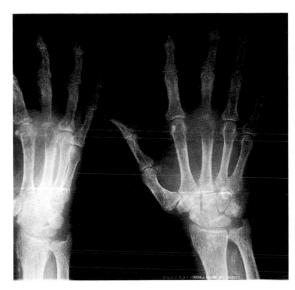

Figure 9.51 Renal osteodystrophy: generalized demineralization, terminal phalangeal and subperiosteal bone resorption and vascular calcification.

Box 9.13 Systematic approach to musculoskeletal imaging

- Bone density
- Soft tissues
- Joints
- Bone
- Periosteum

Box 9.14 Benign and malignant bone lesions

Benign	Malignant
Young person	Older age
Single lesion	Multiple lesions
Well-defined margin	Poorly defined margin
Intact cortex	Destroyed cortex
No periosteal reaction	Periosteal reaction
No growth	Soft tissue extension of lesion
Asymptomatic	Lesions painful

Box 9.15 Bone metastases

- Expansile – thyroid, kidney, breast, bronchus, melanoma and myeloma
- Sclerotic – prostate and breast
- Lytic – breast, bronchus, kidney, thyroid and melanoma
- Mixed – breast, bladder, or previously treated (irradiated) bone lesions

In joint disease MRI is the imaging method of choice because it can visualize all the soft tissue components of the joints. Osteopenia is a non-specific feature of disuse, but occurs in relation to affected joints in rheumatoid arthritis and Still's disease of children. Involvement of the distal interphalangeal joint is a feature of psoriatic arthropathy. In rheumatoid disease the involvement of joints is usually symmetrical, and the wrist is particularly susceptible.

Only radiographs likely to yield specific information should be requested. However, in unilateral

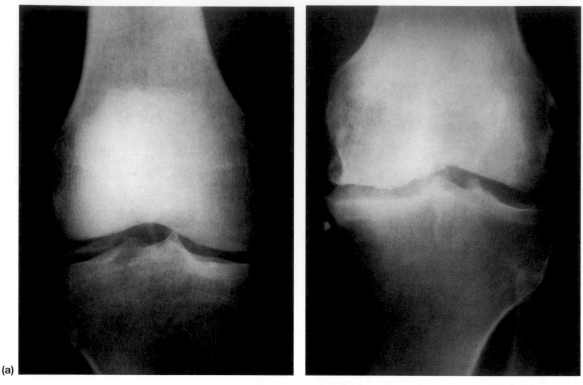

(a)   **(b)**

Figure 9.52   Left and right knee joints. The X-rays show normal joint anatomy but with chondrocalcinosis **(a)** and osteoarthritic change **(b)** on the opposite side. Note the increased bone density and narrowing of the joint space.

joint disease it is useful to examine both sides for comparison (Fig. 9.52(a) and (b)). In patients with inflammatory polyarthritis three routine films are helpful in the diagnosis and assessment of progression: *both hands and wrists* on one plate, *both feet* on another, to compare bone density and to look for periosteal reaction or erosive change, and one of the full *pelvis* (Fig. 9.53) to show the sacroiliac and hip joints. In the absence of so-called 'red flag signs', e.g. weight loss, night pain, fevers, neurological signs, most spinal radiographs are unnecessary.

ARTHROGRAPHY

Injection of contrast medium into the knee joint can be used to confirm the diagnosis of a ruptured popliteal cyst, although ultrasound will demonstrate this non-invasively as well as demonstrating the patency of the popliteal venous system when distinguishing a popliteal cyst from deep venous thrombosis. A double-contrast technique can be used to demonstrate abnormalities of the knee menisci. MRI has largely superseded this technique.

SPECIALIZED RADIOLOGY

The following imaging techniques can provide precise information about localized pathology but are dependent on the clinician making a clear diagnostic request:

- *High-resolution ultrasound* is of value in defining soft tissue structures, including muscles and tendons, and provides an excellent means for guiding aspiration and biopsy procedures. It is also being used in the early detection of bone oedema and erosions in rheumatoid arthritis.
- *Computed tomography (CT).* The combination of superior tissue contrast and tomographic technique permits definition of soft tissue structures obscured by overlapping structures, including intervertebral discs and other joints normally difficult to visualize, such as sacroiliac (Fig. 9.54), sternoclavicular and subtalar.
- *MRI* has unique advantages in evaluating the musculoskeletal system, but it is vital that the clinician define the pathology suspected, as correct positioning and sequence selection (T weighting) are vital in optimizing image quality. MRI is increasingly used to image the major joints in the limbs, especially the knee (see Fig. 9.40), hip, shoulder and elbow. Enhancement by the use of intravenous paramagnetic contrast (e.g. gadolinium) has further improved definition in spinal imaging and in documenting early synovitis. It is of particular value in the non-invasive investigation of disc disease (Fig. 9.55), including spinal infection, and is generally felt to be the most sensitive technique for the diagnosis of avas-

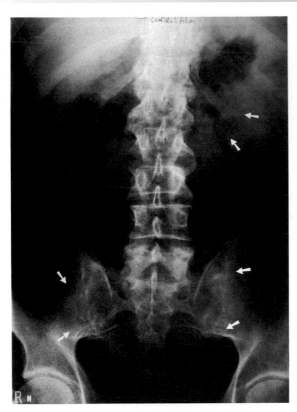

Figure 9.53 X-ray of lumbosacral spine and upper pelvis. There is fusion of several vertebrae, and of the sacroiliac joints (arrows) from ankylosing spondylitis. The renal papillae on the left are calcified, evidence of previous papillary necrosis from analgesic abuse.

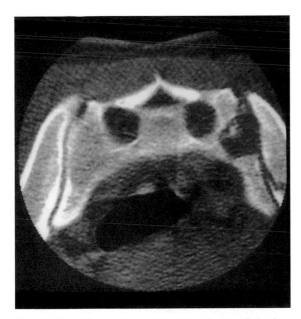

Figure 9.54 CT scan of sacroiliac joints, showing distinctive lesion on the left side with a sequestrum due to tuberculosis.

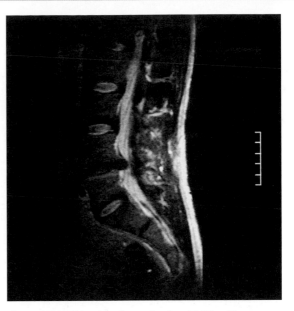

Figure 9.55 There is a disc protrusion at L4/5, with degeneration of the disc itself, shown by the less bright signal in the intervertebral disc at this level.

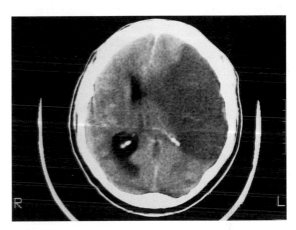

Figure 9.56 CT head showing left middle cerebral artery (MCA) territory infarction. There is a large wedge of low attenuation extending through white and grey matter and involving the basal ganglia, indicating an infarct of at least 24–48 hours' duration. Such infarcts may occur in the antiphospholipid syndrome.

cular necrosis. MR scanning of the brain and spine is the single most important investigation in neuroimaging, as the neural tissues themselves, together with supporting tissues, are well visualized. Bone is less well seen with this technique, however. As a rule of thumb, most abnormalities appear dark on T_1-weighted images and white on T_2-weighted images. Some common problems are

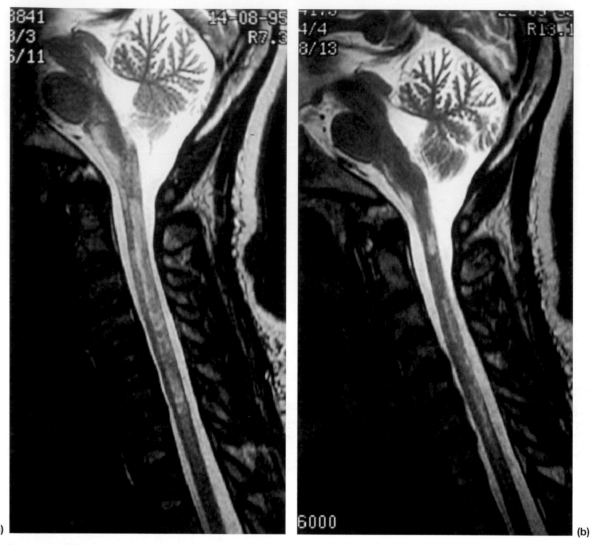

(a)   **(b)**

Figure 9.57   MRI of cervical spine in a patient with transverse myelitis due to SLE **(a)** before and **(b)** after immunosuppression.

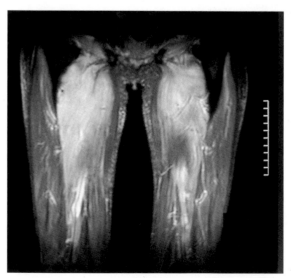

Figure 9.58   MRI scan of thigh muscles showing high signal lesions of inflammatory myositis.

shown in Figures 9.56, 9.57. In inflammatory myopathies, MRI may guide muscle biopsy to increase the diagnostic yield. (Fig. 9.58)

- *Isotopic scanning* (scintigraphy) can be used in the diagnosis of acute (e.g. infection or stress fracture) or multiple (e.g. metastases) bone lesions by use of the first 2-minute (dynamic blood flow) phase, second 10-minute (blood pool) and third 3-hour late phase (osteoblastic) (Fig. 9.59) following intravenous injection of diphosphonate compounds. Tomographic scintigraphy can further refine definition of the isotope uptake (e.g. in stress fracture of the pars interarticularis).

- *DEXA (dual energy X-ray absorptiometry)* is widely used to assess bone mineral density in metabolic bone disease and osteoporosis. Interval scans may be used to assess the effects of therapy.

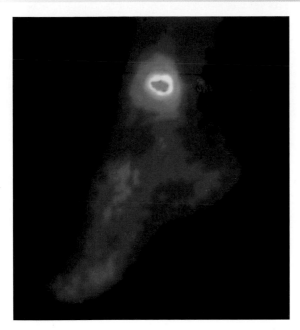

Figure 9.59 Technetium bone scan in a distance runner, showing focally increased uptake in the lower tibia owing to a stress fracture.

- *Positron emission tomography (PET)* scanning is becoming more widely available but remains expensive. It is extremely sensitive in detecting malignancy and is also proving useful in documenting large vessel inflammation in disorders such as Takayasu's arteritis, and more recently in giant cell arteritis.

10 Nervous system

J. McAuley, M. Swash

INTRODUCTION

The variety of presentations of neurological disease requires a rigorous technique to allow diagnostic analysis. The bedside examination provides objective data that can be used to *localize* pathology, and the clinical history gives clues as to the *nature* of this pathology. Many medical specialties use a 'pattern recognition' approach to diagnosis, in which groups of symptoms and signs are considered together as a *disease syndrome*. This is less reliable in neurological practice. As in any medical consultation the clinical history is taken first, thereby setting the scene, and the examination follows. However, it is often important subsequently to review the history and to reinterpret it in relation to the physical findings.

Clinical method in neurology is a three-stage process, designed to formulate a plan of investigation and management:

1. Take a careful and comprehensive *history*.
2. Perform a physical *examination*, focusing on the relevant nervous system function as determined by the history. Then carry out a basic screening examination of the nervous system and a brief general examination.
3. In *formulating* a diagnosis, a more focused history may suggest the nature of the pathology.

The approach is illustrated in Table 10.1. The presenting complaints may direct the clinician to a subsystem, the examination localizes the lesion and the pattern of the history of the presenting complaints suggests the nature of the underlying pathology. In other instances, the presenting symptoms suggest a distinct disease syndrome that may be corroborated by features found on examination. A potential pitfall of the pattern recognition approach is illustrated by the first instance in Table 10.1. The appearance of a weak face involving the eye closure muscles, cheek and lips might suggest Bell's palsy, but focused examination here also reveals a partial sixth-nerve palsy; review of the history revealed an abrupt onset and hence a likely vascular aetiology. The diagnosis in this case was localized haematoma due to a brainstem vascular malformation.

This deductive, focused approach to the clinical problem should be combined with a screening examination of the rest of the nervous system – and indeed of the other body systems – to look for additional clues, e.g. hypertension, perhaps unnoticed by the patient. Sometimes the presenting complaint is unhelpful in directing the examination. A general neurological examination is then particularly important in delineating the responsible lesion or lesions. The clinician should always seek to explain all the clinical manifestations by a single lesion, or by as few separate lesions as possible – the principle of 'Occam's razor'.

Sometimes, despite accurate identification of a functional lesion, it is not possible to make a definite diagnosis. A full differential diagnosis should then be used to generate a plan of investigation and management. A good differential diagnosis always lists the most likely diagnoses first. The neurological history and examination should identify the lesion site; for example, a spastic paraparesis implies spinal cord pathology, and the history will suggest the most likely pathology (see Table 10.1). MRI and CT scanning have transformed neurological diagnosis and refined clinical method. As imaging is rarely available instantly, however, decisions on treatment must usually be made on clinical information alone. Furthermore, it is essential to use clinical information appropriately in deciding which part of the body to image. For example, it is a common mistake to image the lumbosacral spine in a patient with gait problems which, on examination, reflect pyramidal weakness: the spinal cord terminates at T12. A poor clinical examination may result in a differential diagnosis that is wide, unfocused or wrong.

Finally, when assessing patients the clinician must always bear in mind that the objective is treatment, not simply diagnosis. Assessment of the patient's level of disability and handicap is therefore important. For example, rather than simply recording visual acuity and funduscopic appearance, the doctor must consider whether the patient is entitled to be registered blind or whether their vision satisfies driving regulations. Can the patient communicate effectively verbally or in writing? Is swallowing sufficient for nutritional requirements? Can they walk freely outdoors or indoors, and can they

Table 10.1 History and examination in neurological diagnosis

Presenting complaint	Focus upon subsystem	Examination	History of complaint	Diagnosis
Weak right face	→ Cranial nerves	Right lower motor neuron seventh-nerve palsy, partial right sixth-nerve palsy ⇒ right pontine lesion	Sudden onset at age 60 Subacute onset at age 30	→ Brainstem stroke (vascular lesion) in right pons → Demyelinating lesion in right pons
Unilateral visual loss	→ Eye	Disc swelling, impaired colour vision	Gradual onset over several days at age 20 Sudden onset at age 70	→ Optic neuritis → Giant cell arteritis
Weakness of left arm and leg	→ Motor system	Left spastic hemiparesis	Sudden onset at age 70 Gradual onset at age 50	→ Right hemisphere or capsular stroke → Right hemisphere tumour
Walking difficulty	→ Motor and sensory systems of limbs	Spastic paraparesis with mid-cervical motor, sensory and reflex levels	Gradual onset at age 70 Subacute, relapsing and remitting disease at age 30	→ Cervical spondylotic myelopathy, cervical spine tumour → Multiple sclerosis
Weak left foot	→ Left leg	Weak left ankle in plantarflexion, absent ankle jerk, absent sensation left sole	Sudden onset at age 30, back pain Sudden onset after intramuscular injection to buttock	→ Acute left S1 root lesion, probably L5/S1 disc prolapse → Trauma to left sciatic nerve
Intermittent ptosis and swallowing problems	→ Suggests *pattern* of myasthenia	Fatiguability confirms	Variable severity	→ Myasthenia gravis
Familial progressive ptosis, cramping and weakness of hand muscles	→ Suggests *pattern* of myotonic dystrophy	Myopathic facies and percussion myotonia confirm	Slowly progressive over several years	→ Myotonic dystrophy
Slowness of gait and small handwriting	→ Suggests *pattern* of parkinsonism	Bradykinesia, rigidity and tremor confirm	Gradually progressive	→ Parkinson's disease

transfer from bed to commode? Can they attend to their toileting needs? Is activity limited by pain or depressed mood? All these questions are important in directing ongoing management, particularly as long-term neurological disability is common.

THE NEUROLOGICAL HISTORY

The history sets the scene. First, it identifies the likely region or neurological subsystem involved. Second, a more detailed history is helpful (Box 10.1). The temporal development of the complaint, assessed in the context of age, past history and family history, is often helpful in revealing the nature of the pathology localized by examination. For example, a pattern of deterioration followed by steady improvement argues against progressive pathology such as a brain or spinal tumour, whereas acute deterioration suggests the need for rapid investigation and intervention. Thus, certain clinical patterns suggest certain pathologies (Box 10.2). In some circumstances, particularly when the history is of disturbed consciousness or disturbed cognition, or when the patient's main complaint is difficulty with communication, it may be important to *talk to an observer or family member* to find out more. In the case of cognitive disturbance, a patient complaining of poor memory often simply has poor concentration owing to mood problems, whereas if a relative is complaining of a patient's poor memory this more usually suggests that the patient has dementia. Finally, a series of screening questions should be asked once all the presenting complaints have been discussed in case an important aspect was forgotten or not considered.

The general guidelines shown in Box 10.3 can be applied with flexibility in most circumstances. In two common neurological syndromes, headache and seizures, the history is especially important as the examination may be normal. These syndromes have therefore been chosen to provide examples of the use of such guidelines in practice (Tables 10.2, 10.3).

Box 10.1 Key points in neurological history

- Cognitive disturbance
- Episodes of loss of consciousness
- Vision
- Hearing
- Speech, swallowing
- Arms, handwriting
- Legs, walking
- Involuntary movements
- Bladder, bowel function
- Pain

THE NEUROLOGICAL EXAMINATION

The physical examination is much more likely to be efficient and thorough if a strict routine is followed. It is traditional for the examiner to start rostrally and proximally, and to work caudally and distally. Thus, the examination may start with conscious level and cognitive state, and end with walking or assessment of sphincters. What really matters is to use a method that is familiar. The 'focused examination', directed by the particular presenting complaints found on history taking, should not disturb this routine. When the focused part of the examination is finished, switch into 'screening mode' and check the remaining aspects of the nervous system. The recommended minimum screening examination performed in a traditional sequence is shown in Box 10.4.

A neurological examination requires practice and experience. The examination should be reliable and the examiner must know the range of normality:

Box 10.2 Various pathologies suggested by clinical pattern

Pattern of onset and development	Pathology
Sudden	Traumatic, vascular, psychogenic
Acute on chronic	Exacerbation of pre-existing pathology (e.g. cervical spondylosis and disc prolapse, syringomyelia, bleeding into an intrinsic brain or spinal tumour)
Subacute	Infective, inflammatory
Chronic and steadily progressive	Malignant tumours
Chronic and indolent	Benign tumours, degenerative (e.g. spondylotic, neurodegenerative), genetic
Relapsing–remitting	Inflammatory, rarely infective
Stepwise	Vasculitic, inflammatory, multiple strokes
Previous episodes in other neurological systems	Multifocal inflammatory (e.g. multiple sclerosis), hysterical

---

Box 10.3 Scheme of neurological history-taking

Aspect of history	Examples
1. Region(s) or subsystem(s) involved	Vision, swallowing, limbs, gait and stance. (Once listed, screen for other subsystems (Box 10.4))
2. Temporal aspects	Onset, duration, improving or progressing?, periodicity (More detail in Box 10.2)
3. Character, severity	Negative symptoms (e.g. numbness, paralysis) or positive symptoms (e.g. pain, jerking), a pulsing or tight headache, mild urgency or frank incontinence
4. Causative and relieving factors	Headache on coughing, leg pain relieved by rest
5. Associated factors	Symptoms that occur together in attacks, e.g. nausea, sweating, diarrhoea
6. Disability resulting from symptom	Unable to work, unable to feed oneself
7. General health, past history	Other symptoms, weight change, mood
8. Family history	Autosomal dominant pattern of inheritance
9. Medication history, substance abuse, social history	Medication side effects, alcohol, cigarette smoking

only by identifying what is normal can one accurately identify what is abnormal. Clinical examination involves not only eliciting physical signs but also *interpreting* them. For example, carefully grading strength in every muscle group is of no diagnostic value, but the pattern of weakness observed is essential information. Is the weakness proximal, distal, corticospinal or radicular in distribution? There is no real substitute for a knowledge of neuroanatomy when interpreting signs and thereby localizing neurological disease.

LEVEL OF CONSCIOUSNESS

First consider the patient's level of consciousness, as this may determine what can be done with the rest of the examination or, in a head injury, indicate the need for urgent management. A number of terms referring to conscious level require definition to avoid ambiguity:

- *Coma* is an imprecise term, describing a state in which the patient's response to external stimuli or inner needs is grossly impaired. It is described

Table 10.2 History of seizures

Aspect of history	Feature	Diagnosis, classification and management
Region/subsystem	Twitching of one limb	Focal motor
	Positive sensory aura, e.g. flashing lights, taste	Focal, e.g. occipital, mesial temporal
	Generalized twitching and complete loss of consciousness	Generalized tonic–clonic
	Generalized twitching without loss of consciousness	Myoclonic, non-epileptic (hysterical)
	No loss of consciousness	Simple partial (focal)
	Partial loss of consciousness	Complex partial
Temporal aspects	Aura	Hallucinations of taste or smell may suggest complex partial seizures (temporal lobe epilepsy)
	Sudden onset	Suggests diagnosis of seizure
	Prolonged postictal tiredness, confusion	Suggests generalized tonic–clonic
	Evolving from focal to loss of consciousness	Focal onset, then generalized tonic–clonic seizure – suggests a focal lesion
Severity	Sustained or repeated without fully regaining consciousness between attacks	Status epilepticus
Causative factors	Flashing lights	Photosensitive epilepsy
	Dehydration, postural	Suggests faint or syncope, not seizure
	Intercurrent infection, illness	Pyrexia, metabolic insults
	Early morning occurrence	Idiopathic generalized epilepsy
	Night-time occurrence in childhood	Benign rolandic seizures
General health and past history	Weight loss, systemic features	Brain metastasis
	Focal fixed neurological symptoms	Focal onset symptomatic epilepsy
	Penetrating head injury	Known predisposing factor
	Febrile convulsions in infancy	Mesial temporal sclerosis
Family history	Autosomal dominant, frontal	Autosomal dominant nocturnal frontal lobe epilepsy
	Various patterns, no other features	Other idiopathic epilepsies
	Usually recessive, other features	Symptomatic epilepsies of metabolic diseases
Drug and social history	Stopping alcohol consumption	Alcohol withdrawal seizures
	Tricyclics, SSRIs, theophylline	Known predisposing agents
	Antiepileptic drugs	Record correct drugs, doses, compliance
	Pregnancy	Issues with antiepileptic drug side effects

Table 10.3   History of headache (more than one type may coexist)

Aspect of history	Feature	Diagnosis and classification
Region	Unilateral	Migraine or cluster headache
	Top of head	Tension-type headache
	Frontal	Sinusitis
Temporal aspects	More than 50% of days	Chronic daily headache
	Attacks of hours	Migraine
	Attacks of half an hour	Cluster headache
	Attacks of minutes	Paroxysmal hemicrania
	Attacks of seconds	Trigeminal neuralgia
	Worse on wakening	Raised intracranial pressure, sleep apnoea
	New subacute onset	Brain abscess, meningitis, encephalitis
	New explosive severe onset	Subarachnoid haemorrhage
Character and severity	Tight band around head	Tension-type headache
	Throbbing	Migraine
	Boring	Cluster headache
	Stabbing, shooting	Trigeminal neuralgia
Causative/relieving factors	Certain food, alcohol	Migraine
	Relieved by sleep	Migraine
	Certain time of day or night	Cluster headache
	Sudden head movements	Paroxysmal hemicrania
	Touching the face, chewing	Trigeminal neuralgia
	Coughing	Foramen magnum stenosis (rare)
	Brought on by standing	Low cerebrospinal fluid pressure headache
Associated factors	Focusing difficulty	Tension-type headache
	Fortification spectra in vision, photophobia, nausea	Migraine
	Sympathetic disturbance, tears	Cluster headache, hemicrania
	Photophobia, neck stiffness	Meningitis
	Focal fixed neurological symptoms	Intracranial lesion
Disability	Missed days from work, school	?Merits preventative medication
General health	Weight loss, haemoptysis, breast mass	Brain metastasis
	Fever	Brain abscess, meningitis
Familial history	Attacks of hemiparesis	Familial hemiplegic migraine
Medication, social history	'Stressful work'	Tension-type headache, migraine
	Excessive analgesia	'Analgesia headache'
	Medications already tried	Plan future management

in more detail in Chapter 21. The Glasgow Coma Scale (GCS) is used to assign a numerical value to the patient's responses to defined stimuli (Table 21.1). It is particularly useful for quantifying changes in conscious level over time, and can be assessed by nurses as well as doctors.

- *Stupor* describes a state where the patient, although inaccessible, shows some response to painful stimuli. It is better to use the GCS score.
- *Torpor* is a state of extreme psychiatric disturbance where the patient withdraws mentally from his or her surroundings.
- *Disorientation* means that the person is conscious but muddled in time, place and person.
- *Delirium* refers to disorientation, or dementia, occurring in the context of drowsiness, or clouding of consciousness, in which the patient

is more accessible than in stupor. This functional disorder is better assessed by orientation and by digit span than by GCS score.

- *Dementia* consists of impaired cognitive function in the setting of a normal conscious level – the patient is alert and awake, but with a generalized neuropsychiatric deficit.
- *Confusion* implies disorientation. An *acute confusional state* is a state of acute delirium. Dementia causing disorientation without delirium is often described as confusion.

ASSESSMENT

The conscious level is best assessed by observation while taking the history. Severe disturbance should be quantified by the GCS score, but delirium can be

---

Box 10.4   Comprehensive screening neurological examination

Conscious level and cognitive function (determined during history taking)
- Is the patient's conscious level clouded?
- Is the history given accurately, concisely and with insight? Or is the patient concrete, circumlocutory or vague?
- Is the patient neatly dressed and well cared for?
- Is the patient's behaviour normal?
- Is the patient aphasic or dysarthric?

Vision
- Acuity: For each eye, using normal refractive correction, test ability to read small and large print, or use Snellen chart if available. If this fails, test counting of fingers, perception of light.
- Visual fields: Test all four quadrants for each eye individually.
- Fundi: Check for papilloedema, optic atrophy, retinopathy.
- Pupils: Check equality and consensual and direct reactions to light and accommodation.

Eye movements
- Test both eyes together in 'H' pattern for range of movement and diplopia.
- Test both eyes together in '+' pattern for smooth pursuit and nystagmus.

Remainder of cranial nerves
- Nerve V: Pinprick on left and right in ophthalmic, maxillary and mandibular distributions; clenching of teeth; jaw jerk.
- Nerve VII: Appearance and symmetry; screwing up eyes against pressure, forcing lips closed against pressure, blink reflexes.
- Nerve VIII: Hear whispered numbers in each ear.
- Nerves IX and X: Ask patient to say 'ah' and observe palate.
- Nerve XI: Ask patient to shrug shoulders and move head to either side and flex against resistance while you observe sternomastoids.
- Nerve XII: Inspect tongue. Ask patient to protrude tongue and press against inside of cheek on either side.

Limbs and trunk
- *Inspection* for wasting, fasciculation, skin lesions.
- *Posture* of outstretched arms with wrists pronated and supinated, looking for drift, tremor, abnormal movements.
- *Tone* at wrist, elbows, knees and ankles, ankle clonus.
- *Power* of proximal, axial and distal muscles on both sides.
- *Co-ordination:* Finger–nose test; rapid alternating movements; heel–shin test.
- *Reflexes:* Deep tendon reflexes of biceps, supinator, triceps, fingers, quadriceps, gastrocnemius; plantar responses.
- *Sensation:* Test pinprick distally to proximally up arms and legs medially and laterally; and up trunk bilaterally, anteriorly and posteriorly. Vibration sense or joint position sense at little finger, great toe (moving proximally if failed).

Gait and stance
- Observe walking pattern.
- Standing still with feet together and eyes closed.
- Walking heel to toe.
- Jumping and hopping.

---

gauged objectively by the first parts of the Mini-Mental State Examination (MMSE; see Chapter 3), namely orientation and repetition. Digit span, where the patient must immediately repeat a series of numbers ('a telephone number') called out by the examiner, is a good test for delirium. Even a moderately severely demented patient will be able to repeat a six-digit number successfully. If a wide-awake patient without severe dementia fails this test, he or she may have a specific aphasia in the domain of repetition, or hysterical or depressive pseudodementia. Spelling 'world' forwards (preserved even in severe dementia) and then backwards (requiring concentration, organization and 'internal repetition') is another cognitive test relatively sensitive to mild states of delirium.

INTERPRETATION

Clouding of consciousness may result from acute diffuse cerebral dysfunction, e.g. in cerebral hypoperfusion, metabolic disease or encephalitis. Focal lesions of the thalamus, especially if medial and bilateral, can also cause delirium, and lesions of the brainstem reticular activating system cause a markedly impaired conscious level. Altered conscious level makes cognitive assessment largely redundant. There is little point in going through the whole MMSE if the patient cannot hold enough mental focus to repeat a six-digit number.

BEHAVIOUR AND EMOTIONAL STATE

During neurological history taking and examination attention should be paid to the patient's behaviour, demeanour and emotional state, not only because these may colour many of the neurological findings but because many psychiatric states are manifestations of organic brain disease.

COGNITIVE FUNCTION

ASSESSMENT

Cognitive function is tested clinically by means of the MMSE (Table 4.2). However, this test score (maximum 30) gives an indication of severity of dementia rather than the type of cognitive impairment. To investigate the latter, the framework of the MMSE should be expanded with further tests in the different domains of cognitive function. Some domains are *distributed* between different cerebral structures, whereas others tend to be *localized* to particular lobes of the hemispheres.

SPEECH AND LANGUAGE

Although speech may be dysarthric with cranial nerve or brainstem disease the assessment of speech and language is so important for understanding other aspects of cognitive function that it is better done first. It should be obvious while talking with the patient whether or not there is a major communication problem, and whether this is *dysphasia* (speech language problem), *dysarthria* (speech articulation problem) or *dysphonia* (impaired control of air flow). Ask the patient to recite the months of the year. If this simple request is not understood, it is likely there is a major dysphasia or cognitive problem. The large number of long words in the months, with their simple meaning, allows easy detection of a dysarthria or dysphonia.

Dysarthria

There are four main types of speech pronunciation problem:

- *Bulbar palsy.* Pronunciation of consonants is difficult. Ask the patient to repeat 'p', 't' and 'k' sounds, which respectively test for lip seal, tip of tongue movement against the upper gum, and movement of the back of the tongue to close off the larynx. A 'b' sound tests for vocal cord function. Other tests for unilateral or bilateral cranial nerve palsies (nerves VII, X and XII) may corroborate the abnormality.
- *Cerebellar dysarthria.* Speech is 'scanning' and robotic, with syllables pronounced individually

and slowly. Ask the patient to say 'Eye-ay' repeatedly; this will be abnormally slow in cerebellar disease. Corroborative tests include examination of smooth eye movements and coordination of the limbs.

- *Pseudobulbar palsy.* Speech is 'strangled' and spastic. Rapid changes in speech sounds, as required for tongue-twisters, are particularly difficult. 'British constitution' is pronounced 'Brizh Conshishushon'. There may be associated bilateral spasticity of the limbs, as bilateral lesions of the descending corticopontine (and perhaps the neighbouring corticospinal) pathways are necessary to produce a pseudobulbar palsy.
- *Dysphonia.* This is best tested by repeating a large number of sounds, such as the months of the year as described above. A quiet voice may result from poor ventilatory capacity. A fatiguing voice can occur in myasthenia or in parkinsonism.

Dysphasia

Cognitive assessment is dependent on language function: the different domains of language function require formal testing. Language is usually located in the left hemisphere (85% of people) (Fig. 10.1).

- *Comprehension.* Ask the patient to close their eyes without your making a prompting gesture. Then ask the patient to perform a two-component task not requiring verbal output, such as 'Touch your left elbow with your right index finger', or the three-stage command of the MMSE (see Table 4.2).
- *Fluency and prosody.* During your conversation consider whether the patient's word production is normal. Is word usage smooth and non-hesitant (word-finding disorder), and is there normal expressivity in word usage? It does not matter whether or not their speech makes any sense.
- *Repetition.* The only validated phrase to repeat is that in the MMSE: 'no ifs, ands, or buts'. Any other complex phrase can be used.
- *Naming.* Ask the patient to name common objects, e.g. the parts of a watch, or of a pen, or of clothing.
- *Reading and writing.* Use a written instruction – 'close your eyes' – and then ask the patient to write a sentence; this should be meaningful and should contain a verb and a noun.

Comprehension is an input function that localizes to the superior and lateral surfaces of the left temporal lobe. Output language functions, e.g. fluency and naming, localize to the adjacent lateral and inferior surfaces of the left frontal lobe (Fig. 10.2). Lesions in *Wernicke's area*, the posterior left perisylvian region (consisting of posterosuperior tem-

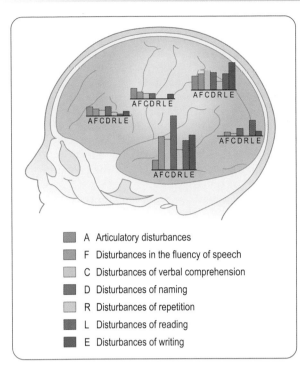

A Articulatory disturbances

F Disturbances in the fluency of speech

C Disturbances of verbal comprehension

D Disturbances of naming

R Disturbances of repetition

L Disturbances of reading

E Disturbances of writing

Figure 10.1 The average degree of disturbance of various language modalities that occurs when there is an isolated lesion of various lobes (frontal, rolandic, parietal, temporal and occipital).

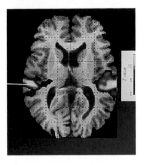

Figure 10.2 fMRI. Listening to words. When the subject listens to words both temporal lobes are activated, but the dominant left temporal lobe (to the right of the picture) is the more active.

poral, opercular, angular and posterior insular gyri), are associated with:

- Impaired comprehension of spoken and written language
- Fluent speech that is devoid of meaning (*jargon aphasia*)
- Hesitant speech, but typically only when the patient searches for the central word in the phrase essential for meaning. Other words and phrases are uttered fluently but often inappropriately (*paraphasia*)
- Unawareness of the speech deficit is characteristic
- Deficits in naming parallel the deficits in comprehension.

Broca's area consists of the posterior part of the inferior frontal gyrus; an ischaemic lesion here produces a more or less pure motor aphasia. There is inability to articulate word sounds even though the lips, tongue and pharynx function in other tasks. Writing is also impossible (*agraphia*). The aphasia improves to a state of effortful articulation (*speech dyspraxia*) and sometimes to complete recovery. In *speech dyspraxia* motor 'programmes' that encode the orofacial and bulbar muscular coordination for speech cannot be activated; this is sometimes called '*cortical dysarthria*'. The term *Broca's aphasia* is often also applied to a more severe motor aphasia *accompanied by subtle but definite compre-*

hension difficulties. The outcome in this syndrome is less good: there is only partial recovery, with persistent non-fluent dysphasia, a tendency to repeat utterances, and agrammatism (lack of use of small grammatical words but relatively preserved meaning). This dysphasia is accompanied by poor repetition and poor writing. The lesion here is larger, involving the inferior frontal gyrus and anterior insula and the deeper frontal white matter.

Global aphasia is a state of *mutism* or preserved ability to speak only a few stock phrases, combined with an inability to understand all but a few simple phrases. Partial recovery may occur. If it is due to stroke, the lesion is in the left middle cerebral artery territory.

Conduction aphasia is a specific inability to repeat phrases with normal fluency and comprehension. The causative lesion is in the interconnecting pathway between anterior frontal and temporal speech areas, in the arcuate fasciculus.

Transcortical aphasia leads to problems with comprehension or conveying meaning in speech. However, the patient can repeat phrases or song lyrics parrot-fashion. It occurs in severely brain-injured patients and with white matter lesions in vascular watershed territories that undercut the perisylvian language areas, isolating them from the rest of the brain.

Nominal aphasia is a component of many aphasias but is a rare isolated deficit. It tends to be a feature of tumours.

Organization and concentration

Spelling the word 'world' backwards is a good test of working memory.

MEMORY

Use the patient's history to test autobiographical memory, and specific questions, such as 'What did you do this morning?'; 'What did you last have to eat?'. You may feel the need to verify their responses, e.g. from a relative, to check that they are not confabulating (making up answers from retained islands of memory, often with an air of apparent certainty). However, this can usually be checked by assessing the internal consistency of the patient's answers. Remote memory, such as autobiographical events from the distant past or national historical events, is important because in all organic dementias remote memory is relatively preserved.

Memory deficits often relate to temporal lobe disease and are sometimes modality specific. Verbal memory is more impaired in dominant temporal disease and visual memory in non-dominant hemisphere disease. Bilateral mesial temporal lobe damage leads to memory loss, visual agnosia for objects, a tendency to explore objects by putting them in the mouth, indiscriminate sexual behaviour, especially to inanimate objects, and a flat affect (Kluver–Bucy syndrome), illustrating the importance of the temporal lobes in memory, language function and emotional behaviour. The latter is mediated through subcortical connections with the limbic system.

FRONTAL LOBE FUNCTIONS
The frontal lobes are important in the internal generation of ideas and actions, and in functions that computer programmers might term 'fuzzy logic', as opposed to generating responses to modality-specific external cues.

Tests of higher frontal lobe function include:

- *Abstractional ability*. Ask the patient the meaning of a well-known proverb, such as 'Too many cooks spoil the broth'. A *concrete interpretation*, characteristic of frontal lobe disease, might be 'too many cooks getting in each other's way', rather than 'a task is best performed by just the right people'.
- *Estimation*. With frontal disease judgemental estimates are inaccurate, e.g. guessing the distance to the nearest city or to another continent, or the height of famous buildings or mountains.
- *Self-cued lists*. 'How many animals whose names begin with the letter "c" can you recite in a minute?'. A normal person should achieve more than six.

The frontal areas are also important in high-level programming of motor tasks, termed *praxis*. Unilateral abnormalities generally lateralize to the contralateral frontal lobe, although certain *apraxias* on the opposite or both sides of the body can also result from a lesion in the dominant parietal lobe, or, if restricted to the non-dominant side, a lesion of the corpus callosum isolating this hemisphere from the opposite, dominant parietal lobe (*disconnexion syndrome*). Apraxia has major practical implications for neurological rehabilitation and is assessed in detail by occupational therapists.

Tests for frontal motor function include:

- *Simultaneous simple motor tasks*. Ask the patient to have one hand open, the other in a fist, and alternate the two positions simultaneously.
- *Limb-kinetic apraxia*. Ask the patient to copy various orientations of the fingers and thumb. A patient with frontal lobe disease may perform poorly despite the fact that there is little spasticity or incoordination on motor testing.
- *Ideomotor apraxia*. This refers specifically to gestures that have a meaning in terms of language. Ask the patient how they would blow a kiss, or thumb for a lift.
- *Ideational apraxia*. Sequencing of complex motor tasks is abnormal. Tests include the three-stage hand test (copying a sequence of hand gestures), performing a mime of a two-handed sequenced activity such as lighting a cigarette, or the three-stage command of the MMSE (provided language comprehension is normal). Finally, deficits of frontal function release primitive motor behaviours, including:
  - *Pout reflex*. Rubbing the chin causes pouting or 'suckling' lip movements; this is a polysynaptic reflex that is released by frontal lobe disease or diffuse degenerative brain disease.
  - *Facial reflex jerks*. Gently pull the patient's lip to the side with a finger over the cheek and tap the finger. There is pouting of the lip. These reflexes may be seen in upper motor lesions of the corticopontine pathways. They are analogous to a brisk jaw jerk.
  - *Palmomental reflex*. Scratching the palm produces a unilateral reflex contraction of the mentalis muscle of the chin. This is a very non-specific sign, present in many normal people.
  - *Grasp reflex*. The patient tends to grasp objects, such as your fingers, when they are placed in the palm, especially with contact between thumb and index finger. The patient's hand may reach for yours even as you move your hand away, or may continually grasp the bedclothes.
  - *Utilization behaviour*. When given common objects the patient will use them out of context. For example, when given someone else's glasses, the patient may attempt to put them on even if he is already wearing his own.

PARIETAL SENSORY LOBE FUNCTIONS
The parietal lobes subsume higher-level sensory perception and sensorimotor integration. Tests include:

- *Drift*. When the patient holds the arms outstretched, palms upwards with eyes closed, lightly displacing the ulnar border of the hand results in a lateral drift of the arm.
- *Astereognosis*. The patient has difficulty identifying coins placed in the hand when the eyes are closed, although there is no defect of primary sensation.

- *Agraphaesthesia.* Without looking, the patient cannot identify digits drawn on the palm or fingertips.
- *Disturbed oculomotor smooth pursuit.* There is a disorder of smooth conjugate following eye movement away from the side *ipsilateral* to a parietal lesion. This is often tested by assessing *optokinetic nystagmus.*

DOMINANT PARIETAL LOBE FUNCTIONS

Higher-level movement (praxis) requires the dominant parietal lobe. Bilateral idiomotor or ideational apraxia may therefore follow lesions here. Other deficits may include loss of numeracy (*dyscalculia*), of reading (*dyslexia*) and of comprehensional aspects of language, especially logical comparisons, e.g. 'A is bigger than B but smaller than C'. The rare Gerstmann's syndrome reflects aspects of these functions and consists of an inability to name body parts; confusion of the left and right sides of the body; acalculia; and agraphia (inability to write).

NON-DOMINANT PARIETAL LOBE FUNCTIONS

Non-dominant parietal function especially involves spatial cognitive domains. These may be assessed from the history, e.g. *dressing apraxia*, where the patient neglects to dress one half of their body, or loss of geographical orientation, e.g. inability to find one's way back home. *Constructional praxis* is tested by copying two intersecting irregular pentagons (see MMSE). Tests for *hemisensory neglect* specifically reflect non-dominant parietal function; a lesion on the dominant side is less likely to produce a deficit. The patient may ignore the affected (left) side (*asomatognosia*), perhaps denying any weakness of the limb or even that the limb belongs to them (*anosognosia*). Tests for neglect include:

- *Bisecting a drawn line.* The patient chooses a point closer to the non-neglected side.
- *Drawing a clock face.* The patient may cluster all the numbers on one side (usually the right), ignoring the abnormal side.
- *Extinction.* Present two stimuli simultaneously to either side, e.g. fingers in the visual fields or touching both limbs; the stimulus on the affected (left) side is ignored.

OCCIPITAL LOBE FUNCTIONS

Cognitive disorders with occipital lobe lesions generally involve *visual agnosia* (failure to recognize objects despite preserved acuity). Such disorders may therefore be picked up during history taking or examination. Examples include:

- *Visual anosognosia (Anton's syndrome).* The patient denies or is indifferent to his blindness even though he collides into objects and fails all visual tests. Rarely, the converse occurs – 'blind sight'; the patient complains of blindness but can navigate 'automatically' and can catch a ball. The responsible lesions are bilaterally located in the visual association cortex.
- *Visual illusions and hallucinations.* These are positive phenomena, reflecting distortion of images or false perceptions of images that do not exist.
- *Prosopagnosia.* Inability to recognize faces, usually due to bilateral occipitotemporal lesions.
- *Colour agnosia.* Failure to recognize colours, which may appear 'washed out', or to name colours, owing to visual association cortex lesions.
- *Balint's syndrome.* This consists of oculomotor apraxia (failure to look around at objects in the visual field); optic ataxia (failure of hand–eye coordination); and visual inattention to the periphery of the visual field without corresponding sensory inattention. The responsible lesion is bilateral and parieto-occipital in location. Detection of this disorder thus also requires eye movement examination, finger–nose pointing tests and visual field testing.

INTERPRETATION

In general, cognitive language functions lateralize to the dominant hemisphere whereas visuospatial functions lateralize to the non-dominant hemisphere. Almost all right-handed individuals have left-sided hemisphere dominance, as do around half of left-handers. Many different cognitive functions follow a lateralizing trend to a greater or lesser extent. For example, lesions of the mesial temporal lobes more usually affect verbal memory if left-sided and spatial memory if right-sided. However, apart from cognitive deficits resulting from stroke or mass lesions, most pathologies causing cognitive deficit are bilateral and often generalized. There are certain localizing features that suggest certain types of dementia (Table 10.4), but making a pathological diagnosis on the basis of the severity of deficits in different cortical domains is unreliable. Perhaps the most important practical information to be gained from cognitive examination is:

- The presence of any cognitive dysfunction; this reliably localizes pathology to supratentorial structures.
- Determining whether the pattern of dysfunction can all be lateralized to one hemisphere, or whether it can be explained only by multifocal or generalized brain disease.

These conclusions will direct subsequent clinical investigation.

THE CRANIAL NERVES

Examination of the cranial nerves is important and relatively objective. The third to twelfth cranial nerves arise from the brainstem and innervate facial,

Table 10.4 Clinical features that may distinguish different types of dementia

Alzheimer's disease	Frontotemporal dementia	Subcortical dementia
Early loss of autobiographical memory	Early personality deterioration	Early apathy, bradyphrenia (slow thought)
Early loss of spatial memory, e.g. getting lost	Behavioural stereotypies – repetitive routines of behaviour	Early signs of spasticity, apraxia, extrapyramidal signs
Early visual agnosia, constructional apraxia	Subtype with early non-fluent dysphasia and phonemic errors ('cat', 'cap')	Stepwise progression if multi-infarct dementia
Early loss of numeracy	Subtype with semantic dementia; non-phonemic errors ('cat', 'dog') and visual agnosia	

cranial and cervical tissues. The first and second cranial nerves actually consist of central nervous tissue rather than peripheral nerve. All the cranial nerves may be involved in disease processes in their intracranial and extracranial courses (*extrinsic lesions*) or at their sites of origin within the brain and brainstem (*intrinsic lesions*). An important aspect of cranial nerve examination is not only to identify lesions in particular nerves but to refine the differential diagnosis by considering whether such lesions are extrinsic or intrinsic.

THE OLFACTORY NERVE (I)

The central processes of the bipolar sensory cells in the olfactory epithelium pass up through the cribriform plate to the second olfactory neurons in the olfactory bulb. These in turn project to the olfactory centres in the uncus and parahippocampal gyrus.

TESTING SMELL

Start with the history: are the senses of smell and taste normal (much of the latter is dependent on smell)? Test smell with pungent, non-irritative odours, such as oil of cloves, oil of peppermint or tincture of asafoetida. You can also use common bedside substances such as soap, fruit or scent. Present these to each nostril separately and ask the patient to name them. Do not use irritating substances such as ammonia, which also stimulate the trigeminal nerve. Smell may be absent (*anosmia*) with subfrontal meningioma or following head injury or craniotomy. Always exclude local disease in the nose itself, such as catarrh. *Hallucinations of smell* may occur as an aura in temporal lobe seizures.

THE OPTIC NERVE (II)

From the retina, the fibres of the *optic nerve* (Fig. 10.3) project to the *optic chiasm*, located just above the pituitary gland, and thence to the *optic tract*. Fibres from the nasal (inner) half of each retina, representing the temporal (outer) field, cross over in the optic chiasm to join the contralateral optic tract, and those from the temporal retina stay on the same side. Thus the optic tracts, and all downstream visual areas, are segregated according to left and right visual fields, rather than left and right eyes. A few fibres pass into the superior colliculus in the brainstem to control the pupillary light reflex. After synapsing in the lateral geniculate body the majority project back through the posterior limb of the internal capsule to the calcarine cortex in the occipital lobe. Fibres in the optic radiation subserving the lower visual field take a direct route through the deep parietal white matter, but those subserving the upper fields pass around the temporal horn of the lateral ventricle (Meyer's loop). This is why upper visual field defects may complicate temporal tumours or follow temporal lobectomy in epilepsy surgery. The most peripheral part of the visual field is represented anteriorly in the calcarine fissure on the inside surface of the occipital lobe, whereas the macular field is represented at the occipital pole (Fig. 10.4). An ischaemic lesion of the posterior cerebral artery results in contralateral visual field loss but may spare the macula because the occipital pole receives blood supply from branches of the middle cerebral artery.

Further visual processing takes place in other parts of the occipital lobe and in the posterior parietal lobe (see Cognitive examination). Irritative lesions of the occipital lobe may result in positive symptoms, such as *fortification spectra* (jagged lines) in migraine, and blobs of light and colour in visual hallucinations resulting from occipital epileptic foci. Lesions in association areas of the visual cortex can result in illusions such as *micropsia*, where everything looks much smaller than in real life. *Complex visual hallucinations* generally arise from the temporal lobe, especially the uncal gyrus, or as a result of more diffuse organic brain disease, as in certain dementias. A common positive visual symptom is of 'floaters' – specks of material in the vitreous; these are of no pathological significance.

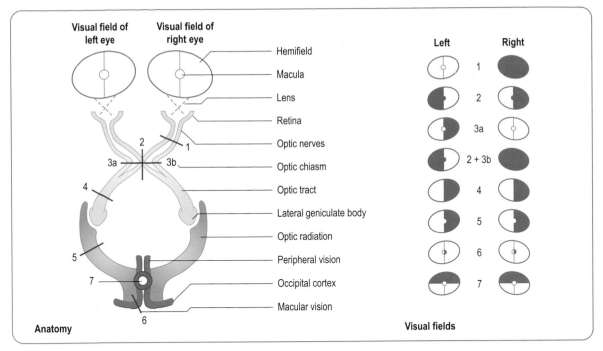

Figure 10.3 The visual pathways. A lesion at 1 produces blindness in the right eye with loss of the direct light reflex. A lesion at 2 produces bitemporal hemianopia. Lesions at 3a and 3b produce binasal hemianopia (a rare disorder). A lesion at 4 produces right homonymous hemianopia with macular involvement. A lesion at 5 produces right homonymous hemianopia with sparing of the macular field. Finally, a lesion at 6 produces right homonymous central (macular) hemiscotoma.

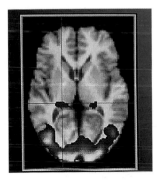

Figure 10.4 PET scanning. Functional segregation in the visual system. Activation of the visual system during a visual task. The occipital cortex and its association cortex, and the lateral geniculate bodies, are visible.

TESTING VISION

Visual acuity (see Chapter 18)

This should be tested while correcting any refractive error by using appropriate glasses. Refractive errors can also be eliminated by testing vision through a pinhole. Formal testing ideally involves a Snellen chart held 6 m (20 ft in the USA) from the patient, examining each eye in turn and if necessary testing close-up vision using standard print sizes. Acuity better than 6/60 is dependent on central (macular) vision. Thus optic neuritis typically reduces acuity down to this level but no further. Lower levels of acuity may be tested by counting fingers held in front of the eye, or by perceiving a pen light switching on and off.

Visual fields (see Chapter 18)

The visual field is the whole extent of the field of vision in each eye (Fig. 10.5). It is limited by the size of the retina and by the margins of the orbit, nose and cheek. The visual field is wider when larger, brighter or moving objects are used for testing. The extreme temporal non-binocular periphery of the visual field, called the *unpaired temporal crescent*, is particularly specialized for the detection of moving objects. There are therefore different ways to test the visual fields at the bedside, depending on what is being looked for:

- *Moving finger test.* Sit or stand in front of the patient. The patient covers one eye and fixes his gaze on your eye. Bring your wiggling finger slowly into view from out of the patient's view. The finger should be kept more than midway between you and the patient. Each of the upper temporal, lower temporal, upper nasal and lower nasal quadrants is tested separately. This test sensitively detects mild partial temporal field defects, such as would result from a pituitary tumour slowly growing into the optic chiasm and affecting the crossing temporal field fibres.
- *Red pin confrontation test.* This test uses a large red hatpin (head 0.5 cm in diameter) held equidistant

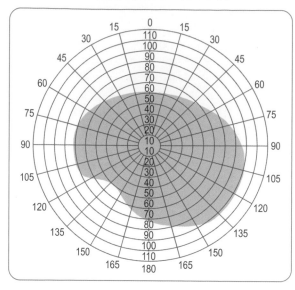

Figure 10.5 The extent of the right field of vision with a white target of 20 mm diameter mapped on to a perimeter at a distance of 330 mm.

between yourself and the patient, using exactly the same conditions as above. The patient again covers the eye not to be tested while you face them about 1.5 m away and cover your own eye. Determine the field limit by checking whether you and the patient see the pin at the same time. This test is accurate in detecting paracentral scotomas or paracentral colour desaturation in optic neuritis, and for comparing the size of the patient's blind spot with your own. The blind spot corresponds to the point of entry of the optic nerve into the retina about 15° lateral to central vision on the horizontal meridian.

- *Binocular testing*. This is useful for detecting visual extinction resulting from a right hemisphere lesion (see cognitive examination).

The visual field can be quantitatively mapped by an optician or ophthalmologist using *perimetry* (see Chapter 18). Common patterns of visual field abnormality are described in Box 10.5 and Figure 10.6.

Colour vision   (see Chapter 18)

This is tested using coloured plates that have patterns of coloured spots, some forming numbers and others a random background. Colour vision is mainly confined to the macular field; acquired abnormalities in colour vision are therefore a sensitive test for optic neuritis and certain retinal diseases.

Funduscopy

This technique is described in Chapter 18. The neurological examination focuses on papilloedema, optic atrophy, or pigmentary retinal degeneration and vascular disease.

Box 10.5   Visual field abnormalities

- *Central scotoma.* A defect in the whole of the central field is best gauged by visual acuity testing, and usually reflects optic nerve or optic nerve head disease.
- *Paracentral scotoma.* This results from disease of the choroid or retina near the macula. When unilateral, paracentral scotoma is often due to *vascular disease*, such as retinal embolism or *retinal artery branch occlusion*. When bilateral, paracentral scotomata may be due to toxic causes, especially alcoholism or vitamin B_{12} deficiency. *Glaucoma* can cause a paracentral *'arcuate' scotoma*; this has a characteristic comma-like shape and is due to damage to a nerve fibre bundle in the retina or optic nerve.
- *Homonymous hemianopia.* The right or left half of the visual field is lost in either eye, the same half in each eye. When the extent of visual loss in the homonymous fields of the two eyes is similar (*congruous hemianopia*) the lesion is likely to be postgeniculate, e.g. a posterior cerebral artery lesion resulting in a contralateral homonymous hemianopia. *Incongruous hemianopia* is more likely to be due to a lesion in the optic tract, chiasm or lateral geniculate. Blindness limited to one quadrant of a field is termed a *quadrantanopia*.
- *Bitemporal hemianopia.* Loss of vision in the temporal (outer) halves of both fields is due to a lesion of the optic chiasm caused by a pituitary tumour or a perichiasmal inflammatory or traumatic lesion extending out of the sella turcica (Fig. 10.6).
- *Altitudinal hemianopia.* The upper or lower half of the visual field is lost. This may occur unilaterally following damage to one optic nerve by ischaemia (e.g. posterior ciliary artery occlusion) or trauma to the optic nerve in a head injury. Occasionally it occurs bilaterally following bilateral partial occipital ischaemia.
- *Concentric constriction* of the visual fields sometimes occurs in long-standing papilloedema, in bilateral lesions of the striate (visual) cortex and in some retinal disorders (e.g. retinitis pigmentosa). It is also found in hysterical patients, where the absolute (not angular) size of the deficit may remain unchanged when testing at different distances from the patient (tunnel vision is not an organic disorder).

EYE MOVEMENTS AND PUPILS (CRANIAL NERVES III, IV, VI)

The external ocular movements and the pupils are controlled by the paired oculomotor, trochlear and abducens nerves (cranial nerves III, IV and VI, respectively). These arise from nuclei in the brainstem and function as a physiological unit; they

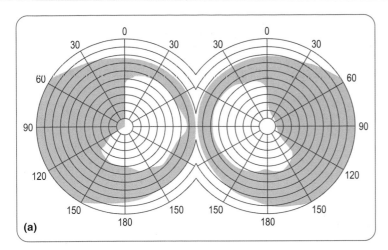

(a)

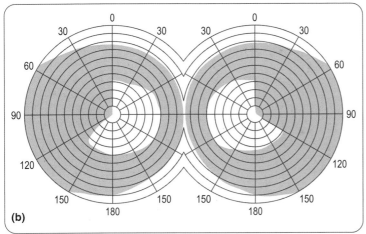

(b)

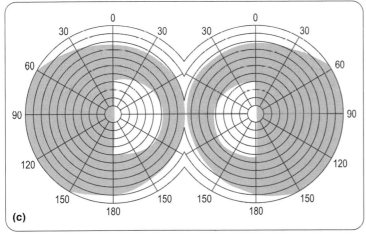

(c)

Figure 10.6 Fields of vision in a patient with a pituitary tumour (chromophobe adenoma), showing the development of bitemporal hemianopia. These fields were plotted many years ago; in the modern era of safe neurosurgery, operative decompression of the optic chiasm by hypophysectomy would have been carried out at the time of initial diagnosis in May. **(a)** May: VA (visual acuity) Lt 6/12, Rt 6/18. **(b)** August: VA Lt 6/12, Rt 6/12. **(c)** October: VA Lt 6/12, Rt 6/12. The fields were plotted at a distance of 2 m from the eye to the point of fixation at the centre of the Bjerrum screen, using a 10-mm white object. The coloured areas show the average normal field of vision and the white areas show the patient's field.

are interconnected by the medial longitudinal fasciculus (MLF).

The nucleus of the *third nerve* lies within the midbrain (Fig. 10.7). Its most superior neurons (*Edinger–Westphal nucleus*) supply parasympathetic innervation via the ciliary ganglion to the ciliary muscle and iris to mediate the light reflex. The afferent arc of the light reflex utilizes fibres from the retina that synapse in the tectum (see above), before relaying to the Edinger–Westphal nucleus. The third-nerve motor neurons innervate all the external ocular muscles except the lateral rectus (VI) and the superior oblique (IV). The nerve emerges from the brainstem on the inner aspect of the cerebral peduncle and passes forward in close relation to the *posterior communicating artery* before entering the lateral wall of the *cavernous sinus*. It enters the orbit through the superior orbital fissure with the sixth and fourth nerves.

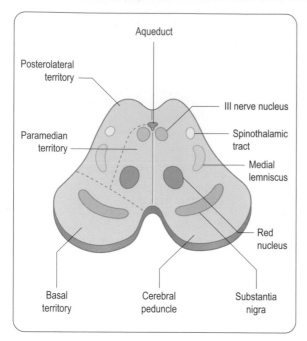

Figure 10.7   Anatomy of the midbrain showing the third-nerve nucleus. Vascular territories are shown on the left.

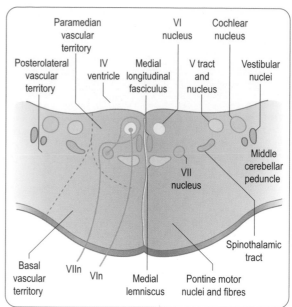

Figure 10.8   Anatomy of the pons, showing fifth-, sixth- and seventh-nerve nuclei. Vascular territories are shown on the left.

The *fourth nerve* nucleus lies in the lower midbrain. This nerve, uniquely, *decussates* in the brainstem and emerges from its *dorsal* surface. It then curls round the midbrain and enters the lateral wall of the cavernous sinus below the third nerve, to innervate the superior oblique muscle.

The *sixth nerve* nucleus is situated in the pons within the floor of the fourth ventricle (Fig. 10.8). It has a long course, passing over the surface of the clivus to enter the inferior petrosal sinus, then forward, laterally to medially, across the cavernous sinus just lateral to the internal carotid artery and entering the orbit to supply the lateral rectus muscle. This long course makes it particularly susceptible to displacement and damage from raised intracranial pressure of any cause.

EXAMINATION OF EYE MOVEMENT

Eye movement abnormalities are important in neurological diagnosis.

TERMINOLOGY

Horizontal movement of the eye outwards (laterally) is termed *abduction* and inwards (medially) is termed *adduction*. Vertical movement upwards is termed *elevation* and downwards is *depression*. The eye is also capable of *diagonal* movements (*version*) at any intermediate angle. *Rotary* movements, in which the eye twists on its anterior–posterior axis, occur automatically during head movements in either *internal* or *external rotation*. Voluntary rotary movements are not possible but are under vestibular control. They are best detected by looking at the movement of blood vessels on the sclera. *Convergence* refers to both eyes moving medially towards each other when fixing on a close-up object. A squint (the eyes point in different directions) is described as *convergent* or *divergent strabismus*, depending on whether the eyes point towards or away from each other.

EXAMINATION

Ask the patient to follow a finger held about 1 m away. Move the finger slowly in a large 'H' pattern while asking the patient if double vision (two separate images) is noted at any point. The patient keeps both eyes open. If diplopia is identified and its nature is not obvious, look at the point of reflection of light on the curved corneal surface to see if it is in the same place relative to the pupil in the two eyes. Ask the patient to close one eye and ask which image disappears. The defective eye is generally the one with the image appearing further out from the primary (straight-ahead) gaze position, simply because the eye has not moved over as far. An alternative to covering one eye completely is to cover it with tinted glass (red glass test) so that the different-coloured images indicate to which eye they belong.

A latent strabismus may be discovered by covering and then uncovering each eye. A 'lazy eye' will then tend to drift off in one direction, as there is no visual image to lock it together with the other eye.

Examination of quality of eye movements

Test *smooth pursuit* by asking the patient to follow a *slowly* moving finger held 1 m in front of them.

Move the finger in a '+' pattern through about a 30° arc from primary gaze while observing whether pursuit is smooth or jerky. Hold your finger still at each of the four end points to look for *nystagmus* (a repetitive jerky oscillatory movement when the eye should be stationary) in either or both eyes. The direction of jerky nystagmus is defined as the direction of its fast phase, not the slow drift.

Test *voluntary saccades* (sudden eye movements directed to a target or position) by asking the patient to look up, down, left and right. Then hold up two fingers, one to the left of centre and one to the right, or above and below, and ask the patient to look from one to the other. These tests reflex saccadic movements. In disease, saccades may be slowed or interrupted.

Interpretation of eye abnormal movement

Impaired movement of one or both eyes may reflect disease of the extraocular muscles, the cranial nerves supplying these muscles, or the nuclear or internuclear brainstem structures that relay signals to these nerves (Box 10.6).

Strabismus (squint) and diplopia (double vision)

In strabismus the eyes are not conjugate: they are directed in slightly different directions. Paralytic strabismus is due to impaired movement of one eye. The patient will experience diplopia, *worse in the direction of action of the weak muscle*, because of the mismatched images received by the two eyes (Box 10.7). Sometimes, if the disparity between the eyes is small, diplopia will occur without an obvious squint.

In congenital strabismus, or strabismus beginning in infancy, binocular vision does not develop properly. The affected person tends to ignore the image from the weaker or non-dominant eye, so there is no diplopia. This causes permanently reduced acuity in that eye – *amblyopia*. Congenital squint is often non-paralytic, meaning that the disparity is the same in all directions of gaze and that each eye individually has a full range of movement. Non-paralytic strabismus may be associated with *pendular nystagmus* (see below). A mild squint (*latent strabismus*) may be suppressed by preserved binocular drive, but may break down, causing diplopia in later life. The 'weaker' eye will be revealed by the cover test.

Monocular diplopia (double vision persisting with one eye closed) is not usually an organic disorder, although rarely it may occur with refractive distortion from a cataract. Sometimes patients report double vision when they are really experiencing blurred margins of objects owing to refractive errors or 'eye strain'.

EXTRAOCULAR MUSCLE AND CRANIAL NERVE LESIONS

Figure 10.9 illustrates the actions of the various muscles. The actions of the rectus muscles are

---

Box 10.6   Disturbances of ocular movement

Infranuclear lesions
- Sixth-nerve palsy
- Third-nerve palsy
- Fourth-nerve palsy

Supranuclear lesions
Conjugate gaze palsies
- Lateral gaze palsy
- Upward gaze palsy
- Downward gaze palsy
- Internuclear gaze palsy

Complex supranuclear gaze palsies
- Convergence nystagmus

Cerebellar lesions
- Nystagmus

Extrapyramidal lesions
- Slowed and interrupted smooth pursuit movements

Box 10.7   Charting diplopia in the nine cardinal directions of gaze in paralytic diplopia

The muscles used in each direction of gaze are listed

Upwards to the left	**Upwards**	**Upwards to the right**
left SR	left and right SR	right SO
right IO	left and right IO	left IO
To the left	**Straight ahead**	**To the right**
left LR	contraction of all	right LR
right MR	extraocular muscles	left MR
Downwards to the left	**Downwards**	**Downwards to the right**
left IR	left and right IR	right IR
right SO	left and right SO	left SO

SR, superior rectus; IR, inferior rectus; LR, lateral rectus; MR, medial rectus; SO, superior oblique; IO, inferior oblique.

straightforward, but note that the sixth nerve supplies the lateral rectus and that all the other ocular muscles, including the levator palpebrae component of the superior rectus, are supplied by the third nerve, except the superior oblique, which is innervated by the fourth nerve.

A *sixth-nerve palsy* will cause failure of abduction on the ipsilateral side. Patients may report double vision on looking to that side, and sometimes also on looking straight ahead in the distance because the eyes are relatively more diverged than on looking close-up.

A complete *third-nerve palsy* affects so many muscles that the eye cannot maintain primary gaze (Fig. 10.10). The eye is tonically deviated inferiorly and laterally ('down and out') owing to unopposed action of the lateral rectus and superior oblique, but this displacement will not be seen immediately because the failure of the levator palpebrae fibres means that a complete ptosis (drooping eyelid) will result. In addition, a complete lesion will result in parasympathetic failure, so the pupil will be large and unreactive (see under Pupil responses, below).

The effects of inferior and superior oblique muscle palsies are complicated by the fact that their direction of action is so different from the axis of the eye. When the eye is in the primary position looking straight ahead, the superior oblique muscle, which hooks round the trochlea on the inside of the orbit and inserts backwards into the upper surface of the globe, acts to pull the eye anteriorly, depress it, and also twist it into internal rotation (vergence). However, when the eye is adducted within the orbit, the vertical plane of action of the superior oblique is now close to the vertical plane of the eye, and the muscle depresses the eye. Thus, a *fourth-nerve palsy* causes failure to intort the eye on tilting the head towards the side of the lesion. In fact, the patient's head is usually tilted away from the side of the lesion to bring the image from a tonically extorted eye back to the vertical. There may also be partial failure of depression of the eye when in an adducted position (the inferior rectus will still be working), for example when reading a book (looking down and focusing on a close-up object).

Because of their proximity within the cavernous sinus and superior orbital fissure, third-nerve palsies are often accompanied by fourth-nerve palsies. The additional involvement of a fourth-nerve palsy is ascertained by failure of depression of the adducted eye, and by lack of intortion movement when the eye is in the primary position and the patient attempts to look downward.

Impaired range of movement may also result from muscle disease. Tethering in Graves' disease often first affects the inferior rectus, causing impaired elevation. Tethering may also be congenital (Brown's syndrome). Extraocular muscle weakness occurs in ocular myasthenia and in certain mitochondrial diseases. Myasthenia causes complicated and *variable* patterns of diplopia that cannot be interpreted on the basis of involvement of particular muscles or cranial nerves.

NUCLEAR AND INTERNUCLEAR LESIONS

The three extraocular muscle nerve nuclei are coordinated in the brainstem to convert supranuclear signals for desired ocular movements into appropriate commands to the two eyes so that they move in concert (Fig. 10.11). Characteristic patterns of gaze abnormality can be recognized with intrinsic brainstem lesions.

Conjugate lateral gaze failure. A lesion in the *ipsilateral sixth-nerve nucleus* interrupts relay fibres controlling adduction of the contralateral eye, as well as fibres running through the ipsilateral sixth nerve. There is therefore failure of abduction of the ipsilateral eye and of adduction of the contralateral eye, rather than just failure of ipsilateral abduction, as occurs with a sixth-nerve lesion.

Internuclear ophthalmoplegia (INO). The m*edial longitudinal fasciculus (MLF)* carries fibres relaying from the sixth- to the third-nerve nucleus that integrate horizontal gaze. A lesion in the MLF causes failure of adduction (on the same side as the lesion) during horizontal gaze away from the side of the lesion. Most patients have an incomplete syndrome; this is best detected by testing saccadic movements, which reveal slow adduction rather reduced range,

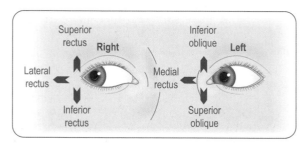

Figure 10.9 The action of the external ocular muscles with the patient facing the examiners.

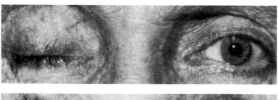
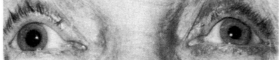

Figure 10.10 Right third-nerve palsy. Note the right ptosis, the dilated pupil and the external strabismus. This was due to a berry aneurysm of the right posterior communicating artery.

and nystagmus in the abducting eye. There is no gaze palsy. The nystagmus may result from involvement of vestibular pathways that run close to the MLF. A lesion more rostrally in the MLF, near both third-nerve nuclei, may cause an INO with additional tonic divergence of both eyes and failure of convergence.

'One-and-a-half' syndrome. A larger MLF lesion may involve the sixth-nerve nucleus. The resultant deficit is therefore a combination of the deficits described above, with failure of conjugate gaze to the side of the lesion and a failure of adduction

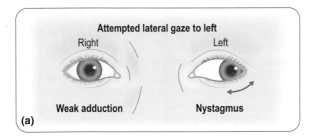

(a)

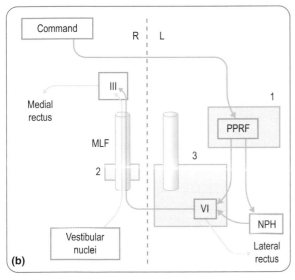

(b)

Figure 10.11 **(a)** Right internuclear ophthalmoplegia, a frequent feature of multiple sclerosis. **(b)** The connections for horizontal gaze. Descending commands for left saccades cross the midline, are processed in the cerebellum, paramedian pontine reticular formation (PPRF) and nucleus prepositus hypoglossi (NPH), and then pass to the VI nerve nucleus to activate the lateral rectus to move the left eye to the left. Signals also relay up the medial longitudinal fasciculus to the right III nerve nucleus to activate the right medial rectus and generate a conjugate movement of the right eye to the left. A lesion of the left PPRF (area 1) will cause conjugate failure of horizontal saccades to the left (smooth movement commands to the VI nerve nucleus bypass the PPRF). A lesion in area 2 will cause failure of adduction of the right eye on looking to the left (internuclear ophthalmoplegia). A lesion in area 3 will cause failure of conjugate left gaze with failure of adduction of the left eye when looking to the right ('one-and-a-half' syndrome).

to the opposite side. The only remaining horizontal movement possible is therefore abduction of the eye contralateral to the lesion. Vertical movements are unaffected.

Parinaud's syndrome. This consists of failure of upgaze, sometimes with convergence–retraction nystagmus on attempted upgaze (*sylvian aqueduct syndrome*). The latter is due to asynchronous adducting saccades and co-contraction of all the rectus muscles so that the eye is retracting jerkily into the orbit. The pupil reactions (see below) are often absent. It is associated with a lesion near the colliculi on the posterior surface of the midbrain. In general, impairments of conjugate upgaze or downgaze localize rather poorly, but may respectively reflect dorsal midbrain or lower medulla lesions.

Skew deviation. One eye is directed upwards and the other downwards. In an unconscious subject this suggests thalamomidbrain haemorrhage, but it may also occur in other midbrain or vestibular disorders.

NYSTAGMUS

The vestibular structures reflexly maintain gaze during head movements. They generate conjugate movement of the eyes in the opposite direction to head movement. If there is a continued head movement *vestibulo-ocular reflex nystagmus* may develop, consisting of sudden conjugate ocular jerks in the opposite direction to the slow drift. Visual perception is suppressed during these saccadic jerks, so there is no loss of visual function. In lower vertebrates the eyes are positioned on the sides of the head, so that torsional eye movements are appropriate to compensate when the head moves up or down. In humans the semicircular canals and 'wiring' of the vestibular nuclei still reflect this vertebrate anatomy, so that pathological nystagmus of vestibular origin often occurs in complex torsional directions (*rotary nystagmus*). Large movements of the visual field without head movement generate following movements (*pursuit movements*) of the eyes to keep the image stable on the retina. Continued field movement, e.g. walking past a fence of vertical railings or looking out of a speeding train, will produce a continued drift stimulus in the same way as continued head movement and will therefore induce a correctional 'physiological nystagmus' – *optokinetic reflex nystagmus*. Several syndromes of pathological nystagmus are recognized:

- *Peripheral vestibular nystagmus.* There is dysfunction in the semicircular canals or vestibular portion of the eighth cranial nerve. Normally, the peripheral vestibular apparatus fires tonically on each side. If there is a lesion on one side, the resultant imbalanced input is interpreted as head movement to the side opposite that of the lesion. A 'compensatory' eye movement drift therefore occurs to the same side as the lesion, whereas fast 'rewind' nystagmus develops *in the direction opposite the lesion*. Because *vestibular nystagmus* relates to head movements rather than eye movements, it may be induced by briskly moving the patient's head from side to side while asking them to fixate ahead ('doll's head movements'). When the head is moved to the lesioned side the patient may make a visible saccade to look back at the examiner instead of a fully compensatory smooth movement. Hallpike's test (see Chapter 19) produces an *adapting* nystagmus when the head is tilted down *towards* the side of the defective posterior semicircular canal.

- *Central vestibular nystagmus.* When the deficit is within the brainstem the nystagmus often has a rotary component. Its severity may vary when the eyes are in different positions, although the direction may remain the same. Hallpike's test may be positive or negative and, if positive, has a very short latency and will not fatigue.
- *Cerebellar nystagmus.* As well as controlling smooth pursuit, cerebellar structures (with the nucleus prepositus hypoglossi in the brainstem) calibrate saccades and convert saccadic signals to a form understood by the eye movement nuclei. Cerebellar pathway lesions cause overshooting of small saccades and an inability to maintain gaze in a non-primary position. There is a drift back towards primary gaze and repeated corrective saccades to the desired position, resulting in *gaze-evoked nystagmus*.
- *Downbeat nystagmus.* This is a feature of cerebellar and cervicomedullary junction lesions, e.g. foramen magnum meningioma or a Chiari malformation.
- *Gaze-paretic nystagmus.* Gaze-evoked nystagmus in only one eye is likely to be due to an INO. Extraocular muscle weakness due to ocular myasthenia can also produce gaze-paretic nystagmus, perhaps because the internuclear yoking pathways cannot compensate for the different strengths of the extraocular muscles.
- *Pendular nystagmus.* This is a regular to-and-fro eye movement, often in the primary gaze position. It is usually due to failure of ocular fixation due to long-standing blindness or to a developmental defect in the brainstem nuclei that control conjugate gaze.

OTHER INVOLUNTARY EYE MOVEMENTS

There are several infrequent involuntary eye movements, such as square-wave jerks, opsoclonus and ocular myorhythmia, that generally reflect brainstem pathology. On examination, it is best simply to make a descriptive record of what was observed.

SUPRANUCLEAR SMOOTH PURSUIT

The voluntary intention to *fixate* upon a moving object is converted into *pursuit* signals by automatic cerebellar and brainstem systems. Lesions here will result in broken jerky pursuit as catch-up saccades are made to keep up with the target.

SUPRANUCLEAR LESIONS AFFECTING SACCADES

Saccades may be reflexive, induced by targets in the visual or auditory field, or voluntary to look at a desired position with no target. Supranuclear lesions are distinguished by affecting the latter more than the former. Because eye movement control is binocular, supranuclear deficits are always conjugate. For example, in Steele–Richardson disease (progressive supranuclear palsy) there is a conjugate progressive supranuclear gaze palsy especially for voluntary downward movements. Saccades to targets, downward pursuit, and especially downward vestibular movements in response to moving the head upward are all less impaired. Impaired upgaze is common in the elderly.

Lesions in the *frontal eye fields* may cause a supranuclear deficit of conjugate voluntary gaze to the opposite direction, and the eyes may tonically deviate ipsilaterally. They may also deviate ipsilaterally when testing optokinetic nystagmus, e.g. by holding a drum with painted vertical strips in front of the eyes and rotating it slowly towards the side of the lesion. An irritative lesion, e.g. in focal epilepsy, may produce contralateral nystagmoid jerks. Lesions of the *posterior parietal cortex* affect reflexive saccades to visually perceived targets more than voluntary saccades. However, both cortical areas innervate the brainstem nuclei bilaterally; unilateral lesions are thus subtle and transient. A *bilateral posterior parietal lesion* results in the much more dramatic eye movement deficit of Balint's syndrome (see Cognitive examination).

In parkinsonism saccades are hypometric, so that a number of slowed, small saccades are made to a target instead of a single rapid, large saccade. There is also slowing of pursuit speed. Hyperkinetic extrapyramidal diseases, such as Huntington's chorea, show a failure of voluntary suppression of undesired saccades to objects appearing in the peripheral field.

EXAMINATION OF THE PUPILS

The pupils should first be examined for size and regularity. *Reaction to light* is assessed by asking the patient to look ahead at a distant object in a shady room and shining a bright pen-light into the eye from the side, so that the patient is not actually looking directly at it. The pupil should constrict over about half a second. The test is done twice for each eye, once checking the reaction of that eye (*direct response*) and once checking the reaction to illumination of the opposite eye. The *accommodation reaction* is assessed by asking the patient to look ahead into the distance and then at a finger brought up close to the eye. The pupil should constrict as part of the 'triple response' when focusing upon close objects (pupil constriction, convergence of the eyes, and thickening of the lens by the ciliary muscles to shorten its focal length). Pupil constriction during accommodation helps focusing via the pinhole camera effect.

INTERPRETATION OF PUPILLARY EXAMINATION

Slight inequality of the pupils may be present in perfectly healthy subjects. If one pupil is larger than the other, the one that changes the least between dark and light conditions is usually the abnormal one. Irregularities are usually due to adhesion of the iris to the lens as a result of old iritis.

Visual lesion. Severe disruption of the afferent visual arc of the light reflex due to a prechiasmal lesion cause an absent direct but preserved consensual light reflex. The affected eye is blind.

Third-nerve palsy. This disrupts the efferent arc of the light reflex and so produces both direct and consensual failure. The pupil is dilated.

Relative afferent pupillary defect. When there is a partial defect of one afferent pathway and a light is shone in the two eyes alternately at a rate of about one per second, the affected pupil *dilates* a little or oscillates when the light falls upon it because the direct response is weaker than the consensual response (Marcus Gunn pupil). This is a feature of optic neuritis; it is difficult to detect when there is bilateral optic neuritis.

Light-near dissociation. Constriction to accommodation is better than to light. This is noted in most partial third-nerve lesions because accommodation is in general a more robust stimulus than light. Extremely rare cases of the opposite have been described in midbrain syndromes, e.g. in encephalitis lethargica, presumably because accommodatory fibres to the Edinger–Westphal nucleus were selectively involved.

Argyll Robertson pupil. This is the classic pupillary abnormality in neurosyphilis. The pupil is small and irregular, reacts briskly to accommodation, but does not react to light either directly or consensually. The abnormality is typically bilateral but is usually more marked on one side. The pupil dilates slowly and irregularly to conjunctival atropine instillation, which blocks postsynaptic receptors in the pupil muscle, but there is no constriction with 2% methacholine. The lesion is thought to be in the pretectal region of the mesencephalon.

Adie's tonic pupil. This is usually unilateral and characterized by absent or delayed pupillary constriction to light or to accommodation. Once constricted, the pupil dilates only very slowly. The pupil may thus variably appear small or large (more usually larger). If smaller, it may be confused with the Argyll Robertson syndrome. Like the latter, it is sometimes associated with absent tendon reflexes, often on the same side as the pupillary abnormality (Holmes–Adie syndrome) and, unlike the Argyll Robertson pupil, is of little clinical significance. The distinction may be confirmed by constriction following the instillation of sterile 2% methacholine owing to parasympathetic denervation hypersensitivity in the Adie syndrome.

Horner's syndrome (see Fig. 18.7). A lesion in the ipsilateral central or peripheral sympathetic pathway results in a *tonically constricted pupil* with failure to dilate on shading the eye, partial *ptosis* and *enophthalmos* (eyeball retraction). *Sweating* on the upper face may be absent. The central sympathetic tract synapses with preganglionic sympathetic neurons in the spinal cord which outflow through the first thoracic nerve roots and to the sympathetic ganglia by the rami communicantes. From the cervical sympathetic chain the postganglionic pupillary nerve fibres pass up along the internal carotid artery to the cavernous plexus, and thence via the ophthalmic division of the trigeminal nerve to the eye, where they cause pupillary dilatation and elevation of the upper lid, the latter through contraction of the smooth muscle fibres in the levator palpebrae superioris. As opposed to a pathological dilatation of the other eye from an Adie pupil or a third-nerve lesion, the small pupil of Horner's syndrome can be confirmed by its failure to dilate on instillation of conjunctival cocaine, which blocks noradrenergic reuptake and enhances the sympathetic response *only if the sympathetic pathway is intact*. Epinephrine (adrenaline) will still work because it directly stimulates the pupillary radial muscles postsynaptically.

Ciliospinal reflex. The normal pupil dilates when the skin of the neck is pinched owing to a sympathetic 'stress' response. However, the test is unreliable and physiologically rather than clinically relevant.

THE TRIGEMINAL NERVE (V)

SENSORY FUNCTION

Somatosensory afferents from the skin and the facial muscles enter the trigeminal (gasserian) ganglion via three branches: the *ophthalmic* division, the *maxillary* division and the *mandibular* division (Table 10.5).

Trigeminal sensory neurons project into the pons through its lateral surface. Fibres subserving light touch synapse in the nucleus near the floor of the fourth ventricle, and proprioceptive projections from the muscles of mastication and the extraocular

Table 10.5 Motor, sensory and autonomic innervation of the three divisions of the trigeminal nerve

Division	Innervation	Course
Ophthalmic V_1	Upper face, nose, cornea and eyelid Scalp to vertex Lachrymal gland via vidian nerve	Via superior orbital fissure to cavernous sinus, to Meckel's cave
Maxillary V_2	Middle face, nasal mucosa, upper teeth, pharynx, tonsils, and inner quadrant of cornea	Via inferior orbital fissure to sphenopalatine fossa and foramen rotundum into cavernous sinus, to Meckel's cave Autonomic fibres (nervus intermedius) form greater petrosal nerve, fusing with deep petrosal nerve to form Vidian nerve
Mandibular V_3 sensory	Lower face (not angle of jaw), lip and teeth, tongue Part of external ear Parasympathetic fibres innervate parotid gland	Via infratemporal fossa through skull base and foramen ovale to Meckel's cave.
Mandibular V_3 motor	Muscles of mastication: masseter, digastric, pterygoids and temporalis	Via V_3

muscles reach the mesencephalic (midbrain) fifth-nerve nucleus. Fibres subserving pain and temperature descend and synapse within the spinal tract of the fifth nerve, and descend as low as the second cervical segment. After synapsing, second-order pain fibres decussate and ascend again within the quintothalamic tract next to the spinothalamic tract, in parallel with the spinothalamic pain pathways.

EXAMINING FACIAL SENSATION

Loss of sensation in the face is best tested using a pin. Test within each of the three divisions separately (Fig. 10.12), checking for symmetry of perceived pinprick intensity between the two sides. Testing for light touch is less discriminatory. If there is reduced sensation, delineate its extent by testing from a normal to an abnormal area. Patients with trigeminal pain, e.g. trigeminal neuralgia, will be reluctant to allow sensory testing. The *corneal reflexes* should be tested by touching – not rubbing – a wisp of cotton wool on the corneal surface at its margin with the conjunctiva. This is quite unpleasant for the patient. There should be a brisk bilateral blink response. The reflex should be interpreted together with facial nerve function, as the latter carries the efferent arc of the reflex.

MOTOR FUNCTION

The motor root of the trigeminal nerve (Table 10.5) originates from a small nucleus medial to the main sensory nucleus, emerges just anterior to the sensory division, and joins the mandibular division of the sensory fifth nerve.

EXAMINING TRIGEMINAL MOTOR FUNCTION

Ask the patient to clench their teeth while you palpate both masseter muscles above the angles of the

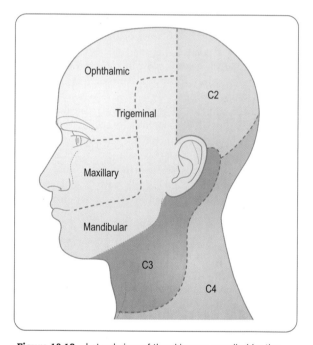

Figure 10.12 Lateral view of the skin area supplied by the trigeminal (V) nerve branches and the second, third and fourth cervical segments.

jaw and then while you palpate both temporalis muscles over the temples. Test the pterygoid muscles by forceful opening of the jaw against resistance: with unilateral lateral pterygoid weakness the jaw deviates to the ipsilateral side as it opens. The jaw jerk is a fifth-nerve stretch reflex. Place your finger on the chin below the lower lip and tap it lightly with a tendon hammer while the patient maintains the jaw half open and relaxed. The reflex is increased in corticobulbar tract (upper motor neuron (UMN) disease.

INTERPRETATION

Sensory abnormality restricted to one of the sensory divisions suggests an extrinsic lesion localized to the skull base or deep facial tissues. In an intrinsic lesion of the spinal tract of the trigeminal nucleus there is 'onion bulb' loss to pinprick that spreads concentrically and bilaterally from the nose. The lesion involves the decussating pain fibres, and is often due to syringomyelia or syringobulbia.

Isolated motor lesions are uncommon. There is often associated mandibular sensory loss. When mandibular weakness is combined with total trigeminal sensory loss the lesion involves the proximal trigeminal nerve or is intrinsic within the ipsilateral pons. The absence of salivation and lacrimation ipsilaterally, trophic changes inside the mouth and corneal ulceration may occur.

THE FACIAL NERVE (VII)

The facial nerve arises from its nucleus lateral to the nucleus of the sixth nerve (see Fig. 10.8), winds round the sixth-nerve nucleus and emerges from the front of the pons medial to the vestibulocochlear nerve. It passes laterally through the petrous bone in the internal auditory meatus. In the middle ear it turns sharply posteriorly at the geniculate ganglion to run back along the medial wall of the middle ear and then vertically downward through the facial canal. In its bony course the facial nerve is vulnerable to basal skull fracture and oedema. It emerges from the facial canal at the stylomastoid foramen anterior to the mastoid process and spreads out within the parotid gland to supply all the superficial muscles of the face, neck and scalp, apart from the levator palpebrae superioris.

Along its course, the nerve gives and receives many branches:

- The *nervus intermedius* is a secretomotor nerve derived from the superior salivary nucleus in the pons. It passes through the internal auditory canal with the facial nerve and then joins it. Some of these autonomic fibres leave the facial nerve at the geniculate ganglion to form the greater petrosal nerve, which joins the trigeminal nerve (see above).
- *Sensation* from a small medial part of the tragus of the pinna, the external auditory meatus and the tympanic membrane is relayed in tympanic branches of the facial nerve to the geniculate ganglion. Central projections travel in the seventh nerve to the trigeminal nucleus. Geniculate herpes, which may cause facial paralysis, may thus appear as vesicles in this sensory distribution.
- The *nerve to the stapedius muscle* leaves the seventh nerve within the facial canal.
- *Taste* fibres from the anterior two-thirds of the tongue pass along the lingual nerve and are then carried within the *chorda tympani*. This nerve passes through the middle ear, near the tympanic membrane, and joins the seventh nerve within the facial canal. It leaves the seventh nerve again as part of the nervus intermedius, eventually to reach the nucleus of the tractus solitarius within the upper medulla. Central projections of these taste fibres pass via the thalamus to the temporal part of the postcentral gyrus and to the amygdala. The chorda tympani also distributes secretomotor fibres from the nervus intermedius to the submandibular and minor salivary glands via the lingual nerve.

EXAMINATION

Look for facial asymmetry and for abnormal involuntary facial movements. Watch the patient smile, bare their teeth, and attempt to whistle. Test the following:

- *Frontalis.* Ask the patient to raise their eyebrows while you look for asymmetry of the forehead skin creases.
- *Orbicularis oculi.* Ask the patient to screw their eyes shut while you try to prevent this with your finger and thumb. In severe weakness the eye may not close at all. A preserved Bell's phenomenon causing elevation of the eye during attempted closure indicates that the patient is trying hard.
- *Orbicularis oris.* Ask the patient to purse the lips shut and stop you from opening them.

ASSESSMENT OF TASTE

Test the sense of taste using strong solutions of sugar and common salt, and weak solutions of citric acid and quinine, as tests of 'sweet', 'salt', 'sour' and 'bitter' respectively. Apply these solutions to the surface of the protruded tongue with a small swab on a spatula. The patient should be asked to indicate perception of the taste *before* the tongue is withdrawn in order to decide whether taste is disturbed anteriorly or posteriorly. After each test the mouth must be rinsed. The bitter quinine test should be applied last, as its effect is more lasting than that of the others.

Positive taste symptoms, e.g. taste hallucinations, may constitute the aura of temporal lobe epilepsy. The chorda tympani supplies taste to the anterior two-thirds of the tongue.

INTERPRETATION

The localization of a facial nerve lesion depends on the distribution of facial weakness and any involvement of other structures. Decide first whether the pattern of facial weakness is characteristic of an upper (UMN) or lower motor neuron (LMN) lesion.

UPPER MOTOR NEURON FACIAL WEAKNESS

This includes lesions anywhere in the UMN distribution, from the contralateral cerebral hemisphere through the internal capsule, corticopontine tract and pontine decussation to (but not including) the facial nerve nucleus. Because corticopontine fibres to the muscles of the upper face (frontalis and orbicularis oculi) pass *bilaterally* to the facial nerve nuclei, a unilateral UMN lesion causes weakness of the cheek, mouth and platysma, but much less weakness of the upper face. At rest, tonic overactivity of weak muscles tends to pull the lips across to the affected side. Thus, tests of voluntary facial contraction are a much better guide to the side of weakness. Facial reflexes, elicited by lightly tapping the muscles around the mouth, are often increased in supranuclear lesions. In thalamic UMN lesions corticobulbar fibres concerned with emotional movement may be especially affected, so that facial weakness is more evident during smiling. Bilateral UMN lesions may result in emotional lability owing to the uncontrolled activity of such pathways. Thus emotional release (*pseudobulbar affect*) should be considered separately. Taste is not affected in supranuclear lesions.

LOWER MOTOR NEURON FACIAL WEAKNESS

Nuclear and infranuclear lesions cause flaccid paralysis and atrophy in the whole nerve distribution. *Intrinsic* brainstem seventh-nerve lesions may be distinguished from extrinsic lesions as in the former the ipsilateral sixth nerve or nucleus is usually also involved, causing diplopia, as it lies so close to the path of the seventh-nerve fascicle within the pons. An *extrinsic* lesion in the proximal part of the nerve, e.g. an acoustic schwannoma at the cerebellopontine angle, may spare taste but be associated with deafness or vestibular disturbance – dizziness. With lesions in the petrous temporal bone, sounds may be heard abnormally loudly (*hyperacusis*) owing to loss of tympanic membrane damping because of involvement of the nerve to stapedius. If the lesion is distal to the entry point of the chorda tympani, taste is preserved. Finally, disease in the parotid gland may selectively affect nerve fibres to certain facial muscles. *Ageusia*, or loss of taste, occurs with lesions of the chorda tympani and lingual nerve. Intrinsic brainstem lesions rarely cause loss of taste without other more serious clinical features.

ABNORMAL FACIAL MOVEMENTS

Synkinesis, e.g. movement of the lip on eye closure, indicates faulty reinnervation following an LMN lesion, especially with Bell's palsy. *Hemifacial spasm*, which involves the whole of one side of the face, is due to an irritative lesion of the facial nerve. *Myokymia*, a rhythmic twitching movement, when it involves the eyelid, is usually associated with anxiety, but it also occurs in multiple sclerosis. Supranuclear disorders, such as *orofacial dyskinesia* due to neuroleptic drugs (extrapyramidal), *myoclonic or focal epileptic jerks* (motor cortex) and *tics* (habit spasms) should also be considered.

THE VESTIBULOCOCHLEAR NERVE (VIII)

Afferents subserving hearing arise from the cochlear ganglion, enter the middle fossa via the internal auditory canal and reach the brainstem at the lower border of the pons, where they project to the dorsal and ventral cochlear nuclei. The secondary auditory tract, after partial decussation, enters the lateral lemniscus and synapses in the inferior colliculus and the medial geniculate body of the thalamus. From the thalamus the auditory pathway projects to the first and second temporosphenoidal gyri. Although sounds received in one ear reach the opposite hemisphere of the brain because there is only partial decussation of the secondary auditory tracts, unilateral cerebral or brainstem lesions do not cause unilateral deafness.

Vestibular eighth-nerve fibres subserving balance originate in the vestibular ganglion and terminate in a group of nuclei in the pons and medulla. Like hearing, perceptual aspects of balance are mediated by the temporal lobe.

ASSESSMENT OF HEARING

In addition to deafness (see Chapter 13), patients may present with a number of positive auditory symptoms:

- *Tinnitus* is a persistent 'ringing in the ears'. The sound is quite variable, including humming, buzzing, hammering, whistling or pulsatile sensations. It is common, but apart from acoustic nerve tumours is almost never due to neurological disease. Pulsatile tinnitus merits investigation for abnormal flow within the cerebral or great neck vessels.
- *Hyperacusis*, a disorder in which even slight sounds are heard with painful intensity, may occur in facial nerve palsy.
- *Auditory hallucinations, or delusions of voices*, are common in the non-organic psychoses (e.g. schizophrenia), but may also occur in organic psychoses. Other complex auditory hallucinations, for example music, sometimes arise as epileptic auras when there is a lesion in the temporal lobe.

ASSESSMENT OF VERTIGO

True vertigo – a sensation of lurching or rotation of the environment or, less specifically, of self – must be distinguished from a feeling of light-headedness, near-fainting or tension headache. Terms that the patient may use, such as dizziness and giddiness, require clarification. Establish whether the vertigo is *positional*, i.e. related to certain head movements or postures, indicating a canal or nerve lesion; or *non-positional*, suggesting an intrinsic brainstem lesion. Tests to distinguish these features in a patient with vertigo are described in Chapter 13. *Visual vertigo* describes a sensation in individuals who experience vertigo from large-scale movements of the visual field, e.g. standing near speeding cars or trains, or walking past vertical railings. This is normally due to constitutional oversensitivity to such stimuli, but is sometimes precipitated by a previous peripheral vestibular lesion.

THE GLOSSOPHARYNGEAL NERVE (IX)

The ninth nerve subserves somatic sensation from the back of the tongue, pharynx and palate. Glossopharyngeal fibres pass through the jugular foramen and travel with the vagus and accessory nerves to enter the lateral side of the medulla and synapse in the nucleus of the fifth nerve. *Taste* fibres from the posterior third of the tongue project to the nucleus of the tractus solitarius. Somatic efferent fibres in the ninth nerve arising in the nucleus ambiguus supply the stylopharyngeus. Autonomic fibres from the inferior salivary nucleus reach the lesser petrosal nerve, travel through the ninth nerve via its tympanic branch, synapse in the otic ganglion lying below the foramen ovale next to the mandibular division of the trigeminal nerve, and innervate the parotid gland through the auriculotemporal branch of the mandibular nerve.

EXAMINATION

The glossopharyngeal nerve is rarely damaged alone; examine the following:

- *Taste* on the posterior part of the tongue.
- *Pharyngeal reflex* contraction after tickling the back of the pharynx with a small cotton-covered stick. The efferent component requires vagal innervation of the palatal musculature.

THE VAGUS NERVE (X)

The vagus nerve emerges from the medulla and leaves the cranial cavity through the jugular foramen. Below the foramen it gives off auricular, pharyngeal, superior laryngeal and recurrent laryngeal branches before entering the mediastinum. The organization of its medullary nuclei is similar to that of the glossopharyngeal nerve; the nucleus ambiguus mediates the somatic muscles of the larynx and pharynx, the nucleus and spinal tract of the fifth nerve receives sensory afferents from the larynx and pharynx, and the dorsal nucleus mediates

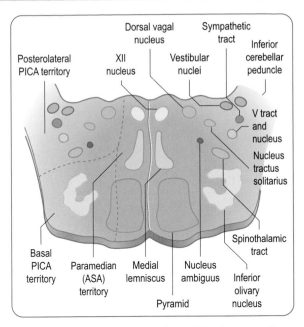

Figure 10.13 Medulla, showing the nuclei and tracts on the right and the vascular territories on the left.

parasympathetic visceral efferents and afferents relating to most of the body (Fig. 10.13). As with the glossopharyngeal nerve, the vagus nerve's somatic sensory ganglia lie in the jugular foramen.

ASSESSMENT

Damage to the vagus nerve is clinically evident only through its *palatine* (pharyngeal) and *laryngeal* branches.

PALATE
- *Nasal regurgitation.* Weakness of the soft palate leads to failure of palatal elevation, failure of closure of the nasopharynx and nasal regurgitation of fluids during swallowing.
- *Palatal dysarthria.* The patient cannot pronounce words requiring complete closure of the nasopharynx, e.g. 'egg' pronounced as 'eng'. In unilateral paralysis these symptoms are less obvious.
- *Palatal elevation.* Ask the patient to open the mouth and say 'aah'. Use a tongue depressor to obtain a good view of the soft palate and uvula. Unilateral paralysis results in elevation only of the normal side and *deviation of the uvula towards the normal side*. In a UMN lesion the palate may be tonically elevated more on the affected side and may move less on phonation.

LARYNX
Unilateral damage to the *superior laryngeal branch* of the vagus nerve is usually symptomless, but bilateral involvement causes paralysis of the cricopharyngeus. This reduces tension on the vocal cords,

preventing singing or speaking higher notes. *Recurrent laryngeal nerve palsy* causes vocal cord paralysis; there is inability to phonate normally (a '*breathy voice*'), and the cough is loose and 'bovine' because the vocal cords cannot properly come together to seal off the airway. In bilateral paralysis these features are much more pronounced; the paralysed cords tend to lie in an adducted position and there is a risk of stridor and respiratory obstruction. Breathing is noisy and partially obstructed.

THE ACCESSORY NERVE (XI)

The cranial part of this nerve resembles a component of the motor root of the vagus nerve; fibres arise in the nucleus ambiguus just below the vagus nerve and travel with it through the jugular foramen, then join the vagal branches that innervate the pharynx and larynx. The spinal part emerges from the lateral column of the spinal cord, perhaps beginning as low as the sixth cervical root. It passes up intradurally through the foramen magnum to join the cranial part, but instead of joining the vagus like the cranial portion, it continues separately to supply the sternomastoid and upper trapezius muscles.

EXAMINATION

Upper trapezius muscle fibres: ask the patient to shrug their shoulders while you press downward on them. The shrug may be weak on the affected side. *Sternomastoid*: ask the patient to turn the head while you resist with a hand on the side of the face. Note contraction of the activated sternomastoid muscle on the side *opposite* to the direction of movement. Because UMN fibres code for movements, not muscles, the innervation of the sternomastoid is *ipsilateral*. This is necessary in order to effect head rotation contralateral to the descending central motor pathway.

THE HYPOGLOSSAL NERVE (XII)

The nucleus of this purely motor nerve is near the midline of the medulla in the lower part of the floor of the fourth ventricle. The nerve emerges from the ventral medulla and passes out of the cranial vault through the hypoglossal canal near the foramen magnum. It travels downwards superficial to the internal and external carotid arteries, and then forward on the hyoglossus to supply the tongue musculature. Motor fibres from upper cervical roots join the nerve at its exit from the skull and leave again as the ansa cervicalis and other branches to supply the depressors of the hyoid bone.

EXAMINATION

Note any *wasting* (Fig. 10.14), *fasciculation* or *tremor* of the tongue. Wasting and fasciculation,

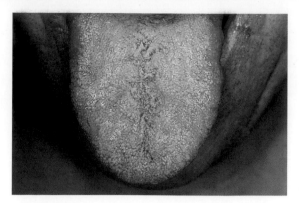

Figure 10.14 Bilateral fasciculation and wasting of the tongue in motor neuron disease. The tongue was fasciculating.

assessed with the tongue relaxed inside the mouth, indicate an LMN lesion involving the nucleus or nerve, whereas a small pointed stiff tongue suggests an upper motor neuron lesion. Bilateral fasciculation of the tongue is almost pathognomonic of *motor neuron disease (amyotrophic lateral sclerosis)*. Unilateral wasting fasciculation occurs with skull base tumours. *Tremor* of the tongue, either at rest or when protruded, is common in Parkinson's disease. Ask the patient to put out their tongue as far as possible. With a unilateral hypoglossal lesion the tongue is protruded more on the normal side, so that it deviates towards the paralysed side instead of being straight. Verify that this is tongue weakness, rather than mouth asymmetry, by asking the patient to push the tongue sideways against the inside of the cheek while you press on this point from the outside.

THE MOTOR SYSTEM OF THE LIMBS AND TRUNK

The 'desire' to make a movement is processed in the brain to generate a sequence of instructions that are transmitted to the effector muscles. This motor pathway starts in cortical association areas and is relayed in the motor cortex. Parallel processing both upstream and downstream of the motor cortex takes place in the basal ganglia and cerebellum. From the motor cortex, *corticospinal* neurons pass down through the anterior two-thirds of the posterior limb of the internal capsule, those to the upper body travelling more anteriorly than those to the lower body. The anterior limb of the capsule carries frontopontine fibres and corticobulbar motor fibres to the cranial nerve nuclei. The posterior third of the posterior limb carries ascending sensory fibres from the thalamus to the sensory cortex. Below the internal capsule, corticospinal fibres are grouped into the cerebral peduncles in the anterior midbrain and then spread out into the anterior bulk of the pons, thence to pass down through the medullary pyramids, which give the corticospinal motor pathways their other name – the *pyramidal tracts*. The corticospinal fibres then cross the midline in the *pyramidal decussation* at the lower medulla and pass into the lateral and anterior *corticospinal tracts* of the spinal cord. These fibres terminate on interneurons or motor neurons in the anterior horn of the spinal grey matter. The motor neuron axons pass out of the cord through the motor roots, join with dorsal sensory roots to form anterior and posterior rami, and finally pass through peripheral nerves to the neuromuscular junctions of the effector muscles. At spinal segments that innervate the limbs the anterior rami become grouped after their exit from the spinal canal into the brachial plexus (levels C5 to T1) and the lumbar plexus (L1 to sacral), in which the segmental roots are reorganized into peripheral nerves.

Within the brainstem corticospinal axons are joined by axons from other motor pathways that travel independently from brainstem nuclei into the spinal cord to reach *interneurons* that indirectly influence motor neurons. These pathways include the midbrain tectospinal and rubrospinal tracts; the former mediates versive movements of the head to visual or auditory stimuli, and the latter is of dubious existence in humans. The vestibulospinal and reticulospinal tracts mediate posture and alerting or startle reactions, respectively. These tracts have complex excitatory and inhibitory effects on the motor neuron pool. The *upper motor neuron* functionally groups all these pathways and is defined as all the components of the central motor pathway from the motor cortex to its terminations on motor neurons. A UMN lesion is synonymous with a *pyramidal tract lesion*. It can be seen that a UMN lesion is *not* synonymous with a corticospinal neuron lesion. The latter is usually only found in isolation in a lesion of the hand area of the motor cortex and does not give the classic UMN features of overactivity, but instead a rather localized deficit of the hand, with impairment of fine finger movements and no increase in tone. Only about 3% of neurons in the corticospinal tract are direct, fast-conducting axons to α motor neurons. The precise nature of a UMN lesion in terms of severity and location of spasticity and weakness is also dependent on the particular pattern of damage to the corticospinal and other descending motor tracts.

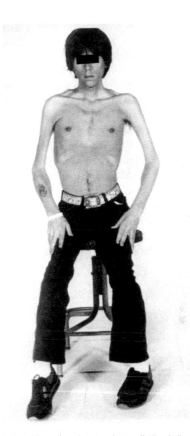

Figure 10.15 Muscular atrophy due to limb-girdle muscular dystrophy. Note the atrophy of the limb and shoulder muscles, especially the biceps and deltoids. Thinning of the thigh musculature can be recognized even through the trousers.

The *lower motor neuron* is the pathway of the motor neurons from the anterior horns to their neuromuscular junctions.

EXAMINATION

Follow a regular sequence (Box 10.8).

INSPECTION
Muscle wasting occurs in a distribution characteristic of particular conditions (Fig. 10.15). *Muscle wasting* develops rapidly over a couple of weeks following peripheral nerve section. Wasting is also a feature of primary muscle disease such as muscular dystrophy, in cachexia of any cause, or with disuse, e.g. due to injury or disease of a joint. *Disuse*

atrophy occurs rapidly in the quadriceps when there is immobility or pain in the knee. In disuse atrophy strength is comparatively well preserved in relation to the degree of muscular wasting. If wasting is due to a motor nerve or motor neuron lesion, *fasciculations* – spontaneous contractions of portions of individual motor units – may occur. Fasciculations are more typical of motor neuron disease and root lesions than of distal motor neuropathies.

Long-term motor deficits acquired during childhood may lead to skeletal changes, such as pes cavus in childhood onset distal motor neuropathy (Fig. 10.16), or a shortened limb following cerebral palsy or polio. Some patients, especially boys with Duchenne muscular dystrophy (Fig. 10.17), develop large muscles (*pseudohypertrophy*) owing to fibrosis and fatty replacement in the affected muscles. The calves, buttocks and infraspinati are particularly affected in Duchenne disease. These enlarged muscles are weak in spite of their size. True hypertrophy of muscles occurs in response to continued excessive workloads in heavy occupations, or following athletic training. It may also occur in certain myotonic disorders. Hypertrophy and atrophy can be quantitatively assessed by transverse CT or MR imaging of muscles (Figs 10.18, 10.19), or by ultrasound studies.

POSTURE AND ABNORMAL MOVEMENTS
Postural control of the upper limbs is assessed by asking the patient to hold the arms outstretched with the eyes closed. Posture of the trunk and lower limbs is assessed separately with gait.

- *Pyramidal drift* describes a tendency for the hand to move upward and supinate if the hands are held outstretched in a pronated position (palms downward), or to pronate downward if the hands are held in supination.
- *Cerebellar drift* is generally upward, with excessive rebound movements if the hand is suddenly displaced downward by the examiner.
- *Parietal drift* is an outward movement on displacing the ulnar border of the supinated hand (see Cognitive examination above).

Take a moment to check for any abnormal movements while the patient is in repose, then during posture, and then during movements such as finger–nose pointing (see Cerebellar system). There are several common types of tremor (Box 10.9):

- *Rest tremor* occurs in Parkinson's disease and is typically a 'pill-rolling' tremor of one or both hands, where the thumb is moved repetitively back and forth across the tips of the fingers at a frequency of 3–6 Hz.
- *Postural tremor: essential tremor* is usually relatively symmetrical and involves the upper limbs more than the legs. It may also affect the head and tongue. A typical parkinsonian tremor may

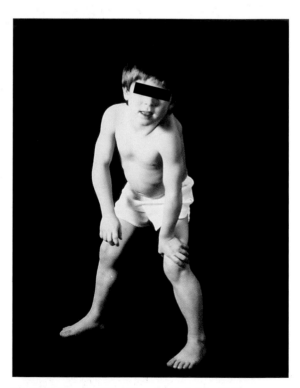

Figure 10.17 Duchenne muscular dystrophy (Xp21 dystrophy). There is pseudohypertrophy of the weak muscles, e.g. the calves and deltoids. The child is 'climbing up himself' with legs widely placed as he gets up from the sitting position to the standing position. This is Gowers' sign.

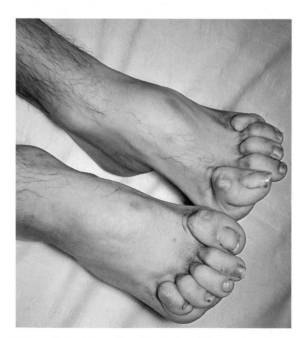

Figure 10.16 Pes cavus, with clawing of the toes in a patient with familial neuropathy. This patient had Refsum's disease and the peripheral nerves were slightly enlarged.

also be worse during posture. Postural tremor also typifies adrenergic tremors, e.g. physiological or anxiety tremor and thyrotoxicosis. Tremor may also occur in sensory ataxic neuropathy.

- *Action tremor*, a terminal tremor in which the finger overshoots and oscillates when approaching a visual target, is indicative of cerebellar ataxia or sensory ataxia.
- *Hysterical tremor* tends to involve a limb or the whole body, to occur at rest and be fast and violent. During distraction by the examiner it disappears.
- *Rubral tremor* is unilateral or bilateral and occurs in rest, posture and action, sometimes building

up over a few seconds of posture. It reflects brainstem disease, including paraneoplastic limbic encephalitis.

- *Pseudoathetosis* describes fidgety movements of the fingers when in posture with the eyes closed and is due to a proprioceptive deficit, including a large fibre sensory neuropathy (Fig. 10.20) or a lesion of the nucleus cuneatus at the synaptic termination of the dorsal columns, e.g. from foramen magnum stenosis. Similar small finger movements can be the result of fasciculatory contractions of pathologically large motor units in motor neuron disease.
- *Myoclonus* is involuntary jerky movement of a body part or parts, or sometimes of the whole body. When rhythmic, it may appear as a rest or action tremor. Its origin can be cortical, e.g. focal epilepsy or, if ongoing, *epilepsia partialis continua*. Myoclonus of body segments is usually spinal in origin, whereas that of the whole body usually originates in the brainstem and can occur normally on falling asleep, or pathologically as an exaggerated startle or shivering response or as part of a generalized epileptiform disorder. When a muscle is voluntarily tonically activated, brief myoclonic relaxation may interrupt the activation. This is called *negative myoclonus*. An example is *asterixis* of liver disease, in which maintained wrist extension is irregularly interrupted, producing a 'flapping' motion. Rarely, negative myoclonus in the quadriceps muscles while standing may result in collapse.
- *Chorea* is a translation of the word 'dance', which accurately portrays its fidgety, fluid, random and semipurposeful quality. The involuntary movements tend to embellish voluntary movements, such as walking, or picking up a cup and saucer. Voluntary actions are performed surprisingly well

Box 10.9 Common causes of tremors

- Anxiety
- Essential tremor
- Physiological tremor
- Thyrotoxicosis
- Parkinson's disease
- Heavy metal poisoning, e.g. mercury, manganese, thallium

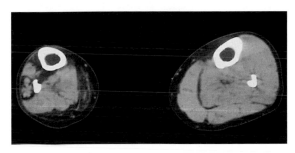

Figure 10.18 Old poliomyelitis. CT scan. Wasting of the muscles of the right leg (to the left of the picture). Note that all the muscles are wasted compared with the normal left side. Also the tibia and fibula are smaller, indicating that the wasting must have been present since childhood.

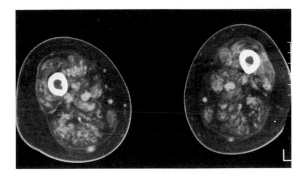

Figure 10.19 Type 3 spinal muscular atrophy. CT scan. There is atrophy, fibrosis and fat replacement of most of the muscles of the thighs and the abnormality is symmetrical. The patient is immobile and has become obese.

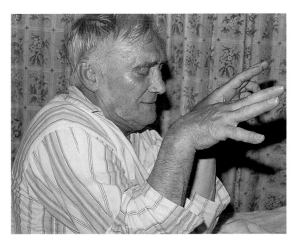

Figure 10.20 Paraneoplastic sensory neuropathy due to small cell carcinoma of the lung. With the eyes closed the patient's outstretched arms become flexed and abnormal postures develop in the fingers.

despite the constant interruption. Its causes include *Huntington's disease*, *Sydenham's chorea*, lupus and pregnancy, and it may also occur idiopathically in the elderly. Finally, chorea and other involuntary movements may arise as side effects of dopaminergic or antidopaminergic drugs; in this context the involuntary movement is termed *dyskinesia*.

- *Ballism* is a violent movement of the proximal limb and trunk. *Hemiballismus* (unilateral ballism) is almost always due to a stroke affecting the contralateral subthalamic nucleus in the midbrain.
- *Athetosis* is a complex, writhing involuntary movement, usually more pronounced in distal than in proximal muscles and of lower amplitude than chorea.
- *Dystonia* describes any abnormal posturing of the body. Its origin may be symptomatic of underlying disease, such as cerebral palsy, pyramidal lesions or generalized inherited or metabolic extrapyramidal diseases. Often, however, dystonia is idiopathic, probably inherited, generalized, limited to particular body segments (e.g. *torticollis*), or focal and perhaps task specific (e.g. *writers' cramp* or *musician's dystonia*).
- *Tics* are simple, normal movements that become *repeated* unnecessarily to the point where they become an embarrassment. They often occur in the context of psychiatric disorders. In contrast to other involuntary movement disorders they can be readily imitated and voluntarily suppressed, albeit briefly. Head nodding and facial twitching are common examples. In *Tourette's syndrome* tics manifest as embarrassing scatological vocalizations.
- *Tetany* is due to hypocalcaemia or alkalosis. There is a characteristic cramped posture of the affected hand (Fig. 10.21) so that fingers and thumb are held stiffly adducted and the hand partially flexed at the metacarpophalangeal joints; the toes may be similarly affected (*carpopedal spasm*). Ischaemia of the affected limb, produced by a sphygmomanometer cuff inflated above the arterial pressure for 2 or 3 minutes, will augment this sign or produce it if it is not already present (*Trousseau's sign*). Another useful test is to tap lightly with a patellar hammer at the exit of the facial nerve from the skull, about 3–5 cm below and in front of the ear. The facial muscles twitch briefly with each tap (*Chvostek's sign*).
- *Cramp* is a spontaneous contraction of part or the whole of a muscle. It is common in healthy people, especially in the calf, and may occur with neurogenic muscle weakness. Other causes of cramp include motor neuron disease or metabolic disorders, e.g. hyponatraemia and hypomagnesaemia. Poor relaxation of muscle, *myotonia*, is a feature of primary muscle disease due to abnormal ion transport across the muscle cell mem-

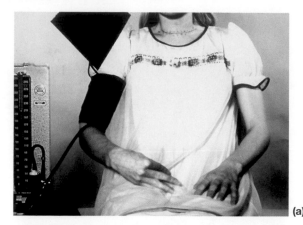

(a)

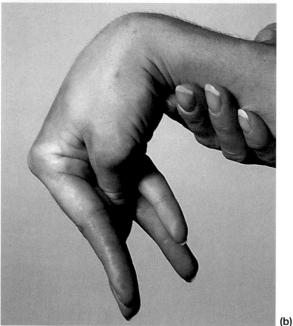

(b)

Figure 10.21   Tetany. Reproduced with permission from Mir M.A. (1995) Atlas of Clinical Diagnosis. London: WB Saunders.

brane, often as the result of a genetic channelopathy such as congenital myotonia, paramyotonia or myotonic dystrophy. Myotonia in some types of hereditary muscle channelopathy is worsened in the cold or induced by active contraction, such as hand gripping; the patient is unable to let go again immediately. Similar difficulty in opening the eyes occurs after forceful closure. *Percussion myotonia* is an enhanced myotatic response elicited by tapping the thenar eminence or the surface of the tongue. *Neuromyotonia* is a continuous muscular activity caused by dysfunction in nerve fibres; as part of a generalized acquired neuropathy it is called *Isaac's syndrome*.

PALPATION

Wasted or atrophic muscles are not only smaller, but softer and more flabby than normal when they are contracted. When muscular wasting is accompanied by fibrosis, as in muscular dystrophy, polymyositis or eosinophilic myositis, the muscles feel hard and inelastic.

TONE

Muscular tone refers to the state of muscle tension or contraction. Increased tone is called *hypertonia* and reduced tone *hypotonia*. In *spasticity* tone is increased in proportion to the speed of passive stretch, whereas *rigidity* is an increase in tone at rest. Tone is assessed by taking a limb and moving it passively back and forth at different rates. Important joints to test include pronation and supination at the wrist, and flexion and extension at the elbow and knee. Ankle tone can be assessed by briskly rolling the relaxed leg from side to side at the knee and observing whether there is a normal loose floppiness at the ankle. The *clasp-knife* phenomenon is a progressive increase in tonic resistance during passive movement, followed by the sudden letting-go of tone characteristic of spasticity. The term *spastic catch* is often used to describe this. *Ankle clonus*, an indication of overactivity of the ankle stretch reflex, is tested by suddenly dorsiflexing the foot with the leg slightly flexed; a series of beats of oscillatory plantarflexion of the ankle is produced at about 3/s.

Rigidity is characteristic of *extrapyramidal disease*. Sometimes it resembles a lever engaging on the teeth of a cogwheel (*cogwheel rigidity*). It can be enhanced by asking the patient to contract another muscle, e.g. to clench the fist, or to move the hand up and down on the opposite side (*Jendrassik manoeuvre*); however, to an extent this enhancement may occur in normal individuals. When rigidity is discovered, especially in association with rest tremor, the examiner should consider whether the features of parkinsonism or idiopathic Parkinson's disease are present. The classic triad of idiopathic Parkinson's disease consists of *bradykinesia, the specific tremor, and cogwheel rigidity*. There is also loss of postural reflexes. Ask the patient to make rapid large-amplitude movements bringing the fingers and thumb together and apart. Parkinsonism produces a characteristic diminishing of amplitude after a few movements (Fig. 10.22). A similar test involves rapid alternating pronation and supination of the cupped hands 'as if screwing and unscrewing a light bulb'. Other features of parkinsonism and related conditions, normally parts of other aspects of examination, may also be brought together (Box 10.10).

In *frontal lobe disease* and *obtunded states* an almost voluntary active resistance to movement develops in which the patient seems to actively oppose your introduced joint displacements, consciously pulling in the opposite direction. This is called *gegenhalten* (literally 'go–stop'). Of course, joint pain or anxiety can also increase muscle tone. Long-term increased tone, especially spasticity, can

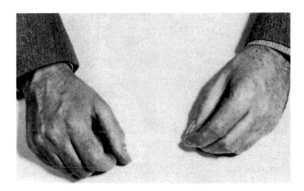

Figure 10.22 Parkinson's disease. The left hand is held partially flexed and immobile. This has resulted in slight oedema of the skin, causing the joints and tendons to appear indistinct. Because the hand is not used, its venous return is not as prominent as in the other hand.

Box 10.10 Features of parkinsonian syndromes to check in suspected Parkinson's disease and in Parkinson 'plus' conditions, such as Steele–Richardson syndrome (also called progressive supranuclear palsy, PSP), dementia with Lewy bodies (DLB) and multiple system atrophy (MSA)

Parkinson's disease	Parkinson's Plus syndromes
Rest tremor	Action tremor and impotence (MSA), myoclonus
Rigidity	Marked axial rigidity (PSP)
Bradykinesia	
Bradyphrenia (slow thought)	
Hypophonia	Cognitive impairment (PSP, DLB)
Slightly jerky saccades and pursuit eye movements	Dysarthria (PSP, MSA)
	Vertical supranuclear saccade palsy (PSP), broken pursuit (MSA)
Facial hypomimia (lack of facial expression)	
Small handwriting	
Stooped posture and festinant gait	Falls early in disease course, ataxic gait (MSA)
Mild autonomic dysfunction	Severe autonomic dysfunction (MSA)

result in a fixed limitation of movement called *contracture*. Reduced muscle tone occurs if the spinal stretch reflex arc is interrupted, e.g. in *tabes dorsalis* or *peripheral neuropathies*, although this sign is difficult to elicit.

POWER

The strength of individual muscle groups is tested by comparing them with the examiner's own strength or by comparison with what the examiner judges to be normal in a person of comparable build to the patient. This requires practice and experience. In testing muscle strength use very simple requests and avoid long explanations: a demonstration or gesture is often most effective. In order to avoid injurious or embarrassing sudden movements, it is generally better for the examiner actively to resist the patient maintaining a certain position (isometric contraction) rather than having the patient actively overcome the examiner; the examiner can then more easily control the build-up and release of force. Most muscles are tested with the patient supine on an examination couch, although the proximal shoulder girdle muscles are usually more conveniently examined with the patient sitting up.

The Medical Research Council (MRC) Scale is used internationally to grade muscle strength (Box 10.11). This scale is clinically based and easy to reproduce, although it is subjective and non-linear. Grade 4 encompasses widely varying degrees of impaired power because many muscles can normally develop far more power than that required to resist gravity. Normal power is different in people of different ages, gender and physical development.

Remember that some muscles are normally much stronger than your arm. For example, the deltoids, gluteus maximus and quadriceps are always very strong in healthy subjects, and you should never be able to overcome them. Test them by actively exercising the patient, e.g. in jumping and hopping. It is always more important to consider the *pattern* of weakness than its severity in reaching a diagnosis (Box 10.12).

ASSESSING THE POWER OF UPPER AND LOWER LIMB MUSCLES

See Tables 10.6 and 10.7 and Figures 10.23–10.45.

ASSESSING THE POWER OF TRUNK AND AXIAL MUSCLES

Examination of the axial musculature of the neck and trunk implies that both range of movement and force should be assessed.

Neck flexion: The cervical musculature is innervated by cranial nerves and cervical roots. Neck flexion is a particularly sensitive marker for the proximal weakness of myopathy. Ask the patient to flex the neck a little and resist your pushing it backwards.

Truncal movements: Severe weakness of the hip flexors and of the muscles of the abdomen is usually evident because the patient is unable to sit up in bed from the supine position without the aid of his arms. *Babinski's 'rising up sign'* is shown by a

---

Box 10.11   The Medical Research Council Scale for grading muscle function (NB: the grades are *not* linear)

Grade 0	Complete paralysis
Grade 1	A flicker of contraction only
Grade 2	Power detectable only when gravity is excluded by appropriate postural adjustment
Grade 3	The limb can be held against the force of gravity, but not against the examiner's resistance
Grade 4	The limb can be held against gravity and against some resistance, but is not normal (a percentage estimate, or a grade of 4+, 4 or 4– is often applied)
Grade 5	Normal power

Box 10.12   Patterns of limb weakness that convey diagnostic information

• *Proximal and axial*	Indicates primary muscle disease.
• *Pyramidal (unilateral or bilateral)*	Worse in the leg flexors than leg extensors. In the arm, shoulder abduction and small hand muscles may be weaker than other muscles. Found in stroke and other focal CNS disease.
• *Distal*	Indicates a polyneuropathy.
• *Focal*	In the distribution of a single peripheral nerve or nerve root.
• *Global or random*	Suggests non-organic illness. Try to describe the pattern and check it for consistency in repeated examinations. Consider additional clinical evidence, such as reflex or sensory findings. Often a rather random pattern actually reflects multiple nerve root involvement.

Table 10.6   Muscles of the upper limb, their nerve supply and examination. Nerve roots printed in bold indicate the major nerve root supply

Action	Muscle	Nerve supply	Examiner's method of testing
Shoulder			
Shoulder abduction, extension	**Deltoid**	Axillary N.; C5	The patient abducts arms with elbows bent. Press down on the upper arms (Fig. 10.23).
Shoulder abduction	Supraspinatus	Suprascapular N.; **C5**, C6	The patient rests the arm down by the side. Grip at the elbow and resist abduction (Fig. 10.24).
Shoulder external rotation	Infraspinatus	Suprascapular N.; **C5**, C6	The patient rests the arm down by his side with the forearm pointing anteriorly at 90° to the arm. Resist external rotation of the shoulder (Fig. 10.25).
Shoulder internal rotation	Rhomboids	Dorsal scapular N.; C4, C5	The patient brings the hand to the small of the back with the palm facing posteriorly. Press against the palm of the patient's hand to resist movement of the hand posteriorly.
Shoulder flexion	Pectoralis major (clavicular head)	Lateral pectoral N.; **C5**, C6	The patient brings the arm up laterally with the forearm pointing superiorly. Hold at the elbow and resist shoulder flexion forwards.
Shoulder adduction	Pectoralis major (sternocostal head)	Medial and lateral pectoral N.; C6, C7, C8	The patient brings the arm just a little away from the side. Hold at the elbow and resist shoulder adduction. Observe the muscle contract on the anterior chest wall (Fig. 10.26).
Shoulder adduction	Latissimus dorsi	Thoracodorsal N.; C6, **C7**, C8	The patient brings the arm up laterally to horizontal. Hold at the elbow and resist shoulder adduction. Observe the muscle contract on the side of the chest wall (Fig. 10.27).
Shoulder adduction	Teres major	Subscapular N.; C6, **C7**, C8	As for latissimus dorsi, but observe teres major on the superior dorsal chest wall.
Stabilization of scapula	Serratus anterior	Long thoracic C5, C6, C7	The patient brings the hands anteriorly to push against a vertical wall. In paralysis, the free medial edge of the scapula 'wings' posteriorly away from the rib cage (Fig. 10.28 (a),(b)).
Elbow			
Elbow flexion	**Biceps brachii**	Musculocutaneous N.; C5, C6	The patient flexes the elbow with the forearm supinated. Hold the wrist, stabilize at the elbow and resist flexion (Fig. 10.29).
Elbow flexion	Brachioradialis	Radial N.; C5, **C6**	The patient flexes the elbow with the forearm mid-pronated. Hold the wrist, stabilize at the elbow and resist flexion. Observe the muscle belly along forearm.
Elbow extension	**Triceps**	Radial N.; C6, **C7**, C8	The patient holds the arm out with the elbow half-extended. Hold at the wrist, stabilize at the elbow and resist extension (Fig. 10.30).
Forearm			
Forearm supination	Supinator	Radial N.; C6, C7	Grasp the patient in a handshake with the patient's elbow extended and resist supination.
Forearm pronation	Pronator teres	Median N.; C6, C7	Grasp patient in a handshake with his elbow extended and resist pronation.
Wrist and hand			
Wrist extension and abduction	Extensor carpi radialis longus	Radial N.; C5, **C6**	The patient cocks the wrist up. Press over the dorsum of the hand at the second metacarpal head and resist extension and abduction of the wrist. Stabilize with your other hand at the base of the forearm near the wrist (Fig. 10.31).

continued

Table 10.6   Muscles of the upper limb, their nerve supply and examination. Nerve roots printed in bold indicate the major nerve root supply – *cont'd*

Action	Muscle	Nerve supply	Examiner's method of testing
Wrist and hand – *cont'd*			
Wrist extension and adduction	Extensor carpi ulnaris	Posterior interosseous N.; **C7**, C8	The patient cocks the wrist up. Press over the dorsum of the hand at the fifth metacarpal head and resist extension and adduction of the wrist. Stabilize with your other hand at the base of the forearm near the wrist.
Wrist flexion and abduction	Flexor carpi radialis	Median N.; C6, C7	Hold the fingers of your hand against the upturned palmar aspect of the patient's second metacarpal head and resist wrist flexion and abduction, stabilizing at the dorsal forearm with your other hand. Observe the flexor tendon at the wrist (Fig. 10.32).
Wrist flexion and adduction	Flexor carpi ulnaris	Ulnar N.; C7, **C8**, T1	Hold the fingers of your hand against the patient's upturned hand at the hypothenar eminence and resist wrist flexion and adduction, stabilizing at the dorsal forearm. Observe the tendon over the ulnar border of the wrist.
Finger flexion	**Flexor digitorum longus**	Median N.; C7, **C8**, T1	Stabilize the patient's proximal phalanx between your thumb and finger and use a finger of your other hand to resist flexion of the proximal interphalangeal joint (Fig. 10.33(b)). (Does not exclude flexor digitorum profundus.)
Finger flexion	Flexor digitorum profundus I, II	Anterior interosseous N.; C7, **C8**	Stabilize the patient's index middle phalanx between your thumb and finger and resist finger flexion by pulling against the flexed distal phalanx (Fig. 10.33(c)).
Finger flexion	Flexor digitorum profundus III, IV	Ulnar N.; C7, **C8**	As for above, but with the patient's little finger (Fig. 10.33(a)).
Thumb flexion	Flexor pollicis longus	Anterior interosseous N.; C7, **C8**	The patient flexes the thumb at the interphalangeal joint. Press against the distal phalanx and resist flexion at this joint (Fig. 10.33(d)).
Thumb abduction	**Abductor pollicis brevis**	Median N.; C8, **T1**	The patient holds the palm upward and brings his thumb away from his hand at 90° to the palm. Hold your thumb against the side of the patient's thumb and resist abduction. Observe the thenar eminence (Figs 10.34, 10.35).
Thumb abduction	Abductor pollicis brevis	Median N.; C6, C7	Figure 10.36.
Index finger abduction	**First dorsal interosseous**	Ulnar N.; C8, **T1**	The patient holds the hand out palm downwards with the fingers apart. Hold your finger against the side of the index finger and resist abduction (Fig. 10.37).
Phalanges extension	Lumbricals	Lateral median and medial ulnar, C8, **T1**	Stabilize the patient's metacarpophalangeal joint in hyperextension by pressing your finger against the palmar surface of the middle phalanx so that the long extensors cannot act, and resist extension of the distal phalanx (Fig. 10.38).
Index finger adduction	First ulnar interosseous	Ulnar N.; C8, **T1**	The converse movement to testing the dorsal interosseous muscle (Fig. 10.39).

similar manoeuvre; in *paralysis* of *a leg*, the affected limb will tend to rise owing to lack of stabilization of the joints, but in *hysterical paralysis* this does not occur (*Hoover's sign*). With weakness of spinal extensor muscles there is excessive lumbar lordosis, and thoracic kyphoscoliosis may develop if the disorder is of childhood onset. In the *dropped head syndrome* there is inability to raise the head to the erect posture because of weakness of neck extensors; this develops in certain myopathies.

Table 10.7 Muscles of the lower limb, their nerve supply and examination. Nerve roots printed in bold indicate the major nerve root supply

Muscle	Action	Nerve supply	Examiner's method of testing
Hip			
Hip flexion	**Iliopsoas**	Spinal branches and femoral N.; **L1**, **L2**, L3	The patient flexes the thigh at the hip near 90°. Resist this by pressing on the anterior aspect of the thigh just proximal to the knee.
Hip extension	**Gluteus maximus**	Inferior gluteal N.; **L5**, **S1**, S2	The patient lies supine with legs extended. Slightly flex the hip by placing your hand under the knee. Ask the patient to extend the hip to support the weight of the pelvis off the couch (Fig. 10.40).
Hip adduction	Hip adductors	Oburator N.; **L2**, **L3**, L4	The patient lies supine with legs extended. Resist adduction of the hip by pressing against the medial surface of the knee, stabilizing with your other hand against the side of the pelvis.
Hip abduction	Gluteus medius and tensor fasciae latae	Superior gluteal N.; **L4**, **L5**, S1	The patient lies supine with legs extended. Resist abduction of the hip by pressing against the lateral surface of the knee, stabilizing with your hand against the opposite side of the pelvis (Fig. 10.41).
Knee			
Knee extension	Quadriceps	Femoral N.; L2, **L3**, **L4**	The patient lies supine with legs extended. Use one hand to lift the patient's leg from underneath the knee to about 20° knee flexion and ask the patient to extend the knee, resisting with your other hand over the patient's lower shin (Figs 10.42, 10.43).
Knee flexion	**Hamstrings**	Sciatic N.; L5, **S1**, S2	The patient lies supine with the knee flexed at 90°. Hold the leg at the ankle and resist pulling of the heel in towards the buttock (Fig. 10.44).
Ankle and foot			
Ankle extension	**Gastrocnemius**	Tibial N.; S1, S2	The patient lies supine with legs extended and plantarflexing the foot. Hold the foot at the metatarsal heads and resist plantarflexion (extension).
Ankle dorsiflexion	**Tibialis anterior**	Deep peroneal N.; **L4**, **L5**	The patient lies supine with legs extended and the foot dorsiflexed. Hold the foot over the dorsal surface and resist dorsiflexion.
Ankle inversion	Tibialis posterior	Tibial N.; L4, L5	Hold the patient's foot medially at the first metatarsal and resist inversion.
Ankle eversion	Peronei	Superficial peroneal N.; L5, S1	Hold the patient's foot laterally at the fifth metatarsal and resist eversion (Fig. 10.45(b)).
Toe flexion	Flexor digitorum longus	Tibial N.; L5, **S1**, **S2**	Hold the patient's toes with your fingers over the plantar surfaces and resist flexion.
Great toe extension	**Extensor hallucis longus**	Deep peroneal N.; **L5**, S1	The patient dorsiflexes the distal phalanx of the great toe. Press against the dorsal surface of the distal phalanx to resist dorsiflexion (Fig. 10.45(a)).
Toe extension	Extensor digitorum brevis	Deep peroneal N.; **L5**, S1	The patient dorsiflexes the proximal phalanges of the toes and attempts to 'spread' the toes. Alternatively, press against the dorsal surfaces of the middle phalanges. Observe and palpate the muscle belly 4 cm distal to the lateral malleolus (Fig. 10.45(a)).
Cupping foot	Small foot muscles	Medial and lateral plantar N.; S1, S2	Ask the patient to cup the foot, palpating the small muscles on the plantar surface (Fig. 10.45(c)).

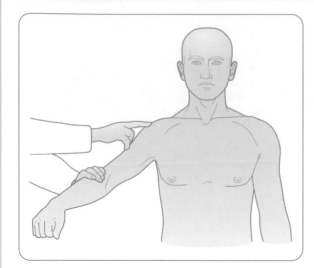

Figure 10.23   Testing the deltoid.

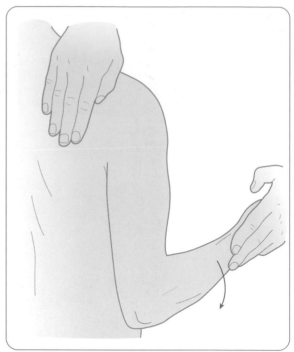

Figure 10.25   Testing the infraspinatus.

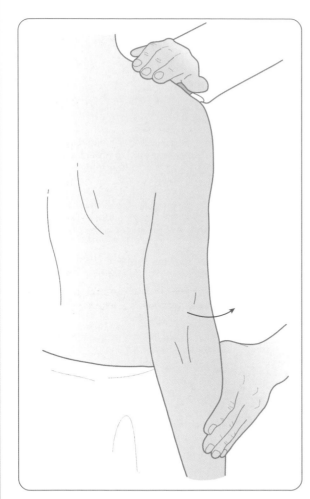

Figure 10.24   Testing the supraspinatus.

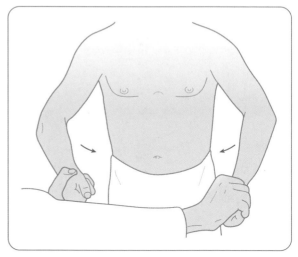

Figure 10.26   Testing the pectoralis major (sternocostal head).

against resistance. With paralysis of the lower segment the umbilicus moves upwards (*Beevor's sign*), and when the upper segment is affected the umbilicus is pulled downwards. This is useful in deciding the level of a thoracic spinal cord lesion.

Diaphragm: The diaphragm is innervated by the upper cervical segments and is vulnerable in C3/4 level traumatic cord transection. It may also be involved in motor neuron disease, certain muscle diseases (e.g. acid maltase deficiency), and sometimes in brachial neuritis. *Diaphragmatic weakness prevents a brisk sniff* – a respiratory movement

Abdominal musculature: Paralysis of part of the anterior abdominal wall can be detected by the displacement of the umbilicus that occurs when the patient attempts to lift his head up from the pillow

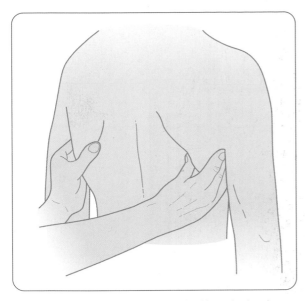

Figure 10.27 Testing the latissimus dorsi by palpating the two posterior axillary folds as the patient coughs.

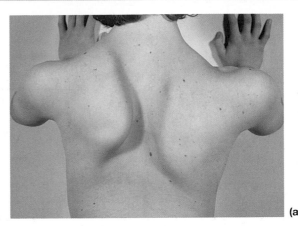

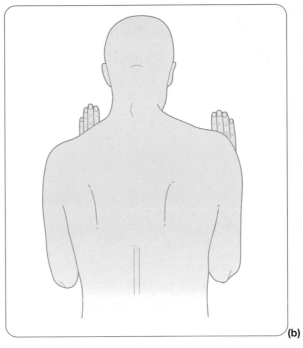

(a)

(b)

Figure 10.28 **(a)** Testing for winging of the scapulae. The left side is affected. **(b)** Testing the serratus anterior.

that requires a sudden maximal diaphragmatic contraction. Diaphragmatic weakness prevents easy breathing when lying flat and in sleep because the abdominal contents now press freely against the lungs. Another simple bedside test is to ask the patient to take a deep breath and then to count aloud slowly – most people can easily reach 20 or more with a single breath.

DEEP TENDON REFLEXES

When the tendon of a lightly stretched muscle is struck a single sharp blow with a soft rubber hammer, thereby suddenly stretching the muscle and exciting a synchronous volley of afferent impulses from the primary sensory endings of the muscle spindles, the muscle contracts briefly. This is called the *deep tendon reflex*, or the *monosynaptic stretch reflex*. These tendon reflexes have only a single synapse between Ia afferent and motor efferent axons. In general the afferent loop is much more critical for reflex function than the efferent loop, so that unless the muscle is almost paralysed, *loss of reflexes* suggests a sensory nerve or root lesion rather than a motor nerve lesion. Increased tendon reflex activity suggests increased excitability of the anterior horn cells in the spinal segment of the stretched muscle due to loss of descending inhibition with a UMN or corticospinal tract lesion. Brisk reflexes alone, however, are not necessarily pathological and usually result from anxiety. It is important to become skilled in the technique of eliciting tendon reflexes (Fig. 10.46):

- Put the patient at ease sitting or lying supine on the examination couch and make sure the genitalia are covered.

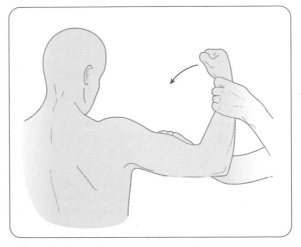

Figure 10.29 Testing the biceps brachii.

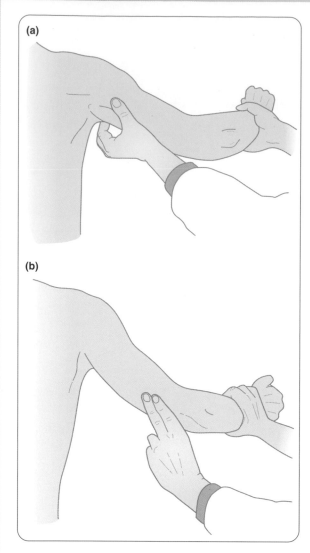

Figure 10.30 Testing the triceps: **(a)** long head; **(b)** whole muscle.

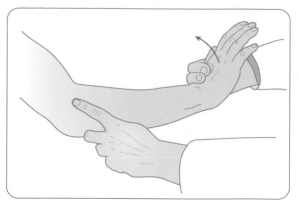

Figure 10.31 Testing the extensor carpi radialis longus.

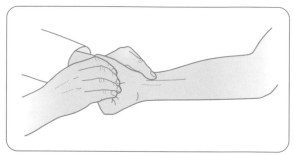

Figure 10.32 Testing the flexor carpi radialis.

- Always make sure the patient is warm and comfortable.
- Always use the same type of tendon hammer in the same manner, standing on the same side of the bed – *standardize your technique*.
- Reassure the patient that the hammer is soft.
- Repeat the test if necessary.

The briskness of deep tendon reflexes varies according to the individual and can sometimes only be elicited in normal individuals by applying *reinforcement* (Jendrassik's manoeuvre). This increases anterior horn cell excitability. Ask the patient to make a strong voluntary muscular effort, e.g. hooking the fingers of the two hands together and then pulling them against one another as hard as possible, making a fist with one hand, or clenching the teeth. Reinforcement is greatest for only a fraction of a second after the onset of contraction, so

the examiner must explain the request beforehand and test the reflex as soon as the patient starts. Compare each reflex side to side: even subtle asymmetry can be very important.

Grade tendon reflexes as follows:

0 Absent
1 Present (as a normal ankle jerk)
2 Brisk (as a normal knee jerk)
3 Very brisk
4 Clonus.

In *hypothyroidism* both the contraction and the relaxation phases of the tendon reflex may be prolonged, resulting in 'hung-up' reflexes. In cerebellar ataxia the reflexes may be '*pendular*': there are oscillatory limb movements after the initial reflex associated with 'loose' tone. This is an unreliable sign.

Method of testing reflexes (see Fig. 10.46)

- *Jaw jerk* (see Trigeminal nerve, above).
- *Biceps jerk C5, 6.* Flex the patient's elbow to almost a right-angle with the forearm in semi-pronation, with your index finger on the biceps tendon, and strike it firmly with the patellar hammer. The biceps contracts.
- *Supinator jerk C5, 6.* A blow on the styloid process of the radius stretches the supinator, causing supination of the forearm. The patient's

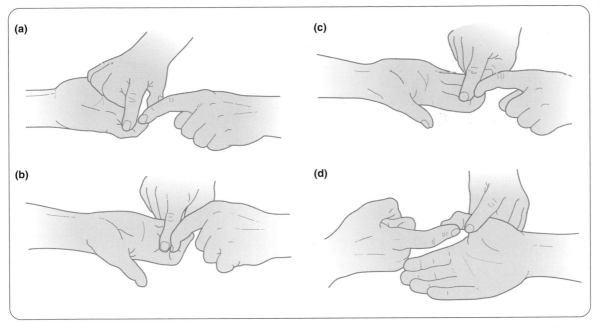

Figure 10.33 Testing **(a)** flexor digitorum superficialis; **(b)** flexor digitorum profundus I and II; **(c)** flexor digitorum longus; **(d)** flexor pollicis longus.

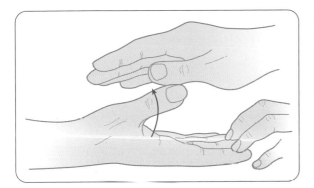

Figure 10.34 Testing the abductor pollicis brevis.

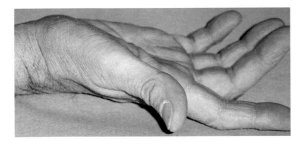

Figure 10.35 Thenar eminence atrophy.

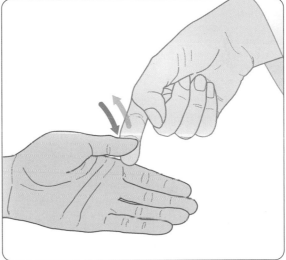

Figure 10.36 Testing the opponens pollicis.

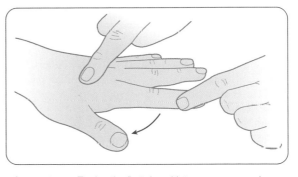

Figure 10.37 Testing the first dorsal interosseous muscle.

elbow should be slightly flexed and slightly pronated, in order to avoid contraction of brachioradialis. With midcervical lesions (*cervical myelopathy*) the supinator or biceps jerks may be absent but brisk flexion of the fingers may occur instead. This is *inversion* of the reflex and suggests

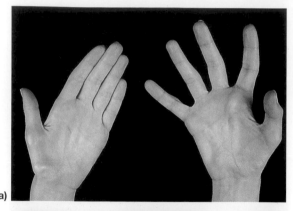

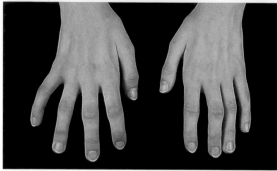

(a)

(b)

Figure 10.38 Wasting of the small hand muscles in a chronic neuropathy. **(a)** There is marked wasting of the abductor pollicis brevis and **(b)** guttering of the dorsal surface of the hand, indicating atrophy of the dorsal interossei.

hyperexcitability of anterior horn cells below the affected level.

- *Triceps jerk C6, 7.* Flex the patient's elbow with the forearm resting across the chest or in their lap. Tap the triceps tendon just above the olecranon. The triceps contracts. Do not strike the belly of the muscle itself, as this generates a direct myotactic response.
- *Knee jerk L2, 3, 4.* The patellar hammer is named from its invention for eliciting the patellar reflex, the first tendon reflex to become a regular part of the neurological examination. The quadriceps contracts when the patellar tendon is briskly tapped. With the patient supine, pass your hand under the knee to be tested so that it supports the relaxed leg with the knee flexed at a little less than 90°. Strike the patellar tendon midway between its origin and its insertion. Look for a contraction of the quadriceps. The knee jerk can often more easily be elicited with the patient sitting up with the legs dangling freely over the edge of the bed.
- *Ankle jerk S1, 2.* Slightly dorsiflex the ankle so as to stretch the Achilles tendon and, with your other hand, strike the tendon on its posterior surface, or the sole of the foot. A quick contraction of the calf muscles results. This reflex can

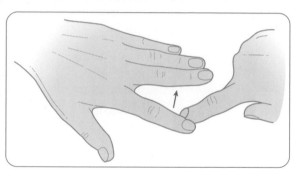

Figure 10.39 Testing the first palmar interosseous muscle.

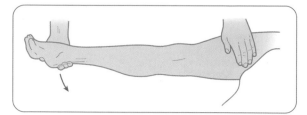

Figure 10.40 Testing the adductors of the thigh.

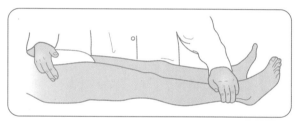

Figure 10.41 Testing the hip adductors (gluteus medius and minimus), and the tensor fasciae latae.

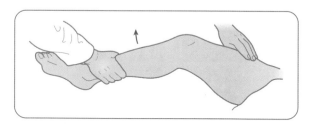

Figure 10.42 Testing the quadriceps femoris.

also be elicited when the patient is kneeling on a chair.

SUPERFICIAL REFLEXES (Table 10.8)
These are polysynaptic reflexes elicited in response to cutaneous stimuli. They do not depend on muscle stretch receptors. The abdominal and plantar reflexes are particularly important.

- *Corneal and palatal reflexes.* See Cranial nerves, above.
- *Scapular reflex (C5–T1).* Stroke the skin between the scapulae. The scapular muscles contract.

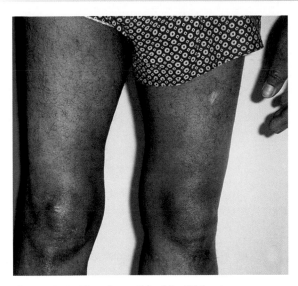

Figure 10.43 There is wasting of the thigh extensor muscles, particularly evident in the medial component of the quadriceps group. The small scar on the left side is from a muscle biopsy. The patient had limb girdle muscular dystrophy.

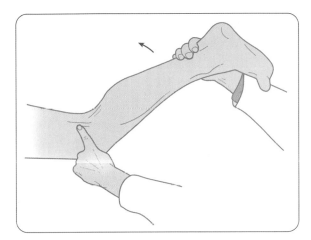

Figure 10.44 Testing the hamstring muscles – knee flexion.

- *Superficial abdominal reflexes (T7–12).* The patient lies relaxed and supine, with the abdomen uncovered. A thin wooden stick or the reverse end of the tendon hammer is dragged quickly and lightly across the abdominal skin in a dermatomal plane from the loin towards the midline. A ripple of contraction of the underlying abdominal musculature follows the stimulus. Abdominal reflexes, like all supraspinal long-latency reflexes, are absent in UMN lesions above their spinal level, as well as in lesions of the local segmental thoracic root or the spinal cord. Abdominal reflexes are difficult to elicit in obese or multiparous women. An anxious patient will have brisk abdominal reflexes as well as brisk tendon reflexes.

- *Cremasteric reflex (L1/2).* Stroke the skin at the upper inner part of the thigh. The testicle moves upwards.
- *The plantar reflex (L5, S1)* (Fig. 10.47). The plantar reflex (the *Babinski response*) is important in identifying a UMN lesion; it is an objective response that can be compared by various observers. To elicit it, the muscles of the lower limb should be relaxed. The outer edge of the sole of the foot is stimulated by firmly scratching a key or a stick along it from the heel towards the little toe. (A final medial movement across the sole of the metatarsus was not used by Babinski.) In healthy adults even a slight stimulus also produces early contraction of the tensor fascia lata, often accompanied by a slighter contraction of the adductors of the thigh and of the sartorius. With a slightly stronger stimulus flexion of the four outer toes appears, which increases with the strength of the stimulus until all the toes are flexed on the metatarsus and drawn together, the ankle being slightly dorsiflexed and inverted. This is called the flexor plantar response. With still stronger stimuli withdrawal of the limb occurs.

  Babinski's extensor plantar response is pathognomonic of an UMN lesion. Instead of the normal flexor response, dorsiflexion (the anatomical nomenclature calls this movement extension) of the great toe precedes all other movement. This is followed by spreading and extension of the other toes, by marked dorsiflexion of the ankle, and by flexion withdrawal of the hip and knee. This response represents the release of a primitive segmental nociceptive flexion withdrawal response. Note that the muscles involved in the Babinski extensor response are those that are clinically weak to volitional effort in corticospinal lesions. Like the normal flexor plantar response, this so-called extensor plantar response is best elicited from the outer edge of the sole of the foot; more medial stimuli elicit foot flexion as part of the grasp response, a different phenomenon. With major corticospinal lesions the area (receptive field) from which the extensor plantar reflex can be elicited enlarges, spreading inwards and over the sole of the foot, and then upwards along the leg to the knee or even higher. For this reason, extension of the great toe, generally associated with some dorsiflexion of the foot, can sometimes also be obtained by squeezing the calf or pressing heavily along the inner border of the tibia (Oppenheim's sign), or by pinching the calcaneus tendon (Gordon's reflex). In infants under 1 year of age the extensor response is the normal response. The flexor response appears in the subsequent 6–12 months as myelination of the corticospinal pathways is completed.

  Flexor spasms may occur when testing the plantar reflex. These consist of an exaggerated

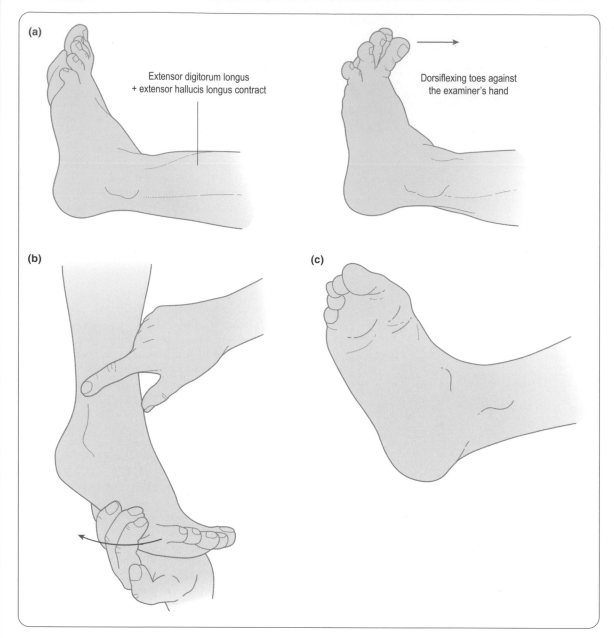

(a) Extensor digitorum longus + extensor hallucis longus contract

Dorsiflexing toes against the examiner's hand

(b)

(c)

Figure 10.45 Testing **(a)** the extensor digitorum longus and extensor hallucis longus; **(b)** peroneus longus and brevis; **(c)** small muscles of the foot.

extensor plantar response, the whole limb being suddenly drawn up into flexion and the large toe extended. They occur in severe bilateral upper motor neuron lesions, especially spinal lesions that involve the more dorsal reticulospinal and vestibulospinal pathways, and in circumstances where generally increased sensory input from bedsores or urinary infection excite the motor neuron pool still further. Extensor spasms, conversely, are more likely to occur in patients with spinal lesions affecting the more ventral (spinothalamic) descending pathways.

- *Sphincteric reflexes*. These are the reflexes concerned with swallowing, micturition, defecation and sexual function. They depend upon complex muscular movements excited by increased tension in the wall of the viscus, and involve both striated and smooth muscles.
- *Swallowing*. Is there difficulty in swallowing (dysphagia)? Note any regurgitation of food through the nose (see cranial nerve examination). Swallowing requires coordinated activity of the lips, tongue, pharynx and oesophagus to seize food, masticate it, progress the bolus across the

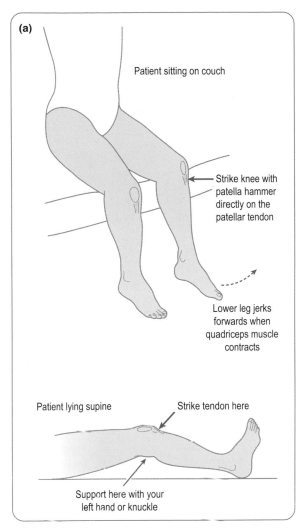

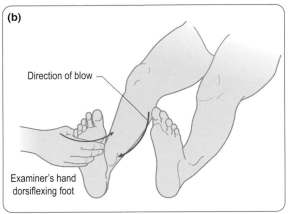

Figure 10.46 Methods for testing tendon reflexes (see text). The words 'jerk' and 'reflex' are interchangeable. **(a)** Knee jerk; **(b)** ankle jerk.

tongue toward the pharynx and initiate the pharyngeal phase of swallowing, in which the airway is closed by the soft palate. In general, patients with neurological dysphagia usually report difficulty in swallowing liquids, whereas those with mechanical obstruction to the oesophagus or pharynx cannot swallow solids.

- *Micturition*. Ask about holding or initiating urination, and whether bladder and urethral sensations are normal. Note any retention, incontinence or urgency of micturition. Urinary incontinence in neurological disorders may be due to overflow from an atonic distended bladder in which sensation has been lost. In this case the bladder will be enlarged to palpation or percussion, and suprapubic pressure may result in the expulsion of urine from the urethra. Incontinence may also be due to an unstable bladder or urge incontinence, when micturition occurs either at regular intervals as the bladder partially fills, or abruptly and unexpectedly in response to a sudden noise, to movement or to exposure to cold. Urge incontinence is often idiopathic, but also occurs as an early feature of prostatism and in intrinsic disease of the spinal cord. Stress incontinence – when urine leaks on coughing – is due to weakness of the sphincter mechanism, to sphincter tears in childbirth, or to denervation of the sphincter.

- *Defecation*. Ask about defecation and faecal continence to formed and liquid stool, and to flatus. Is anorectal sensation normal? Assess the voluntary anal sphincter by introducing a lubricated gloved index finger into the anus and noting whether the voluntary squeeze contraction of the sphincter is normal. In patients with weakness of the pelvic floor, usually due to damage to the innervation of the pelvic floor musculature, coughing is accompanied by descent of the pelvic floor by several centimetres toward the examiner's finger. This is often associated with stress incontinence of faeces or of urine.

- *Anal reflex*. Gently scratch the skin on either side of the anus. A brisk contraction of the sphincter

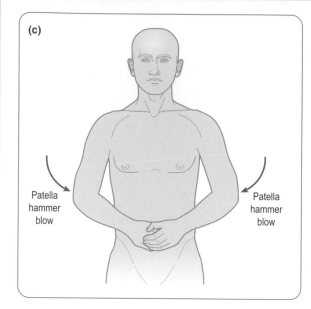

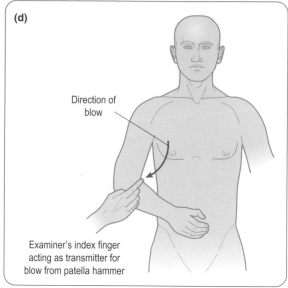

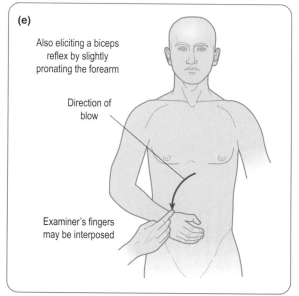

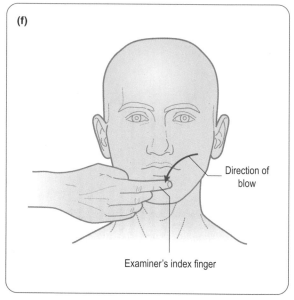

Figure 10.46 – cont'd   **(c)** triceps reflex; **(d)** biceps reflex; **(e)** supinator reflex; **(f)** jaw jerk.

should immediately occur – the anal reflex. The anal sphincter also contracts briskly in reflex response to a sudden cough – the anal cough reflex.

- *Sexual function.* When there is urinary or faecal incontinence associated with neurological disease, e.g. cauda equina lesions, erectile failure, ejaculatory failure or, in both sexes, anorgasmia, may be noted.

COORDINATION

Motor acts require the orderly recruitment of muscles or groups of muscles. If coordination is impaired, motor performance becomes difficult or even impossible (*ataxia*). The cerebellum learns, stores and outputs patterns of signals that enable motor activity in response to sensory afferent infor-

mation from the periphery. Lesions of the efferent corticospinal pathway will prevent signals from reaching the spinal cord to generate muscle activity. These lesions cause specific clinical syndromes, although information from other sensory pathways can be used to compensate for functional defects. For example, *sensory ataxia*, which typically results from sensory neuropathies or dorsal column lesions, is best tested with the patient's eyes closed, and corroborative evidence is gained by testing vibration sense or joint position sense. Clumsiness of the fingers, for example while bringing the tip of the thumb in contact with those of each of the fingers in succession, is as much a feature of *corticospinal tract dysfunction* as of *cerebellar disease*, *extrapyramidal disease* or *sensory ataxia*, because

Table 10.8 Superficial spinal reflexes

Reflex	How excited	Clinical result	Level of cord
Anal	Stroking or scratching skin near anus	Contraction of anal sphincter	3rd and 4th sacral segments
Bulbocavernosus	Pinching dorsum of glans penis	Contraction of bulbocavernosus	3rd and 4th sacral segments
Plantar response	Stroking sole of foot and toes, or leg	Flexion of toes and of foot	5th lumbar and 1st sacral segments
Cremasteric	Stroking skin at upper and inner part of thigh*	Upward movement of testicle	1st and 2nd lumbar segments
Abdominal	Stroking abdominal wall below costal margin and in iliac fossa	Contraction of abdominal muscles	7th and 12th thoracic segments
Scapular	Stroking skin in interscapular region	Contraction of scapular muscles	5th cervical to 1st thoracic segment

*The cremasteric reflex can often be more easily elicited by pressing over the sartorius in the lower third of Hunter's canal.

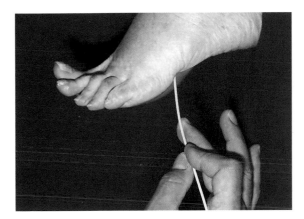

Figure 10.47 The Babinski plantar response. A firm, stroking stimulus to the outer edge of the sole of the foot evokes dorsiflexion (extension) of the large toe and fanning of the other toes.

Box 10.13 Clinical signs of cerebellar lesions

- Cerebellar ataxia
- Intention tremor
- Involvement of limbs, trunk and external ocular movement (nystagmus)
- Past-pointing
- Rebound
- Impaired ability to generate alternating rhythmic movements

such fine voluntary movements require discrete motor cortical control. This is therefore a sensitive but non-specific test of coordination. In anxiety any errors of movement tend to occur in the direction of the movement, rather than at right-angles to the intended direction of movement as in cerebellar ataxia. Accurate movements require a stable base, so *proximal weakness* can also mimic cerebellar ataxia; always formally check muscle strength (Box 10.13).

Testing coordination in the upper limbs
Several different tests can be used.

Finger–nose test. Ask the patient to touch the point of the nose and then the tip of your finger, held at arm's length in front of the patient's face, using their index finger. Cerebellar lesions particularly affect the last, visually guided phase of this test, as the cerebellum integrates different afferent inputs. Ask the patient to repeat the test with the eyes closed; any additional irregularity suggests impairment of position sense in the limb.

Dysdiadochokinesis. Ask the patient to tap your palm with the tips of the fingers of one hand, alternately in pronation and supination, as fast as possible. Minor degrees of incoordination can be both felt and heard. All normal people can do this very rapidly, but usually slightly less rapidly with the non-dominant than with the dominant hand. Dysdiadochokinetic movements are slowed, *irregular*, incomplete, and may be impossible. Parkinsonism may also impair rapid movements, with slowing, reduced amplitude and prominent fatigue, but without irregularity.

Fine movements. Watch the patient dressing or undressing, writing, handling a book or picking up pins. These complex and practised everyday movements offer a very sensitive way of assessing coordination.

Testing coordination in the lower limbs
Several tests are used.

Heel–shin test. While the patient is lying supine on the couch, ask them to lift one leg and then to bend the knee, place the heel on the opposite knee and slide this heel down the shin towards the ankle under visual guidance. In cerebellar ataxia, a characteristic, irregular, side-to-side series of errors in the speed and direction of movement occurs. Also, watch the patient draw a large circle in the air with the toe. The circle should be drawn smoothly and accurately, but in ataxia it is 'squared off' irregularly. Rapid alternating movements of the foot are difficult to assess.

Stance and gait. This important aspect of coordination is described below, as it is usually tested at the end of examination when the patient is asked to stand. *Truncal ataxia* occurs in cerebellar disease, especially in degeneration of the vermis in alcoholism, and is an important aspect of assessment of lower limb and whole-body coordination.

Segmental motor innervation. The several segments innervating the muscles are shown in Figures 10.48 and 10.49. These are important for localization of cord, riot and peripheral nerve disease.

THE SENSORY SYSTEM OF THE LIMBS AND TRUNK

A sensory modality is a sensory experience recognized by individuals as unique. This practical psychophysical definition accords with general experience. Apart from the special senses of vision, hearing, taste and smell, there are six main sensory modalities that can be tested at the bedside:

- Pain
- Temperature
- Tactile sensibility. This includes light touch and pressure, and tactile localization and discrimination
- Vibration
- Position sense – the appreciation of passive movement
- Stereognosis – recognition of the size, shape, weight and form of objects (see under parietal cortex examination).

Sensory perception depends on the physiological interactions between afferent inputs at different levels in the nervous system. The perception of vibration, for example, is not carried by a special set of nerve fibres but is the perception of touch, rapidly applied. The particular receptor combination and the temporal and spatial pattern of afferent signals results in a characteristic sensation. There are specialized receptors in the skin and other tissues that are sensitive to brief or maintained pressure, touch, pain

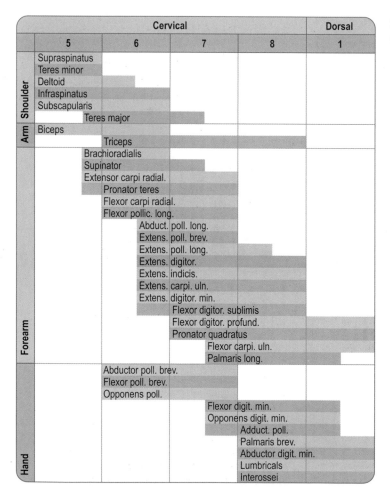

| | | Cervical | | | | Dorsal |
		5	6	7	8	1
Arm	**Shoulder** Supraspinatus	█	█			
	Teres minor	█	█			
	Deltoid	█	█			
	Infraspinatus	█	█			
	Subscapularis	█	█			
	Teres major		█	█		
	Biceps	█	█			
	Triceps		█	█	█	
Forearm	Brachioradialis	█	█			
	Supinator		█	█		
	Extensor carpi radial.		█	█		
	Pronator teres		█	█		
	Flexor carpi radial.		█	█		
	Flexor pollic. long.		█	█	█	
	Abduct. poll. long.			█	█	
	Extens. poll. brev.			█	█	
	Extens. poll. long.			█	█	
	Extens. digitor.			█	█	
	Extens. indicis.			█	█	
	Extens. carpi. uln.			█	█	
	Extens. digitor. min.			█	█	
	Flexor digitor. sublimis			█	█	█
	Flexor digitor. profund.			█	█	█
	Pronator quadratus			█	█	█
	Flexor carpi. uln.				█	█
	Palmaris long.				█	█
Hand	Abductor poll. brev.				█	█
	Flexor poll. brev.				█	█
	Opponens poll.				█	█
	Flexor digit. min.			█	█	█
	Opponens digit. min.			█	█	█
	Adduct. poll.				█	█
	Palmaris brev.				█	█
	Abductor digit. min.				█	█
	Lumbricals				█	█
	Interossei				█	█

Figure 10.48 Segmental innervation of the muscles of the upper limbs.

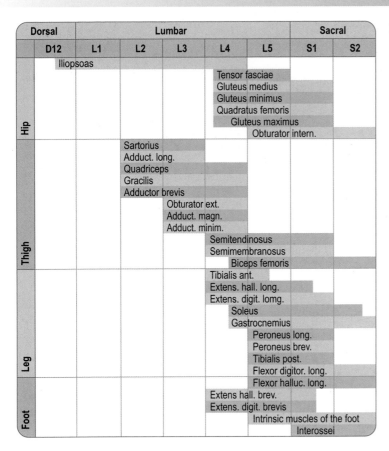

Figure 10.49 Segmental innervation of the muscles of the lower limbs.

| | Dorsal | Lumbar | | | | | Sacral | |
	D12	L1	L2	L3	L4	L5	S1	S2
Hip	Iliopsoas							
					Tensor fasciae			
					Gluteus medius			
					Gluteus minimus			
					Quadratus femoris			
					Gluteus maximus			
						Obturator intern.		
Thigh			Sartorius					
			Adduct. long.					
			Quadriceps					
			Gracilis					
			Adductor brevis					
				Obturator ext.				
				Adduct. magn.				
				Adduct. minim.				
					Semitendinosus			
					Semimembranosus			
					Biceps femoris			
Leg					Tibialis ant.			
					Extens. hall. long.			
					Extens. digit. lomg.			
					Soleus			
					Gastrocnemius			
						Peroneus long.		
						Peroneus brev.		
						Tibialis post.		
						Flexor digitor. long.		
						Flexor halluc. long.		
Foot					Extens hall. brev.			
					Extens. digit. brevis			
						Intrinsic muscles of the foot		
						Interossei		

and temperature. These are found at different densities in different portions of the skin. For example, the fingertips are very sensitive to minor skin deformation, and therefore to light touch and discrimination. There is a historical description of sensation into epicritic and nociceptive modalities, respectively meaning discriminatory sensibility and pain detection. Broadly speaking, the epicritic sensory modalities enter the nervous system via large myelinated peripheral nerve fibres and nociceptive modalities via small, thinly myelinated or unmyelinated fibres. For clinical purposes, vibration sense and position sense belong to the former division and pain and temperature detection to the latter. Light touch belongs to both, and so is not helpful in distinguishing large fibre versus small fibre disease or dorsal column versus spinothalamic disease.

The central processes of large myelinated fibres pass up the ipsilateral *dorsal column* of the spinal cord to the nucleus cuneatus (arm) or nucleus gracilis (leg). After synapsing, they cross the midline and pass up the *medial lemniscus* to the thalamus. Small nociceptive fibres, on the other hand, pass only a few segments *up or down* the cord in Lissauer's tract before crossing the midline and synapsing. Second-order fibres pass up the *spinothalamic tract* of the cord and brainstem to the thalamus. Sorting of afferent inputs occurs in the *substantia gelatinosa* of the dorsal root entry zone of the cord, at each segmental level, so that sensory input can be directed to the appropriate sensory pathways in the cord – the *gate hypothesis* of modulation of sensory input.

EXAMINATION

In sensory testing the examiner must be aware of the whole dermatomal and peripheral nerve distribution of sensation in the body (Figs 10.50 and 10.51). This knowledge is necessary to appreciate that a certain distribution of abnormal sensation results from a lesion of a particular peripheral nerve, nerve root or spinal segmental level. Normality can be established by testing a colleague, but especially by clinical experience of the examination of many patients, and in an individual by establishing clear differences between homologous body parts.

PINPRICK (SMALL FIBRES/SPINOTHALAMIC PATHWAY)

Use a pin that is sharp enough to cause a painful 'pricking' sensation rather than just localized pressure. Use disposable pins. Do *not* use disposable hypodermic needles – these are designed to painlessly penetrate the skin! Delineate areas of abnormality by moving from an area of reduced sensation to a normal zone, not the other way round. Thus, as distal sensory loss is more common than proximal,

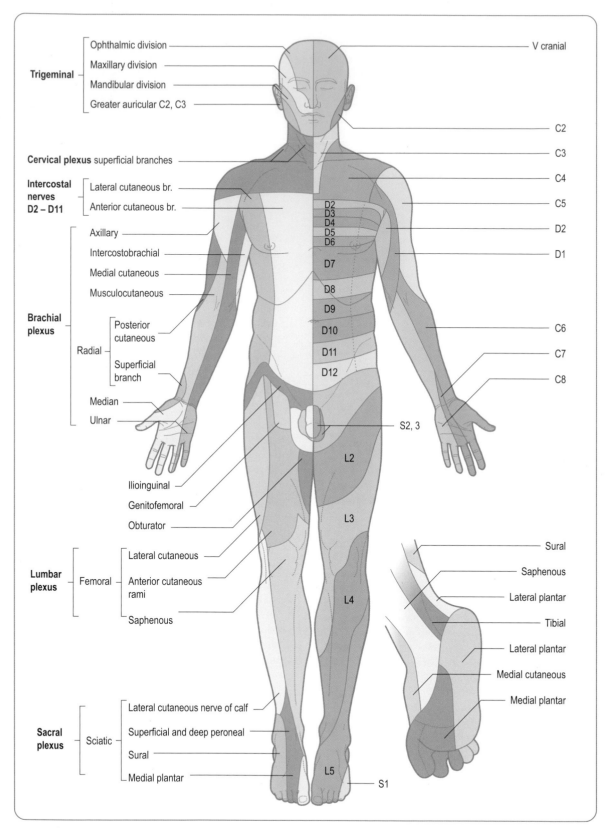

Figure 10.50   Anterior view to show the segmental innervation of the skin (left) and the peripheral nerve supply (right).

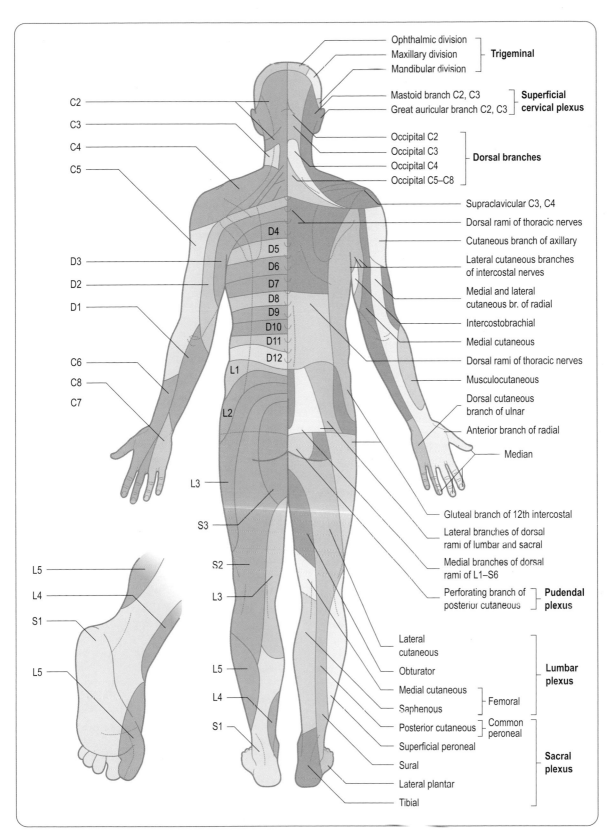

Ophthalmic division ⎤
Maxillary division   ⎬ **Trigeminal**
Mandibular division ⎦

Mastoid branch C2, C3   ⎤ **Superficial**
Great auricular branch C2, C3 ⎦ **cervical plexus**

Occipital C2   ⎤
Occipital C3   ⎬ **Dorsal branches**
Occipital C4   ⎪
Occipital C5–C8 ⎦

Supraclavicular C3, C4

Dorsal rami of thoracic nerves

Cutaneous branch of axillary

Lateral cutaneous branches of intercostal nerves

Medial and lateral cutaneous br. of radial

Intercostobrachial

Medial cutaneous

Dorsal rami of thoracic nerves

Musculocutaneous

Dorsal cutaneous branch of ulnar

Anterior branch of radial

Median

Gluteal branch of 12th intercostal

Lateral branches of dorsal rami of lumbar and sacral

Medial branches of dorsal rami of L1–S6

Perforating branch of ⎤ **Pudendal**
posterior cutaneous ⎦ **plexus**

Lateral cutaneous ⎤
Obturator   ⎪
Medial cutaneous ⎬ **Lumbar**
Saphenous — Femoral ⎪ **plexus**
                  ⎦

Posterior cutaneous ⎤ Common
Superficial peroneal ⎬ peroneal
Sural   ⎪ **Sacral**
Lateral plantar   ⎬ **plexus**
Tibial   ⎦

C2
C3
C4
C5
D3
D2
D1
C6
C8
C7
L5
L4
S1
L5

D4
D5
D6
D7
D8
D9
D10
D11
D12
L1
L2
L3
S3
S2
L3
L5
L4
S1

Figure 10.51   Posterior view to show the segmental innervation of the skin (left) and the peripheral nerve supply (right).

in the sensory examination it is sensible to start testing distally and work proximally.

Follow a standard system of sensory testing and test fairly quickly. People rapidly lose concentration during sensory testing and start to report spurious observations. First, demonstrate on a likely normal area, such as the base of the neck, to establish what you mean by 'sharp'. Then start at the side of the tip of a digit, e.g. the large toe, and test skin points progressively up that side of the limb while it is in the anatomical position (e.g. the arm supinated), asking the patient each time if it feels the same or different as you progress proximally or across dermatomal peripheral nerve boundaries. Only you will have knowledge of the latter. The patient should have their eyes open: pain cannot be 'seen'. If the eyes are closed, the patient may become anxious that you may hurt them, or assume that the test is to detect any sensation rather than just sharpness. Repeat the test for the other side of the limb, noting a possible symmetrical glove or stocking distribution of sensory loss, and visualizing the asymmetrical medial–lateral pattern of the dermatomes along the two sides. Each limb should take no more than 15 seconds to examine both medially and laterally. Avoid repeating the test more than once, as repetition causes fatigue.

If the patient does manual work the skin of the palmar surface of the hand may be thickened and insensitive, so it is important to test the sides and not the palmar surfaces of the fingers. In the leg, pay attention to the rear of the thigh, which unlike the medial and lateral aspects is supplied by sacral roots. Test the anterior surface of the trunk bilaterally, and check the posterior trunk with the patient sitting forward. Remember that dermatomal levels are higher on the trunk posteriorly than anteriorly. Simulated or hysterical (functional) sensory loss usually presents with a horizontal level from back to front. Truncal testing for *suspended sensory loss* (a distribution affecting a number of thoracic levels with normal sensation below, as opposed to a *sensory level*, below which all sensation is lost) is particularly important for the detection of cord lesions such as *syringomyelia*. Such areas are unlikely to have been noted by the patient. Finally, lower sacral sensation around the perineum may be tested by moving the patient on to their side, as for a rectal examination.

Pressure pain may be tested by squeezing the Achilles tendon. This was a popular test when late syphilis was more common, typified by tabes dorsalis, and it is still used to determine the level of response in coma.

Pain is a common *positive symptom. Spontaneous pain* due to nervous dysfunction, a form of *neuropathic pain*, is distinguished from *nociceptive pain*, the normal painful sensation following tissue injury. A lesion of CNS pain pathways, especially the spinothalamic tracts, the thalamus or even the sensory cortex, may lead to an increased pain threshold, with increased intensity of pain perception once this threshold is surpassed. Neuropathic pain may be chronic, unremitting and very distressing. Pain occurring in response to cutaneous stimulation is usually peripheral in origin and usually, as in the small fibre neuropathy of diabetes mellitus, has a lowered threshold. Specific terms are used to describe various positive and negative pain symptoms and signs:

- *Analgesia* – the absence of sensibility to pain
- *Hypoalgesia* – reduced pain sensibility
- *Hyperalgesia* – an increased pain sensibility to mildly painful stimuli
- *Allodynia* – pain perception from a normally non-painful stimulus
- *Hyperpathia* – pain perception that spreads out from the point of the stimulus or outlasts the stimulus in time
- *Paraesthesiae* – tingling sensations sometimes so intense as to be painful, occurring spontaneously or in response to light cutaneous stimuli.

TEMPERATURE (SMALL FIBRES/SPINOTHALAMIC PATHWAY)

The sensation of warmth or cold is normally poorly localized. Thermal testing is useful in corroborating a spinothalamic-type area of deficit delineated by pinprick testing. Hot and cold metal, e.g. the cold end of a tuning fork, lightly applied to the skin is an easy test. The patient should report differences between different body parts.

LIGHT TOUCH (MODERATELY MYELINATED FIBRES/COMBINED PATHWAYS)

This can be tested using the same anatomical scheme as for pinprick, using your fingertip or a strand of cotton wool. However, this may miss mild sensory abnormalities; pinprick testing is more sensitive.

VIBRATION SENSE (LARGE MYELINATED FIBRES/DORSAL COLUMN PATHWAY)

First, demonstrate the test by plucking a lower C (128 Hz) tuning fork and pressing its base over the patient's sternum, then repeating without the vibration. Test bony prominences, starting distally at the side of the tip of the index finger. If this is abnormal, establish a level by repeating over the knuckle, the elbow and the clavicle. In the leg, test the side of the great toe and, if abnormal the knee, the iliac crest and perhaps the ribs. Asking when the perception of vibration fades makes the test semiquantitative.

JOINT POSITION SENSE (LARGE MYELINATED FIBRES/DORSAL COLUMN PATHWAY)

Teach the patient the test by passively moving the terminal phalanx of their little finger while they watch. This is the only sensory test for which it is necessary for the patient to be looking away or have their eyes closed. Take the sides of the index (C6) or little (C8) finger between your thumb and forefinger. Then test 'up' and 'down' movements at various amplitudes and ask the patient to respond. It is not necessary first to make several bizarre rapid movements to confuse the starting position: the test is for direction. Normal subjects detect very small movements. Repeat the test more proximally if it is abnormal distally. In the lower limb, use the great toe.

TWO-POINT DISCRIMINATION

This is a useful, sensitive, quantitative test of fingertip sensory discrimination that requires intact distal sensory function and also intact dorsal columns and primary sensory cortex function. Use a pair of blunt dividers (*two-point discriminator*) and ask whether one or both points can be felt. Normally 2 mm separation of the points can be recognized as two separate stimuli on the fingertips, and rather wider separation – about 1 cm – on the pulps of the toes.

STANCE AND GAIT

The bipedal stance requires the integration of a great deal of sensory information and ongoing adjustment of activity in postural muscles. It is therefore often abnormal in neurological diseases. Posture is dependent on vestibular input related to head position and movement, proprioception from neck and leg and axial muscles, and joint position and deep pressure information from the trunk, legs and feet. This information is synthesized with visual information on position in space. Integration into an overall picture of posture occurs largely unconsciously in the brainstem and midline cerebellum. The effector muscles compensate for sway in different directions, and include many leg, trunk and even arm muscles.

Gait is dependent on the same vestibular, proprioceptive and integrative systems as stance and balance, but in addition requires direction from central gait mechanisms in the frontal lobes, basal ganglia and brainstem, their efferent corticospinal and extrapyramidal tracts, and the motor nerves, muscles and joints of the trunk, arms and legs.

ASSESSMENT OF STANCE

- First evaluate the stance with the patient's feet firmly together and their eyes open. Then ask the patient to close their eyes and note whether the balance is *much* worse (*Romberg's test*). A positive test indicates that the patient is excessively reliant upon vision and suggests a defect in the vestibular pathway or the proprioceptive pathway (*sensory ataxia*). In cerebellar disease the balance is likely to be poor even with the eyes open.

- If a *vestibular lesion* is suspected, ask the patient to jump up and down quickly and repeatedly with the eyes closed. A destructive peripheral lesion falsely indicates body sway in the opposite direction and the effector systems will attempt to compensate. Thus the patient will steadily rotate in the direction of such a lesion (*Unterberger's test*).

- Test *postural reflexes* by asking the patient to stand; then pull them abruptly backwards (or forwards) from the shoulders. Be careful to protect the patient from overbalancing. The normal response is to arch the back and make compensatory arm and leg movements to keep the centre of gravity in line with the feet. This postural response is defective with lesions of the descending outputs from the frontal lobes and basal ganglia to brainstem centres, as in frontal disease, including multi-infarct cerebrovascular disease, in idiopathic Parkinson's disease and, especially, in 'Parkinson-plus' syndromes.

ASSESSMENT OF GAIT

Observe the patient walking at a brisk pace, including turning. Pay particular attention to:

- Reduced arm swing
- Stooped posture
- Lurching to one side
- Asymmetry and loss of smoothness of steps
- Increased breadth of base (transverse distance between steps)
- Excessive stiffness or floppiness at the ankle or knee joints
- Associated involuntary movements
- Apparent pain.

Various specific adjectives are used to describe different abnormal gaits (Box 10.14). These suggest particular neurological abnormalities, and so care should be taken not to apply them inappropriately if the nature of the abnormality is not clear. If you are uncertain, simply describe what you observe. The following patterns are recognized:

- *Frontal (apraxic) gait.* This may be excessively erect and the patient tends to make small stamping steps, called '*marche à Petipa*' after the Russian ballet master of 100 years ago.
- *Parkinsonian gait* (Fig. 10.52). This is a characteristically stooped gait, with small rapid steps: the patient tries to 'catch up' with the centre of gravity. There may be reduced arm swing and a distal pill-rolling tremor. Gait initiation and turns are slow. Sensory distraction or task complication, such as walking through a doorway, adversely affects the gait. Walking to an auditory rhythm, or regular visual cues such as stripes marked on the floor, improves the gait. The gait of Steele–Richardson syndrome can

Box 10.14   Gait disorders

Upper motor neuron
- *Hemiplegia*. Circumduction of leg with inability to flex hip and dorsiflex foot against resistance (or gravity)
- *Paraplegia and quadriplegia*. Scissoring, stiff-legged gait and flexed posture

Lower motor neuron
- *Foot drop*. Weakness of dorsiflexion and eversion of the foot leads to excessive hip flexion to compensate; due to common peroneal nerve palsy or L5/S1 root lesion, or to peripheral neuropathy
- *Quadriceps weakness*. Knee extension weak, leading to sudden falls, difficulty rising from chair or descending stairs
- *Proximal weakness*. Rolling gait, with difficulty climbing stairs. Arms cannot be lifted above shoulder height. Axial weakness may be present
- *Peripheral neuropathy*. Distal weakness and sensory loss

Cerebellar syndrome
- *Ataxia*. Unsteadiness and inability to walk on a narrow base, or to turn quickly

Extrapyramidal syndromes
- *Parkinson's disease*. Shuffling festinant gait, with flexed posture, tremor of hands and face
- *Dystonia*. Involuntary movements and rigid postures
- *Involuntary movements*. Chorea, athetosis, ballismus

Sensory ataxia
- Cerebellar-like ataxia associated with distal loss of position sense:
- *Apraxic gait*. Loss of concept of walking, often associated with tiny rapid steps
- *Hysteria*. Bizarre 'functional' gait disorder; miraculously the patient does not fall

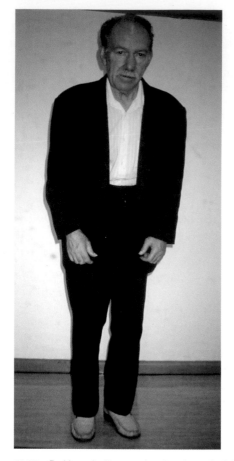

Figure 10.52   Parkinson's disease, showing the typical rigid, flexed posture involving the trunk and limbs. The face is impassive.

combine the features of a parkinsonian (slow gait) with a frontal (erect) gait, whereas in multiple system atrophy there are cerebellar features.
- *Vestibular gait*. A peripheral vestibular lesion, if acute and not yet compensated, causes the patient to lurch to one side (see Unterberger's test).
- *Cerebellar gait*. The gait is unsteady ('drunken') and irregular, with a wide base. The latter feature is brought out by asking the patient to walk on a narrow base by walking one heel directly in front of the toe of the other foot.
- *Spastic gait*. The patient walks on a narrow base with the knees slightly flexed and ankles plantarflexed so that the toes scuff on the floor, and the hip circumducts while the stepping leg is being lifted forward. It occurs in spinal cord disease or bilateral pyramidal tract disease in the brain.
- *Hemiplagic gait*. This is a spastic gait affecting one leg. The ipsilateral arm may be held in a decorticate posture with the hand near the chest. It occurs after a contralateral hemispheric stroke or other cerebral corticospinal tract lesion.
- *Sensory ataxic gait*. This is unsteady like a cerebellar gait, but may have a stamping quality, as if the patient cannot accurately place his foot upon the floor. It is much worse in the dark.
- *High-stepping gait*. In isolation this indicates foot drop, usually either from a common peroneal nerve palsy or from an L5 root lesion. The ankle joint seems excessively loose. Slight weakness may be tested by asking the patient to stand and walk on his heels. Similarly, test for weakness of ankle extension by asking the patient to walk on their toes.
- *Waddling gait*. This is characteristic of proximal muscle disease involving the pelvic girdle, especially the gluteal hip abductors. The muscles on the stance leg can no longer support the

pelvis against the tendency to drop down under the influence of gravity towards the stepping foot as the latter is lifted from the floor. This can be corroborated by observing the patient from behind as he stands still and lifts one foot (*Trendelenburg's sign*). Hip joint disease may result in a similar gait. Associated weakness of axial muscles causes an increased lumbar lordosis.

THE AUTONOMIC NERVOUS SYSTEM

The autonomic nervous system subserves physiological functions mediated by efferent and afferent innervation of cardiac muscle, gastrointestinal smooth muscle and glandular tissue. Autonomic feedback loops are also modulated by descending influences from the hypothalamus and higher centres via the central sympathetic tract in the brainstem and spinal cord, although autonomically innervated structures are not under direct voluntary control.

Parasympathetic autonomic efferent neurons lie within cranial nerve and sacral nuclei. The axons of the preganglionic cranial parasympathetic neurons travel with the cranial nerves and synapse in ganglia that typically lie close to their end-organs, such as the pupil, the lacrimal and salivary glands, most of the gastrointestinal tract and the heart. Short postganglionic fibres then reach these organs. Preganglionic parasympathetic fibres to the bladder, distal colon and rectum, and genitalia, including the uterus, arise from cell bodies within the anterior horns of the sacral spinal cord.

Sympathetic preganglionic neurons arise from thoracic and lumbar spinal segments. They synapse with postganglionic fibres before reaching their target end-organs. The sympathetic ganglia lie near the spinal canal and are interconnected by relays running up and down the sympathetic chain, allowing postganglionic fibres to innervate all parts of the body rather than just thoracic and lumbar segments. In the trunk, both postganglionic sympathetic and parasympathetic fibres are grouped into large plexuses, such as the cardiac and splanchnic plexuses, before supplying the viscera. The adrenal glands receive preganglionic fibres directly. Sweating is a sympathetic function.

The clinical presentation of autonomic dysfunction varies greatly depending on the distribution of abnormality in the central or peripheral sympathetic or parasympathetic components of this neuronal system. For example, in the rare syndrome of progressive *primary autonomic failure* there is degeneration of both pre- and postganglionic neurons, leading to several *autonomic abnormalities*:

- Constipation and other disorders of gastrointestinal motility
- Incontinence of urine
- Impotence

Box 10.15   Clinical assessment of autonomic function

- Check the pupillary responses to light and accommodation
- Is the skin normal? If dry, suspect absence of sweating
- Is there a resting tachycardia?
- Does the pulse rate slow with deep inspiration?
- Are there trophic changes in distal skin, e.g. absence of hair growth?

- Pupillary areflexia
- Disturbances of sweating
- Orthostatic hypotension, causing *syncope* (fainting) in the erect posture
- Loss of cardiovascular reflexes.

Loss of cardiovascular reflexes causes:

- Tachycardia at rest
- Absence of the normal slowing of the pulse in response to the Valsalva manoeuvre
- Absence of the normal slight increase in pulse rate and blood pressure on standing
- Absence of the normal increase in blood pressure during hand gripping
- Absence of the blood pressure increase with stressful tasks such as mental arithmetic.

These functional autonomic disturbances may also develop in peripheral neuropathies that involve the small autonomic fibres, e.g. diabetic neuropathy and other small fibre neuropathies, such as hereditary autonomic and sensory neuropathies and the familial amyloid polyneuropathy.

ASSESSMENT

Several simple clinical tests can be carried out at the bedside. A preliminary assessment is described in Box 10.15.

STANDING TEST FOR ORTHOSTATIC HYPOTENSION

- *Blood pressure.* Record the supine blood pressure after the patient has been resting quietly on a couch for 15 minutes. Then ask the patient to stand. This will reduce the recorded blood pressure, but sympathetic mechanisms should correct this over the next minute or so. Thus, measure the blood pressure 1 and 3 minutes after standing. A fall of over 20 mmHg systolic compared to the supine pressure suggests autonomic failure.
- *Pulse.* Record the R-R interval on the ECG and use it to determine the instantaneous heart rate, at rest and then on the 15th and 30th beats after standing. The heart rate should normally rise after about 30 seconds as part of the response to return the blood pressure to normal. The normal

30th:15th pulse heart rate ratio is >1.03 in normal subjects, and <1.0 when there is autonomic disturbance. This is a selective test for cardiac sympathetic innervation as opposed to vasomotor innervation, and may suggest that sympathomimetic medication such as midodrine and ephedrine could be helpful to control syncopal symptoms.

DEEP BREATHS TEST
Lie the patient flat. When the pulse has steadied, record the pulse rate during six slow *maximal* deep breaths. In normal subjects the pulse rate should slow by >15 beats/min; with autonomic disturbances the pulse rate slows <10 beats/min.

HANDGRIP TEST
With the patient lying flat, measure the maximal handgrip force by having the patient grip a semi-inflated sphygmomanometer cuff as hard as possible. Then, with a second sphygmomanometer, measure the rise in diastolic blood pressure after a 30% handgrip sustained for 5 minutes. The diastolic pressure should rise >16 mmHg; in autonomic disorders it will rise <10 mmHg.

VALSALVA TEST
The patient closes the glottis and attempts maximal expiratory effort for 15 seconds. The resultant reduced venous return should reflexly lower the pulse rate via the vagal parasympathetic. The ratio of the highest pulse rate in a preliminary rest period to the lowest pulse rate during the test is >1.5 in normal subjects and <1.1 in patients with autonomic disturbances. The test may be repeated up to three times if the initial result is equivocal.

OTHER TESTS
Tests of bowel motility and of bladder and urethral function using cystometry are also useful in evaluating the extent of autonomic dysfunction. Quantitative pupillometry, and the response to conjunctival application of parasympathomimetic and sympathomimetic drugs can also be used (see Chapter 18).

INTERPRETING CLINICAL SIGNS

For the student, as well as for the experienced clinician initially baffled by a complex array of abnormal examination findings, a good approach to localization is that espoused by Sir Arthur Conan Doyle: starting from the top and working downward, eliminate all the possible sites where the lesion *cannot* be, until you are left with the remaining probable location. On the other hand, it is a long-established axiom that a lesion should be suggested at the most peripheral location possible, as this is the simplest explanation of the pathophysiology.

ASSOCIATION CORTEX
Lesions at this highest level producing motor or sensory symptoms will be associated with cognitive deficits such as difficulties with praxis or perception (see under Cognitive examination).

MOTOR HEMISPHERE
The large volume of the motor system within the motor cortex and deep white matter, including the internal capsule of the hemisphere, compared to the lower part of the CNS, implies that the functional consequences of lesions here produce more localized deficits. For example, a laterally placed lesion might affect just the face and hand, whereas a lesion on the mesial surface (Fig. 10.53) deep within the central sulcus might only affect the leg (Fig. 10.54).

There are two important features to note in relation to lesions of this area and other CNS motor areas. First, the hemispheres, as well as the lower structures of the diencephalon, are paired and lateralized, so that single structural lesions are more likely to be *unilateral* than bilateral (this applies somewhat less to the thalami and to the motor cortex subserving the leg, because these paired structures lie close together). In contrast, lesions in motor structures below the internal capsule are more likely to cause *bilateral* features. Complicating this is the fact that a few motor structures are bilaterally innervated by one hemisphere. Thus *the upper face is much less weak than the lower face*

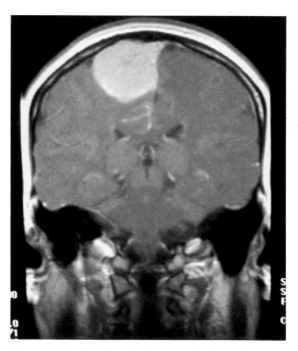

Figure 10.53   MRI. There is a large parasagittal meningioma arising from the meninges close to the sagittal sinus and deforming the brain. The patient presented with a major generalized seizure and headache. The left plantar response was extensor.

following a unilateral lesion between the hemisphere and upper brainstem because the remaining side can still exert ipsilateral control (see Cranial nerve VII). However, in degenerative processes such as amyotrophic lateral sclerosis (motor neuron disease), bilateral but asymmetrical features are likely, whereas multifocal lesions, such as the demyelinating plaques of multiple sclerosis, will affect the two sides at random (Fig. 10.55).

Second, lesions in the hemispheres and other CNS structures cause a *UMN* pattern of deficit. Many of these descending inputs to the motor neuron pool are inhibitory rather than excitatory. After a delay of hours to weeks this lack of inhibitory input results in increased motor neuron excitability. Afferent stimulus to the segmental reflex arc causes major muscle activation. A UMN lesion, after an initial period of 'cerebral' or 'spinal shock' when the affected limbs are flaccid and paralysed, but with extensor plantar responses, shows a number of characteristic features:

- *Increased tone.* There is spasticity (velocity-dependent increased tone) because the muscle spindle stretch responses that are most responsible for overexcitability signal stretch velocity.
- *Spastic posture and pyramidal weakness.* Lesions at different levels of the UMN pathway will cut off the influences of different descending pathways. A hemispheric or capsular lesion will preserve reticulospinal and vestibulospinal pathways

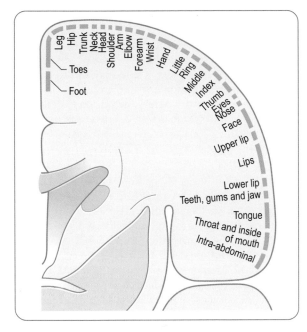

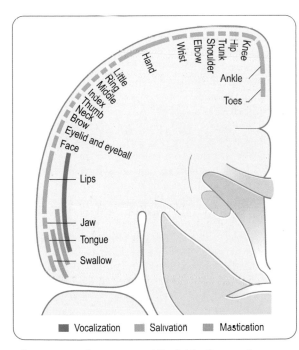

Figure 10.54 Rasmussen and Penfield's diagram of localization in the sensory (top) and motor (bottom) cortices.

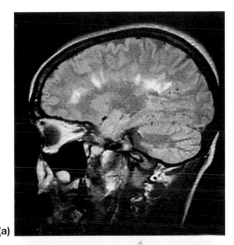

(a)

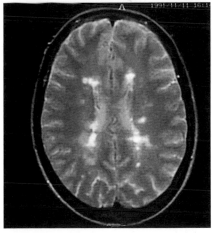

(b)

Figure 10.55 T$_2$-weighted MRI **(a)** sagittal and **(b)** axial images in multiple sclerosis, showing bright periventricular white matter lesions. In the sagittal image the high signal areas have a finger-like appearance (Dawson's fingers).

so that primitive activation and posture-maintaining influences are still preserved, resulting in a tendency for antigravity muscles to be relatively more active. The leg is therefore held out stiffly with hip extended, the knee straight and the ankle plantarflexed. Even in spinal lesions this antigravity pattern of preservation in the legs is maintained because these segmental stimulatory influences are well developed. In the bipedal human the effects of a UMN lesion on the upper limb are more complex. A hemispheric or capsular lesion tends to result in an arm posture flexed at the elbow and wrist so that the hand is held against the chest. A lower-level lesion sometimes results in the more typical lesioned quadriped posture, where the arm is held in against the side with the shoulder pronated and the elbow extended. The pattern of weakness closely parallels these postural effects. In the arm, whatever the level of lesion shoulder abduction tends to be weak. In the legs, the *hip flexors are weaker than the extensors*, the *knee flexors are weaker than the extensors* and *ankle dorsiflexion is weaker than plantar extension* – the pattern of corticospinal weakness.

- *Brisk tendon reflexes and extensor plantars*. These, and other signs such as absent superficial abdominal muscle responses, are indicative features of UMN lesions.
- *UMN bladder weakness*. Bilateral, or bifrontal hemisphere, lesions typically result in an automatic bladder with a tendency to overactivity of the bladder wall muscle – 'spastic' bladder.

A superficial motor cortex lesion might not result in a typical UMN picture because so much of the remainder of the descending motor pathway is intact. Instead, deficits in the hand area of the cortex relate to the specific fine voluntary finger muscle control mediated by corticospinal neurons – the 'cortical hand'.

SENSORY HEMISPHERE

This is discussed separately from the motor hemisphere as the structure's large size means a lesion often affects one part without the other, as distinct from what is generally found following a lesion in the diencephalon. Perhaps surprisingly, *numbness* – loss of sensation – is not typical of a hemispheric sensory lesion. Even central pain from such a lesion is a rare finding. Instead, the thalamus should be considered the 'top' of the pathway of sensory detection, whereas the primary sensory cortex subserves further processing of sensory information, such as that required for two-point discrimination and stereognosis, and the association sensory cortex mediates higher functions, such as planning and execution of tasks and multimodal sensory and sensorimotor integration.

DIENCEPHALON

These deep brain areas include the basal ganglia, internal capsule and thalamus. A functional lesion of the *basal ganglia* presents with generalized (or lateralized) excess or paucity of movements, rather than total failure of a particular aspect of function. A focal absence of function, e.g. a paralysed limb, an absent reflex or a cranial nerve palsy, argues against a diencephalic lesion. However, the basal ganglia lie close to the internal capsule and thalamus, and so a structural or vascular lesion often involves these structures together. An *internal capsule* lesion generally causes a widespread contralateral hemiparesis as the motor fibres are packed so closely together at this site. A *thalamic* lesion may cause a variety of effects. There may be *lateralized* features, such as dystonia, hemiparesis, incoordination, tremor or sensory disturbance, or *non-lateralized* features such as speech arrest, confusion or memory disturbance.

CEREBELLUM

A single lesion here may be bilateral as well as unilateral in its effects, because the cerebellum is both a paired structure (cerebellar hemispheres) and a midline structure. Lesions will typically result in irregularly irregular unsteadiness of limb or trunk movement and posture, with eyes open or shut. There is no tremor at rest but on postural adjustment ataxic movement, described as an 'intention' tremor, develops (Box 10.13). Nystagmus is usually present on attempted lateral gaze.

Because the cerebellum is rather close to the brainstem there may be associated brainstem signs.

BRAINSTEM

Descending and ascending pathways are closely grouped in the brainstem and so structural lesions are often bilateral, though asymmetrical. Because the brainstem is supplied by a single basilar artery, vascular lesions also tend to produce bilateral deficits (see following section). The key feature of either type of brainstem lesion is that there are likely also to be cranial nerve deficits, which in different nerves may be supranuclear or nuclear depending on the exact level of the lesion (see Figs 10.7, 10.8, 10.13).

- *Medial lesions* tend to affect the somatic cranial motor nerves, which are medially placed, and, at least in the pons and upper medulla, medial lesions may also affect the medial lemniscal sensory pathway.
- *Lateral lesions* tend to affect sensory cranial nuclei, other sensory pathways and the cerebellar peduncles. The *superior peduncle* largely transmits efferents and lesions result in ipsilateral ataxic tremor; the *middle peduncle*

transmits afferents from frontopontine projections and lesions result in general clumsiness, sometimes mistaken for a contralateral frontal lesion, and the *inferior peduncle* largely transmits ascending proprioceptive afferents and lesions result in failure of motor adaptation (quantitatively changing the parameters of a motor task, e.g. throwing a ball at a target, based on a review of performance in previous trials).

- *Ventral lesions* affect the descending corticospinal pathway.
- *Low medullary lesions* may be bilateral or may result in ipsilateral weakness or sensory disturbance because the main pathways decussate at this level.

A possible error in concluding that hemiparesis or quadriparesis associated with cranial nerve involvement indicates brainstem disturbance is the presence of *false localizing signs*. Raised intracranial pressure from any cause may result in unilateral or bilateral sixth-nerve palsy, whereas tentorial herniation from a hemisphere lesion may cause a contralateral pupil-involving third-nerve palsy. The latter can also result from a posterior communicating artery aneurysm.

SPINAL CORD

The spinal cord is so compact that upper motor neuron involvement is nearly always bilateral, i.e. paraparetic rather than hemiparetic. It is much more important to localize the *level of the lesion* in the cord than its cross-sectional extent. This is done using different aspects of examination:

- *Power level.* Each muscle has a segmental myotomal origin from the spinal cord. A lesion will result in UMN pattern weakness of all muscles innervated from segmental levels below the lesion, and perhaps LMN pattern weakness at the segmental level of the lesion if the exiting motor root fascicles are involved.
- *Reflex level.* Stretch reflexes have a similar segmental pattern, so knowledge of reflex levels helps to delineate the level of a lesion. The reflexes will be normal above the lesion level and brisk below. If all the limb reflexes are brisk, an upper cord lesion can be distinguished from a bilateral hemisphere lesion by the presence of a normal rather than a brisk jaw jerk, as well as by the lack of UMN or LMN problems such as swallowing or speech deficits. At the actual level of the reflex damage to the sensory root entry zone may interrupt the sensory reflex arc, so that the reflex may be absent at this level. However, this sign is limited by the fact that there are only a few testable reflex levels. Superficial abdominal reflexes can help to localize the level of a thoracic lesion. Finally, some cord lesions extend longitudinally, so that here there may be a number of levels of reflex loss as well as multiple levels of lower motor neuron-type weakness.

- *Sensory level.* Knowledge of the segmental dermatomal distribution of pinprick sensation also allows determination of the level of a lesion. The sensory pathway to the brain will be interrupted below the level of the lesion. Unfortunately, such sensory localization is made somewhat inaccurate by the fact that the central processes may synapse with second-order spinothalamic neurons as many as four levels *above or below* their level of root entry.

Cross-sectional patterns of *spinal cord lesion* include:

- *Dorsal cord lesions.* These primarily affect the medial lemniscal tracts running up the dorsal columns and will therefore cause joint position and vibration sense loss and sensory ataxia, but there will be preserved deep tendon reflexes (unlike in a sensory peripheral neuropathy).
- *Lateral and ventral cord lesions.* These affect the descending motor tracts bilaterally to cause spastic paraparesis or quadriparesis. Common causes include distortion of the cord by cervical spondylosis, which results in shear damage affecting both lateral sides of the cord simultaneously, and anterior spinal artery thrombosis, which causes ischaemia of these areas.
- *Central lesions.* These will damage deep structures such as bladder control pathways and decussating spinothalamic sensory fibres. A classic cause is syringomyelia.
- *Unilateral lesions.* Because the pyramidal tracts and medial lemnisci decussate in the brainstem, but the spinothalamic tracts do so at segmental levels, in the rare cases where there is a unilateral lesion the weakness, brisk reflexes, upgoing plantar response, absent abdominal reflexes and vibration sense loss will be ipsilateral, whereas pinprick loss will be contralateral or suspended and bilateral. This is called the *Brown–Séquard syndrome* (Fig. 10.56, Box 10.16). Thus, in the rare case of hemiparesis resulting from a cord lesion, if there is widespread pinprick loss it *must* be present on the opposite side to the weakness.

Finally, an important differential is between extrinsic and intrinsic cord lesions. *Extrinsic lesions* may result in root pain and other root symptoms (see below) and result in paraplegia followed by a progressively ascending sensory level (Fig. 10.57, Box 10.17). *Intrinsic lesions* may have early incontinence and an early *suspended*, perhaps dissociated, sensory deficit as a result of the involvement of spinothalamic fibres from neighbouring dermatomes decussating at this level. Suspended sensory loss is defined as an area of involvement of one or several dermatomal levels, with normal sensation below, as

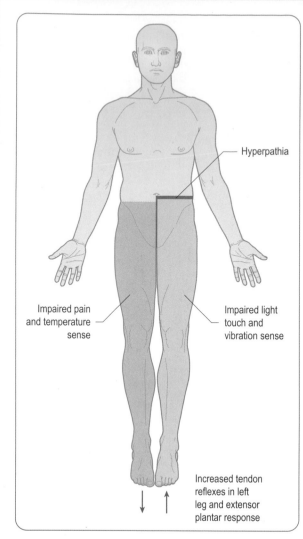

Figure 10.56 Brown–Séquard syndrome. Note the distribution of corticospinal, posterior column and lateral spinothalamic tract signs. The cord lesion is on the left side.

Labels in figure:
- Hyperpathia
- Impaired pain and temperature sense
- Impaired light touch and vibration sense
- Increased tendon reflexes in left leg and extensor plantar response

opposed to a sensory *level*, which has absent sensation everywhere below the level.

MOTOR NEURONS

The motor neurons lie in the anterior horns of the grey matter of the spinal cord. Diseases that selectively affect the motor neurons are generally degenerative rather than structural, such as motor neuron disease and spinal muscular atrophy. However, a syrinx or other central cord pathology may affect the motor neurons at a number of segmental levels (Fig. 10.58); a typical presentation of syringomyelia is with a wasted hand and dissociated suspended sensory loss.

Involvement at the motor neuron or at more distal levels produces LMN impairment:

- Wasting
- Fasciculation (if neuron or proximal nerve)
- Flaccid paresis or paralysis
- Loss of reflexes (especially if sensory arc is interrupted).

NERVE ROOTS

Motor fascicles at spinal levels pass out of the cord as nerve roots that leave the spinal canal through small lateral intervertebral foramina. Sensory nerves have a similar organization, except that the sensory cell bodies lie in ganglia outside the spinal canal and the sensory roots carry the sensory processes more posteriorly into the spine. This difference has a useful consequence for electrical nerve conduction testing. A root lesion giving weakness, loss of deep tendon reflexes and sensory loss will reveal impaired motor conduction, but *sensory conduction will be normal* as the axon and cell body distal to the lesion remain as a viable unit isolated from afferent pathways mediating reflexes or perception.

During childhood the spinal column grows more than the spinal cord, so that by adulthood the terminal sacral cord levels (called the conus) are located at the level of the T12 vertebra. The roots, however, exit at their anatomical vertebral level. This has two consequences. First, a spinal column lesion at lower thoracic levels will affect a cord level that is significantly lower. Second, the lumbar level roots must travel down the lumbar canal, where they are collectively called the *cauda equina* ('horse's tail'), so a lumbar spinal canal lesion will not cause a UMN cord syndrome but instead will present with multiple lumbar root lesions.

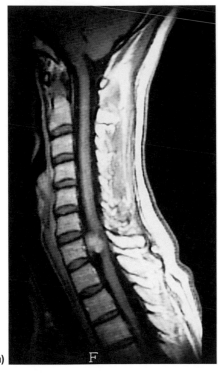

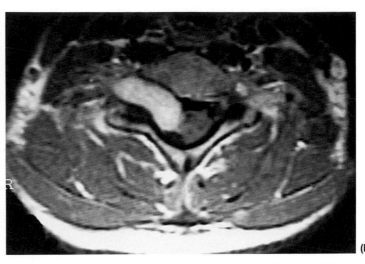

(a)

(b)

Figure 10.57 **(a)** MRI scan of the cervical spine with gadolinium enhancement. There is a neurofibroma at the C6 level which is compressing the spinal cord, causing progressive paraparesis. **(b)** The tumour enhances slightly and can be seen as a sausage-shaped mass arising in the intervertebral foramen and compressing the spinal cord in the axial view.

> **Box 10.17** Features of progressive intrinsic and extrinsic spinal cord disease, in their order of development
>
> This sequence is particularly characteristic of tumours arising within the spinal cord, or compressing it from without.
>
> **Intrinsic disease**
> - Urge incontinence/retention of urine
> - Dissociated sensory loss
> - Spinothalamic pain
> - Bilateral corticospinal tract signs
> - Paraplegia and sensory level
>
> **Extrinsic disease**
> - Root pain, worsened by movement
> - Progressive asymmetrical paraparesis
> - Brown–Séquard syndrome
> - Paraplegia with sensory level
> - Incontinence/retention of urine and faeces

Nerve roots are frequently affected by structural lesions because of their constrained course through the intervertebral foramina, and the fact that rheumatological disease is common at the mobile cervical and lumbar spinal levels. A lesion involving the root exit, such as a posterolateral disc prolapse (Fig. 10.59) or neurofibroma, will result in a unilateral lesion at a single nerve root level. On the other hand, an extra-axial lesion within the canal may affect nerve roots bilaterally or extend vertically to affect multiple levels. If it is in the cervical or thoracic canal such a lesion may also grow inward to compress the cord, giving mixed cord and root signs; in the lumbar canal it may affect multiple root levels even if it is at a single canal level. Physical constraint of nerve roots also means that root disease is often associated with *mechanical* symptoms and signs. Thus, flexion and rotatory movements of the lumbar spine in lumbosacral nerve root syndromes, rotation of the trunk or coughing in thoracic disc lesions, and stretching of the arms and neck in cervical root disease will cause a shooting pain that radiates into the territory of the sensory innervation of the affected root. *Straight-leg raising* involves passively flexing the patient's hip while keeping the knee straight and dorsiflexing the ankle. This stretching of the sciatic nerve will cause sciatic pain and limit movement if the root (L5 or S1) is tethered. In L'hermitte's phenomenon sudden neck flexion causes electric tingling running down the arms and down the spine, due to hyperexcitability of the posterior columns to mechanical displacement, associated with demyelination.

A further anatomical point relates to the precise level of root disease. The first cervical level (which

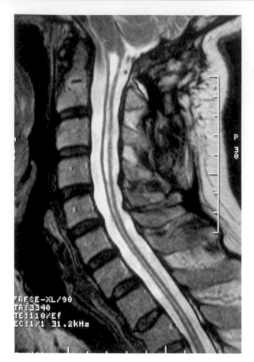

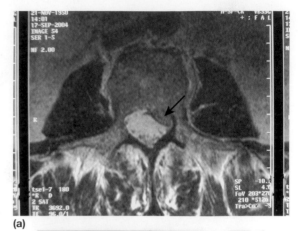

Figure 10.58 Sagittal MRI scan showing an extensive syrinx, extended through the cervical and upper thoracic cord. In this T$_2$-weighted image the syrinx shows similar attenuation to CSF.

carries only motor fibres) exits between the occiput and C1, so *cervical roots* always exit *above* the vertebra with the same number. Thus a left C5/6 disc prolapse will result in left C6 root neurological signs. The C8 root exits between C7 and T1. Because of this C8 naming system, *thoracic and lumbar roots* exit *below* the vertebra with the same number. There is a further complication in the case of lumbar disc prolapse. A far lateral disc prolapse will affect the root as it exits the interspace, so this kind of L4/5 prolapse would affect the L4 root level. However, disc prolapse is much more commonly posterolateral than lateral and actually presses within the canal on the next root down as it swings laterally towards its exit at the spinal level below. So a typical L4/5 prolapse usually in fact affects the L5 root!

BRACHIAL AND LUMBOSACRAL
PLEXUS   (Box 10.18)

These structures are separated side to side, and so structural lesions will be unilateral. A multiroot-level unilateral lesion of an arm or leg that is LMN in type will probably involve the plexus; if it is a UMN type it will involve the hemisphere. The brachial plexus is susceptible to idiopathic localized inflammation, called brachial neuralgia, which usually presents with severe unilateral arm pain, followed rapidly by weakness and then eventual recovery. It may also suffer *radiation necrosis* as a

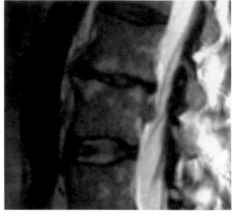

(b)

Figure 10.59 **(a)** MRI scan, transverse image, showing lumbar disc protrusion (arrow). Disc material has ruptured through the annular ligament and is compressing the thecal sac on the left (right of image), impinging on nerve roots. Note the psoas muscles to either side of the vertebral body, and the paraspinal muscles at the lower part of the image on either side of the posterior spinous process. **(b)** Sagittal MRI scan showing lumbosacral disc protrusion with displaced material in the spinal canal that is displacing nerve roots. Note the dark, low attenuation, image of the aorta anterior to the spine.

late complication of radiotherapy for breast or bronchial carcinoma. The lower brachial plexus may be affected by a cervical band or rib or by a *Pancoast lesion* (a bronchial carcinoma at the apex of the lung). Lower plexus lesions may present with small hand muscle weakness and a Horner's syndrome, the latter due to involvement of the T1 sympathetic ganglion. The lumbosacral plexus may be involved in infiltrative malignant disease, such as lymphoma or metastatic prostate carcinoma.

PERIPHERAL NERVES

- *Mononeuropathy.* Most nerves are mixed sensory and motor, and so traumatic, ischaemic, infiltrative or inflammatory lesions will typically result in muscle weakness and sensory loss in the distribution of the nerve involved (Fig. 10.60, Box 10.19).

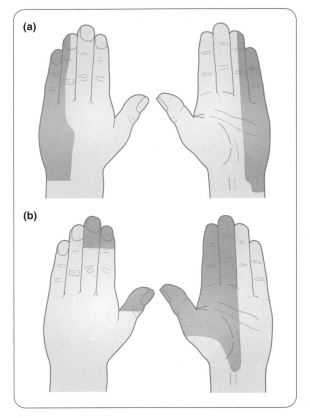

Figure 10.60   Cutaneous sensory loss: **(a)** after the division of the ulnar nerve above the elbow; **(b)** after division of the median nerve in the arm. A lesion of the median nerve at the carpal tunnel may spare the palm.

- *Mononeuritis multiplex*. Some conditions, especially inflammatory disorders and diabetes mellitus, affect multiple nerves in a patchy manner to give a complex clinical picture of deficits in multiple motor and sensory nerve distributions. Sometimes this can be difficult to distinguish from widespread root disease, as the overlapping nerve and root patterns become confused.
- *Polyneuropathy*. This typically occurs in a disease process – usually hereditary, metabolic or inflammatory – that has metabolic effects on nerve tissue so that the severity of involvement depends largely on the length of the nerve. The resulting neuropathy has distal motor involvement, widespread areflexia and a 'glove-and-stocking' distribution of sensory loss, with the legs more extensively involved than the arms.
- *Mixed neuropathy*. Weakness is usually the main disabling complaint, but many acquired inflammatory neuropathies, as opposed to hereditary motor and sensory neuropathies, produce unpleasant dysaesthesiae. *Axonal neuropathies*, where the whole axon is destroyed, are more likely to result in early muscle wasting than are primarily *demyelinating neuropathies*, where the nerve sheath is primarily damaged, because axoplasmic flow of trophic factors to the muscle may be preserved in the latter type. In some neuropathies, for example hereditary motor and sensory neuropathy type III, there may be palpable thickening of nerves. Sensory loss in any neuropathy rarely extends beyond the mid forearm or much above the knees. If this does occur, such as sensory loss on the trunk in an acute inflammatory neuropathy (Guillain–Barré syndrome), it signifies that the process also involves the nerve roots.
- *Motor neuropathy*. Occasionally a widespread process may be selective for motor nerves. Because reflexes are more dependent on the afferent arc, a very selective motor nerve disease needs to cause very severe weakness before reflex loss results. Thus reflexes are preserved until late in spinal muscular atrophy, and are sometimes preserved in the inflammatory disorder called multifocal motor neuropathy.
- *Sensory neuropathy*. When a selective sensory neuropathy primarily affects small fibres, e.g. in diabetes or alcohol toxicity, it causes painful or painless distal sensory loss and distal areflexia. When it affects large fibres, sensory ataxia and widespread areflexia result. *Sensory neuronopathy* affecting the cell bodies in the dorsal root ganglia, often the result of paraneoplastic disease from small cell bronchial carcinoma, also presents with ataxia and areflexia.

NEUROMUSCULAR JUNCTIONS

Disorders affecting the cholinergic neuromuscular junctions (motor endplates) are strictly motor

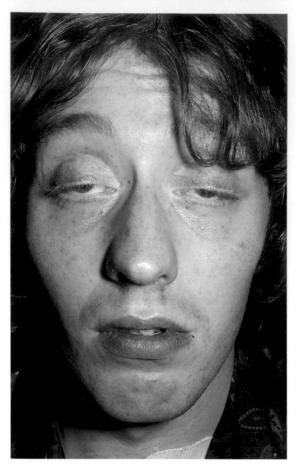

Figure 10.61 Myasthenia gravis. There is bilateral ptosis with resting divergence of the eyes and lower facial weakness, so that the mouth and jaw hang open. There is compensatory overactivity of the frontalis muscles in an effort to open the eyelids.

MUSCLES

Muscle disorders typically produce symmetrical proximal weakness, seen especially in the neck flexor muscles, the shoulder abductors and pelvic girdle muscles. Some muscle disorders, such as certain types of congenital myopathy and muscular dystrophy, have a predilection for particular muscles, proximal or otherwise, such as restriction at first to the upper body in facioscapulohumeral dystrophy, or involvement of the extraocular muscles in oculopharyngeal myopathy and certain mitochondrial cytopathies. Hyporeflexia occurs only when the muscle is almost completely atrophic. Wasting may occur out of proportion to weakness. Pseudo-hypertrophy suggests Duchenne's muscular dystrophy, and a woody hardness may be found in eosinophilic myopathy.

VASCULAR ANATOMY OF THE NERVOUS SYSTEM

Every nervous structure requires a blood supply for normal function. The anatomical complexity of this vascular supply rivals that of the nervous system itself. Because of this special mutually localizing relationship, and because vascular disease in the form of stroke represents one of the most common neurological conditions, the clinical localization of vascular lesions of the nervous system merits special consideration.

ARTERIAL SUPPLY TO THE BRAIN

The brain receives its arterial supply from the paired internal carotid and vertebral arteries that rise up through the neck. These arteries form a large anastomosis within the skull at the base of the brain – the *circle of Willis* (Fig. 10.62). The sharing of vascular supply through this anastomosis means that cerebral infarction does not generally result from occlusion, thrombotic or otherwise, of these four arteries. Instead, a stroke results when a thrombus becomes dislodged and embolizes (Fig. 10.63) in an artery distal to the circle of Willis, or when a thrombus forms de novo in one of these distal arteries. Thus, a patient with a 90% stenosis of the internal carotid artery and a vascular event in the corresponding territory is considered a good candidate for carotid endarterectomy to clear the stenosis, whereas a patient with a 100% occlusion, and therefore no potential for emboli to flow up the vessel, is at a lower risk for stroke and does not warrant surgery.

The anatomy of the circle of Willis means that carotid emboli tend frequently to pass to the *ipsilateral* ophthalmic artery (which branches directly off the carotid in the cavernous sinus), the anterior choroidal artery (which also branches directly off the carotid and supplies the choroid plexus, optic

disorders without sensory features. Myasthenia gravis, involving postsynaptic receptors, has a predilection for the laryngeal, pharyngeal, external ocular and facial muscles, producing a typical myopathic facies (Fig. 10.61). In the limbs, muscle involvement has a distribution typical of a proximal myopathy. There is fatiguability, no wasting and preserved reflexes.

Presynaptic involvement is typified by the Eaton–Lambert syndrome, which has a more uniform limb distribution. It may also affect parasympathetic cholinergic terminals to result in difficulty in focusing and dry eyes and mouth. The condition is typified by the converse of fatiguability: in order to generate sufficient transmitter release, the neuromuscular junction must rely on tetanic and post-tetanic potentiation mechanisms activated by maintained contraction. In fact, the response to a brief phasic nerve impulse is so poor that areflexia is common. When the muscle is exercised the reflexes may then appear.

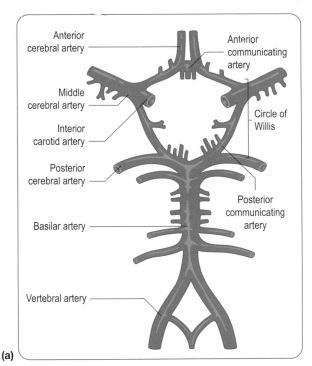

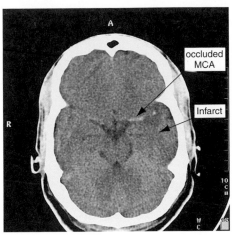

Figure 10.63 CT scan, early cerebral infarction. There is occlusion of the left middle cerebral artery due to embolism from traumatic dissection of the wall of the left carotid artery, causing infarction in the left middle cerebral artery territory, causing slight hypointensity of the affected area.

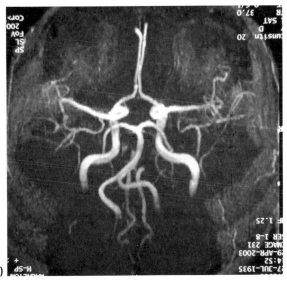

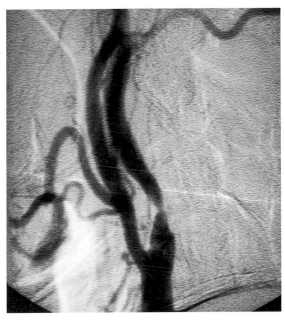

Figure 10.62 **(a)** The blood supply to the brain and the circle of Willis. **(b)** Magnetic resonance angiogram showing the same as the diagram. The basilar artery and the two vertebral arteries join the posterior communicating arteries to form the circle of Willis with the two carotid arteries and the anterior communicating artery. The middle cerebral, anterior cerebral and posterior cerebral arteries can be seen.

Figure 10.64 Carotid artery stenosis, presenting with transient ischaemic attacks (hemiparesis).

tract and sometimes lateral geniculate and posterior internal capsule), the anterior cerebral artery or the middle cerebral artery, the last being most commonly affected (Fig. 10.64). Vertebrobasilar emboli tend to pass to *either* the posterior cerebral, superior cerebellar, anterior inferior cerebellar or ipsilateral posterior inferior cerebellar arteries. A

detailed knowledge of the territory supplied by these arteries will allow the vascular site of a stroke to be identified based on its clinical features (Fig. 10.65). However, in practice these vascular territories are somewhat variable and overlap.

ANTERIOR CEREBRAL ARTERY
This artery courses near the midline and loops up and back over the front of the corpus callosum. It supplies the leg area of the motor cortex and the micturition and cognitive areas of the medial frontal lobe. Occasionally it gives off a branch called the

239

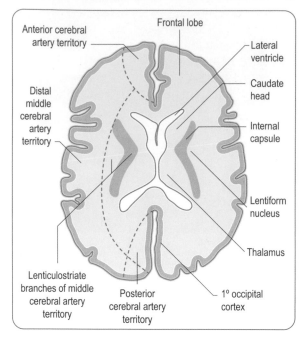

Anterior cerebral
artery territory

Distal
middle
cerebral
artery
territory

Lenticulostriate
branches of middle
cerebral artery
territory

Posterior
cerebral artery
territory

Frontal lobe

Lateral
ventricle

Caudate
head

Internal
capsule

Lentiform
nucleus

Thalamus

1° occipital
cortex

Figure 10.65   Anatomy of the circle of Willis, showing the vascular supply on the left and the anatomy on the right.

recurrent artery of Heubner, and if this is the case an occlusion will also involve the anterior internal capsule and result in proximal arm and facial pyramidal weakness as well as leg weakness.

MIDDLE CEREBRAL ARTERY

This artery arises from the carotid and during its lateral course through the sylvian fissure it gives off a number of lenticulostriate branches that supply the basal ganglia and internal capsule. More distally, the middle cerebral artery trifurcates into superior and inferior superficial branches that supply most of the outer surface of the cortex, and a deep branch that runs posteriorly to supply the cortical radiation.

An occlusion of the terminal branch causes hemiparesis affecting the face and arm, and perhaps the leg mildly, with cognitive signs depending on whether the infarct is on the left or the right. Some lesions may be more distal still and affect only either the face or the arm (see Fig. 10.63).

Occlusions of the lenticulostriate vessels are often lacunar in aetiology and result in hemiparesis without cognitive deficit, and usually without sensory loss (the posterior tip of the internal capsule is normally supplied by the posterior cerebral artery).

Finally, occlusion of the main trunk of the middle cerebral artery results in a lesion representing a combination of the above. The fact that both the cortical and the capsular face and arm regions are involved (called an 'undercut' stroke) means that recovery is especially poor. The area involved is extensive and the initial oedema from infarction can result in potentially fatal brain swelling in the early stages following a stroke.

POSTERIOR CEREBRAL ARTERY

This artery constitutes the terminal division of the basilar artery in front of the midbrain. It first gives off branches to the cerebral peduncle and midbrain and to the posterior temporal lobe, and then curls back around the midbrain, giving thalamogeniculate branches to the thalamus and posterior internal capsule. Finally, the artery divides into terminal branches supplying the inner surface and deep parts of the occipital lobe.

A terminal occlusion of the posterior cerebral artery therefore affects the visual cortex. However, macular sparing often occurs because the occipital pole receives a dual blood supply from middle and posterior cerebral artery branches. Thalamogeniculate branch lesions may result in a variety of thalamic and capsular features, ranging from contralateral sensory loss to central pain, hemianopia, dystonia, speech arrest, hemiparesis and tremor. Sometimes memory loss may occur, especially of verbal memory if the occlusion is left-sided. A main posterior cerebral trunk lesion (Fig. 10.66) may result in all these effects, with additional hemiparesis or hemiballismus from midbrain involvement, and occasionally memory loss from temporal lobe involvement, although, as with thalamic lesions, memory loss more usually results only from bilateral involvement.

SUPERIOR CEREBELLAR ARTERY

This artery arises from the central basilar artery and winds around the midbrain parallel to and just below the posterior cerebral artery. Perforating branches supply the midbrain. The midbrain also receives branches from the posterior cerebral artery (see above). The pattern of cerebellar artery perforators is such that branch occlusions cause infarcts that are paramedian, anterolateral (basal) or posterolateral in distribution. A number of classic stroke syndromes therefore result.

- *Paramedian infarction.* Red nucleus and third-nerve nucleus, giving contralateral ataxia and third-nerve palsy (see Fig. 10.7).
- *Basal infarction (Weber's syndrome).* Third-nerve fascicle and cerebral peduncle, giving ipsilateral third-nerve palsy and contralateral hemiplegia (face and body) (see Figs 10.7, 10.8).
- *Posterolateral infarction.* Spinothalamic, medial lemniscal and sympathetic tracts and superior cerebellar peduncle, giving total contralateral sensory loss, ipsilateral Horner's syndrome, and sometimes ipsilateral ataxia (see Figs 10.7, 10.8).

The terminal part of the superior cerebellar artery then goes on to supply the superior surface of the cerebellum and some midline cerebellar structures.

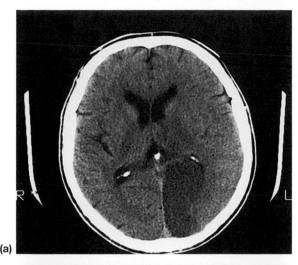

(a)

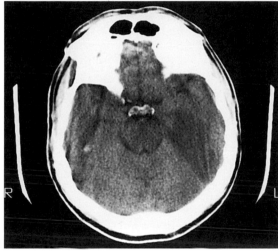

(b)

Figure 10.66 CT scan, showing **(a)** infarction in the left posterior cerebral artery territory to involve the occipital lobe and its deep white matter. On a lower axial slice **(b)** the infarct extends anteriorly into the posterior part of the temporal lobe.

All the cerebellar arteries anastomose over its surface, so that vertebrobasilar territory lesions resulting in cerebellar features tend to be better characterized by the involvement of particular cerebellar peduncles than of individual cerebellar structures.

ANTERIOR INFERIOR CEREBELLAR ARTERY
This lies below and follows the same pattern as the superior cerebellar artery, supplying the pons.

- *Paramedian infarction.* Sixth- and seventh-nerve nuclei and medial lemniscal tract, giving lateral gaze failure, lower motor neuron facial weakness and loss of contralateral body position sense.
- *Basal infarction* (see Fig. 10.8). Sixth- and seventh-nerve fascicles and the pyramidal pathways, giving diplopia, lower motor neuron

facial weakness, and contralateral upper motor neuron facial weakness and body weakness. Because the pontine motor nuclei and fibres are rather diffusely distributed, the contralateral hemiplegia may be localized.

- *Posterolateral infarction.* Sympathetic pathway, spinothalamic tract, middle cerebellar peduncle, fifth-nerve nucleus, and vestibular, cochlear and eye movement control nuclei, giving ipsilateral sensory loss in the face, perhaps ipsilateral clumsiness of the body, and loss of contralateral pinprick sensation in the body, often combined with nystagmus and Horner's syndrome.

The artery also gives off a vestibulocochlear branch, so that an embolus here may result in *peripheral* vertigo and deafness, and terminates over the anterior part of the large inferior surface of the cerebellum.

POSTERIOR INFERIOR CEREBELLAR ARTERY
This artery comes laterally off the vertebral artery before the latter joins with its partner to form the basilar artery. At about the same level, the vertebral artery gives off a medial branch that joins with a similar one on the other side to form a single central anterior spinal artery that descends down the spinal cord. The posterior inferior cerebellar artery follows a tortuous course, winding up around the medulla. Unlike the upper brainstem, the medial part of the medulla is not supplied by paramedian perforators but by branches from the anterior spinal artery. This means that central medullary infarcts are often *bilateral*, as they may derive from this single unpaired artery. Posterior inferior cerebellar artery perforators supply the basal and posterolateral portions.

- *Paramedian infarction* (see Fig. 10.13). Twelfth-nerve nucleus, medial lemniscus (or nucleus gracilis and nucleus cuneatus lying more posteriorly and inferiorly and involved ipsilaterally) and medullary pyramid, giving tongue weakness, paralysis and absent position sense, *either unilateral or bilateral.*
- *Basal infarction* (not well described). Inferior olive and perhaps pyramid, giving contralateral ataxia and motor adaptation failure, and perhaps contralateral hemiplegia.
- *Posterolateral infarction (Wallenberg's syndrome).* Sympathetic tract, spinothalamic tract, nucleus and tract of the fifth nerve, lower vestibular nuclei, inferior cerebellar peduncle and ninth- and tenth-nerve nuclei, giving ipsilateral Horner's, facial numbness and ataxia, loss of contralateral body pinprick sensation, and vestibular disturbance and speech and swallowing difficulty.

The posterior inferior cerebellar artery goes on to supply the posterior inferior part of the cerebellum.

TEMPORARY ISCHAEMIA

A few minutes' ischaemia in a vascular territory, often due to embolism, may result in a temporary stroke-like episode lasting up to a few hours, called a transient ischaemic attack (TIA). The symptoms correspond to the territories of the various cerebral and brainstem vessels described above, but are often more or less widespread and less well defined. Anterior (carotid) territory TIAs typically give left or right hemisphere symptoms, whereas posterior (vertebrobasilar) territory TIAs may present with bilateral limb features, brainstem features, blindness, and most importantly a reduction in conscious level as a result of generalized ischaemia of the brainstem reticular activating formation or thalami. Minor TIAs may be more focal, such as isolated dysphasia from a transient left distal middle cerebral artery occlusion, left face and hand weakness from a similar branch occlusion on the right, or *transient global amnesia* from a posterior territory transient occlusion or hypoperfusion of small vessels bilaterally supplying the thalami or posterior temporal lobes.

There is some controversy as to whether TIA should be defined to encompass a duration of up to 24 hours, or even longer. The essential feature is complete recovery without evidence of infarction on subsequent MRI scanning of the brain (Fig. 10.67).

CEREBRAL HYPOPERFUSION

Cerebral ischaemia may result from general hypoperfusion as well as from occlusion of a particular vessel. Thus temporary states of low cardiac output, such as arrhythmia, may present with neurological features, including episodes of disorientation, delirium or loss of consciousness. Prolonged hypoperfusion may result in infarction that typically occurs in watershed areas on the borders between the territories of cerebral arteries. Such sites include sections of the frontal lobes and posterior parietal lobes, extending outward respectively from the frontal and occipital horns of the lateral ventricles, as well as the diffuse white matter territories underlying the cortex. Patients with coronary disease susceptible to low cardiac output states often also have atherosclerotic stenosis of the great neck vessels or cerebral vessels, making them more susceptible to neurological consequences. Sometimes, pre-existing stenosis in a particular vessel may result in corresponding focal symptoms if the overall cardiac output is reduced.

VENOUS DRAINAGE OF THE BRAIN

The major clinical difference between the arterial supply and the venous drainage of the brain is that the latter is much more variable and often midline, resulting in bilateral involvement. *Venous infarction*

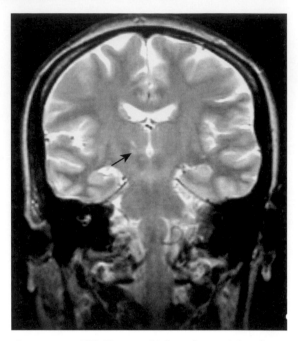

Figure 10.67   MRI. Three small infarcts (lacunar infarcts) are shown in the right basal ganglia area (arrow).

is often accompanied by small haemorrhages because of the raised capillary pressure. The hemispheres are drained by the superior and inferior sagittal sinuses running posteriorly, whereas the deeper structures are drained by the internal cerebral vein and the great vein of Galen. All these sinuses and vessels drain into the paired transverse and sigmoid sinuses and eventually into the jugular veins. However, even thrombosis of the basal sinuses may present bilaterally, because one transverse sinus is often dominant. The brainstem has an excellent diffuse venous drainage through its surface, and venous infarction here is extremely rare.

Venous sinus thrombosis is an important clinical diagnosis and should be suspected in any stroke with an unusual presentation, especially if there are risk factors such as pregnancy, dehydration, vasculitis or abnormal clotting, and if the features include papilloedema, obtundation, bilateral signs, headache or a grumbling course.

CEREBRAL HAEMORRHAGE

Bleeding into different brain compartments may result in different clinical features.

Extradural haemorrhage is generally an early complication of head trauma and results in a mass effect pressing on one hemisphere to cause contralateral signs or a false localizing third-nerve palsy due to tentorial herniation.

Subdural haemorrhage is often venous, and because the subdural space is more open tends to

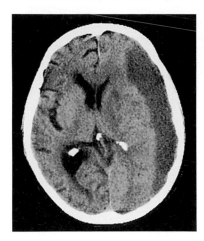

Figure 10.68 CT of a patient presenting with confusion, showing a left chronic subdural haemorrhage with concave distribution of low-density broken-down blood and midline shift. In an acute bleed the haemorrhage would be hyperdense compared to the neighbouring brain tissue.

result in a long, thin concave haemorrhage (Fig. 10.68) rather than the more localized convex extradural haemorrhage. These factors often make the presentation more vague and subacute, with obtundation as well as lateralized hemispheric signs. The trauma resulting in the haemorrhage may have been a mild and forgotten event weeks earlier. Subdural haemorrhage may occur spontaneously, especially if the patient has a bleeding diathesis, or occasionally as a result of low cerebrospinal fluid pressure from a dural tear.

Intracerebral haemorrhage within the brain substance may also be traumatic, but more often occurs spontaneously. Lacunar haemorrhages of small diencephalon vessels have an atherosclerotic aetiology while larger hemispheric haemorrhages in the elderly relate to vascular changes of chronic hypertension, known as cerebral amyloid angiopathy. In younger patients, causes include arteriovenous malformations, venous cavernomas, vasculitis or venous thrombosis (see above). Intracerebral haemorrhages typically present as a stroke with or without headache. Seizures are more likely to accompany such haemorrhages than those of subdural origin. Sometimes blood also enters the subarachnoid space.

Subarachnoid haemorrhage typically presents with an explosive-onset severe headache owing to the rupture of an intracerebral berry aneurysm or arteriovenous malformation. In a few cases no cause can be found. The blood seeps through the diffuse subarachnoid spaces and is more likely to cause meningeal and diffuse brain irritation (e.g. seizures, obtundation) than focal deficit. When the latter does occur, it usually results from irritative vasospasm of an intracerebral vessel.

BLOOD SUPPLY OF THE SPINAL CORD

The spinal cord receives supply from both a single anterior spinal artery and paired posterior spinal arteries. The anterior spinal artery derives from the vertebral arteries and receives branches from the costocervical trunk and aorta via segmental feeders. The posterior arteries receive segmental supply from the aorta via radicular feeders, and also via numerous anastomoses wrapping around the cord's surface and connecting them with the anterior spinal artery. Small perforators from the anterior and posterior spinal arteries supply the cord substance. One would think this rich anastomosing supply would be more than adequate to protect from infarction, but in fact the segmental supply is rather deficient at the midthoracic levels, being dependent on a single *artery of Adamkiewicz* coming off a left T10–12 intercostal vessel. Occlusion (atherosclerotic or iatrogenic) may result in anterior spinal artery thrombosis. This tends to affect the descending motor tracts more than the posteriorly located dorsal columns, so that a spastic paraparesis is the typical clinical picture.

Venous drainage from the cord is diffuse. Sometimes mild compressive lesions are said to result in ischaemia via venous obstruction. For example, the direction of drainage of the cervical cord is normally upwards, so that a high cervical lesion may sometimes result in a T1 root level deficit, such as weak and wasted hands.

BLOOD SUPPLY OF PERIPHERAL NERVES

Even peripheral nerves and the lumbar and cervical plexuses require an adequate blood supply: this is delivered by the vasa nervorum. Many causes of mononeuritis multiplex, such as diabetes, vasculitis and haematological malignancies, are in fact at least partly ischaemic in pathogenesis.

SIGNS OF MENINGEAL IRRITATION

The main feature is neck stiffness, or increased resistance to passive flexion of the neck. It should be tested whenever there is a clinical possibility of meningeal irritation. It is a more sensitive test than Kernig's sign. These signs are nearly always due to *meningitis* (Fig. 10.69) or to *subarachnoid haemorrhage*.

NECK STIFFNESS

Passively but gently flex the patient's neck. The chin should normally touch the chest without pain. In meningeal irritation neck flexion causes pain in the posterior part of the neck, sometimes radiating down the back, and the *movement is resisted* by spasm in the extensor muscles of the neck. In addition to meningeal irritation, neck rigidity is also

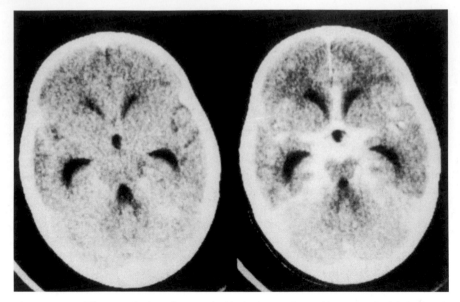

Figure 10.69   CT scans of tuberculous meningitis. In the unenhanced image on the left the basal cisterns are obliterated. On the right the inflamed meninges and the inflammatory exudate have been visualized (enhanced) following intravenous injection of iodine-based contrast. The white central areas represent the abnormality. The clinical sign of neck stiffness represents reflex spasm in the neck extensors caused by inflammation of the basal meninges.

caused by diseases of the cervical spine, and by raised intracranial pressure due especially to a posterior fossa tumour, with rostral–caudal displacement of the vermis in the foramen magnum, leading to local dural irritation. *Head retraction*, now rare, represents an extreme degree of neck rigidity, especially in untreated tuberculous meningitis.

KERNIG'S SIGN

Kernig's sign is elicited with the patient supine on the bed. Passively extend the patient's knee on either side when the hip is fully flexed. In patients with meningeal irritation affecting the lower part of the spinal subarachnoid space this movement causes pain and spasm of the hamstrings.

SPECIAL INVESTIGATIONS

There are many methods for the clinical investigation of patients with neurological disorders. Investigation must be planned to yield relevant results in a timely manner and at reasonable clinical risk and financial cost.

LUMBAR PUNCTURE

This procedure is used to obtain samples of cerebrospinal fluid (CSF), which 'bathes' CNS tissues and is therefore often a more specific marker for neurological disease than is blood. The lumbar meninges are punctured using a long hollow needle inserted between the spines of two lumbar vertebrae below the level of the termination of the conus medullaris.

TECHNIQUE

First examine the fundi to exclude raised intracranial pressure and, in the acute situation, consider CT scanning of the brain. Except in acute bacterial meningitis, lumbar puncture is almost always contraindicated in the presence of raised intracranial pressure because of the risk of consequent transtentorial or tonsillar herniation.

Locate the third and fourth lumbar spines. The fourth lumbar spine usually lies in the transverse plane of the iliac crests. The puncture may be made through either the L3/4 or the L4/5 interspace. Lie the patient on his or her left side on a firm couch or on the firm edge of a bed, with the trunk flexed so that the knees and chin are as nearly approximated as possible and the trunk's transverse axis – i.e. a line passing through the posterior superior iliac spines – is perfectly vertical. Local anaesthesia is produced by injecting about 1 mL of 1% or 2% sterile lignocaine at the chosen site, first raising a bleb under the skin, and then, when this is insensitive, anaesthetizing the whole dermis, but not the deep ligaments.

Push a special lumbar puncture needle, with the central retractable solid stylet firmly in place and the bevel pointing upward, through the skin in the midline and press it steadily *forwards and slightly towards the patient's head*, keeping it *exactly horizontal throughout*. When the needle 'gives' as it is felt to enter the spinal cavity, withdraw the central stylet. CSF will then drip slowly from the hollow outer end. Collect CSF in three sterilized stoppered test tubes. If any blood is present, a marked difference in the amount in the first and subsequent tubes indicates that the blood is due to trauma from the puncture. For similar reasons, lumbar puncture in suspected subarachnoid haemorrhage is best delayed by 6 hours to allow *xanthochromia* (yellow staining from blood breakdown) to develop; the presence of xanthochromia in the CSF thus helps distinguish hours-old aneurysmal bleeding from fresh lumbar puncture trauma. The patient should lie flat for 8–24 hours afterwards, in order to reduce the chance of post-lumbar puncture low CSF volume headache developing.

The CSF pressure can be measured at the time of lumbar puncture using a manometer. For this measurement, the patient should be lying with his head on a pillow at the same level as the sacrum, breathing quietly and with muscles relaxed. The neck and legs should not be too intensely flexed. The normal CSF pressure is 60–150 mm of CSF. Correct location of the tip of the needle in the subarachnoid space is indicated by pressure fluctuations with pulse, respiration and coughing.

Queckenstedt's test, a crude method to detect a block in the circulation of CSF in the spinal canal, e.g. from spinal tumours, is no longer recommended. The diagnosis of spinal tumour, if suspected, should be confirmed by MR imaging *without previous lumbar puncture*, as the latter may cause clinical deterioration.

DIFFICULTIES WITH LUMBAR PUNCTURE

The commonest cause of a 'dry tap' – the failure to obtain CSF – is an incorrectly performed puncture, usually because the patient is not in the correct position. The needle is therefore not introduced at right-angles to the transverse axis of the back, and misses the spinal canal. Frequently, the needle is introduced too deeply, so that it traverses the spinal canal and wedges against the posterior margin of the intervertebral disc; if the needle is withdrawn slightly, CSF will begin to flow. Occasionally, however, a 'dry tap' is due to complete blockage of the flow of CSF through the spinal canal. In this circumstance, urgent MRI or other imaging of the spinal canal is required.

ABNORMALITIES OF THE CSF

Normal CSF is clear and colourless, like water.

- *Yellow coloration*. Yellowness (*xanthochromia*) is pathological and is due to either old haemorrhage, jaundice or an excess of protein. In *Froin's*

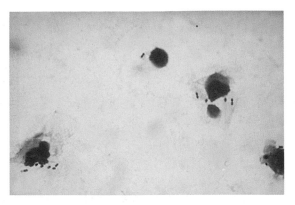

Figure 10.70 Smear from cellular deposit in CSF from a patient with acute meningitis showing Gram-positive diplococci, many located intracellularly in polymorphonuclear leukocytes.

syndrome a pronounced yellow colour is associated with a great excess of protein and the formation of a coagulum. It is almost always due to spinal tuberculosis with a spinal block to the flow of CSF, but is now a very rare phenomenon. Even slight increases in CSF protein, however, cause a noticeable increase in viscosity of the fluid and an excessive frothiness of its surface when it is gently shaken.

- *Turbidity*. This may be due to the presence of white blood cells, either as a result of infection or following subarachnoid haemorrhage. If this does not clear on standing it is due to microorganisms.
- *Bloodstaining*. The presence of *blood* may be due to needle injury to a vessel or to subarachnoid haemorrhage (see above).
- *Cytology*. A centrifugal deposit should be examined with Leishman's stain in order to obtain an idea of the character of the cells present, and by the Gram and Ziehl-Neelsen methods for bacteria (Fig. 10.70), and perhaps India ink stain for cryptococcus. Cell counts are performed in a counting chamber and must be done immediately the fluid has been collected. The normal white cell count is 0–2/mL. An increased count (*pleocytosis*) may consist of polymorphonuclear cells or lymphocytes. In a *polymorphonuclear* CSF more than 75% of the cells are polymorphs; in a *lymphocytic* CSF more than 98% are lymphocytes. Bacterial meningitis is associated with a polymorphonuclear pleocytosis, viral meningitis and syphilis with a lymphocytic CSF, and tuberculous meningitis with either a lymphocytic or a mixed type. Cytological examination of the centrifugal deposit may reveal malignant cells in patients with secondary neoplastic invasion of the meninges from lymphoma or carcinoma (Fig. 10.71).
- *Biochemistry*. Normal CSF contains only a trace of albumin and hardly any globulin, the *total protein* being not more than 0.4 mg/L. In TB

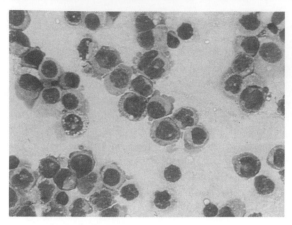

Figure 10.71 Cerebrospinal fluid cytology. Cell deposit from cerebrospinal fluid comprising almost exclusively carcinoma cells shed from the leptomeninges. Metastasis to the meninges from a primary carcinoma of the breast. May–Grünwald–Giemsa stain ×160.

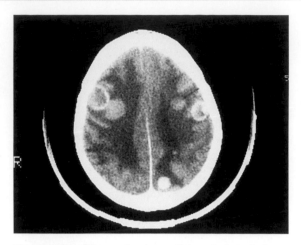

Figure 10.72 CT scan showing multiple metastases in the brain from primary carcinoma of the breast. There is marked oedema of the white matter.

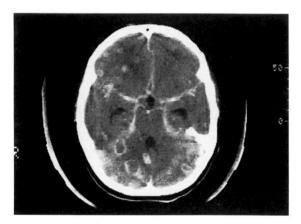

Figure 10.73 Enhanced CT scan showing multiple tuberculomas in the brain. The lesions show enhancement of their capsules. They vary in size. Note that there is effacement of the cortical pattern, suggesting widespread meningeal inflammation.

meningitis and in CSF obstruction the total protein may be very high. In some neurological diseases, particularly multiple sclerosis, and in many acute and subacute virus infections, the globulin fractions in the CSF are increased. *The CSF IgG concentration* can be measured directly by immunoelectrophoresis. In *multiple sclerosis* the abnormal IgG may be *oligoclonal*. It is compared with the blood IgG to verify that the raised CSF IgG level is due to endogenous local IgG synthesis within the central nervous system. *Glucose* is present in normal CSF in a concentration of 2.5–4.2 mmol/L, which is about a half to two-thirds of the blood glucose concentration. In purulent tuberculous or fungal meningitis and rarely in carcinomatous meningitis the CSF sugar is *reduced to less than half of the blood glucose*. Remember that the brain scan is important in patients with suspected intracranial infections (Figs 10.72, 10.73).

- *Culture and serology*. Culture identifies bacterial infection and, after 4–6 weeks, tuberculous infection, and the antibiotics to which they are sensitive. Many serological tests for viral, bacterial and parasitic infections are available.

The typical changes in the CSF in various neurological diseases are summarized in Table 10.9.

ELECTROENCEPHALOGRAPHY (EEG)

Electrodes applied to the patient's scalp pick up small changes of electrical potential which, after amplification, are recorded on paper or displayed on a video monitor and recorded electronically. The EEG is of particular value in the investigation of epilepsy; it is also used in the diagnosis of encephalitis, and sometimes in the assessment of patients with dementia.

THE ELECTROMYOGRAM (EMG), NERVE CONDUCTION STUDIES (NCS) AND EVOKED POTENTIALS

Electrical activity occurring in muscle during voluntary contraction, or in denervated muscles at rest, can be recorded with needle electrodes inserted percutaneously into the belly of the muscle, or with surface electrodes (silver discs attached to the skin overlying the muscle using a salty paste). This electrical activity is amplified and displayed as an auditory signal through a suitable loudspeaker and as a visual signal on an oscilloscope. It may be recorded on magnetic tape, or selected potentials may be printed. Online quantitative analysis of the EMG is useful in the diagnosis of primary diseases of muscle (*myopathies*, *dystrophies* and *myasthenia*) and of lower motor neuron lesions (*denervation*).

Table 10.9 Typical changes in the cerebrospinal fluid (CSF) in various diseases

Disease	Physical characteristics	Cytology (cells/μL)	Protein (g/L)	Glucose* (mmol/L)	Stained deposit	Culture
Normal	Clear and colourless	Lymphocytes 0–2	0.1–0.4	2.5–4.2	No organisms	Sterile
Bacterial meningitis	Yellowish and turbid	Polymorphs 200–2000 Lymphocytes	0.5–2.0 5–50	<2.0	Bacteria	Positive
Tuberculous meningitis	Colourless, sometimes viscous or yellow	Polymorphs 0–100 Lymphocytes 100–300	May be 5.0–15	<2.0	Tubercle bacilli in CSF in most cases	Usually positive
Viral meningitis	Usually clear	10–100 mixed cells at first, becoming lymphocytic in 36 hours	0.1–0.6	2.5–4.2	No organisms	Sterile
Multiple sclerosis	Clear and colourless	Rarely 5–20 lymphocytes IgG level raised with monoclonal bands	0.1–0.6	2.5–4.2	No organisms monoclonal IgG bands shown by several methods	Sterile
Neoplastic meningitis (infiltration)	Clear or yellowish	5–1000 cells of mixed type	0.5–2.0	<3.0	Inflammatory and malignant cells usually present	Sterile

*CSF glucose is usually more than half the blood glucose. Therefore, simultaneous blood and CSF glucose measurements should always be performed.

The speed of conduction of afferent impulses (*sensory nerve conduction velocity*) and efferent impulses (*motor nerve conduction velocity*) in peripheral nerves can be calculated by techniques using electrical nerve stimulation and recording electrodes with amplifying or digital averaging equipment. These methods are useful in the diagnosis of peripheral nerve disorders, particularly those due to local compressive lesions, for example carpal tunnel syndrome, and in the clinical assessment of nerve plexus or radicular disease.

Similar investigations of sensory conduction in the central nervous system can be achieved by averaging scalp recordings triggered by sensory stimulation (*somatosensory evoked potentials*), reversing chequered visual patterns (*visual evoked potentials*), or clicks in the ears (*auditory or brainstem evoked potentials*). It is also possible to study *motor unit evoked potentials* from stimulation of the brain using magnetic impulses.

SECTION 4

Clinical specialties

Section contents

Skin, nails and hair

R. Cerio

11

INTRODUCTION

The skin is the largest organ of the human body. Forming a major interface between man and his environment, it covers an area of approximately $2\,m^2$ and weighs about $4\,kg$. The structure of human skin is complex (Figs 11.1, 11.2), consisting of a number of layers and tissue components with many important functions (Box 11.1). Reactions may occur in any of the components of human skin and their clinical manifestations reflect, among other factors, the skin level in which they occur.

Dermatology is a visual specialty. The accurate diagnosis of most skin lesions requires an adequate history, careful examination of the patient and, occasionally, laboratory investigation.

HISTORY

Detailed information should be sought concerning the present skin condition. This should include the site of onset, mode of spread and duration of the disorder. Any personal history or family history of skin disease, including *atopy* (an allergic skin reaction becoming apparent more or less immediately on contact), is important. Previous medical conditions should be noted and a full drug history obtained, including use of over-the-counter preparations. The social and occupational history and, in some circumstances, details of recent travel and sexual activity, may be important.

EXAMINATION

The whole skin, including hair, nails and assessable mucosae, should be fully exposed, preferably in natural light. Sometimes a magnifying lens is useful.

COLOUR AND PIGMENTATION

Before inspecting any rash or lesion note the *colour* of the skin. Normal skin colour varies, depending on lifestyle and light exposure as well as constitutional and ethnic factors.

Pallor can have many causes. It may be:

- Temporary, due to shock, haemorrhage or intense emotion

- Persistent, due to anaemia or peripheral vasoconstriction.

Vasoconstriction is seen in patients with severe atopy – an inherited susceptibility to asthma, eczema and hay fever. Pallor is a feature of *anaemia*, but not all pale persons are anaemic; conjunctival and mucosal colour is a better indication of anaemia than skin colour. A pale skin resulting from diminished pigment occurs with *hypopituitarism* and *hypogonadism*.

Normal skin contains varying amounts of brown *melanin* pigment. Brown pigmentation due to deposited *haemosiderin* is always pathological. *Albinism* is an inherited generalized absence of pigment in the skin; a localized form is known as *piebaldism*. Patches of white and darkly pigmented skin (*vitiligo*) (Fig. 11.3) are due to a complete absence of melanocytes. Several autoimmune endocrine disorders are associated with vitiligo.

Abnormal redness of the skin (*erythema*) is seen after overheating, extreme exertion, sunburn and in febrile, exanthematous and inflammatory skin disease. *Flushing* is a striking redness, usually of the face and neck, which may be transient or persistent. Local redness may be due to telangiectasia, especially on the face. *Cyanosis* is a blue or purple-blue tint due to the presence of excessive reduced haemoglobin, either locally, as in impaired peripheral circulation, or generally, when oxygenation of the blood is defective. The skin colour in methaemoglobinaemia is more leaden than in ordinary cyanosis; it is caused by drugs, such as dapsone, and certain poisons.

Jaundice varies from the subicteric lemon-yellow tints seen in pernicious anaemia and acholuric jaundice to various shades of yellow, orange or dark olive-green in obstructive jaundice. Jaundice, which stains the conjunctivae, must be distinguished from the orange-yellow of *carotenaemia*, which does not. Slight degrees of jaundice cannot be seen in artificial light.

Increased pigmentation may be racial, due to sunburn, or connected with various diseases. In *Addison's disease* there is a brown or dark-brown pigmentation affecting exposed parts and parts not normally pigmented, such as the axillae and the

251

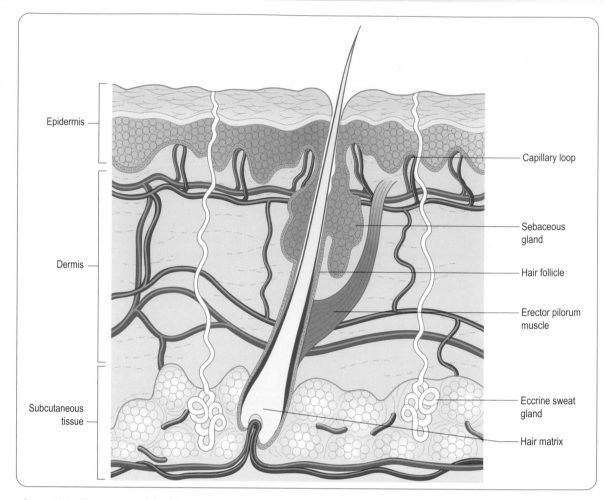

Figure 11.1 The anatomy of the full thickness of the skin in section.

Epidermis

Dermis

Subcutaneous tissue

Capillary loop

Sebaceous gland

Hair follicle

Erector pilorum muscle

Eccrine sweat gland

Hair matrix

palmar creases; the lips and mouth may exhibit dark bluish-black areas. Note, however, that mucosal pigmentation is a normal finding in a substantial proportion of negroid people.

More or less generalized pigmentation may also be seen in:

- *Haemochromatosis*, in which the skin has a peculiar greyish-bronze colour with a metallic sheen, due to excessive melanin and iron pigment
- *Chronic arsenic poisoning*, in which the skin is finely dappled; affects covered more than exposed parts
- *Argyria*, in which the deposition of silver in the skin produces a diffuse slate-grey hue
- The *cachexia* of advanced malignant disease.

In *pregnancy* there may be pigmentation of the nipples and areolae, of the linea alba, and sometimes a mask-like pigmentation of the face (*chloasma*). Chloasma may also be induced by oral contraceptives containing oestrogen. A similar condition, *melasma*, may be seen in Asian and African males.

Localized pigmentation may be seen in pellagra and in scars of various kinds, particularly those due to X-irradiation therapy. *Venous hypertension* in the legs is often associated with chronic purpura, leading to haemosiderin pigmentation. The mixture of punctate and fresh purpura and haemosiderin may produce a golden hue on the lower calves and shins. Pigmentation may also occur with chronic infestation by *body lice. Erythema ab igne*, a reticular pattern of pigmentation of the legs of women who habitually sit too near a fire, used to be common. When seen on the belly or back it indicates prolonged use of a hot-water bottle to relieve pain, for example from malignant disease. *Livedo reticularis*, a web-like pattern of reddish-blue discoloration, mostly involving the legs, occurs in autoimmune vasculitis, especially in systemic lupus erythematosus (SLE) and antiphospholipid syndrome, when it is associated with cerebral infarction. The lesions of *lichen planus* are slightly raised, flat-topped papules and have a violaceous hue (Fig. 11.4). Psoriasis usually presents as a symmetrical plaque on extensor surfaces (Fig. 11.5). *Keloid* con-

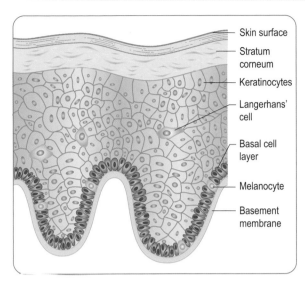

Figure 11.2 The anatomy of the epidermis.

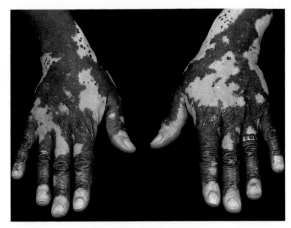

Figure 11.3 Vitiligo: a disorder of cutaneous pigmentation that is often autoimmune in origin and associated with other autoimmune disorders.

Box 11.1 Functions of the human skin

- Protection: physical, chemical, infection
- Physiological: homoeostasis of electrolytes, water and protein
- Thermoregulation
- Sensation: specialized nerve endings
- Lubrication and waterproofing: sebum
- Immunological: Langerhans' cells, lymphocytes, macrophages
- Vitamin D synthesis
- Body odour: apocrine glands
- Psychosocial: cosmetic

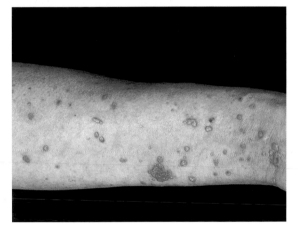

Figure 11.4 Flat-topped papules of lichen planus.

---

sists of raised and slightly pigmented, overgrown scar tissue (Fig. 11.6).

SKIN LESIONS AND ERUPTIONS

Skin eruptions and lesions should be examined with special reference to their morphology, distribution and arrangement. The terminology of skin lesions is summarized in Boxes 11.2 and 11.3. *Colour, size, consistency, configuration, margination* and *surface characteristics* should be noted.

MORPHOLOGY OF SKIN LESIONS

Inspection and palpation

Assessment of morphology requires *visual and tactile examination*. Do not be afraid to feel the lesions. You will rarely be exposed to any danger in doing so, with the exception of herpes simplex, herpes zoster, syphilis and human immunodeficiency virus (HIV) disease. If infections such as these are suspected it is wise to wear disposable plastic gloves

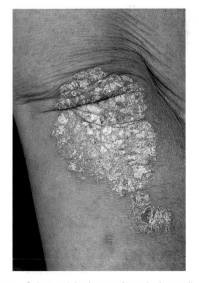

Figure 11.5 Salmon-pink plaque of psoriasis on elbow covered in characteristic silver scale.

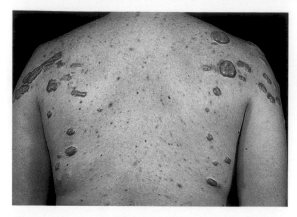

Figure 11.6 Multiple keloid scarring of the back due to acne vulgaris. There is a genetic predisposition to the formation of keloid in scar tissue.

when examining open or bleeding cutaneous lesions. Begin with palpation of the skin. Pass the hand gently over it, pinching it up between the forefinger and thumb, and note the following points:

- Is it smooth or rough, thin or thick?
- Is it dry or moist?
- Is there any visible sweating, either general or local?

The *elasticity* of the skin should be investigated. If a fold of healthy skin is pinched up, it immediately flattens itself out again when released. Sometimes, however, it only does so very slowly, remaining creased for a considerable time. This is found frequently in healthy old people but may be an important sign of dehydration, for example after severe vomiting and diarrhoea, or in uncontrolled diabetes mellitus.

Box 11.2   Primary skin lesions: a glossary of dermatological terms

Macule	Non-palpable area of altered colour
Papule	Palpable elevated small area of skin (<0.5 cm)
Plaque	Palpable flat-topped discoid lesion (>2 cm)
Nodule	Solid palpable lesion within the skin (>0.5 cm)
Papilloma	Pedunculated lesion projecting from the skin
Vesicle	Small fluid-filled blister (<0.5 cm)
Bulla	Large fluid-filled blister (>0.5 cm)
Pustule	Blister containing pus
Wheal	Elevated lesion, often white with red margin due to dermal oedema
Telangiectasia	Dilatation of superficial blood vessel
Petechiae	Pinhead-sized macules of blood
Purpura	Larger petechiae which do not blanch on pressure
Ecchymosis	Large extravasation of blood in skin (bruise)
Haematoma	Swelling due to gross bleeding
Poikiloderma	Atrophy, reticulate hyperpigmentation and telangiectasia
Erythema	Redness of the skin
Burrow	Linear or curved elevations of the superficial skin due to infestation by female scabies mite
Comedo	Dark horny keratin and sebaceous plugs within pilosebaceous openings

Box 11.3   Secondary skin lesions that evolve from primary lesions

Scale	Loose excess normal and abnormal horny layer
Crust	Dried exudate
Excoriation	A scratch
Lichenification	Thickening of the epidermis with exaggerated skin margin
Fissure	Slit in the skin
Erosion	Partial loss of epidermis which heals without scarring
Ulcer	At least the full thickness of the epidermis is lost. Healing occurs with scarring
Sinus	A cavity or channel that allows the escape of fluid or pus
Scar	Healing by replacement of fibrous tissue
Keloid scar	Excessive scar formation (see Fig. 11.6)
Atrophy	Thinning of the skin due to shrinkage of epidermis, dermis or subcutaneous fat
Stria	Atrophic pink or white linear lesion due to changes in connective tissue

Subcutaneous oedema

When *oedema* (see Chapter 2) is present, firm pressure on the skin with a finger produces a shallow pit that persists for some time. In some cases, especially when the oedema is of very long standing, pitting is not found. The best place to look for slight degrees of oedema in cardiac disease is behind the malleoli at the ankles in patients who are ambulant, and over the sacrum in those who are confined to bed. The finger pressure should be maintained for 20–30 seconds, or slight degrees of oedema will be overlooked. Pitting is minimal or absent in oedema due to lymphatic obstruction, where the skin is usually thickened and tough.

Subcutaneous emphysema

Air trapped under the skin gives rise to a characteristic crackling sensation on palpation. It starts in, and is usually confined to, the neighbourhood of the air passages. On rare occasions it may result from the clostridial infection of soft tissues after injury (*gas gangrene*).

DISTRIBUTION OF SKIN LESIONS

Consider the distribution of an eruption by looking at the whole skin surface.

- Is it *symmetrical* or *asymmetrical*? Symmetry often implies an internal causation, whereas asymmetry may imply external factors.
- Is the eruption *centrifugal* or *centripetal*? Certain common diseases such as chickenpox and pityriasis rosea are characteristically centripetal, whereas erythema multiforme and erythema nodosum are centrifugal. Smallpox, now eradicated, was also centrifugal.
- A disease may exhibit a *flexor* or an *extensor* bias in its distribution: atopic eczema in childhood is characteristically flexor, whereas psoriasis in adults tends to be extensor.
- Are only exposed areas affected, implicating sunlight or some other external causative factor?
- If sunlight is suspected, are areas normally in shadow involved?
- Are the genitalia involved?
- Localized distributions may point immediately to an external contact as the cause, for example contact dermatitis from nickel earrings, lipstick dermatitis etc.

Swelling of the eyelids is an important sign. Without redness and scaling, bilateral periorbital oedema may indicate acute nephritis, nephrosis or trichinosis. If there is irritation, contact dermatitis is the probable diagnosis. *Dermatomyositis* often produces swelling and heliotrope erythema of the eyelids without scaling of the skin. In *Hansen's disease* (leprosy) the skin lesions may be depigmented or reddened, with a slightly raised edge; they are also anaesthetic to pinprick testing (Fig. 11.7) and mainly

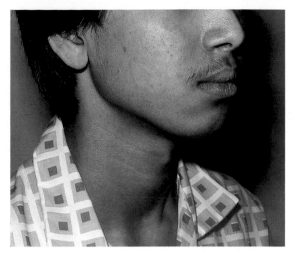

Figure 11.7 Hansen's disease. There is a depigmented area of anaesthetic and slightly pink skin on the exposed cheek. In this lepromatous lesion acid-fast bacilli were found in scrapings.

Box 11.4 Configuration of individual lesions	
Nummular/discoid	Round or coin-like
Annular	Ring-like
Circinate	Circular
Arcuate	Curved
Gyrate/serpiginous	Wave-like
Linear	In a line
Grouped	Clustered
Reticulate	Net-like

located in skin that is normally cooler than body temperature.

CONFIGURATION OF SKIN LESIONS

Once the morphology of individual lesions and their distribution has been established, it is useful to describe their configuration on the skin (Box 11.4).

THE HAIR

Hair colour and texture are racial characteristics that are genetically determined. The yellow-brown Mongol race has black straight hair, negroid people have black, curly hair, and white Caucasians have fair, brown, red or black hair. *Secondary sexual hair* begins to appear at puberty and has characteristic male and female patterns. Common baldness in men is genetically determined but requires adequate levels of circulating androgens for its expression. It occurs in women only in old age.

GROWTH

Unlike other epithelial mitotic activity that is continuous throughout life, the growth of hair is cyclic

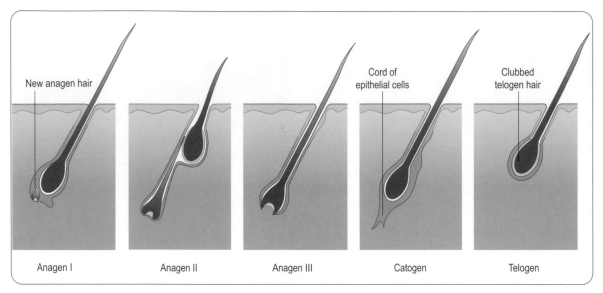

Figure 11.8 Hair follicle growth stages.

(Fig. 11.8), the hair follicle going through alternating phases of growth (*anagen*) and rest (*telogen*). *Anagen* in the scalp lasts 3–5 years; *telogen* is much shorter, at about 3 months. *Catogen* is the conversion stage from active to resting and usually lasts a few days. The duration of the anagen phase determines the length to which hair in different body areas can grow. On the scalp there are about 100 000 hairs. As many as 100 may be shed from the normal scalp every day as a normal consequence of growth cycling. These proportions can be estimated by looking at plucked hairs (trichogram): the 'root' of a telogen hair is non-pigmented and visible as a white, club-like swelling. Normally 85% of scalp hairs are in anagen and 15% in telogen.

ALOPECIA

Hair loss (*alopecia*) has many causes. It is convenient to subdivide alopecia into localized and diffuse types. In addition, the clinician should determine whether the alopecia results in scarring and hence permanent hair loss (Box 11.5).

Any inflammatory or destructive disease of the scalp skin may destroy hair follicles in its wake. Thus, burns, heavy X-ray irradiation or herpes zoster infection in the first division of the trigeminal nerve may cause scarring and alopecia. Alopecia in the presence of normal scalp skin may be patchy and localized, as in traction alopecia in nervous children, ringworm infections (*tinea capitis*) or auto-immune *alopecia areata*. Secondary syphilis is a rare cause of a patchy 'moth-eaten' alopecia.

Scalp hair loss at the temples and crown, with the growth of male-type body hair, is characteristic of women with virilizing disorders. Metabolic causes of diffuse hair loss in women include hypothyroidism

Box 11.5 Causes of alopecia	
Non-scarring	**Scarring**
Alopecia areata	Burns, radiodermatitis
Trichotillomania	Aplasia cutis
Traction alopecia	Lupoid erythema
Scalp ringworm (human)	Necrobiosis
Sarcoidosis	
Pseudopelade	
Kerion (see Fig. 11.30)	

and severe iron deficiency anaemia. Antimitotic drugs may affect the growing hair follicles, producing a diffuse loss of anagen hairs, which are pigmented throughout their length. Dramatic metabolic upsets, such as childbirth, starvation and severe toxic illnesses, may precipitate follicles into the resting phase, producing an effluvium of telogen hairs 3 months later, when anagen begins again. This is called *telogen alopecia*. In the autoimmune disorder *alopecia totalis* (Fig. 11.9) there is complete loss of hair. Self-inflicted *traction alopecia* (Fig. 11.10) may indicate psychological problems.

THE NAILS

The nails should be examined carefully. The structure of the nail and nailbed is shown in Figures 11.11 and 11.12. The nail consists of a strong, relatively inflexible keratinous nail plate over the dorsal surface of the end of each digit, protecting the fingertip.

NAIL MATRIX ABNORMALITIES

Thimble pitting of the nails is characteristic of psoriasis (Fig. 11.13), but eczema and alopecia areata

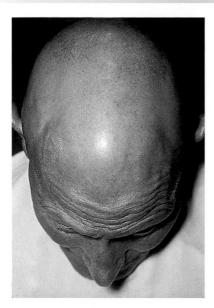

Figure 11.9 Alopecia totalis.

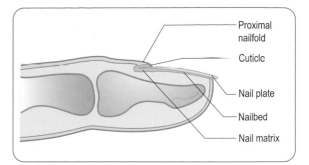

Figure 11.11 Structure of the nail (lateral view).

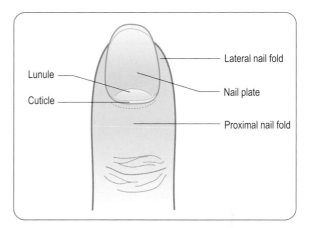

Figure 11.12 Structure of the nail (dorsal view).

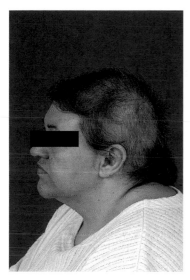

Figure 11.10 Traction alopecia in a psychologically troubled patient.

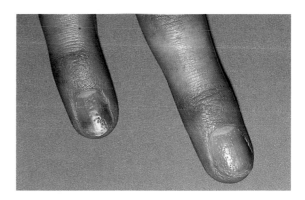

Figure 11.13 Psoriasis of the nailbeds.

may also produce pitting. A severe illness may temporarily arrest nail growth; when growth starts again transverse ridges develop. These are called *Beau's lines* and can be used to date the time of onset of an illness. Inflammation of the cuticle or nailfold (*chronic paronychia*) may produce similar changes. The changes described above arise from disturbance of the nail matrix.

NAIL AND NAILBED ABNORMALITIES

Disturbance of the nailbed may produce thick nails (*pachyonychia*) or separation of the nail from the bed (*onycholysis*). This may occur in psoriasis, but may be idiopathic. Tetracyclines may induce separation when the fingers are exposed to strong sunlight (*photo-onycholysis*). The nail may be destroyed in severe lichen planus (Fig. 11.14) or epidermolysis bullosa (a genetic abnormality in which the skin blisters in response to minor trauma). Nails are missing in the inherited nail–patella syndrome. *Splinter haemorrhages* under the nails may result from trauma, psoriasis, rheumatoid arthritis or other 'collagen vascular' diseases, bacterial endocarditis and trichinosis.

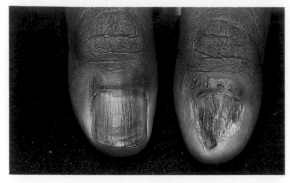

Figure 11.14 Lichen planus, showing longitudinal ridging of the nails and overgrowth of the cuticle on the nail plate (pterigium).

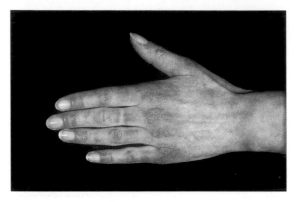

Figure 11.15 Typical erythema seen in dermatomyositis (periungal and Gottron's papules over the knuckles).

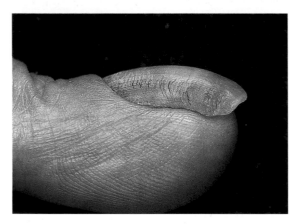

Figure 11.16 Yellow nail syndrome in bronchiectasis.

THE NAILS IN SYSTEMIC DISEASE

In *iron deficiency states* the fingernails and toenails become soft, thin, brittle and spoon-shaped. They lose their normal transverse convex curvature, becoming flattened or concave (*koilonychia*). The 'half and half' nail, with a white proximal and red or brown distal half, is seen in some patients with *chronic renal failure*. Whitening of the nail plates may be related to *hypoalbuminaemia*, as in cirrhosis of the liver. Some drugs, notably antimalarials, antibiotics and phenothiazines, may discolour the nail. *Nailfold telangiectasia* or *erythema* is a useful physical sign in dermatomyositis (Fig.11.15), systemic sclerosis and systemic lupus erythematosus. In dermatomyositis the cuticle becomes ragged. In systemic sclerosis loss of finger pulps may lead to curvature of the nail plates. An impaired peripheral circulation, as in Raynaud's phenomenon, can lead to thinning and longitudinal ridging of the nail plate, sometimes with partial onycholysis. In bronchiectasis the nails may take on a curved, yellow appearance (Fig. 11.16).

CLUBBING

This is probably caused by hypervascularity and the opening of anastomotic channels in the nailbed (see Chapter 2). Rarely, clubbing may be congenital. The distal end of the digit becomes expanded, with the nail curved excessively in both longitudinal and transverse planes. Viewed from the side, the angle at the nail plate is lost and may exceed 180°. In normal nails, when both thumbnails are placed in apposition there is a lozenge-shaped gap, whereas in clubbing there is a reduction in this gap (Schamroth's window test; Fig. 11.17). In hypertrophic pulmonary osteoarthropathy there is clubbing of the fingers and thickening of the periosteum of the radius, ulna, tibia and fibula. (The causes of clubbing are listed in Box 11.6.)

CUTANEOUS MANIFESTATIONS OF INTERNAL DISEASE

GENODERMATOSES (LESIONS OF INHERITED ORIGIN)

White macules shaped like small ash leaves which are present at birth may be the first sign of *tuberous sclerosis*. Sometimes they are difficult to see by natural light but show up under Wood's light (ultraviolet light). They should be looked for in infants with seizures. *Pigmentation of the lips* is a feature of the genetically determined Peutz–Jeghers syndrome, in which multiple polyps of the stomach or colon appear that may later undergo malignant transformation. *Café au lait* type macules are a common sign of *neurofibromatosis (NF1)*; they may be multiple. Another valuable sign in von Recklinghausen's neurofibromatosis is bilateral freckling of the axillary skin. The characteristic soft neurofibromata may be solitary or few, or hundreds may be scattered over the body. *Ichthyosis* (scaly fish skin) is usually present from childhood and is genetic, but if ichthyosis is acquired in adult life a search should be made for malignancy or other underlying disease.

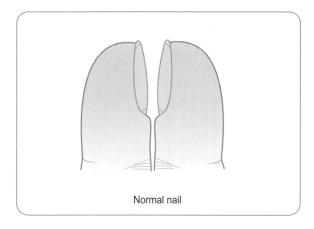

Normal nail

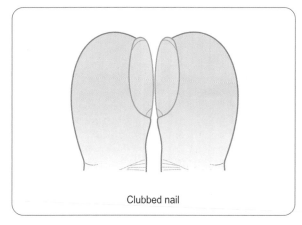

Clubbed nail

Figure 11.17 Schamroth's window test.

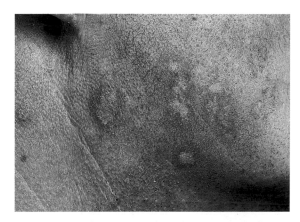

Figure 11.18 Discoid lupus erythematosus, showing atrophic scars.

NON-ORGAN-SPECIFIC AUTOIMMUNE DISORDERS

Several of the so-called collagen vascular diseases show characteristic cutaneous eruptions. *Systemic lupus erythematosus*, seen in women between puberty and the menopause, may show a symmet-

---

Box 11.6   Causes of clubbing of the fingers

Cardiopulmonary disorders
- Severe chronic cyanosis
- Cyanotic congenital heart disease
- Chronic fibrosing alveolitis
- Chronic suppuration in the lungs
  - bronchiectasis
  - empyema
  - lung abscess
- Carcinoma of the bronchus
- Subacute bacterial endocarditis

Chronic abdominal disorders
- Crohn's disease
- Ulcerative colitis
- Cirrhosis of the liver

---

rical 'butterfly' erythema of the nose and cheeks. In *discoid lupus* the cutaneous lesion is localized (Fig. 11.18). In *polyarteritis nodosa*, reticular livedo of the limbs, with purpura, vasculitic papules and ulceration, occurs. In *scleroderma* (systemic sclerosis), acrosclerosis of the fingertips with scarring, ulceration and calcinosis, follows a Raynaud's phenomenon of increasing severity. *Dermatomyositis* often presents with a heliotrope discoloration and oedema of the eyelids, and with fixed erythema over the dorsa of the knuckles and fingers (Fig. 11.15) and over the bony points of the shoulders, elbows and legs. There is usually weakness of the proximal limb muscles. Dermatomyositis in the middle-aged is associated in about 10% of cases with internal malignancy.

SKIN PIGMENTATION

Acanthosis nigricans is a brownish velvety thickening of the axillae, groins and sides of the neck. Sometimes there is thickening of the palms and soles, and warty excrescences may develop on the skin, eyelids and oral mucosa. In the middle-aged, acanthosis nigricans is strongly associated with internal malignancy, but benign minor forms are seen in obese young women, especially Arabs, and in children with endocrinopathies characterized by insulin resistance. Patchy depigmented macules which are hypoanaesthetic and associated with enlargement of the peripheral nerves are a feature of certain types of *leprosy (Hansen's disease)*.

Generalized, severe persistent *pruritus* in the absence of obvious skin disease may be due to systemic disease (Box 11.7). However, in old people with dry skin it is common and of no systemic significance. *Diabetes mellitus* has a number of skin manifestations: of these, pruritus vulvae, pruritus ani, balanoposthitis and angular stomatitis are due to *Candida* overgrowth. Boils, follicular pustules or ecthyma are staphylococcal. Impetigo and erysipelas, a streptococcal infection, are uncommon (Fig. 11.19). *Eruptive xanthomata* are a rare feature of uncontrolled diabetes mellitus. *Necrobiosis lipoidica diabeticorum* (Fig. 11.20) produces reddish-brown plaques, usually on the shins, with central atrophy of the skin. It has to be distinguished from *peritibial myxoedema* (which is hypertrophic, not atrophic), the *dermatoliposclerosis* of chronic venous disease in the legs and the *epidermal hypertrophy* of chronic lymphatic obstruction.

Neuropathic ('perforating') ulcers are found on pressure points of the heel, ball of foot, or toes and are characteristically painless. *Arteriopathic ulceration* resulting from large vessel disease is seen on the foot, and due to small vessel disease on the calves. *Spider naevi* consist of a central arteriole feeding a cluster of surrounding vessels. Many young people have up to seven naevi on the face, shoulders or arms. In older age groups pregnancy, the administration of oestrogens (as in oral contraceptives) and liver disease may cause multiple lesions. Pregnancy and liver disease may also produce erythema of the thenar and hypothenar eminences ('*liver palms*'). *Leukonychia* is also seen in liver disease.

Erythema nodosum is a condition in which tender, painful, red nodules appear, typically on the shins. They fade slowly over several weeks, leaving bruising, but never ulcerate. *Sarcoidosis* and *drug sensitivity* are the commonest causes, but other systemic disorders should be considered (Box 11.8).

Xanthomata are yellow or orange papules or nodules in the skin caused by dermal aggregations of lipid-loaded cells. Different patterns of hyperlipoproteinaemia may induce varying patterns of xanthomatosis. Thus, the *type IIa (hypercholesterolaemia)* pattern typically causes tuberous xanthomata on the extensor aspects of the knees and elbows and on the buttocks, sometimes associated with tendon xanthomata. Widespread eruptive xanthomata are more characteristic of *hypertriglyceridaemia*. White deposits of lipid (*arcus senilis*) in the cornea may

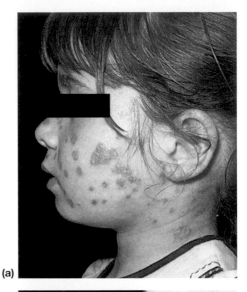

(a)

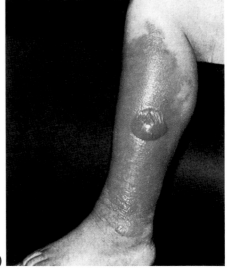

(b)

Figure 11.19   **(a)** Impetigo. **(b)** Erysipelas.

ture in those over 60. Flat lipid deposits around the eyes (*xanthelasma*) may be due to hyperlipidaemia, but are also seen in the middle-aged and elderly without any general metabolic upset.

Carotenaemia produces an orange-yellow colour to the skin, especially of the palms and soles. It

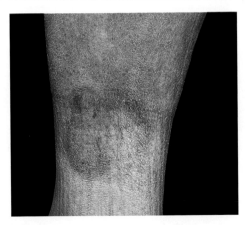

Figure 11.20 Necrobiosis lipoidica diabeticorum.

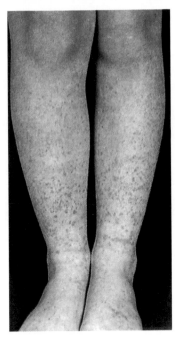

Figure 11.21 Purpura in Henoch–Schönlein disease.

occurs in those who eat great quantities of carrots and other vegetables, in hypothyroidism, in diabetic patients, and also in those taking β-carotene for the treatment of porphyria.

HAEMORRHAGE IN THE SKIN

Aggregations of extravasated red blood cells in the skin cause *purpura* (Fig. 11.21). Purpura may be punctate, from capillary haemorrhage, or may form larger macules, depending on the extent of haemorrhage and the size of vessels involved. The *Hess test* for capillary fragility involves deliberately inducing punctate purpura on the forearm by inflating a cuff above the elbow at 100 mmHg for 3 minutes. Sensitivity to drugs may cause widespread 'capillaritis'.

The term *ecchymosis* implies a bruise, usually with cutaneous and subcutaneous haemorrhage causing a palpable lump. A frank fluctuant collection of blood is a *haematoma*. Unlike erythema and telangiectasia, purpura cannot be blanched by pressure. It must not be confused with *senile haemangioma* (cherry angioma or Campbell de Morgan spot), which is common in later life on the trunk and has no pathological significance. Haemorrhage into the thick epidermis of the palm or sole due to trauma (e.g. *'jogger's heel'*) may induce brown or almost black macules that take weeks to disappear, inviting confusion with melanoma.

THE SKIN IN SEXUALLY TRANSMITTED DISEASES

The skin is involved in various sexually transmitted diseases. The *primary chancre* of syphilis may occur on the genitalia of either sex, at or near the anus, on the lip or, rarely, elsewhere. The rash of *secondary syphilis* is brownish-red, maculopapular, and typically involves the palms and soles. It does not itch. Other manifestations of the secondary stage are condylomata lata around the anogenital area, snail-track ulceration and 'mucous patches' in the mouth. There may be low-grade fever, lymphadenopathy and splenomegaly.

Septicaemia is a rare complication of *gonorrhoea* that occurs particularly in pregnant women, presenting with pustular skin lesions. *Recurrent type II herpes simplex* is common on the penis; it occurs less often on the buttocks, where relapses may be heralded by a radiating neuralgia. *Genital viral warts* are common in both sexes. They are particularly important in females because there is evidence that certain viral subtypes are responsible for chronic cervical dysplasia with malignant potential.

AIDS and other *HIV-related syndromes* have many cutaneous manifestations, including disseminated *Kaposi's sarcoma* candidiasis, molluscum contagiosum, seborrhoeic dermatitis, folliculitis and oral hairy leukoplakia (Fig. 11.22).

VIRAL INFECTION OF THE SKIN

Several of the most common viral infections and illnesses of childhood are characterized by fever and a distinctive rash (*exanthem*), including measles, varicella and rubella. In measles, upper respiratory symptoms are quickly followed by a characteristic maculopapular and erythematous rash. In rubella (German measles) the rash is more transient, micropapular, and associated with occipital lymphadenopathy and only slight malaise. The exanthem of varicella (chickenpox) is papulovesicular and centripetal, and there may be lesions in the mouth. In herpes zoster and herpes simplex (Fig. 11.23) infections there is a non-follicular papulovesicular

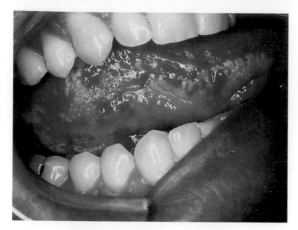

Figure 11.22   Hairy leukoplakia.

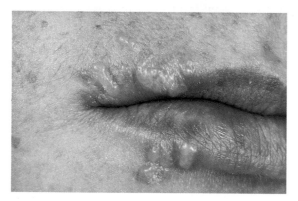

Figure 11.23   Herpes simplex (type I)

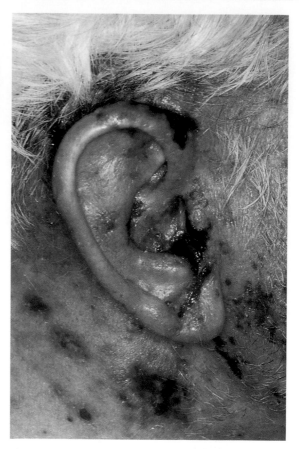

Figure 11.24   Herpes zoster vesicles on the ear lobe involving the C2 dermatome.

rash in which the vesicles are planted in an inflamed base. The rash is painful. In herpes zoster the rash follows a segmental distribution, in the skin of a dermatome. The vesicular lesion becomes encrusted (Fig. 11.24) and, later, secondary infection may occur.

Other less common viral infections associated with a rash include erythema infectiosum, due to a parvovirus, in which the exanthem on the face gives a 'slapped-cheek' appearance, and roseola infantum, a disease of toddlers, which mimics rubella.

DRUG ERUPTIONS

In the last 30 years eruptions caused by drugs have become common. Most such rashes are due to allergic hypersensitivity.

Drug rashes can mimic almost every pattern of skin disease. Thus *urticaria* may be caused by penicillin; a measles-like (*morbilliform*) rash may be induced by ampicillin, especially when given in infectious mononucleosis; *eczema-like* rashes are seen with methyldopa and phenylbutazone therapy; and gold and chloroquine rashes mimic *lichen planus*. Generalized *exfoliative dermatitis* may be induced by sulphonylureas, indomethacin and allopurinol.

Drugs that may sensitize the skin to sunlight (*phototoxic reaction*) include tetracyclines, sulphonamides and nalidixic acid. *Acne-like* rashes may follow high-dose prednisolone therapy, and are common with phenytoin therapy. Certain cytotoxic drugs and sodium valproate cause *hair loss*. Both *erythema nodosum* and *erythema multiforme* may be induced by sulphonamides, including co-trimoxazole. Laboratory tests are of almost no value in the diagnosis of drug eruptions. Careful history taking and knowledge of the common patterns of drug reactions usually allow accurate diagnosis.

TUMOURS IN THE SKIN

Exposure to the sun may, after many years, result in the development of skin tumours, for example *squamous* or *basal cell carcinoma*, or *melanoma*. These tumours are especially common in fair-skinned people. Basal cell carcinoma arises especially on the face, near the nose or on the forehead (Fig. 11.25). The lesion may be ulcerated with a firm, rounded edge, or papular. Melanomas occur especially on skin that has been burned by the sun (e.g. torso, forearms and legs). They may be pigmented or

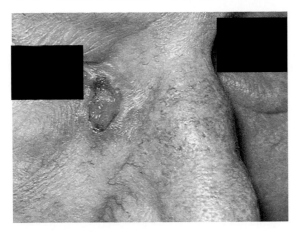

Figure 11.25 Basal cell carcinoma.

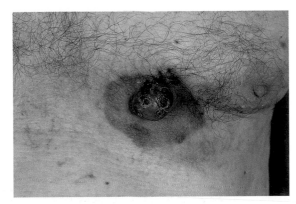

Figure 11.26 Malignant melanoma on a male chest. The nodule is invasive.

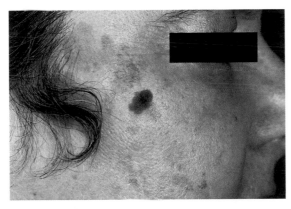

Figure 11.27 A pigmented basal cell papilloma (seborrhoeic keratosis) on the face. This is a benign lesion.

unpigmented, and may develop rapidly in a mole that has been present for many years (Fig. 11.26). *Seborrhoeic keratosis* is a raised pigmented lesion found in the sun-exposed elderly (Fig. 11.27). A symptomatic pigmented skin lesion having an asymmetric, ragged border, three or more colours and diameter of >7 mm, particularly if it is increasing in size or bleeding, and found on sun-damaged skin,

should be regarded as suspicious of *malignant melanoma*.

SPECIAL TECHNIQUES IN EXAMINATION OF THE SKIN

The skin is uniquely available to the examining physician. There are a number of diagnostic procedures.

TZANCK PREPARATION

This technique is useful for rapid diagnosis of vesicular infections or blistering eruptions such as pemphigus. The intact blister is opened and the base gently scraped. The material obtained is smeared on to the microscope slide, allowed to air-dry and then stained. Viral lesions will show typical multinucleated giant cells and pemphigus will show acantholytic cells.

MICROSCOPIC EXAMINATION

Microscopic examination is useful in the diagnosis of scabies, pediculosis and fungal infection (tinea and candidiasis).

SCABIES
Scabies is caused by the mite *Acarus (Sarcoptes) scabei*. The female is larger than the male and burrows in the epidermis, depositing eggs. These burrows should be looked for between the fingers, on the hands or wrists and on the sides of the feet. They can be recognized with the naked eye as short dark lines terminating in a shining spot of skin. The eggs lie in the dark line, the mite in the shining spot. It may be picked out by means of a flat surgical needle and placed on a microscope slide for more detailed examination.

PEDICULOSIS
Three forms of pediculosis or louse infestation occur: *Pediculus capitis* on the head, *Pediculus corporis* on the trunk, and *Pediculus pubis* on the pubic and axillary hairs. The eggs or nits of *P. pubis* and *P. capitis* adhere to the hairs. From their position on the hairs one can judge roughly the duration of the condition, as they are fixed at first near the root of the hair and are carried up as the hair grows, so the higher the nits are, the longer the pediculi have been present. *P. corporis* should be looked for in the seams of the clothes, especially where the clothes come into contact with the skin, for example over the shoulders. The bites of the parasite produce haemorrhagic spots, each with a dark centre and a paler areola. Marks of scratching should be looked for on parts accessible to the patient's nails. *P. pubis* is venereally acquired and causes intense pubic itching. The nits are laid on the pubic hair and the lice themselves are easily visible.

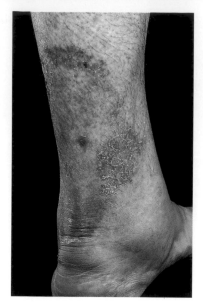

Figure 11.28   Tinea rubrum (ringworm infection).

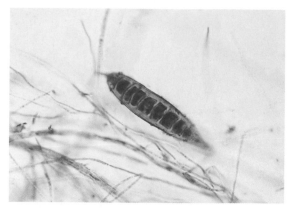

Figure 11.29   Lactophenol blue preparation showing macronidia of *Microsporum* spp. isolated from skin scrapings from a patient with ringworm.

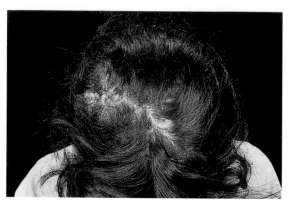

Figure 11.30   Kerion, due to localized deep dermatophyte infection in the scalp.

P. corporis is seen only in the grossly deprived, in vagrants, in those living rough, and in conditions of war and social upheaval. In contrast, *P. capitis* is common in schoolchildren, however clean they and their families may be, and is endemic in many schools.

FUNGAL INFECTIONS
Fungus may grow in the skin, nails or hair and can cause disease (*ringworm* or *tinea*), for example *athlete's foot*.

Skin
The skin between the toes, the soles of the feet and the groin are the commonest sites of fungal infection. The lesions may be scaly or vesicular, tending to spread in a ring form with central healing (Fig. 11.28); macerated, dead-white offensive-smelling epithelium is found in the intertriginous areas, such as the toe clefts.

Nails
Discoloration, deformity, hypertrophy and abnormal brittleness may result from fungus infection.

Hair
Ringworm of the scalp is most common in children. It presents as round or oval areas of baldness covered with short, lustreless broken-off hair stumps. These hair stumps may fluoresce bright green under Wood's light. Some fungi do not fluoresce with Wood's light, however, and these can be detected only by microscopy and culture (Figs 11.29, 11.30).

Microscopic examination for fungus infection
Scales from the active edge of a lesion are scraped off lightly with a scalpel, or the roofs of vesicles are snipped off with scissors. The material is placed in a drop of 10–20% aqueous potassium hydroxide solution on a microscope slide, covered with a coverslip and left for 30 minutes to clear. It is then examined under the light microscope with the 8-mm or 4-mm objective using low illumination. The mycelia are recognized as branching, refractile threads that boldly transgress the outlines of the squamous cells. Nails are examined in much the same way, but it is necessary to break up the snippings and shavings into small fragments. These are either heated in potassium hydroxide or are left to clear in it overnight before being examined.

A scalp lesion is cleaned with 70% alcohol or with 1% cetrimide; infected stumps and scales are removed by scraping with a scalpel. The hairs are cleaned in potassium hydroxide in the same way as skin scales. Examination under the microscope reveals spores on the outside of the hair roots, and mycelia inside the hair substance. The species of fungus responsible may be established by culture on Sabouraud's glucose–agar.

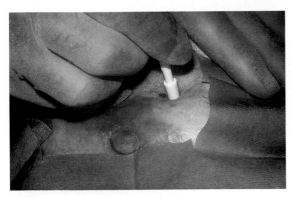

Figure 11.31 Disposable punch skin biopsy, especially useful where minimal scarring is desirable.

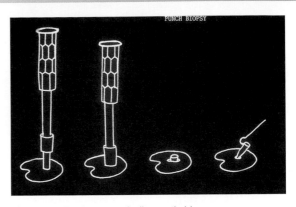

Figure 11.32 4 mm punch diagnostic biopsy.

WOOD'S LIGHT

Wood's light lamp emits long-wave ultraviolet light at a peak of 360 nm. Wood's light examination is performed in a darkened room and is useful to identify the fluorescence of fungi and corynebacterial infection (erythrasma), elevated porphyrins in urine, or in the localization of pigmentary abnormalities.

PATCH TESTING

This is an important and valuable tool for the diagnosis of suspected allergic dermatitis due to contact (contact dermatitis).

The formulation of the allergens is critical, and various standard contact allergen test batteries have been developed in different countries and clinics to include the commonest culprits. Patch testing is simple, but the results are not always easy to interpret. Allergens are placed in shallow aluminium

$1 cm^2$ wells and applied in strips to the patient's back for 48 hours for initial reading and a second reading at 96 hours. This ensures that any delayed-type hypersensitivity (e.g. Coombe's type IV reaction to an allergen) can be identified.

SKIN BIOPSY

Biopsy of the skin is used not only for the excision of benign and malignant tumours but also to identify the nature of expanding or inflammatory lesions. Punch biopsy (Figs 11.31, 11.32) is popular because of its convenience and results in minimal scarring. The biopsy can be studied by conventional histology, often supplemented by immunofluorescence, and sometimes molecular biology, to identify specific proteins or genetic abnormalities. Skin biopsy is increasingly used in diagnosis and in assessing the progress of skin diseases.

12 Endocrine disorders

J. P. Monson, W. Drake

INTRODUCTION

The endocrine system comprises the classic endocrine organs:

- Hypothalamus/pituitary
- Thyroid
- Parathyroid
- Adrenal
- Pancreatic islet cells
- Gonads.

The mode of presentation of endocrine disorders does not fit neatly into a system-based model, the symptoms rarely being specific to a particular system. Frequently, endocrine disease is suggested by a constellation of non-specific symptoms.

THE HISTORY

As in other systems the history consists of presenting symptoms, the history of the development of the illness and the family history.

PRESENTING SYMPTOMS

There are a number of symptom complexes that particularly suggest endocrine disease.

THIRST AND POLYURIA

Excessive thirst (*polydipsia*) and increased urine output (*polyuria*) are the most important presenting symptoms of diabetes mellitus; these are discussed in detail in Chapter 13. Polydipsia and polyuria may also be due to impairment of renal concentrating capacity as a result of a deficiency of antidiuretic hormone (*cranial diabetes insipidus*) or a failure of antidiuretic hormone action (*nephrogenic diabetes insipidus*). The latter may be inherited or may occur secondary to impairment of antidiuretic hormone action by hypercalcaemia or hypokalaemia. Sometimes, apparent polydipsia and polyuria may be due to increased fluid intake, which at its most extreme may be vastly excessive (*psychogenic polydipsia*). The distinction between psychogenic polydipsia and diabetes insipidus is important. Generally, nocturnal polyuria is not a feature of psychogenic polydipsia,

but this is not an absolute distinction and further investigation of urine concentrating capacity is usually required.

WEIGHT LOSS

Loss of weight is a feature of decreased food intake or increased metabolic rate. Sometimes both factors may operate to reduce body weight, as in the *cachexia* of malignant disease. Thyroid overactivity (*hyperthyroidism*) is nearly always associated with a combination of weight loss and increased appetite, although occasionally the latter may be stimulated more than the former so that there is a paradoxical increase in weight. Weight loss is rarely the sole presenting symptom of hyperthyroidism and other clinical features often predominate, particularly in younger patients (Box 12.1). In the elderly, however, hyperthyroidism may be occult or may simulate the gradual weight loss of malignant disease. Cardiac arrhythmias are a frequent feature in the elderly. *Anorexia nervosa*, a psychogenic disorder characterized by a long history of low body weight in the absence of other features of ill-health, must be considered, especially in young women. Any form of weight loss may be associated with amenorrhoea.

Other endocrine conditions in which weight loss is a major feature are listed in Box 12.2. Weight loss with diabetes mellitus is discussed in Chapter 13.

WEIGHT GAIN OR REDISTRIBUTION

An increase in body weight (Box 12.3) is a predictable result of a reduction in metabolic rate. Weight gain is therefore a common feature of *primary hypothyroidism*. However, obesity is rarely a consequence of specific endocrine dysfunction, an exception being the recently described but very rare phenomenon of leptin deficiency. In the majority of patients 'simple obesity' is due to a long-standing imbalance between energy intake and expenditure; it frequently begins in childhood and is often present in more than one family member. Glucocorticoid hormone excess (*Cushing's syndrome*) results in an increase in body fat predominantly involving abdominal, omental and interscapular fat (truncal obesity), with paradoxical thinning of the limbs due to muscle atrophy.

Box 12.1   Clinical features of hyperthyroidism

- Tachycardia
- Atrial fibrillation/heart failure
- Eye signs
- Lid lag
- Lid retraction
- Exophthalmos (Graves' disease)
- Sweating
- Thyroid gland enlargement and bruit (Graves' disease)
- Fine distal tremor
- Thinning of hair
- Proximal weakness; cannot rise from squat
- Chorea

Box 12.2   Endocrine and metabolic diseases in which weight loss is a clinical feature

- Hyperthyroidism
- Type 1 insulin-dependent diabetes mellitus (see Chapter 13)
- Hypopituitarism
- Adrenocortical failure (Addison's disease)
- Anorexia nervosa

Box 12.3   Conditions in which increased body weight is a feature

- Simple obesity: energy intake/expenditure imbalance
- Primary hypothyroidism
- Cushing's syndrome
- Hypothalamic lesions
- Leptin deficiency

Box 12.4   Conditions in which metabolic myopathy is a feature

Painless
- Hyperthyroidism
- Cushing's syndrome, including iatrogenic steroid myopathy
- Acromegaly

Painful
- Vitamin D deficiency
- Osteomalacia
- Hypothyroidism

Box 12.5   Conditions in which temperature intolerance is a feature

- Intolerance to cold
  - hypothyroidism
- Intolerance to heat
  - hyperthyroidism

Box 12.6   Clinical features of hypothyroidism

- Weight gain
- Sallow complexion and dry skin
- Thinning of scalp and lateral eyebrow hair
- Cold intolerance
- Deepened, gruff voice
- Slow physical and mental activity
- Unsteadiness and slightly slurred speech
- Tingling in toes and fingers
- Aching muscles with cramp
- Mild proximal weakness
- Slow pulse and shortness of breath

MUSCLE WEAKNESS

Symptomatic muscular weakness not due to neurological disease is a feature of several metabolic disorders, including thyrotoxicosis, Cushing's syndrome and vitamin D deficiency. In all these conditions the *metabolic myopathy* (Box 12.4) causes symmetrical proximal weakness, mainly involving the shoulder and hip girdle musculature. There is usually associated muscle wasting. The major symptom is difficulty in climbing stairs, boarding a bus or rising from a sitting position. Most patients with hyperthyroidism have proximal weakness. This may be subclinical; it is best demonstrated by asking the patient to rise from the squatting position. The proximal myopathy of *vitamin D deficiency* is often painful, in contrast to other causes. The differential diagnosis of painful proximal muscular weakness includes polymyositis and polymyalgia rheumatica, as well as spinal root or plexus disease.

COLD INTOLERANCE

An abnormal sensation of cold, out of proportion to that experienced by other individuals, may indicate underlying hypothyroidism (Boxes 12.5, 12.6). This symptom differs from the localized vasomotor symptoms in the hands found in Raynaud's phenomenon and is rather non-specific, especially in the elderly.

HEAT INTOLERANCE

The increased metabolic rate of thyrotoxicosis may be associated with heat intolerance in which, at its most extreme, the patient finds comfortable an ambient temperature that others find unpleasantly cold. This is an important symptom, highly specific for thyroid overactivity, which may partly explain some of the seasonal variation in presentation of the condition.

INCREASED SWEATING

Hyperhidrosis (excessive sweating) may be a constitutional abnormality, characterized by onset in childhood or adolescence and, sometimes, by a family history. A recent increase in sweat secretion, on the other hand, may be an early indication of thyroid overactivity. Paroxysmal sweating is a common feature of *anxiety*. Increased catecholamine secretion from a phaeochromocytoma of the adrenal medulla is a rare cause of hyperhidrosis. Intermittent sweating after meals (*gustatory hyperhidrosis*) may occur in patients with autonomic dysfunction. Growth hormone excess (acromegaly) also increases sweating, perhaps because of hypertrophy of the sweat glands, and this feature can be used to assess the activity of the disease in the clinic. Increased sweating should be distinguished from flushing that occurs physiologically at the time of the natural menopause. Flushing may be a presenting feature of serotonin-secreting carcinoid tumours of the gut and usually indicates extensive disease with hepatic metastases.

TREMOR

A fine rapid resting tremor is one of the cardinal clinical features of thyrotoxicosis. This must be distinguished from the coarser and more irregular tremor of anxiety, which is usually associated with a cool peripheral skin temperature, in contrast to the warm skin of the thyrotoxic patient. Tremor due to neurological disease is greater in amplitude, slower in rate, and may be present at rest, as in Parkinson's disease, or on movement, as in cerebellar tremor. It therefore rarely simulates thyrotoxic tremor. Essential tremor is not so rapid as thyrotoxic tremor, is variable, and is worse in certain postures. It often involves the head and neck.

PALPITATIONS

Palpitations are a heightened, unpleasant awareness of the heartbeat. They may be a feature of thyrotoxicosis, but are more likely to be due to anxiety. Awareness of the heartbeat while lying down is normal. Other causes of rapid heart rate include paroxysmal tachyarrhythmias. The sensation of intermittent forceful cardiac contraction, sometimes described by the patient as a missed beat, is often due to a compensatory pause following an ectopic beat, and is usually a normal phenomenon.

POSTURAL UNSTEADINESS

Dizziness, or a sensation of faintness on standing, should prompt measurement of lying and standing blood pressure. Postural hypotension, a fall of diastolic blood pressure on standing, occurs with reduced blood volume. In the absence of obvious bleeding or gastrointestinal fluid loss, adrenal insufficiency should be considered. Postural hypotension is frequently due to autonomic neuropathy, especially in long-standing diabetes mellitus. It is also a common complication of any drug therapy for essential hypertension. The drug history is particularly important in the elderly patient with dizziness.

VISUAL DISTURBANCE

Several endocrine conditions may cause visual symptoms. Decreased visual acuity may be due to space-occupying lesions compressing the optic nerve. For example, severe dysthyroid eye disease and orbital or retro-orbital tumours may present in this way. *Bitemporal hemianopia* (bilateral loss of part or all of the temporal fields of vision), often asymmetrical or incongruous, is a major feature of suprasellar extension of pituitary adenomas compressing the optic chiasm, but may occur in other tumours in this location. Double vision (*diplopia*) on lateral or upward gaze often results from medial or lateral rectus muscle tethering in dysthyroid eye disease (Figs 12.1, 12.2). Apparent magnification of vision (*macropsia*) can occur in hypoglycaemia.

FASTING SYMPTOMS

Tachycardia, sweating and tremor occurring intermittently, especially when fasting, are suggestive of hypoglycaemia. These symptoms resemble those associated with the increased sympathetic drive found in states of fear or with excess secretion of norepinephrine (noradrenaline), as in phaeochromocytoma. In severe persistent hypoglycaemia these symptoms may progress to decreased consciousness. This is a serious emergency implying *neuroglycopenia* sufficient to impair brain function. Spontaneous or fasting hypoglycaemia can be due to:

- Autonomous insulin production due to an insulinoma
- Glucocorticoid deficiency, with or without thyroxine and growth hormone deficiency (e.g. primary adrenal failure or hypopituitarism)
- Inappropriate insulin or excessive sulphonylurea drug administration in a diabetic patient
- Rarer causes of hypoglycaemia, for example hepatic failure and rapidly growing malignant lesions, especially thoracic or retroperitoneal mesothelial tumours secreting proinsulin-like growth factor II.

CRAMPS AND 'PINS AND NEEDLES'

Intermittent cramp and 'pins and needles' (*paraesthesiae*), especially if bilateral, can be due to a decreased level of circulating ionized calcium. This may occur in hypoparathyroidism or be associated with a fall in the ionized component of serum cal-

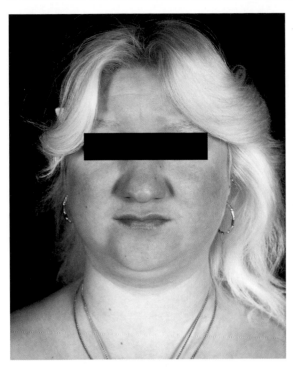

Figure 12.1 Typical facial appearance of Cushing's syndrome. Note the increased fat deposition and the plethoric appearance. The patient presented with a 2-year history of secondary infertility, easy bruising and central adiposity.

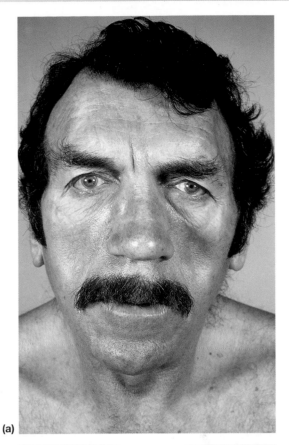

(a)

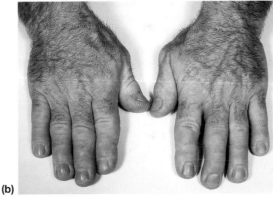

(b)

Figure 12.2 The facial (a) and hand (b) appearance of acromegaly. There is overgrowth of the facial skeleton, coarsening of features and an increase in soft tissues, most obvious in the hands. The patient had a 4-year history of excessive sweating, increased shoe size, frontal headache and 'pins and needles in fingers'.

cium, owing to an increased extracellular pH (*alkalosis*). The latter may occur with any alkalosis, but is particularly well recognized in hyperventilatory states (respiratory alkalosis) and hypokalaemia (metabolic alkalosis). Refractory cramping symptoms after correction of hypocalcaemia can be due to an associated hypomagnesaemia. However, the differential diagnosis of paraesthesiae in the hands includes median nerve compression at the wrist (carpal tunnel syndrome), a syndrome that is usually accompanied by typical sensory and motor disturbance suggestive of a lesion in the median nerve (see Chapter 10).

NAUSEA

This is a rare symptom of endocrine disease. It is an important presenting feature of adrenal insufficiency, in which typically it is maximal in the morning and may be associated with vomiting. Similar symptoms may occur with severe hypercalcaemia and may be the sole manifestation of this condition. These two conditions should be considered early in the differential diagnosis of a patient presenting with upper gastrointestinal symptoms in the absence of demonstrable structural disease. Occasionally, thyrotoxicosis may present with nausea and vomiting, although looseness of stools is the more common gastrointestinal manifestation of this condition.

DYSPHAGIA

Difficulty in swallowing is an unusual manifestation of endocrine disease but may be the presenting feature of multinodular thyroid enlargement with retrosternal extension. Smaller goitres only rarely result in dysphagia. Severe hyperthyroidism with generalized weakness may be associated with a reversible myopathy of the pharyngeal musculature and consequent dysphagia.

NECK PAIN AND SWELLING

Superficial discomfort in the neck may lead to the incidental finding of thyroid enlargement. Modest degrees of thyroid enlargement are very common, whereas pain arising from the thyroid is comparatively unusual. The most common cause of local discomfort and tenderness in the neck is inflammatory lymphadenopathy. Severe tenderness of the thyroid itself, especially when accompanied by fever and signs of thyrotoxicosis, suggests a diagnosis of viral subacute thyroiditis (de Quervain's thyroiditis). Occasionally autoimmune thyroiditis may give rise to pain and tenderness, which mimics a viral thyroiditis but is less severe. The sudden onset of localized pain and swelling in the thyroid is indicative of bleeding into a pre-existing thyroid nodule and is a recognized complication of multinodular goitre. The symptoms are self-limiting. Painless enlargement of the thyroid gland (*goitre*) presents either with pressure effects, resulting in dysphagia progressing to tracheal compression and stridor, or cosmetic disturbance. The underlying cause of thyroid enlargement is often difficult to establish. The family history and subsequent investigation may point to autoimmune thyroiditis or dyshormonogenesis. A history of rapid enlargement of the gland, especially in an elderly patient, suggests an anaplastic thyroid carcinoma. Coexisting severe diarrhoea points towards a diagnosis of medullary carcinoma of the thyroid. In the differential diagnosis goitrogenic drugs, for example lithium, should be considered, as should residence in an iodine-deficient area. Previous exposure to neck irradiation or to radioactive iodine in childhood may also be important.

IMPOTENCE

Reduced erectile potency may be a consequence of primary abnormalities, such as:

- Decreased blood supply to the penis (e.g. atherosclerosis)
- Neural dysfunction (e.g. autonomic neuropathy complicating diabetes)
- Testosterone deficiency (e.g. hypopituitarism and primary testicular failure)
- Hyperprolactinaemia
- Drug therapy (e.g. certain antihypertensives)
- Psychological factors
- A combination of several causes.

It is often difficult to distinguish with certainty between impotence due to organic factors and that which is psychological, although total erectile failure and the absence of nocturnal and morning erections suggest a physical cause. Impotence in a diabetic patient should not be assumed to be inevitably due to autonomic neuropathy, and other causes should be considered. Most importantly, it should be recognized that male impotence is often complicated by a psychological disturbance, which may serve to exacerbate the problem.

GYNAECOMASTIA

Gynaecomastia refers to a smooth, firm, mobile, often tender, disc of breast tissue under the areola in the male. It should be distinguished from the soft, fatty enlargement often seen in obesity. Mild gynaecomastia (sometimes unilateral or asymmetrical) frequently occurs as a temporary phenomenon in normal puberty and may persist for several years, or sometimes indefinitely. In adults, gynaecomastia may result from:

- Excess oestrogen stimulation
- Reduction in circulating androgen
- Antagonism of androgen action
- Androgen insensitivity (Box 12.7).

Clinical assessment of the patient with gynaecomastia should therefore include an enquiry about any change in libido and examination of thyroid status, the genitalia, the muscles, and for stigmata of chronic liver disease (Box 12.7).

AMENORRHOEA

The term amenorrhoea describes absence of menstrual periods (menses). Perhaps the most common cause of failure of onset of menses (*primary amenorrhoea*) is physiological delay of puberty, a diagnosis that can only be made with certainty in retrospect. Important pathological causes include:

- Hypothalamic–pituitary dysfunction, for example due to tumours
- Ovarian failure (e.g. failure of normal ovarian development or cytotoxic chemotherapy)

Box 12.7   Causes of gynaecomastia

Increased oestrogen/testosterone ratio
- Chronic liver disease
- Thyrotoxicosis
- Phenytoin therapy

Androgen receptor antagonists
- Spironolactone; digoxin

Inherited androgen receptor defects
- Testicular feminization syndrome

Testosterone deficiency or oestrogen excess
- Primary and secondary hypogonadism
- Tumour production of human chorionic gonadotrophin (HCG)
- Oestrogen production of Leydig cell tumour of testis

Congenital and hereditary
- X-linked spinal muscular atrophy (Kennedy syndrome)
- Klinefelter's syndrome (karyotype XXY)

- Thyroid dysfunction
- Defects in lower genital tract development.

Important diagnostic pointers in the history include symptoms suggestive of thyroid disease, or any visual disability that might indicate compression of the optic chiasm by a hypothalamic or pituitary tumour. Secondary amenorrhoea (cessation of previously established menses) has similar causes. In addition, marked weight loss may lead to amenorrhoea, as in anorexia nervosa or inflammatory bowel disease. Amenorrhoea, or oligomenorrhoea (infrequent scanty periods), may occur in women subject to excessively rigorous physical training programmes. Normal pregnancy is the most common cause of secondary amenorrhoea.

GALACTORRHOEA
Occasionally physiological lactation may persist after breastfeeding has ceased. Inappropriate lactation is usually bilateral. There are a number of causes, which include:

- Prolactin-secreting tumours of the pituitary gland
- Idiopathic galactorrhoea, in which there is an apparent increased sensitivity to normal levels of serum prolactin
- Hyperprolactinaemia due to hypothyroidism
- Hyperprolactinaemia due to dopamine antagonist drugs
- Hyperprolactinaemia due to lactotroph-disinhibiting lesions of the hypothalamopituitary region.

Inappropriate secretion of breast milk should therefore always prompt enquiry for symptoms referable to the thyroid and pituitary glands, and a thorough drug history should be taken. Even with very high prolactin levels galactorrhoea is rare in men.

EXCESS HAIR GROWTH
An increase in the growth of facial and body hair in adult females is a relatively common symptom and may be due to increased circulating androgens. However, it is most commonly a normal, constitutional characteristic. Pathological causes of hirsutism include:

- Polycystic ovary syndrome
- Late presentation of congenital adrenal hyperplasia
- Androgen-secreting ovarian or adrenal tumours.

The history is vital in the clinical assessment. If the symptoms commenced shortly after the menarche, then a tumour source of androgen is unlikely. A regular menstrual cycle is good evidence against severe androgen excess but does not exclude polycystic ovary syndrome. Increased libido suggests substantially increased androgen secretion, which may be either ovarian or neoplastic in origin.

BOWEL DISTURBANCE
Constipation and abdominal distension may be features of hypothyroidism or panhypopituitarism. Diarrhoea may occur as part of autonomic neuropathy involving the gut in diabetes mellitus. Peptic ulceration may occur in the Zollinger–Ellison syndrome, in which gastrin-secreting tumours of the gut result in increased gastric acid secretion.

SKIN CHANGES
Pallor often occurs in *primary testicular failure* and in *panhypopituitarism*. Excessive pigmentation occurs in ACTH-dependent *Cushing's syndrome*, and increased sebum production causing greasy skin and acne on the face and shoulders may occur in all causes of glucocorticoid excess. In *carcinoid tumours* of the gut or lung increased humoral secretion results in a violaceous cyanosis-like skin discoloration. A variegate, patchy rash is a feature of *porphyria*, an inherited abnormality of haem metabolism. In *primary hypoadrenalism* there is increased pigmentation of the conjunctival membrane beneath the eyelids and of the inside of the mouth, the axillae and the palmar skin creases. In *hypothyroidism* the skin appears dry, pale, sallow or even slightly yellow, scalp hair is coarse and lateral eyebrow hair is thinned. In *hyperthyroidism* the skin is dry and hot, but often not flushed. In *hypocalcaemia* the nails are friable. In *uraemia* the skin is pale, or yellow and slightly pigmented, and in terminal uraemia a 'uraemic frost' may appear on the skin.

Vitiligo, a patchy depigmentation of the skin, is common in association with many autoimmune disorders, particularly autoimmune hypothyroidism and vitamin B_{12} deficiency.

FAMILY HISTORY

The family background of endocrine or metabolic disease may be particularly useful in the evaluation of several of the more common disorders. It is also particularly important in the assessment of less common, inherited disorders of metabolism.

THYROID DISEASE
Autoimmune hypothyroidism and hyperthyroidism frequently show familial aggregation. Dyshormonogenetic goitre is also often inherited. A family history of organ-specific autoimmune disease (e.g. pernicious anaemia, vitiligo, Addison's disease) may also point to an autoimmune aetiology of thyroid disease.

RENAL CALCULI
Primary hyperparathyroidism, an important cause of renal stones, may be familial, occurring either as an isolated disorder or as a part of the syndrome of multiple endocrine neoplasia (type I).

THE EXAMINATION

GENERAL ASSESSMENT

This should begin with observing the general appearance of the patient. Start by assessing the state of nutrition and by measuring weight and height. Calculate the body mass index (BMI) (see Chapter 5). The distribution of fat should be noted. Deposition of fat in the intra-abdominal, thyrocervical and interscapular regions with relative sparing of the limbs (truncal obesity) is characteristic of Cushing's syndrome and is accompanied by a typical moonfaced plethoric appearance (Fig. 12.1) owing to a combination of increased subcutaneous fat and thinning of the skin.

Patients with growth hormone hypersecretion, resulting from somatotroph pituitary adenomas, also demonstrate a classic facial appearance with increased fullness and coarsening of soft tissues, including the lips and tongue, which in patients with long-standing disease may be accompanied by overgrowth of the zygoma, orbital ridges and mandible (prognathism) (Fig. 12.2). Acromegaly in young people occurring before epiphyseal fusion causes abnormally tall stature (gigantism). Increased adiposity in a child who is growing poorly suggests the possibility of growth hormone deficiency hypothyroidism or, rarely, Cushing's syndrome. Simple obesity is associated with normal or increased linear growth velocity.

The skeletal proportions should be noted: a long-limbed appearance may indicate delayed epiphyseal fusion due to hypogonadism (*eunuchoidism*) or the connective tissue abnormality Marfan's syndrome. A eunuchoid body habitus is confirmed by demonstrating that the leg length (top of symphysis pubis to ground) exceeds the sitting height, or that the span exceeds the total height. Shortening of the limbs occurs with a variety of skeletal dysplasias.

The cytogenetic disorder *Turner's syndrome* (karyotype 45 × 0), which is characterized by gonadal dysgenesis and the variable presence of other visceral abnormalities, has a typical phenotypic appearance, including short stature, failure of secondary sexual development, decreased or absent secondary sexual hair, an increase in the normal angulation between the humerus and the lower arm, a low posterior hairline and an exaggerated fold of skin between the neck and shoulder. It is most important that accurate wall-mounted stadiometers be used in the assessment of normal growth and its possible disorders.

The hands should be carefully examined for evidence of finger-clubbing which, among other things, may be a rare manifestation of thyrotoxic Graves' disease (*thyroid acropachy*). Palmar erythema may also be found in thyrotoxicosis of any cause, as well as in patients with chronic liver disease or rheumatoid arthritis, and in pregnancy.

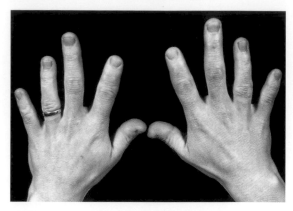

Figure 12.3 The hands in pseudohypoparathyroidism. Note the characteristic shortening of the fourth and fifth metacarpals.

A unique selective shortening of the fourth and fifth metacarpals may be found as the major somatic manifestation of a group of recessively inherited disorders of parathormone action (*pseudohypoparathyroidism*; Fig. 12.3).

THE SKIN

Pigmentation, especially buccal, circumoral or palmar, may indicate the increased secretion of adrenocorticotrophic hormone that occurs with adrenal failure (*Addison's disease*; Fig. 12.4); patches of depigmentation, or vitiligo (Fig. 12.5), may also be found in Addison's disease or other organ-specific autoimmune disorders. Violaceous striae, arising as a result of stretching of thin skin with exposure of the dermal capillary circulation, suggest the possibility of glucocorticoid excess (Fig. 12.6), and abnormal dryness of the skin and coarseness of the hair are found in hypothyroidism (Fig. 12.7). Localized thickening of the dermis due to mucopolysaccharide and inflammatory cell deposition, particularly on the anterior aspects of the legs, when it is known as pretibial myxoedema, is one of the classic but relatively rare extrathyroidal manifestations of Graves' disease.

In females, dermatological examination should also include attention to any abnormality of hair distribution, either excess hair growth in an androgen-dependent distribution (*hirsutism*) or hair loss in a male pattern, both of which may indicate increased circulating androgen and should prompt examination for evidence of virilization (see below).

THE THYROID

EXAMINATION OF THE THYROID   (Fig. 12.8a–e) The anatomical landmarks relevant to inspection and palpation of the thyroid are shown in Figure 12.8(a). Immediately inferior to the thyroid cartilage (with its superior notch) is the cricoid cartilage,

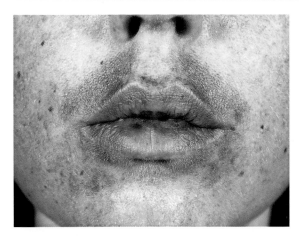

Figure 12.4 Circumoral pigmentation in a patient with hypersecretion of adrenocorticotrophic hormone (ACTH).

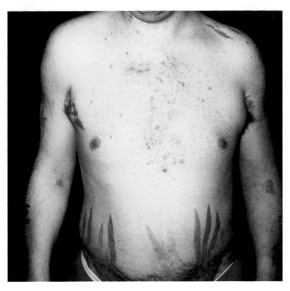

Figure 12.6 Violaceous striae typical of Cushing's syndrome.

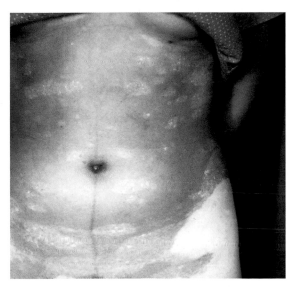

Figure 12.5 Extensive areas of depigmentation (vitiligo) in a patient with organ-specific autoimmune disease.

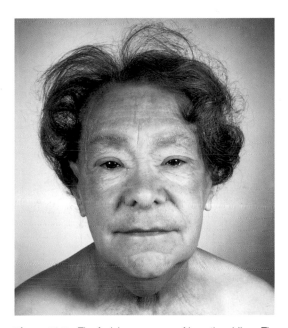

Figure 12.7 The facial appearance of hypothyroidism. The patient demonstrates periorbital puffiness and coarsening of scalp hair. (Courtesy of Professor P.G. Kopelman.)

with the thyroid isthmus lying just below in the midline. The right and left lobes of the thyroid curve posterolaterally round the trachea and oesophagus and are partially covered by the sternomastoid muscles. The attachment of the thyroid to the pretracheal fascia dictates that it moves superiorly on swallowing; absence of this movement raises the possibility of an infiltrative thyroid carcinoma. Remember that the right lobe is slightly larger than the left; hence, diffuse thyroid enlargement, as in Graves' disease (Fig. 12.8(c)) is often apparently asymmetrical. There are several methods for examining the thyroid, but the suggested routine is as follows.

With the patient's neck slightly extended, inspect the area below the cricoid cartilage (Fig. 12.8(a)). Ask him/her to take a sip of water, extend the neck again and swallow. Watch for the superior move-

ment of the gland, carefully noting its contour and any asymmetry.

Thyroid palpation is best carried out from behind, with the patient's neck slightly extended, but not so much that the neck musculature is tightened. This may feel awkward initially, but with time and practice it will become more comfortable. Have a glass of water available throughout the examination, so the patient may take repeated sips and swallow as necessary. Position both hands to encircle the neck (Fig. 12.8(b)), with the fingers

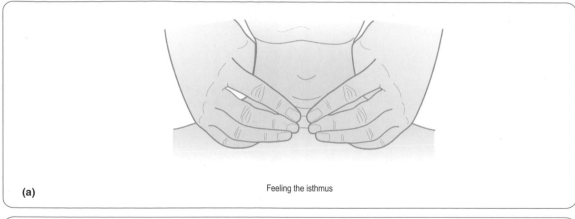

(a)   Feeling the isthmus

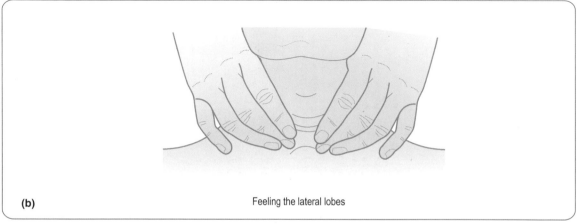

(b)   Feeling the lateral lobes

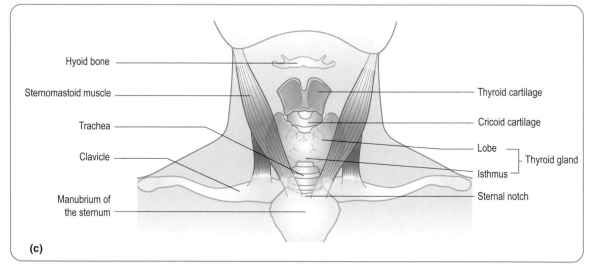

(c)

Figure 12.8   Examination of thyroid. **(a)** Feeling the isthmus; **(b)** feeling the lateral lobes; **(c)** anatomical landmarks.

slightly flexed, such that the tips of the index fingers lie just below the cricoid in order to palpate the isthmus. Now rotate the fingers down and slightly laterally in order to feel the lateral lobes, including the inferior border. The anterior surface of each lobe should be no larger than the terminal phalanx of the patient's thumb.

The following points should be addressed:

- Is the thyroid diffusely enlarged, as in thyroid stimulating hormone (TSH)-mediated or autoimmune enlargement? If so, is it soft (e.g. dyshormogenesis, diffuse goitre of puberty) or firm/hard (e.g. autoimmune thyroiditis). In general, the firmer the texture of an enlarged thyroid, the more likely is the pathology to be autoimmune.

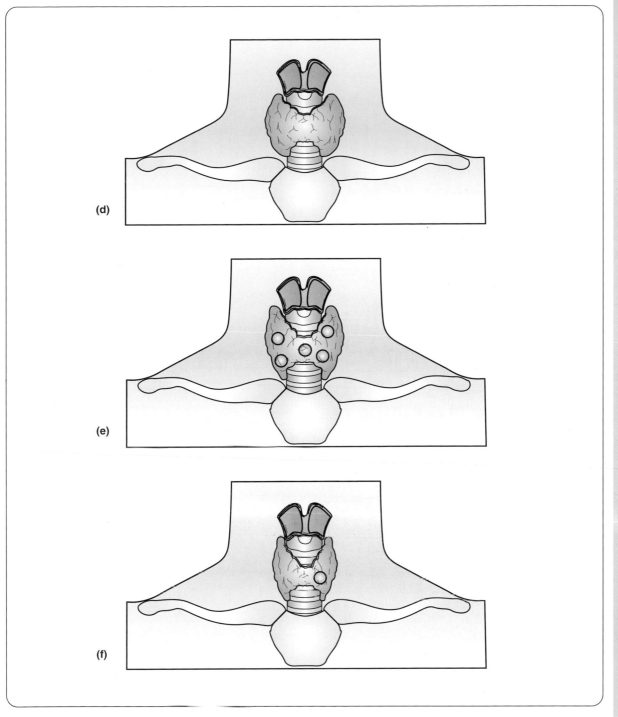

Figure 12.8 – *cont'd* **(d)** diffuse enlargement; **(e)** multinodular gotre; **(f)** single nodule.

- Are there two or more identifiable nodules (Fig. 12.8(d), Fig. 12.9) and, if so, is the patient thyrotoxic and does the gland extend downward behind the sternum? (If the gland is partially or completely retrosternal, the inferior border may not be palpable, or palpable only on swallowing.) Most multinodular goitres are benign, but a history of neck irradiation,

enlarged cervical lymph nodes or progressive enlargement of one of the nodules raises the suspicion of malignancy.
- Is the palpable abnormality a single focal nodule (Fig. 12.8(e)), suggesting a cyst, adenoma or carcinoma? Rapid growth, hard texture, lack of movement on swallowing (see above), enlarged regional lymphadenopathy, male gender and a

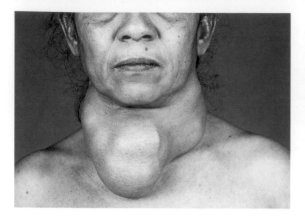

Figure 12.9   A large multinodular goitre. Note the asymmetrical growth of the nodules.

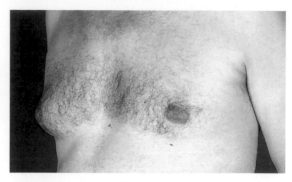

Figure 12.10   Gynaecomastia. There is enlargement of both breasts in this man.

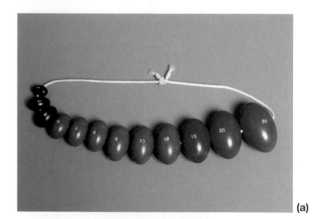

(a)

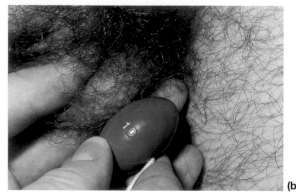

(b)

Figure 12.11   Prader orchidometer. **(a)** Testicular volume (in ml) may be estimated by comparison with calibrated ellipsoids. **(b)** Gently grip the testis in one hand and compare its volume (including the scrotal skin, but excluding the epididymis) with that of the ellipsoids. The patient shown has a reduced testicular volume of 8 mL, due to Klinefelter's syndrome; the normal secondary sexual hair is due to the provision of exogenous testosterone.

history of neck irradiation all increase the probability of malignancy.

- Is the goitre firm and asymmetrical?
- Are there features of local pressure effects or local infiltration (e.g. dysphonia from recurrent laryngeal involvement)?
- Is there weight loss and debility? These suggest anaplastic carcinoma or lymphoma.
- Is there a bruit, indicating increased blood supply? This is frequently found in untreated Graves' disease, but should not be confused with a transmitted bruit from the carotid.

THE CARDIOVASCULAR SYSTEM

Particular attention should be paid to any postural drop in blood pressure. This may indicate a depleted extracellular fluid volume, for example in patients with adrenal insufficiency, or autonomic dysfunction, the commonest cause of which is diabetes mellitus. Additional indicators of the latter include failure of reflex bradycardia during the Valsalva manoeuvre and loss of beat-to-beat variation in cardiac cycle length, as determined by ECG. A hyperdynamic circulation, sinus tachycardia or atrial fibrillation may be found in thyrotoxicosis; this may progress to cardiac decompensation and cardiac failure.

THE BREASTS AND GENITALIA

The breasts should be examined for mass lesions and, if suggested by the history, for galactorrhoea. In males any tendency to gynaecomastia should be noted (Fig. 12.10). This may range from minor degrees of subareolar glandular enlargement to substantial breast prominence; breast enlargement associated with generalized adiposity should not be confused with true gynaecomastia.

Genital examination in the male should document testicular volume. This is particularly important in the assessment of pubertal development,

for which volume should be measured by comparison with calibrated ovoids (Prader orchidometer, Fig. 12.11). Prepubertal testicular volume is less than 4 mL; increased volume implies pubertal gonadotrophin stimulation. Testicular atrophy in the adult male indicates hypogonadism, due either to primary testicular failure, hypothalamopituitary

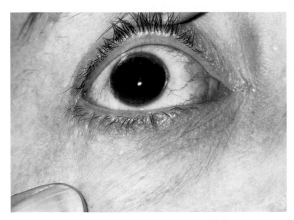

Figure 12.12 Corneal calcification (band keratopathy) in a patient with long-standing hyperparathyroidism.

dysfunction or chronic liver disease. Tumours of Leydig cells are usually palpable and should be sought in any patient with gynaecomastia.

Examination of the external genitalia in the female is important when androgen hypersecretion is suspected. Enlargement of the clitoris is a feature of excess androgen secretion.

Ambiguity of the external genitalia is indicative of fetal androgen excess in the karyotypic female and of testosterone or dihydrotestosterone deficiency or resistance in the male; these conditions are rare and require specialized investigation.

THE EYES

The hypercalcaemic patient should be carefully examined for corneal calcification, evident as a narrow band on the medial or lateral border of the cornea (Fig. 12.12); this usually indicates long-standing hypercalcaemia and a diagnosis of primary hyperparathyroidism.

In patients with thyroid disease the presence of exophthalmos (*proptosis*) should be noted. This may be unilateral or bilateral, and may be associated with apparent ophthalmoplegia due to tethering of the extraocular muscles, particularly the medial and inferior rectus muscles, such that diplopia occurs on upward or lateral gaze (*dysthyroid eye disease*; Fig. 12.13). These ocular signs are especially important in the diagnosis of autoimmune thyroid disease (*Graves' disease*). It must be remembered that unilateral proptosis may also occur with an orbital tumour. Lid retraction, evident as a wide-eyed staring expression, and lid lag, in which depression of the upper lid lags behind the eye in a downward gaze, are due to increased activity of the sympathetic innervation of levator palpebri superioris and are not specific to Graves' disease. Any degree of corneal exposure due to failure of complete lid apposition should be documented.

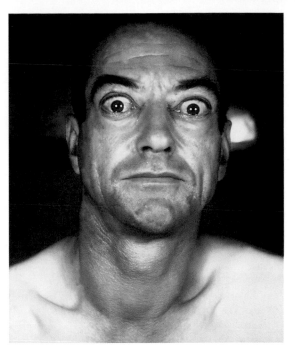

Figure 12.13 Lid retraction and proptosis in a patient with thyrotoxic Graves' disease. In this patient there had been a 6-month history, of effortless weight loss, tremulousness, shortness of breath on exertion and palpitations.

Visual acuity should be measured both with and without a pinhole to correct for any refractive error. Reduced acuity may be a feature of optic nerve compression in severe dysthyroid eye disease or of asymmetrical pressure on the optic chiasm due to hypothalamopituitary space-occupying lesions. In the latter, assessment of the visual fields may reveal a *bitemporal hemianopia*; this is frequently incomplete and incongruous, reflecting the asymmetrical growth of the tumour. Examination of the optic discs with the ophthalmoscope may show papilloedema, indicating recent onset of optic nerve compresson, or pallor, indicating neural atrophy resulting from long-standing pressure. In the context of a pituitary mass lesion, pallor of the optic discs suggests that full visual recovery is improbable.

THE NERVOUS SYSTEM

In *thyrotoxicosis* examination of the nervous system reveals a rapid fine tremor. Proximal weakness with or without wasting of the shoulder and hip girdle musculature (*proximal myopathy*) is a typical feature of thyrotoxicosis, glucocorticoid excess and vitamin D deficiency. Osteomalacic myopathy is often associated with myalgia.

Hypocalcaemia is associated with increased neural excitability, which may be demonstrated by gentle percussion over the proximal part of the facial nerve (as it exits from the parotid gland). The test is positive if this manoeuvre evokes involuntary facial muscular twitching (*Chvostek's sign*).

Tendon reflexes will be abnormally brisk in thyrotoxic patients and may show a slow relaxation phase in hypothyroidism. Both hypothyroidism and acromegaly may give rise to nerve entrapment syndromes, particularly of the median nerve at the wrist (*carpal tunnel syndrome*).

INVESTIGATION

The investigation of endocrine and metabolic disorders usually involves: (a) the measurement of electrolytes, minerals, metabolites or hormones in plasma; and (b) isotopic, ultrasonographic, radiological or magnetic resonance (MR) imaging of specific endocrine glands. In investigating endocrine disease one is usually interested in whether a specific gland is over- or underactive. These questions may be answered by basal hormone measurements, for example serum free thyroxine and thyroid-stimulating hormone in thyrotoxicosis and hypothyroidism, but in many instances the lack of a clear distinction between basal hyposecretion, normal secretion and hypersecretion necessitates the use of stimulation and suppression tests.

ENDOCRINE STIMULATION TESTS

These are designed to demonstrate how much hormone a gland can secrete in response to a near-maximal stimulus. Examples include:

- *Insulin tolerance testing*, in which carefully controlled insulin-induced hypoglycaemia stimulates hypothalamopituitary secretion measured by serum growth hormone, cortisol and prolactin
- *Tetracosactrin testing*, in which an injection of a synthetic adrenocorticotrophic hormone (ACTH) analogue is used to assess adrenocortical reserve
- *Oral glucose tolerance test*, which is an indirect test of insulin secretion and action as determined by the rise and subsequent fall in the plasma glucose level following an oral glucose load.

ENDOCRINE SUPPRESSION TESTS

These test whether a physiological feedback mechanism is intact, or if secretion of the hormone in question has become at least partly autonomous. For example, the suppression of plasma cortisol by the synthetic glucocorticoid dexamethasone is incomplete in Cushing's syndrome, and suppression of serum growth hormone by an oral glucose load fails to occur in acromegaly.

ENDOCRINE IMAGING

Plain X-ray imaging is of limited value in the investigation of endocrine disorders. However, lateral

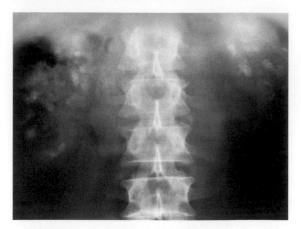

Figure 12.14   Widespread renal calcification typical of nephrocalcinosis in a patient with long-standing hyperparathyroidism.

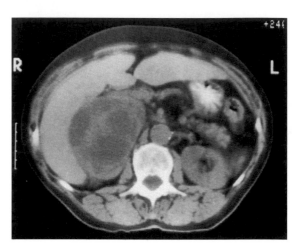

Figure 12.15   Axial CT scan of the abdomen in a patient with a right adrenal medullary phaeochromocytoma. Note the extensive tumour mass, with areas of hypodensity indicating episodes of partial tumour infarction.

and anteroposterior views of the pituitary fossa can be useful in demonstrating abnormal calcification in the fossa, or gross expansion and erosion of the fossa due to large intrasellar or suprasellar tumours. Plain abdominal radiology may show renal calcification (*nephrocalcinosis*; Fig. 12.14) in patients with long-standing hypercalcaemia or renal tubular acidosis.

CT imaging is useful in assessing the pituitary, adrenal glands (Fig. 12.15) and thorax. However, MR imaging of the pituitary (Fig. 12.16), offers definite advantages over CT in terms of improved precision in detecting small intrasellar tumours, and better definition of the lateral border of the pituitary and the cavernous sinus.

Isotopic imaging is particularly useful for demonstrating autonomous function within endocrine tumours. This technique is applicable to the thyroid

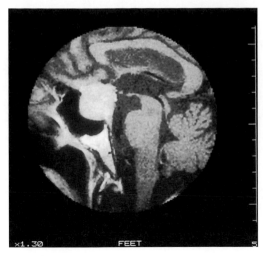

Figure 12.16   Magnetic resonance imaging (sagittal view) of the pituitary, demonstrating a large pituitary adenoma with suprasellar extension.

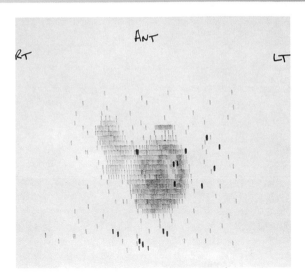

Figure 12.17   Technetium-labelled isotope scan of the thyroid in a patient with a focal thyroid nodule. Note the focal area of uptake corresponding to the palpable lesion, with surrounding inactivity indicating autonomous function within the nodule.

gland (radiolabelled pertechnetate; Fig. 12.17), the adrenal medulla (radiolabelled metaiodobenzyl-guanidine) and parathyroids (combined radio-labelled sesta MIBI and pertechnetate differential scanning).

13 Diabetes and other metabolic disorders

G. A. Hitman, T. A. Chowdhury

INTRODUCTION

The study of *metabolism* (Box 13.1) began as long ago as the 15th century BC, with the first description of diabetes in the Ebers Papyrus. Metabolic diseases comprise a variety of disorders encompassing a number of medical specialties. They contribute significantly to mortality and morbidity, predominantly from cardiovascular disease. Diabetes and metabolic disorders have become more prevalent in both developed and developing countries, leading to a significant burden of chronic disease and complications related to those diseases. This increased prevalence is related to ready access to excessive calorific intake coupled with reduced physical activity. Whereas in the past metabolic diseases such as diabetes were deemed diseases of the rich, in developed countries they are now frequently diseases of lower social class, as access to healthier foods may be expensive and difficult.

The major metabolic disorders considered in this chapter are:

- Diabetes mellitus and the metabolic syndrome
- Lipid disorders.

DIABETES MELLITUS AND THE METABOLIC SYNDROME

Diabetes is a Greek word meaning 'a passer through; a siphon', and *mellitus* derives from the Greek word for 'sweet'. The Greeks named it thus due to the excessive amounts of urine produced by sufferers which attracted insects because of its glucose content. The ancient Chinese tested for diabetes by observing whether ants were attracted to a person's urine.

Diabetes mellitus is the most common metabolic disorder encountered in clinical practice. It is strongly linked to *obesity*. Diabetes mellitus is characterized by abnormal carbohydrate and lipid homoeostasis, leading to elevation in plasma glucose, or *hyperglycaemia*, and abnormality of serum lipids, or *dyslipidaemia*. Glucose homoeostasis is modulated mainly by the release of *insulin* from the *islet cells* (β cells) of the pancreas. Diabetes develops as a result of a variable combination of absolute insulin deficiency as a result of pancreatic islet cell dysfunction, and tissue *insulin resistance* due to reduced cellular responsiveness to insulin.

The World Health Organization (WHO) has developed a classification of diabetes mellitus based on its pathogenesis (Table 13.1). The two predominant classes of diabetes are *type 1* and *type 2*, and clinical differences between the two are listed in Table 13.2. Type 1 is characterized by absolute insulin deficiency due to autoimmune-mediated pancreatic islet cell destruction. In contrast, type 2 diabetes is associated with a variable degree of tissue insulin resistance, leading – at least in the early stages – to high plasma insulin levels, then subsequently to relative insulin deficiency as pancreatic islet cell function fails to overcome this resistance. The diagnostic criteria for disorders of glucose metabolism based on the 75 g oral glucose tolerance test are shown in Table 13.3. Note that glycosuria itself (glucose in the urine) is not a reliable diagnostic test for diabetes mellitus.

It has long been recognized that many people have a clustering of risk factors for cardiovascular disease. Thus the term *metabolic syndrome* has been coined, with various pseudonyms of *syndrome X* or *insulin resistance syndrome*. Clinical and biochemical characteristics of the metabolic syndrome are shown in Box 13.2. People with the syndrome are at high risk of diabetes and cardiovascular disease. The condition is common among certain ethnic groups (African-Americans, Mexican-Americans, Asian Indians, Australian Aboriginals), and features can be present for up to 10 years before hyperglycaemia is detected. Vigorous treatment can reduce mortality and morbidity from cardiovascular disease.

PRESENTING SYMPTOMS OF DIABETES

Many people with type 2 diabetes may be asymptomatic at diagnosis, for example by routine screening of blood or urine, when there may be only mildly increased levels of hyperglycaemia. Once diagnosed, however, many patients do admit to some long-standing, often mild symptoms. Acute metabolic decompensation, leading to marked hyperglycaemia, occurs infrequently.

In contrast, type 1 diabetes is often abrupt in onset, and characterized by severe hyperglycaemia with acute life-threatening decompensation (*diabetic ketoacidosis*).

The cardinal symptoms of diabetes mellitus are *weight loss*, *polyuria* and *polydipsia*, and their presence should always result in an immediate test for blood glucose and urine for *ketones*.

POLYURIA, POLYDIPSIA AND NOCTURIA

Acute hyperglycaemia causes increased urine excretion (*polyuria*) and as a result, excessive thirst and

Table 13.1   The World Health Organization classification of diabetes mellitus

Type	Common subtypes/pathogenesis	Treatment
Type 1	Destruction of pancreatic islet cells leading to insulin deficiency	Insulin
Type 2	Ranges from predominantly insulin resistance with relative insulin deficiency (often associated with obesity) to predominantly insulin deficiency	Diet/oral hypoglycaemic agents/insulin
Other types Genetic defects of β-cell function	Diabetes associated with glucokinase, hepatic nuclear factor (HNF) 1α, HNF1β, HNF4α, Neurod1 and insulin promotor factor mutations (all previously grouped under maturity onset diabetes of the young (MODY)) Mitochondrial diabetes	Tablets or insulin depending upon genetic defect Tablets or insulin
Genetic defects of insulin action	Insulin resistance syndromes (type A insulin resistance, leprechaunism, Rabson–Mendenhall syndrome lipoatrophic diabetes)	Insulin-sensitizing agents and insulin
Diseases of the exocrine pancreas	Fibrocalculous pancreatic diabetes, pancreatitis, trauma/pancreatectomy, neoplasia, cystic fibrosis, haemochromatosis, others	Frequently insulin required
Endocrinopathies	Cushing's syndrome, acromegaly, phaeochromocytoma, glucagonoma, hyperthyroidism, somatostatinoma, others	Treatment of underlying cause
Drug- or chemical-induced	Glucocorticoids, α-adrenergic agonists, β-adrenergic agonists, thiazides, interferon-α therapy	Avoid
Uncommon forms of immune-mediated diabetes	Insulin autoimmune syndrome (antibodies to insulin), anti–insulin receptor antibodies, 'stiff man' syndrome	Variable
Other genetic syndromes associated with diabetes	Down's, Friedreich's ataxia, Huntington's chorea, Klinefelter's, Lawrence–Moon–Biedl, myotonic dystrophy, porphyria, Prader–Willi, Turner's, Wolfram's	Variable
Gestational diabetes		Diet/insulin

Table 13.2   Clinical differences between type 1 and type 2 diabetes

	Type 1	Type 2
Ketosis prone	Yes	Uncommon
Insulin requirement	Yes (absolute insulin deficiency)	Often later in disease (insulin resistance ± deficiency)
Onset of symptoms	Acute	Often insidious
Obese	Uncommon	Common
Age at onset (years)	Usually <30	Usually >30
Family history of diabetes	10%	30%
Concordance in monozygotic twins	30–50%	90–100%

Table 13.3 The oral glucose tolerance test in diagnosing diabetes mellitus

	Fasting plasma glucose (mmol/L)		2 hour plasma glucose (mmol/L)	Random plasma glucose (mmol/L)
Diabetes mellitus	>7.0	or	>11.1	>11.1
Impaired glucose tolerance (IGT)	<7.0	and	Between 7.8 and 11.0	–
Impaired fasting glucose (IFG)	Between 6.1 and 6.9	and	<7.8	–

Oral glucose tolerance test (OGTT) is performed as follows:
- Fast patient from midnight
- Check plasma glucose at time zero
- Give 75 g of glucose solution orally
- Check plasma glucose 2 hours later.

In the absence of symptoms diabetes should only be diagnosed on the basis of **two** abnormal glucose results. **One** abnormal glucose result is sufficient if the patient has symptoms.
These levels apply to a **plasma** (venous) glucose, **not** a capillary glucose (finger prick). These levels do not apply to the diagnosis of gestational diabetes.

Table 13.4 Causes of polyuria

Osmotic diuresis	Diabetes mellitus, chronic renal failure, drugs
Polydipsia	Psychogenic
Lack of ADH	Cranial diabetes insipidus due to: idiopathic, surgery, pituitary/hypothalamic tumour, familial, postpartum
Failure of response to ADH	Nephrogenic diabetes insipidus due to: primary, renal tubular disorders, hypokalaemia, hypercalcaemia, drugs

Box 13.2 The International Diabetes Federation Definition of Metabolic Syndrome

For a person to be defined as having the metabolic syndrome they must have:

Central obesity –

| Waist circumference | >94 cm for Europid men |
| | >80 cm for Europid women |

With ethnic specific values for other groups.

Plus any two of the following four factors:

- *Raised triglyceride level:* >150 mg/dL (1.7 mmol/L), or specific treatment for this lipid abnormality
- *Reduced HDL cholesterol:* <40 mg/dL (0.9 mmol/L) in males and <50 mg/dL (1.1 mmol/L) in females, or specific treatment for this lipid abnormality
- *Raised blood pressure:* systolic BP >130 or diastolic BP >85 mmHg, or treatment of previously diagnosed hypertension
- *Raised fasting plasma glucose (FPG)* >100 mg/dL (5.6 mmol/L), or previously diagnosed type 2 diabetes

water ingestion (*polydipsia*). These presenting symptoms of diabetes mellitus are also termed *osmotic symptoms*. Raised plasma glucose leads to increased renal tubular delivery of glucose, which then exceeds the resorptive capacity of the renal tubule, leading to *glycosuria*. Therefore, despite hyperglycaemia, people with an increased renal threshold for glucose may have no osmotic symptoms. Conversely, people with a low renal threshold for glucose may have *glycosuria* despite being normoglycaemic. It is for this reason that glycosuria is an unreliable feature in the diagnosis of diabetes mellitus. *Nocturia* is also common in patients presenting with osmotic symptoms of diabetes, and enquiry regarding the frequency of passing urine at night can be helpful in evaluating symptoms.

Other conditions can cause polyuria and polydipsia (Table 13.4). *Diabetes insipidus (DI)* is characterized by loss of renal concentrating capacity, owing to either loss of secretion of antidiuretic hormone (arginine vasopressin) from the posterior pituitary gland (*cranial DI*) or to poor renal tubular responsiveness to antidiuretic hormone (*nephrogenic DI*). This leads to loss of free water, which if uncorrected by increased water ingestion can lead to severe dehydration and plasma hypertonicity. Electrolyte disturbance, such as *hypercalcaemia* or *hypokalaemia*, can impair antidiuretic hormone action and hence lead to polyuria and polydipsia. In addition, polyuria and nocturia are common symptoms of chronic renal failure.

WEIGHT LOSS AND LETHARGY

Loss of more than 5% of total body weight should be considered clinically important in a subject not deliberately attempting to lose weight. Weight loss is a common presenting symptom in people with type 1 diabetes, and occasionally in type 2 diabetes with marked hyperglycaemia. Loss of weight in diabetes is predominantly due to renal glucose loss as a result of lack of insulin to enable cellular uptake of glucose. The weight loss usually occurs despite a normal appetite and dietary intake. This is in contrast to the weight loss of malignant disease, which is usually associated with reduced appetite and oral intake, or thyrotoxicosis, which is associated with increased appetite and oral intake.

Lethargy and fatigue are also common presenting symptoms of diabetes mellitus, particularly type 2, where the symptoms may have been present for some time.

SKIN PROBLEMS

Dermatological manifestations of diabetes are common at diagnosis, especially in patients with poor glycaemic control. Skin infections, such as *staphylococcal* infection leading to *boils, carbuncles* or *abscesses*, which are often recurrent, may occur. Severe infection itself can lead to hyperglycaemia, and a new diagnosis of diabetes should be reconsidered once the acute infection has cleared.

Oral and genital *candidiasis* can also be presenting features of diabetes mellitus. The presence of the characteristic white plaques on the tongue and oropharynx in a previously healthy person not on antibiotic therapy should alert the physician to the possibility of diabetes mellitus, although other conditions leading to immune paresis, such as HIV infection or haematological malignancy, can also lead to candidiasis. Genital candidiasis in women leads to a thick white discharge and vaginal soreness. Similarly, in men it can lead to a severe *balanitis* (inflammation of the glans penis). Always check the blood sugar in people with recurrent candidiasis.

VISUAL DISTURBANCE

Hyperglycaemia can lead to blurred vision, owing to osmotic changes within the aqueous humour of the lens of the eye. This can also occur when chronic hyperglycaemia is treated, causing further osmotic shifts in the lens. The symptom usually settles once normoglycaemia is achieved.

OTHER IMPORTANT ASPECTS OF A DIABETIC HISTORY

FAMILY HISTORY

A history of diabetes in first-degree relatives is a potent risk factor for diabetes. Type 2 diabetes appears to have a stronger genetic component than type 1, with around a third of patients having a positive family history compared to around 10% of type 1 diabetic patients.

A family history of premature cardiovascular disease is also important. Patients with diabetes are at risk of cardiovascular disease, and this risk is increased when there is a family history of vascular disease in fathers or brothers aged less than 55 years, or mothers or sisters aged under 65.

DIET AND LIFESTYLE HISTORY

The cornerstone of management of diabetes is lifestyle; accordingly, assessment of the patient's lifestyle is important. Regularity of meals, the quality and quantity of foods eaten and the frequency of snacks should be known. Enquire about:

- Regularity of meals – three meals a day is ideal
- Content of fatty/greasy foods – particularly discourage saturated (animal) fats, as this type of fat is linked to heart disease
- Content of fruit and vegetables – at least five portions a day are recommended
- Content of sugar and sugary foods – avoid carbonated drinks, cakes, sweets and biscuits
- Content of salt – a high salt intake can lead to hypertension
- Alcohol intake – a maximum of two units of alcohol per day for a woman and three units per day for a man.

The smoking history is of paramount importance, as smoking in diabetes is strongly linked to cardiovascular disease. Occupational history may be important, because if insulin therapy is required this may have an impact on legal requirements for driving. Assess physical activity, to ascertain whether increased activity may improve glycaemia and weight. At least 30 minutes of moderate exercise, e.g. brisk walking, per day is recommended.

ASSESSMENT OF OTHER CARDIOVASCULAR RISK FACTORS

Cardiovascular risk is greatly increased in people with diabetes, and additional cardiovascular risk factors multiply the risk. Thus, any history of hypertension, hyperlipidaemia or previous vascular disease (cerebro-, cardio- or peripheral vascular) should be noted. Take a full medication history, including the use of antiplatelet, antihypertensive and lipid-lowering drugs.

HOME GLUCOSE TESTING

In a patient previously diagnosed with diabetes, assess their self-monitoring of glucose. This will enable a reasonable judgement of glycaemic control. Self-monitoring can be done by home capillary blood testing, or by urine testing for glycosuria (Fig. 13.1).

INSULIN INJECTIONS

In patients taking insulin it is important to ascertain whether the patient self-injects, the delivery device (disposable pen, cartridge pen or syringe/vial) used, the sites chosen, and whether they experience any problems.

SYMPTOMS OF COMPLICATIONS OF DIABETES

Chronic complications of diabetes mellitus can be usefully subdivided into large blood vessels (*macrovascular*), small blood vessels (*microvascular*), and others (Table 13.5).

SYMPTOMS OF MACROVASCULAR DISEASE

The features of ischaemic heart disease are described elsewhere (see Chapter 7). People with diabetes have fewer, less severe symptomatic chest pains, possibly due to autonomic neuropathy leading to reduced deep pain sensation – so-called *silent ischaemia*.

Thus, the only symptom of ischaemic heart disease in a diabetic subject may be breathlessness.

Peripheral vascular disease presents with claudication (Chapter 7). In addition, in patients with diabetes, a combination of peripheral neuropathy and peripheral vascular disease can lead to *foot ulceration*, particularly at sites of pressure (Fig. 13.2).

Cerebrovascular disease in diabetic patients can present with any stroke syndrome (Chapter 10). Transient ischaemic attacks are common.

SYMPTOMS OF MICROVASCULAR DISEASE

Diabetic retinopathy is frequently asymptomatic until it causes significant visual loss, which may be acute in onset (e.g. owing to a sudden *retinal haemorrhage*) or insidious (e.g. owing to *cataract* or *maculopathy*). *Diabetic nephropathy* is similarly

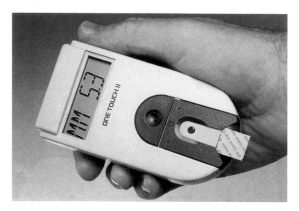

Figure 13.1   Home glucose testing is an important part of diabetes care.

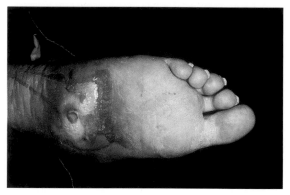

Figure 13.2   Diabetic neuropathic ulcer in a patient with Charcot's neuroarthropathy.

Table 13.5   Chronic complications of diabetes

Macrovascular	Coronary heart disease	
	Peripheral vascular disease	
	Cerebrovascular disease	
Microvascular	Retinopathy	Non-proliferative
		Proliferative
		Maculopathy
	Neuropathy	Peripheral sensory neuropathy
		Autonomic neuropathy
		Mononeuropathy
		Proximal motor neuropathy
	Nephropathy	
Other	Dermatological	Diabetic dermopathy
		Necrobiosis lipoidica diabeticorum
		Bullosis diabeticorum
		Granuloma annulare
		Acanthosis nigricans
	Rheumatological	Diabetic cheiroarthropathy
		Flexor tendinopathy
		Adhesive capsulitis
		Diabetic osteoarthropathy
		Charcot neuroarthropathy
		Diffuse idiopathic skeletal hyperostosis
	Hepatic	Non-alcoholic steatohepatitis

asymptomatic until renal dysfunction becomes so severe that uraemia ensues (see Chapter 14). Uraemic symptoms include fatigue, breathlessness and tachypnoea, pleuritic chest pain due to pericarditis, and pruritus. Heavy proteinuria may lead to the development of a *nephrotic syndrome* (Chapter 14).

In contrast, *diabetic neuropathy* can manifest in a number of ways. Chronic *peripheral sensory neuropathy* is the commonest form, affecting around 5% of patients with diabetes. This can present with symptoms varying from numbness, a feeling of 'walking on cotton wool' and paraesthesiae (pins and needles), to burning, sharp and shooting pains. The latter is a feature of selective involvement of small pain fibres. Typically the symptoms start distally and spread up in a stocking distribution, and are characteristically worse at night, frequently leading to insomnia.

Proximal motor neuropathy (*diabetic amyotrophy*, or *femoral neuropathy*) is uncommon, but is seen predominantly in middle-aged men with type 2 diabetes. The condition is characterized by severe, deep pain and paraesthesiae in the upper anterior thigh, followed by weakness and wasting of the quadriceps muscle. The condition is often unilateral, generally short-lived (around 3 months), and usually resolves spontaneously. Associated weight loss and cachexia are common.

Mononeuropathies, particularly affecting the median nerve of the hand (*carpal tunnel syndrome*; see Chapter 10) are common in patients with diabetes. This frequently presents with paraesthesiae and numbness in the median nerve distribution of the hand (lateral two-and-half digits), and is again worse at night. Similar symptoms may occur in the foot (*tarsal tunnel syndrome*). Cranial mononeuropathies are rare, but palsies of cranial nerves III and VI are seen in patients with diabetes, leading to blurred or double vision due to ophthalmoplegia (Chapter 10). The pupillomotor fibres are usually spared in diabetic third-nerve palsy.

Diabetes can cause *autonomic neuropathy*, the symptoms of which can be very troublesome. They include *impotence*, *gustatory sweating* (severe facial sweating on tasting food), *urinary retention* or *incontinence*, dizziness or syncope due to *postural hypotension*, *constipation or diarrhoea* (so called *diabetic diarrhoea*), and recurrent *nausea and vomiting* due to *diabetic gastroparesis*.

HYPOGLYCAEMIA

Treatment of diabetes is aimed at reducing symptoms and reducing the risk of diabetic complications. In attempting to reduce hyperglycaemia using oral hypoglycaemic tablets or insulin therapy, the patient with diabetes is at risk of *hypoglycaemia*.

Physiological responses to hypoglycaemia start at a plasma glucose of around 3.8 mmol/L, with the release of counter-regulatory hormones such as glucagon or epinephrine (adrenaline). Symptoms of hypoglycaemia normally occur at around this level owing to sympathetic overactivation. Such symptoms include sweating, palpitations, hunger, agitation or blurred vision, and most patients recognize them as hypoglycaemia and are able to treat themselves rapidly. A further drop in blood glucose leads to *neuroglycopenic symptoms*, where cerebral glucose is low, leading to impaired intellectual activity or diminished psychomotor skills. Further drops in glucose levels can lead to severe agitation, confusion, coma and epileptiform siezures. The symptoms of hypoglycaemia can be distressing, and have a significant adverse impact on quality of life. Loss of awareness of hypoglycaemia is sometimes a problem in diabetics with autonomic neuropathy, and in insulin-treated diabetes this can lead to unexpected hypoglycaemia. Patients at risk should be warned against driving motor vehicles, and taught the early symptoms of hypoglycaemia in order to raise their awareness of this potentially serious complication of therapy.

EXAMINATION OF THE DIABETIC PATIENT

GENERAL ASSESSMENT

Patients with diabetes can present with acute metabolic decompensation, leading to *diabetic ketoacidosis* (DKA), *hyperosmolar hyperglycaemic syndrome (HHS)* or, in treated patients, hypoglycaemia. Thus it is mandatory for all patients presenting with coma or reduced conscious level to have their blood glucose checked immediately.

Characteristically, the cardinal symptoms of severe polyuria, polydipsia and weight loss will have been present for some time prior to coma; such symptoms should never be ignored in a diabetic person. Patients with acute hyperglycaemic crises are frequently severely dehydrated, with hypotension (including postural hypotension), tachycardia, dry mucous membranes and reduced skin turgor. Other signs of diabetic ketoacidosis include rapid deep sighing respiration (*Kussmaul* breathing – a respiratory compensation for metabolic acidosis) and *ketones* on the breath (a sweet odour reminiscent of nail polish remover). Diabetic ketoacidosis can occasionally present with symptoms of an acute abdomen.

In the non-acute setting measurement of weight and height to ascertain the *body mass index* (BMI) is of great importance in the assessment of the diabetic patient (Box 13.3). It is desirable for all patients with diabetes to undergo a full medical assessment once a year – the so-called diabetic *annual review* (Box 13.4).

Box 13.3   Body mass index

BMI = Weight (kg)/Height (m)^2

In European racial group
Normal BMI	20–25
Overweight	25.1–30
Obese	30.1–35
Grossly obese	>35.1

In Asians
Normal BMI	18–23
Overweight	23.1–28
Obese	28.1–33
Grossly obese	>33.1

Box 13.4   The diabetic annual review

History
- Patient concerns
- Events – life and medical
- Glucose diary (urine or blood)
- Current treatment
- Hypoglycaemia
- Driving
- Pregnancy/contraception in women
- Impotence
- Symptoms of CHD or PVD
- Smoking habit?

Examination
- Weight/BMI
- Blood pressure – erect and supine
- Injection sites
- Urinalysis
- Eye examination
- Foot examination

Tests
- Renal function, liver function
- Glycated haemoglobin (HbA1c)
- Lipids
- Urine for albumin excretion

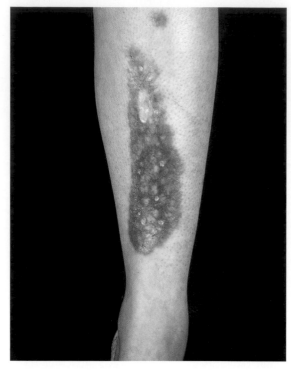

Figure 13.3   Necrobiosis lipoidica diabeticorum.

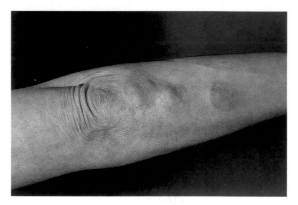

Figure 13.4   Granuloma annulare. (Courtesy of Dr David Peterson.)

SKIN, NAILS AND HANDS

Dermatological manifestations of diabetes are common. Fungal nail infections, particularly of the feet, are common, as are dermatophyte infections of the skin of the feet (*tinea pedis*). Staphylococcal skin infections leading to pustules, abscesses or carbuncles can also be seen. Other skins lesions seen in diabetes include *necrobiosis lipoidica diabeticorum* (Fig. 13.3). This is a rare complication of diabetes, predominantly seen in young women aged 15–40 years. This presents as a painless red macule, usually over the anterior shin, which then heals with scarring to form a yellowish/brown lesion. The condition can be unsightly, and little effective treatment is available. *Vitiligo* is seen a small number of patients with type 1 diabetes, reflecting its autoimmune nature.

Diabetic dermopathy is characterized by brown macules on the lower legs that heal to form atrophic, shiny white scars. A further skin lesion seen in patients with diabetes is *granuloma annulare*, pale, shiny rings and nodules usually seen on the hands (Fig. 13.4). *Bullosis diabeticorum* is a rare manifestation, characterized by tense blistering, mainly on the feet.

Acanthosis nigricans is characterized by a dark velvety appearance in the axillae or neck of people with insulin resistance (Fig. 13.5) and frequently

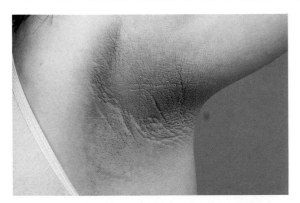

Figure 13.5 Acanthosis nigricans.

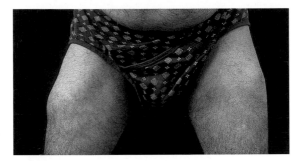

Figure 13.6 Lipohypertrophy. (Courtesy of Dr David Peterson.)

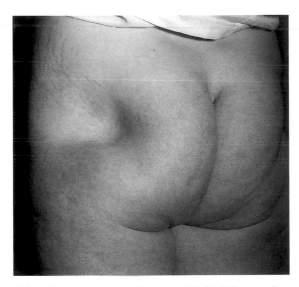

Figure 13.7 Lipoatrophy. (Courtesy of Dr David Peterson.)

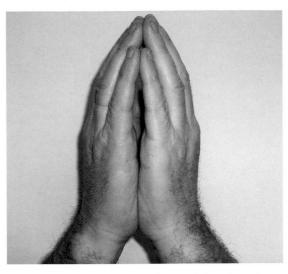

Figure 13.8 The prayer sign in diabetic cheiroarthropathy.

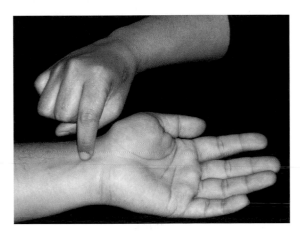

Figure 13.9 Tinel's sign in carpal tunnel syndrome: tapping on the median nerve at the wrist induces pain in the median nerve distribution.

Diabetic cheiroarthropathy, or 'stiff hand syndrome' or 'limited joint mobility', is seen in some patients with long-standing diabetes. It is characterized by skin thickening and sclerosis of the tendon sheaths, leading to reduced joint mobility and the characteristic *prayer sign* (Fig. 13.8). Examination of the hands for signs of carpal tunnel syndrome (Chapter 10) is important if the patient has suggestive symptoms. Thus, the presence of *Tinel's* sign (Fig. 13.9) and *Phalen's* sign (Fig. 13.10) should be sought. Thenar eminence wasting may also be seen.

EYES

Examination of the eyes is mandatory in patients with diabetes. External examination may indicate signs of dyslipidaemia (*corneal arcus* and *xanthelasmata*; Fig. 13.11). A reduced pupillary response to light may indicate autonomic neuropathy. Visual acuity should be assessed yearly with a Snellen

accompanies type 2 diabetes, but may occur in people with insulin resistance in the absence of diabetes.

Diabetic patients treated with insulin should have their injection sites examined for signs of *lipohypertrophy* (a physiological response to insulin injected near fat cells) (Fig. 13.6) or *lipoatrophy* (an allergic response to non-human insulins – now rarely seen) (Fig. 13.7).

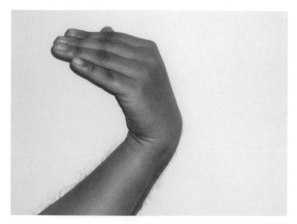

Figure 13.10 Phalen's sign in carpal tunnel syndrome: hyperflexion of the wrist leads to pain in the median nerve distribution.

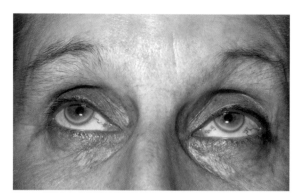

Figure 13.11 Corneal arcus and xanthelasmata in a patient with diabetic dyslipidaemia.

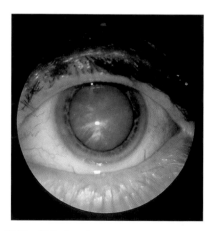

Figure 13.12 Diabetic cataract.

> **Box 13.5 Characteristic features of diabetic retinopathy**
>
> **Non-proliferative retinopathy**
> - Microaneurysms
> - Dot haemorrhages
> - Hard exudates (lipid deposits) not involving the macula
>
> **Mild**
> - <5 microaneurysms
> - Haemorrhages and/or exudates
>
> **Moderate**
> - Extensive (≥5) blot haemorrhages and/or microaneurysms and/or cottonwool spots (retinal ischaemia)
> - Venous beading
> - Looping or reduplication
> - Intraretinal microvascular anomaly (IRMA)
>
> **Severe**
> - Intraretinal deep blocked haemorrhages in four quadrants
> - Venous beading in two quadrants
> - Severe IRMA in one quadrant
>
> **Proliferative retinopathy**
> - New vessels on disc (NVD) or elsewhere (NVE)
>
> **Maculopathy**
> - This is any retinopathy 1 disc diameter around macula
> - *Focal or exudative maculopathy*
> - *Diffuse*
> - *Ischaemic*

carefully examined, starting from the optic disc and radiating into each quadrant of the eye. The macula is examined last, as this can be quite uncomfortable for the patient. The use of green light may aid the detection of microaneurysms. Ideally, all patients with diabetes should have annual fundal photography. A classification of diabetic retinopathy is shown in Box 13.5 (Figs 13.13–13.17).

CARDIOVASCULAR SYSTEM

Examination of the heart and vasculature is important in patients with diabetes. Palpation of peripheral pulses, especially of the feet, is extremely important, as is auscultation of the carotid and femoral arteries to detect bruits. Blood pressure should be measured frequently in patients with diabetes, to detect hypertension (classed at >140/80 mmHg in patients with diabetes) or postural hypotension (drop in systolic BP >20 mmHg on standing). A resting tachycardia, loss of sinus arrhythmia (reflex bradycardia on expiration) and loss of reflex bradycardia during a Valsalva manoeuvre can indicate autonomic neu-

chart, and unexplained loss of acuity should be investigated. Funduscopy should be undertaken with pharmacological dilatation of the pupils in order to obtain an adequate view. Loss of the red reflex on funduscopy may indicate cataract formation, and the lens should be assessed for opacities (Fig. 13.12). The vitreous and retina should be

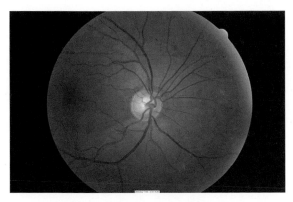

Figure 13.13 Background retinopathy (dot haemorrhages and microaneurysms) in the inferior nasal region. (Courtesy of Dr Paul Dodson.)

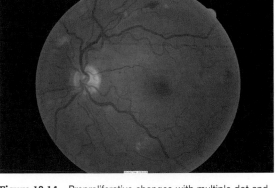

Figure 13.14 Preproliferative changes with multiple dot and blot haemorrhages and cottonwool spots. (Courtesy of Dr Paul Dodson.)

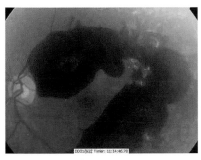

Figure 13.15 Retinal haemorrhage due to new vessel formation in severe proliferative retinopathy. (Courtesy of Dr Paul Dodson.)

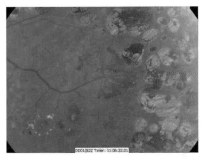

Figure 13.16 New vessel formation and laser photocoagulation burns in severe proliferative retinopathy. (Courtesy of Dr Paul Dodson.)

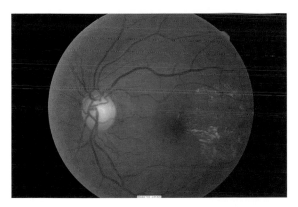

Figure 13.17 Exudative diabetic maculopathy. (Courtesy of Dr Paul Dodson.)

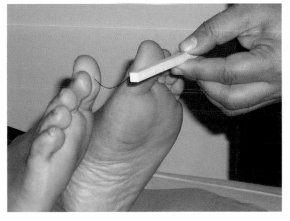

Figure 13.18 Testing for neuropathy using a Semmes Weinstein monofilament giving standard 10 g of fine touch.

ropathy, although these are best assessed by electrocardiography (ECG).

FEET

The feet of patients with diabetes should be examined at least once a year. Signs of *deformity*, *callus* (a sign of excessive pressure at this site), fungal infection especially between the toes, nail care and ulceration should be carefully assessed. Peripheral pulses and nailfold refill should be assessed for signs of peripheral vascular disease. Nerve function should be assessed by testing vibration sense at the great toe, medial malleolus and knee, and testing fine touch on the toes, metatarsal heads, heels and dorsum of the feet with a 10 g monofilament (*Semmes Weinstein monofilament*) (Fig. 13.18).

Loss of ankle jerks is also a sign of early diabetic peripheral sensory neuropathy.

A complication of diabetic peripheral neuropathy is the neuropathic joint – *Charcot neuroarthropathy* (see Fig. 13.2). This usually affects the ankle and presents with a painless, swollen, hot red joint, sometimes with a history of minor local trauma. The natural history is of progressive deformity until the process settles, usually over a few months. Untreated, the joint develops severe deformity, which then puts the foot at high risk of ulceration, infection and amputation. Treatment is with immobilization in a plaster cast boot, and intravenous bisphosphonates.

Diabetic patients with signs of peripheral vascular disease or peripheral neuropathy, even if asymptomatic, should be classified as at high risk for ulceration and be given careful education on foot care by a podiatrist.

INVESTIGATION

Diagnosis of diabetes is based on a fasting plasma glucose or oral glucose tolerance test (OGTT), using the WHO criteria (Table 13.3). Although clinically it is relatively simple to distinguish between type 1 and type 2 diabetes, occasionally the diagnosis is not clear, especially in younger-onset type 2 diabetes without a family history. In these circumstances, the use of immunological tests such as *anti-islet cell* (ICA) or *antiglutamic acid decarboxylase* (GAD) antibody may be helpful. Positivity of either is a good indicator of autoimmune islet cell destruction (and hence probable type 1 diabetes), insulin deficiency and a subsequent requirement for insulin therapy.

In acute hyperglycaemic decompensation of diabetes urgent investigations are required, including a laboratory glucose estimation, assessment of renal function (urea and electrolytes), urinalysis testing for ketones and glucose, and arterial blood gas assessment to determine pH and bicarbonate level. A search for precipitating causes should be undertaken, including a chest radiograph, ECG, white cell count and, in younger women, a pregnancy test.

In order to reduce the risk of chronic complications it is important to ensure a full biochemical assessment is undertaken yearly as part of an annual diabetic review. Renal and liver function should be checked, along with assessment of urine albumin excretion. Glycaemic control can be assessed using the *glycated haemoglobin* (HbA1c), the percentage of which is well correlated to prevailing glycaemic control over the preceding 6–8 weeks. Lipid profile (cholesterol, triglycerides, LDL cholesterol and HDL cholesterol) should be checked at least yearly.

LIPID DISORDERS

The two circulating lipids, *cholesterol* and *triglyceride*, are transported within *lipoproteins* in the circulation. The *apolipoproteins* over the surface of these molecules enable their recognition by cells in organs such as the liver. The different types of lipoprotein are shown in Table 13.6.

Lipid disorders are common and contribute significantly to the burden of cardiovascular disease. They can be conveniently divided into primary and secondary (Table 13.7). Primary lipid disorders are usually inherited, whereas secondary are acquired as a result of other medical disorders.

HISTORY

Lipid disorders rarely cause significant symptoms, unless the patient presents with an acute feature such as acute pancreatitis or myocardial infarction. Thus, any previous history of vascular disease or acute abdominal pain should be sought. Acute pancreatitis is a rare complication of severe hypertriglyceridaemia, and presents with acute severe generalized abdominal pain. Although alcohol and

Table 13.6   Types of lipoprotein

Lipoprotein	Apolipoprotein	Characteristics
Chylomicrons	Apo B48 Apo E Apo C-II	Mainly triglyceride containing Manufactured by gut wall Metabolized in liver/cells by lipoprotein lipase
Very low density (VLDL)	Apo B100 Apo E	Main carrier of triglycerides in circulation Metabolized by lipoprotein lipase to IDL
Intermediate density (IDL)		VLDL remnants which are removed by liver
Low density (LDL)	Apo B100	Main carrier of cholesterol in circulation 50% of circulating LDL is removed by liver each day Small dense LDL highly atherogenic Direct correlation of serum LDL levels with CHD
High density (HDL)	Ap A1	Transports 30% of total circulating cholesterol Inverse correlation of serum HDL levels with CHD

cholelithiasis are the commonest causes of acute pancreatitis, hypertriglyceridaemia is a well recognized and easily overlooked cause of the condition, and any patient presenting with acute pancreatitis should have their serum lipids checked.

In the assessment of patients with lipid disorder it is important to enquire about symptoms of ischaemic heart disease (chest pain history, admissions for ischaemic heart disease and any cardiological/cardiothoracic interventions), peripheral vascular disease (intermittent claudication) and cerebrovascular disease (transient ischaemic attacks, amaurosis fugax and strokes). Other cardiovascular risk factors should also be assessed. The smoking history is very important and a family history of premature vascular disease (under the age of 55 years) should be carefully sought. In familial hypercholesterolaemia, half of men and a fifth of women die before the age of 60 from coronary heart disease. Possible symptoms of secondary causes should also be assessed. Thus symptoms of hypothyroidism (Chapter 12), diabetes (above), renal failure or nephrotic syndrome (Chapter 14), and liver disease (Chapter 8) should be sought. Alcohol intake and dietary history should also be assessed.

EXAMINATION

The diagnostic hallmark of familial hypercholesterolaemia are *tendon xanthomata*. These are localized infiltrates of lipid containing macrophages that resemble atherosclerotic plaques; they develop from the third decade onwards. The commonest sites are the Achilles tendon and the extensor tendons of the hands, particularly over the knuckles (Fig. 13.19). Other sites include the tibial tuberosities, at the site of insertion of the patellar tendon (*subperiosteal xanthomata*) or at the triceps tendon at the elbow.

As the cholesterol deposition is deep within the tendon, and the swelling is fibrous, tendon xanthomata are felt as hard nodules along the length of the tendon. They occasionally become inflamed, and a *tenosynovitis* develops. On the extensor surface of the hands they may overlie the knuckle and be very hard and quite easy to miss.

Xanthelasmata are deposits of lipid in the skin of the eyelids, more commonly the upper rather than

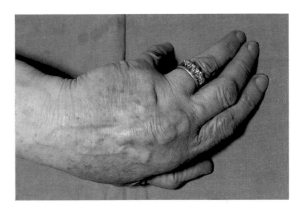

Figure 13.19 Tendon xanthoma of the hands. (Courtesy of Dr David Peterson.)

Table 13.7 Classification of lipid disorders

(a) Primary

Lipid problem	WHO classification	Lipoprotein abnormality	Diagnosis
Hypercholesterolaemia	Type IIa	High LDL	Polygenic hypercholesterolaemia Familial hypercholesterolaemia Familial defective apolipoprotein B100
Hypertriglyceridaemia	Type IV		Familial hypertriglyceridaemia
Mixed hyperlipidaemia	Type IIb	Raised VLDL and LDL	Familial combined hyperlipidaemia
	Type III	Raised chylomicron remnants and IDL	Familial dysbetalipoproteinaemia (type III hyperlipidaemia or broad β disease)
	Type V or type I	Raised chylomicrons and VLDL	Lipoprotein lipase deficiency

(b) Secondary

Mainly cholesterol	High saturated-fat diet Drugs (steroids, thiazides) Hypothyroidism Nephrotic syndrome Chronic liver disease Pregnancy
Mainly triglycerides	Alcohol Hypothyroidism Type 2 diabetes Glucocorticoid excess (steroid therapy or Cushing's) Chronic renal failure

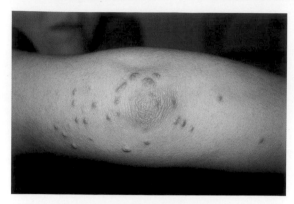

Figure 13.20   Eruptive xanthomata in severe hypertriglyceridaemia. (Courtesy of Dr David Peterson.)

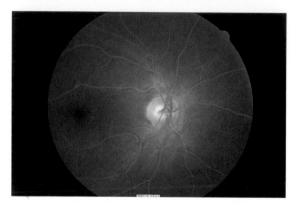

Figure 13.21   Lipaemia retinalis. (Courtesy of Dr Paul Dodson.)

the lower (see Fig. 13.11). Although a dramatic sign they are not present in the majority of patients with familial hypercholesterolaemia.

More common is a *corneal arcus*, seen as a rim of lipid deposit around the iris (Fig. 13.11). This can be seen at any age, although it is more common in older people; only in the minority is this sign associated with hypercholesterolaemia.

The characteristic sign of hypertriglyceridaemia is *eruptive xanthomata* (Fig. 13.20). These are yellow nodules or papules that usually appear on the extensor surface of the elbows, knees, buttocks and back. In severe forms of hypertriglyceridaemia hepatosplenomegaly may be seen. Funduscopy in severe hypertriglyceridaemia may show *lipaemia retinalis*, characterized by optic pallor and the retinal vessels appearing white (Fig. 13.21).

A careful cardiovascular examination should be performed in all patients with significant hyperlipidaemia, including a search for carotid or femoral bruits and signs of peripheral vascular disease.

INVESTIGATION

All patients with lipid disorders should undergo a fasting lipid profile, comprising total cholesterol, LDL cholesterol, HDL cholesterol and triglycerides. In severe hypertriglyceridaemia the serum may become turbid and take on the appearance of milk. Investigations to exclude secondary causes should include thyroid, liver and renal function and fasting glucose. Resting or exercise ECG may be checked to look for signs of ischaemic heart disease. Rarely, genotyping to determine the type of familial lipid abnormality is required, although this is usually only available in specialist centres. Genotyping should be considered, depending on the parents' wishes, to aid in antenatal diagnosis of familial monogenic hypercholesterolaemia.

Acute pancreatitis can be diagnosed using the *serum amylase*, which is frequently very elevated in the condition. In severe hypertriglyceridaemia, however, falsely low serum amylase can lead to diagnostic confusion, as triglycerides interfere with the amylase assay. Severe hypertriglyceridaemia can lead to a *pseudohyponatraemia*, and care should be exercised when interpreting serum sodium levels in the condition.

Kidneys and urinary tract

R. Thuraisingham

14

THE DIAGNOSTIC PROCESS IN NEPHROLOGY AND UROLOGY

These systems are more dependent than most on laboratory, histopathology and imaging techniques to complete the diagnostic process. The basic principles and requirements of clinical assessment often lead to a diagnosis, and even if they do not they direct subsequent laboratory and other technically orientated investigations. Disease of the kidney and urinary tract manifest a somewhat restricted array of symptoms and signs, but almost all patients can be categorized into a well-defined renal or urological syndrome; keeping these in mind informs the clinical diagnostic process. There are many areas of overlap between clinical and pathological processes within a single syndrome, and in general it is not helpful to create artificial distinctions between the two. Once the syndrome has been established, further details of assessment and management objectives become clearer. It is important to emphasize that a number of these syndromes were first described many years ago. They have stood the test of time principally because of their pragmatic value and relative ease of recognition on the basis of clinical assessment and quite simple tests.

SYMPTOMS OF RENAL AND UROLOGICAL DISEASE

PAIN

Pain arising from the urinary tract is a common symptom that is often due to *obstruction, infection* or *tumour*. Renal pain is usually felt in the flank or the loin. When renal pain arises from ureteric obstruction (e.g. a stone) discomfort may additionally radiate to the iliac fossa, the testicle or the labia, the pattern depending to a certain extent on the level of the obstruction. Patients with polycystic kidney disease may suffer chronic flank pain. Exacerbations occur with cyst infection and haemorrhage.

Acute bladder outflow obstruction presents with severe suprapubic pain. However, pain in the suprapubic region and perineum most commonly arises from lower urinary tract infection – *cystitis* or *urethritis*. Such pain is frequently accompanied by

dysuria, frequency or *strangury* (painful micturition). These symptoms comprise the syndrome of *cystitis*. It is nearly always associated with urinary abnormalities on urine stick testing (protein, blood and leukocytes). In men this pain may be associated with severe perineal or rectal discomfort, in which case prostatitis is suggested.

In young children with urinary tract infection and cystitis the symptoms may be much less obvious, but cystitis should be suspected in any child who cries on micturating. Pain from the kidneys, if it results from acute infection or abscess, may occasionally reflect tracking of pus upwards to the diaphragm, causing diaphragmatic pain, or in the retroperitoneal space to the psoas muscle, leading to pain when the muscle is stretched on passive hip extension. Glomerulonephritis is usually painless. Kidney tumours may cause a dull persistent flank pain.

HAEMATURIA

This can be present with or without pain and may be continuous or intermittent. If visible to the naked eye it is termed *macroscopic* or *gross haematuria*; if detected only by stick tests or microscopy it is called *microscopic haematuria*. Haematuria as a result of parenchymal renal disease is usually:

- continuous
- painless
- microscopic (occasionally macroscopic).

Haematuria arising from renal tumours is likely to be:

- intermittent
- associated with renal pain
- macroscopic.

Bleeding from bladder tumours is often intermittent, with associated local symptoms suggesting cystitis.

It is important to decide early in the diagnostic process whether the haematuria originates from the kidneys or elsewhere in the urinary tract (Box 14.1). This decision affects the order in which investigations should be conducted. For example, continuous painless microscopic haematuria with associated

Box 14.1   Causes of haematuria

Systemic
- Purpura
- Sickle cell trait
- Bleeding disorders, including anticoagulant drugs

Renal
- Infarct/papillary necrosis
- Trauma
- Tuberculosis
- Stones
- Renal pelvis transitional cell carcinoma, and other renal tumours
  - Wilms' tumour (in children)
  - Acute glomerulonephritis

Postrenal
- Ureteric stones
- Ureteric neoplasms
- Bladder tumours (transitional cell carcinoma)
- Bladder tuberculosis and bilharziasis
- Radiation cystitis
- Drug-induced cystitis, e.g. ciclophosphamide
- Prostatic enlargement
- Urethral neoplasms
- Bacterial cystitis

proteinuria in a young man or woman is most likely to be the result of glomerulonephritis or other renal pathology. However, haematuria in an older person with risk factors for urothelial malignancy (smoking) is more likely to be caused by a bladder or ureteric tumour and merits a cystoscopy early in the investigative process. It is important to remember that the commonest cause of dipstick haematuria in women is contamination from menstrual blood.

OLIGURIA/ANURIA

Oliguria is the passage of <500 mL urine per day. Anuria is the complete absence of urine flow. A reduction in urinary flow rate to the point of oliguria may be physiological, as in a patient whose fluid intake is low. Physiological reduction of urinary flow rate implies that the glomerular filtration rate (GFR) remains normal, and that the kidney is avidly retaining sodium and water. If inadequate fluid intake leads to a significant reduction in the extracellular fluid compartment (ECF), the resulting decrease in renal blood flow leads to oliguria and reduction of the GFR. Oliguria arising in this fashion is termed *prerenal* and is clearly pathological. *Renal oliguria* implies the presence of intrinsic renal disease, whereas *postrenal oliguria* results from mechanical obstruction at any level, from the collecting system in the kidney to the urethra. Anuria and oliguria may be signs of renal failure.

POLYURIA

Polyuria implies no more than a high urinary flow rate. There will always be an associated increase in the frequency of micturition (*frequency*), and often *nocturia* as well. Polyuria results from *excessive water intake* (psychogenic polydipsia, or beer drinking, for example), from an *osmotic diuresis* (glucose, as in diabetes mellitus, urea as in chronic renal failure, and sodium chloride as in diuretic use), and finally from *abnormal renal tubular water handling*, as seen in pituitary diabetes insipidus or renal resistance to antidiuretic hormone – nephrogenic diabetes insipidus.

FREQUENCY

Increased frequency of micturition results from polyuria, a reduction in functional bladder capacity or bladder/urethral irritation. The commonest cause of polyuria is excessive fluid intake, whereas reduced functional bladder capacity is seen most frequently in patients with prostatic hypertrophy and bladder outlet obstruction. Lower urinary tract infection (cystitis) causes bladder irritation and an increase in urinary frequency. Some patients with neurological diseases, in particular multiple sclerosis, also have frequency of micturition. The detrusor muscle of the bladder contracts at an inappropriately low bladder volume, resulting in a low functional bladder capacity.

NOCTURIA

This term implies the need to empty the bladder during the hours of sleep. In health there is a substantial diurnal variation in urinary flow rate: a night-time reduction in urine flow, together with adequate functional bladder capacity, serves to obviate the need for night-time micturition. Thus polyuria of any cause, or any cause of reduction of functional bladder capacity, may lead to nocturia. In addition, failure of the kidney's urine concentrating ability, as occurs in renal impairment and sickle cell disease, will also lead to nocturia. Obviously, diuretics taken in the evening and at night will lead to this symptom.

DYSURIA

This is a specific form of discomfort arising from the urinary tract in which there is pain immediately before, during or after micturition. The urine is often described as 'burning' or 'scalding', and there is usually associated frequency of micturition and decreased functional bladder capacity. Infection and neoplasia in the bladder or urethra are the most important causes. An extreme form of dysuria, *strangury*, implies an unpleasant and painful desire to void when the bladder is empty or nearly so.

URGENCY OF MICTURITION, INCONTINENCE AND ENURESIS

Urgency is the loss of the normal ability to postpone micturition beyond the time when the desire to pass urine is initially perceived. *Incontinence* is the involuntary passage of urine. In extreme cases urgency may lead to *urge incontinence*, in which the desire to void cannot be voluntarily inhibited. *Stress incontinence*, on the other hand, is leakage of urine associated with straining or coughing, often due to weakened pelvic floor muscles. The term enuresis is usually used to describe *noctural enuresis*, or bed-wetting.

SLOW STREAM, HESITANCY AND TERMINAL DRIBBLING

This triad of symptoms is most frequently seen in elderly men with prostatic hypertrophy. Here the bladder outlet is partially obstructed by the enlarging prostate gland, with the result that the maximum achievable urinary flow rate during micturition is reduced. There is often difficulty in initiating micturition (*hesitancy*) and in completing micturition in a 'clean stop' fashion (*terminal dribbling*). The symptoms are nearly always associated with *frequency* of micturition and *nocturia*, the result of a low functional bladder capacity. In more advanced cases there may be progressive bladder enlargement, with eventual *overflow incontinence* and continuous or intermittent dribbling of urine.

URETHRAL DISCHARGE

This is usually only noticed by men and always requires further investigation. There may be associated symptoms of urethral irritation and the underlying pathology is likely to be urethritis, which is often infective and sexually transmitted.

PHYSICAL SIGNS IN RENAL AND UROLOGICAL DISEASE

These physical signs fall into three principal groups:

- Local signs related to the specific pathology, for example an enlarged palpable tender kidney in renal carcinoma, or a palpably enlarged bladder in a patient with acute or chronic retention
- Symptoms of disturbance of renal salt and water handling, with resulting extracellular fluid volume expansion or contraction: to elicit the appropriate physical signs in this category requires careful assessment of the patient's volume status
- Signs of failure of the kidney's normal excretory and metabolic functions.

In many renal patients, particularly those with advanced chronic renal failure and uraemia, signs from all three of the above categories may be present.

GENERAL FEATURES

Patients with chronic renal failure look unwell. The skin is pallid, the complexion sallow, and a slightly yellowish hue is often evident. The mucous membranes are pale, reflecting the normochromic, normocytic anaemia that is associated with chronic renal failure. There may be *bruises*, *purpura* and *scratch marks* due to uraemic pruritus, and also an underlying disorder of platelet function and capillary fragility. The nails often appear pale and opaque (*leukonychia*) in the nephrotic syndrome, and sometimes in chronic renal failure. Intercurrent episodes of severe illness in the past may have led to the appearance of *Beau's lines*, which appear as transverse ridges across the nails. *Splinter haemorrhages* in the nailbeds point to underlying vasculitis, which may be the cause of the renal failure or be indicative of endocarditis; there may be an associated *purpuric rash* (Fig. 14.1). *Uraemic frost* may be seen on any part of the body and appears as a white powder; it is formed from crystalline urea deposited on the skin via the sweat. The onset of chronic renal failure in childhood is associated with impaired growth, causing *short stature*. Severe bony deformity may be evident in some cases, particularly in children, who may develop rickets (Fig. 14.2). Advanced uraemia is also associated with *metabolic flap*, a coarse tremor which is best seen at the wrists when in the dorsiflexed position. It is similar to the metabolic flap (*asterixis*) seen in patients with

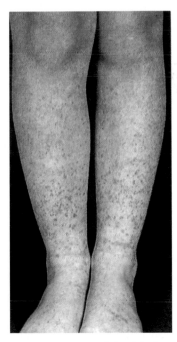

Figure 14.1 Purpura in Henoch–Schönlein disease.

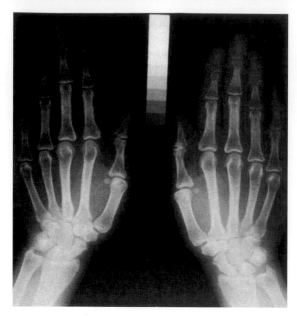

Figure 14.2 X-ray of the hands of a patient with chronic renal failure and secondary hyperparathyroidism, showing renal osteodystrophy. There is a loss of density of the tips of the digits (acro-osteolysis) with loss of density on either side of the interphalangeal joints and subperiosteal bone resorption. The latter is best seen in the middle phalanges of the index and middle fingers.

advanced hepatic disease or respiratory failure. Metabolic acidosis, if present, leads to increased ventilation with an increased tidal volume – *Kussmaul respiration*.

THE CIRCULATION IN THE RENAL PATIENT

Of crucial importance here is the correct assessment of the patient's fluid volume status. It is important to define whether the patient is *euvolaemic, hypovolaemic* or *hypervolaemic*. This is a bedside assessment that, with practice, can usually be made correctly.

Hypervolaemia is associated with some or all of the following:

- Hypertension
- Elevation of the jugular venous pressure
- Peripheral oedema at the ankles or sacrum
- Basal crackles on lung auscultation
- Ascites
- Pleural effusion.

In patients with *nephrotic syndrome* (see below) oedema and salt and water retention are caused by reduced plasma oncotic pressure. Oedema with expansion of the extracellular fluid (ECF) is often accompanied by hypertension and, particularly if the cardiac reserve is poor, may progress to pulmonary oedema and other manifestations of heart failure. The presence of oedema itself, however, can

coexist with intravascular volume depletion, especially in patients with nephritic syndrome.

The diagnosis of *hypovolaemia* requires the absence of any signs of *hypervolaemia*. The hypovolaemic patient may have the following:

- Low blood pressure, often exaggerated in the upright position – *postural hypotension*
- Sinus tachycardia (exaggerated in the upright position)
- Low pulse pressure (exaggerated in the upright position)
- Flat neck veins even when almost supine.

Poor skin turgor, 'sunken eyes' and dry mucous membranes are often cited as signs of volume depletion, but these are generally unreliable features.

ABDOMINAL PALPATION

The detection of the kidneys in the abdominal examination is described in Chapter 8. In slim people with relaxed abdominal muscles it is sometimes possible to feel a normal right kidney (the right kidney is situated slightly lower than the left at the level of T12–L3). More often a palpable kidney can only be felt because it is enlarged, as in hydronephrosis, multiple cysts (polycystic kidney disease), or tumour (generally unilateral). A *distended bladder* is identified in the lower abdomen by a combination of palpation and percussion. *Rectal examination* is an important part of the clinical assessment of the renal patient: bimanual palpation of the bladder is a more reliable way of assessing bladder enlargement than is simple per abdominal examination. Rectal examination also allows evaluation of the *prostate gland*, both for benign enlargement and for the detection of malignant change suggested by hard irregularity of the gland.

AUSCULTATION

Uraemic pericarditis and *pleurisy* may be suggested by pericardial and pleural friction rubs, respectively. Their presence points to either advanced uraemia or a multisystem inflammatory disorder such as systemic lupus erythematosus (SLE), which may have both renal and extrarenal manifestations. Added heart sounds (S3 and S4) suggest, respectively, volume expansion and incipient heart failure, and ventricular hypertrophy, often as a consequence of hypertension. The presence of vascular bruits and/or impairment of the major arterial pulses is an important finding, raising the possibility of renal vascular disease, which may underlie hypertension and/or renal failure if bilateral.

THE EYE IN URAEMIA

Corneal calcification (limbic calcification) occurs in patients with long-standing hyperparathyroidism with elevation of blood calcium and phosphorus concentrations (see Chapter 12). The presence of limbic calcification should not be confused with a *corneal arcus* (*arcus senilis*), which is a broader band at the edge of the cornea and merges with the sclera. Corneal arcus is usually most marked in the superior and inferior positions, whereas limbic calcification is seen medially and laterally or circumferentially. *Retinal changes* are extremely important in uraemic patients, many of whom have hypertension and/or diabetes. Patients with renal disease as part of systemic vasculitis may have manifestations of the latter in the retinae, with haemorrhages and exudates. Patients with chronic renal failure are at greatly increased risk of a range of vascular complications affecting both the macro- and the microvasculature. In the retinae, thrombosis of the central retinal artery or its branches, or of the central retinal vein and its branches, is an important manifestation of this.

THE RENAL AND UROLOGICAL SYNDROMES

These syndromes are listed in Table 14.1. Some are exclusively renal, others exclusively urological, and some fall into both areas. The effects of renal failure on other organ systems are listed in Box 14.2.

ACUTE RENAL FAILURE

This is the abrupt onset of declining renal function occurring over a period of hours or days, usually (but not always) accompanied by a marked reduction of the urinary flow rate – *anuria* or *oliguria*. Central to the diagnosis, however, is a rapid decline in the GFR, leading to nitrogen retention and usually to sodium and water retention as well. An exception is the patient in whom the decline of GFR is not accompanied by reduction of urine flow – so-called *non-oliguric acute renal failure*. The outlook depends on the cause. Many are reversible spontaneously (repair of ischaemic injury as in tubular necrosis) or as a result of therapy (removal of stone or other cause of obstruction).

CHRONIC RENAL FAILURE

Chronic renal failure implies that the GFR has been reduced for a considerable period and that the

---

Box 14.2 Effects of renal failure on other organ systems

Disturbances of water and electrolyte balance
- Breathlessness due to salt and water overload
- Deep sighing breathing (Kussmaul respiration) due to acidosis
- Weakness and postural fainting due to hypotension caused by salt and water depletion
- Lethargy and weakness from hypokalaemia

Disturbances of the haematological system
- Lethargy and breathlessness associated with anaemia owing to impaired production of erythropoietin by the kidneys
- Defective coagulation and excessive bruising (advanced renal failure)
- Haemorrhage from the gastrointestinal tract or lungs

Disturbances of the cardiovascular system
- Cardiac failure or angina associated with fluid overload, hypertension, anaemia, and impaired ventricular function (uraemic cardiomyopathy)
- Precordial chest pain due to pericarditis
- Cardiac arrhythmias associated with left ventricular hypertrophy and hyperkalaemia/hypokalaemia

Disturbances of the respiratory system
- Breathlessness and haemoptysis from fluid overload
- Chest pain due to pleurisy
- Disturbances of the musculoskeletal system
- Muscular weakness and bone pain due to impairment of vitamin D activation and to excessive parathyroid gland activity
- Acute pain due to gout

Disturbances of the nervous system
- Hypertensive stroke and encephalopathy
- Clouding of consciousness, fits and coma in advanced renal failure
- Impaired sensation or paraesthesiae in the feet, due to peripheral neuropathy in long-standing uraemia
- Impaired higher mental/intellectual function
- Entrapment neuropathies

Disturbances of the eyes
- Pain from conjunctivitis caused by local deposits of calcium
- Visual blurring from hypertensive retinal damage or retinal vascular disease

---

Table 14.1 Renal and urological syndromes

Renal	Renal and urological	Urological
Chronic renal failure	Acute renal failure	Urinary tract infection
Acute nephritic syndrome	Asymptomatic urinary abnormality	Urinary tract obstruction
Nephrotic syndrome	Recurrent gross haematuria	Renal and urinary tract stone
Renal hypertension		
Tubular syndromes		

reduction is largely or completely irreversible. It can result from almost any form of renal parenchymal disease, chronic renal ischaemia or unrelieved urinary obstruction. If renal impairment is severe, there may be clinical manifestations of *uraemia*. These are usually evident when the GFR has fallen to one-third of normal or less. The implication of the term *chronic renal failure* is that the timescale of onset and progression is rarely shorter than a few months, and often much longer. A further and crucial implication is an irreversible reduction in the number of functioning nephrons with no prospect of significant recovery. These patients manifest a number of symptoms that are not attributable to specific pathophysiological changes. Lethargy, poor concentration, irritability, and failure of higher mental functions and ability to handle tasks are all commonly reported. In advanced cases there may be confusion, fits and stupor. These are preterminal, but reversible if steps are taken to remove the excess uraemic toxins by dialysis. Nausea, vomiting and diarrhoea are also common in advanced uraemia, and likewise improve following restoration of normal kidney function or treatment with dialysis or transplantation.

THE ACUTE NEPHRITIC SYNDROME

As in acute renal failure, the acute nephritic syndrome implies a fairly brisk onset (days, weeks or months) of reduction in GFR and retention of nitrogenous waste, and usually salt and water also. *Oliguria* is, therefore, common. The underlying pathology is an acute glomerulonephritis which, as well as causing the functional abnormalities described above, also results in florid abnormalities of the urine. *Haematuria* (macroscopic or microscopic), *proteinuria* and *tubular casts* are often present. Many of the causes of acute nephritis are associated with functional abnormalities of the immune system which may be detected by laboratory tests and which may also manifest with disease in other organs, for example the skin, joints or eyes, as in systemic lupus erythematosus, Henoch–Schönlein purpura and systemic vasculitis.

THE NEPHROTIC SYNDROME

This is defined somewhat imprecisely as the presence of *heavy proteinuria* (usually >3 g/day, compared with normal of <150 mg/day), *hypoalbuminaemia*, *hypercholesterolaemia* and *oedema*. It is not generally very helpful to attempt a more precise definition because the clinical response to a given level of proteinuria shows considerable variability from patient to patient. It is, however, unusual for nephrotic syndrome to occur when the proteinuria is <2 g/24 h, and conversely some patients are able to maintain a normal or near-normal serum albumin concentra-

tion despite very heavy proteinuria in excess of 6 g/24 h.

Proteinuria of this magnitude implies glomerular pathology and may coexist with a significant reduction in GFR. Thus a number of the pathological entities capable of causing nephrotic syndrome may also present as acute nephritic syndrome or the syndrome of chronic renal failure in other patients.

ASYMPTOMATIC URINARY ABNORMALITY

This is the presentation that arises in the patient who presents for a routine medical examination, often in the context of employment or life insurance. Urine testing leads to the unexpected finding of *proteinuria, haematuria* or *pyuria* in an otherwise healthy patient. Further assessment may reveal the coexistence of other renal syndromes, but nevertheless it is worth maintaining the operational definition asymptomatic urinary abnormality because this is such a frequent presentation in clinical practice. It should not be forgotten that this syndrome may not only reflect disease of the kidneys, as it can also be a manifestation of malignancy anywhere in the urinary tract, infection or stone (if asymptomatic).

RECURRENT GROSS HAEMATURIA

This implies intermittent – or in some cases continuous – bleeding into the urinary tract to a degree sufficient to alter the macroscopic appearance of the urine. Depending on the circumstances of the bleeding, the urine may be a rusty-brown colour, lightly tinged with red blood, or more heavily bloodstained. The source of the bleeding may be anywhere in the urinary tract, from the glomeruli at the top to the urethra at the bottom. Important causes are certain types of glomerulonephritis, renal tumours and infections (particularly tuberculosis), and tumours of the urinary tract transitional cell epithelium (urothelium) anywhere from the renal pelves to the bladder and urethra.

URINARY TRACT INFECTION

The normal urinary tract is sterile except at its extreme distal end. Infection in the urinary tract leads to a range of symptoms and signs that reflect the location and severity of the infection. By far the most frequent site is the bladder, and the local symptoms reflect bladder irritation, with *frequency of micturition, low functional bladder capacity* and pain on passing urine – *dysuria*. The presence of urinary tract infection is defined importantly by the presence of a significant number of infecting organisms in the urine – a working definition would be more than 10^5 colony-forming units/mL urine in a carefully collected midstream specimen (MSU). For less common infections this definition may not be appropriate. For example, in tuberculosis of the urinary tract the number of organisms being excreted may be extremely low, and formal identification on the basis of urine culture is sometimes difficult or impossible.

URINARY TRACT OBSTRUCTION

This syndrome may conveniently be divided into lower and upper tract obstruction. Lower urinary tract obstruction is defined by residual urine in the bladder after micturition, or in more extreme forms by urinary retention with inability to empty the bladder at all. The most common causes relate to prostatic hypertrophy (benign hyperplasia or carcinoma), and a characteristic array of symptoms and signs arises (*frequency, nocturia, poor stream, hesitancy, terminal dribbling*). All of these are a consequence of a low functional bladder capacity, inability to empty the bladder completely, and impairment of the urinary flow rate.

The presence of upper urinary tract obstruction is established in most cases by the demonstration of a dilated renal collecting system (renal pelvis and/or calyces), often seen to be proximal to a specific obstructing lesion. These features may be demonstrated by a number of imaging techniques, including ultrasound and intravenous urography (IVU). Upper and lower urinary tract obstruction may coexist, most frequently when the lower urinary tract obstruction is severe and/or of long standing, and leading to progressive dilatation of the upper urinary tract with consequent renal damage. It is important to remember that unilateral renal obstruction should not result in a rise in the serum creatinine. Therefore, if the creatinine is elevated there is also dysfunction of the contralateral kidney.

RENAL AND URINARY TRACT STONES

The operational definition is largely observational, depending on the demonstration of one or more stones in any part of the urinary tract. Resulting symptoms and signs depend much on the location of the stone(s) and on size. For example, small stones in the kidneys are frequently asymptomatic, or they may lead to subtle urinary abnormalities, presenting initially with *asymptomatic urinary abnormality*. Larger stones in the kidneys frequently lead to renal pain, whereas stones in the ureter are particularly likely to cause acute obstruction and very severe ureteric and renal pain. Bladder stones are usually associated with symptoms suggestive of cystitis: frequency, haematuria and pain are all common, and urinary tract infection is often associated.

RENAL HYPERTENSION

By far the most common cause of sustained blood pressure elevation is essential hypertension. However, in a minority of patients with raised blood pressure renal disease will be found to be the cause, and the likelihood of this is greatly increased in patients with coexisting renal disease of any kind. Hypertension may be one of the presenting features of virtually any disease of the renal parenchyma, including all forms of glomerulonephritis, many forms of tubulointerstitial disease, renal vascular disease, renal stone disease and obstruction. Renal tumours and renal infections may occasionally present with hypertension, which in some cases can be the only presenting feature. Thus, in any patient with newly identified hypertension the possibility of underlying renal disease should be considered. Conversely, the exclusion of renal disease as a cause of hypertension is generally straightforward, comprising the absence of symptoms and signs of renal disease, the absence of urinary abnormalities on simple stick testing, and the presence of a normal GFR as judged by serum creatinine concentration or other surrogate for GFR.

RENAL TUBULAR SYNDROMES

The majority of patients with parenchymal renal disease or obstructive renal damage manifest disordered tubular function, although in only a few of these are the tubular defects responsible for specific clinical manifestations. Tubular syndromes arising in this context are generally unobtrusive and are certainly common. Much less common is the patient in whom the tubular defect dominates the clinical picture. These defects may be inherited or acquired, and are seen mainly in children. They usually require careful laboratory testing to characterize them fully. Proximal tubular abnormalities include renal phosphate wasting, aminoaciduria (of these, cystinuria with cystine stone formation is the most important), and renal tubular acidosis leading to chronic metabolic acidosis. Distal tubular defects are also associated with metabolic acidosis and with disturbances of potassium metabolism, sodium-losing nephropathy and nephrogenic diabetes insipidus, with resulting failure, respectively, of salt and water conservation.

LABORATORY ASSESSMENT AND IMAGING OF THE KIDNEYS AND URINARY TRACT: ASSESSMENT OF STRUCTURE AND FUNCTION

THE URINE

The urine should be tested as part of every general medical examination and not just in patients with known renal or urinary tract disease. Not only may the testing lead to the discovery of hitherto unsuspected diseases, such as diabetes or renal disease, but also documentation of normal urine often provides a very useful historical yardstick in the event of the later development of renal disease or urinary abnormalities. The urine specimen should be passed into a clean container without additives. Testing should normally be conducted as soon as possible, and if delayed more than 2 hours the urine should be refrigerated (not frozen) and returned to room temperature before testing. A midstream specimen is essential for microbiological assessment and desirable for microscopic examination.

QUANTITY

Normal adults in temperate climates usually pass between 750 and 2500 mL of urine every 24 hours. The minimum daily urine output compatible with normal renal excretory function varies from person to person, and also with other factors such as diet. Abnormally low urine output (oliguria or anuria) implies that the flow rate is below the minimum required to allow excretion of the daily solute load (usually <500 mL/day in an adult). Polyuria is an imprecise term implying no more than the passage of a large volume of urine, but implying nothing about the reasons for this.

COLOUR

Urochrome and uroerythrin are pigments that contribute to the natural yellow tinge of urine. Darkening occurs on staining as a result of oxidation of urobilinogen to coloured urobilin. The colour of urine is also heavily influenced by the urinary flow rate: high flow leads to dilute urine and hence a pale colour. Bile pigments in excess colour the urine brown, with a characteristic yellow froth on shaking. Small to moderate quantities of blood impart a smoky appearance, with larger amounts leading to progressive brown or, in the case of brisk bleeding, bright red discoloration. Free haemoglobin from intravascular haemolysis (e.g. in severe malaria – blackwater fever) produces a darker red

colour, verging on black in severe cases. Myoglobin may appear in the urine after acute muscle necrosis (rhabdomyolysis), causing a brown-red discoloration. Certain drugs discolour the urine – examples include rifampicin (red), anthraquinone purgatives such as senna (orange), nitrofurantoin (brown) and methyldopa (grey). Urine is normally transparent when freshly passed and still warm, but may be cloudy if there are large numbers of red blood cells or leukocytes, or if phosphates have precipitated in significant amounts.

SPECIFIC GRAVITY AND OSMOLALITY

These measurements yield similar information, and in the absence of significant glycosuria are functions of the urinary concentrations of sodium, chloride and urea. The range of specific gravity is 1.001–1.035, which is equivalent to 50–1350 mOsmol/kg water (Fig. 14.3). The presence of renal insufficiency leads to a reduction in the range of osmolality that the kidneys can generate, and in advanced renal disease the osmolality becomes relatively fixed at about 300 mOsmol/kg water – close to that of the glomerular filtrate (Fig. 14.4). This is termed *isosthenuria*, and predisposes the patient to sodium and

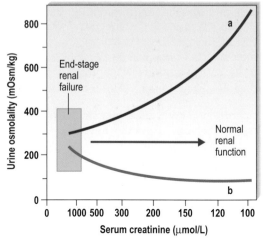

Figure 14.4 Relationship between renal concentration and diluting capacity, and serum creatinine concentration. The serum creatinine is plotted on a logarithmic scale. This therefore represents linear changes in glomerular filtration rate, such as might occur in progressive renal failure. End-stage renal failure is shown on the left, and normal renal function on the right. Curve (a) represents maximum concentrating capacity, e.g. in water deprivation, when the normal kidney can maintain the serum creatinine in the normal range by increasing urine osmolality. In renal failure the urine cannot be concentrated and the serum creatinine rises. Curve (b) represents the maximum diluting capacity, e.g. after the ingestion of large volumes of water. The normal kidney excretes urine of low osmolality. In end-stage renal failure urine osmolality cannot be reduced and the water load is not adequately handled. There is also isosthenuria, i.e. the urine tends towards an iso-osmolar state (specific gravity 1.010).

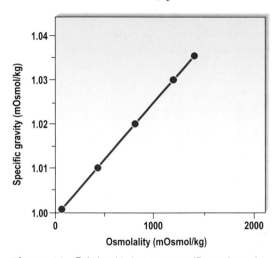

Figure 14.3 Relationship between specific gravity and osmolality.

water overload if intake is high, and to salt and water depletion if intake is low.

pH

This varies from 4 to 8 and can be measured crudely using paper strips impregnated with an indicator. If more accurate measurements are needed, as in suspected renal tubular acidosis, a pH electrode is used. Most people pass acid urine most of the time, exceptions being some vegetarians, certain types of renal tubular acidosis, rapid water diuresis, metabolic alkalosis, and urine infection with urea-splitting organisms.

GLUCOSE

Glucose oxidase-impregnated dipsticks provide a quick and semiquantitative test for glucose in urine. By far the commonest causes of abnormal glycosuria are elevation of the plasma glucose to a point where the tubular reabsorptive capacity for glucose is exceeded (usually seen in people with diabetes), and during pregnancy, in which glycosuria occurs with normal plasma glucose concentrations. Very rarely, tubular transport defects may be associated with glycosuria at normal plasma glucose concentrations, and more frequently – but less predictably – patients with acquired chronic renal diseases may exhibit glycosuria at normal plasma glucose concentrations. Collectively these disorders are termed *renal glycosuria*.

PROTEIN

The normal daily urine protein output is <150 mg. Dipsticks reactive to urine albumin provide a simple semiquantitative test. They are sensitive to 200–300 mg protein/L and have almost completely superseded the more cumbersome sulphosalicylic acid test. The urinary protein excretion rate generally rises in the upright posture and with activity, and in some normal individuals this may lead to apparently abnormal proteinuria on spot urine specimens in ambulant patients, and even in 24-hour urine collections (*orthostatic proteinuria*). Measurement of protein in an early-morning urine, however, reveals no protein, and this serves to distinguish abnormal proteinuria from orthostatic proteinuria. A further refinement is the specific measurement of urine albumin, which is increasingly used and should be <20 mg/day. Albumin excretion in the range 20–200 mg/day is termed *microalbuminuria*. Although this range is frequently too low to be detectable by stick testing, it is an important finding, particularly in diabetics, in whom it predicts the later onset of overt diabetic nephropathy. The albumin:creatinine ratio is a useful surrogate marker for proteinuria and is used instead of the 24 hour urine collection for quantification of protein excretion.

The diagnostic implications of proteinuria depend greatly on its magnitude (Table 14.2). Heavy proteinuria (>1.5 g/24 h) is nearly always glomerular in origin and albumin predominates over larger proteins such as globulins. Other proteins, rarely measured, arise from the renal tubules and include Tamm–Horsfall protein, retinol-binding protein and nephrocalcin, the latter helping to prevent the formation of urinary stones.

MICROSCOPY (Figs 14.5–14.8)

This is performed after slow spinning (at not more than 1000 *g*) of a fresh urine specimen for approximately 2 minutes. The pellet is resuspended in 0.5 mL of urine and examined unstained on a microscope slide under a coverslip. Important findings include leukocytes (suggestive of infection), *red blood cells* and various types of *tubular casts*. The presence of tubular casts is indicative of parenchymal renal disease. They may be red cell casts or white cell casts, in which Tamm–Horsfall protein matrix has solidified and is studded with red or white blood cells. Granular casts probably represent degenerate cellular casts and have a grainy appearance. Hyaline casts contain no elements or debris and may be seen in small numbers in normal urine. It is usual to express the number of cells or casts seen per high-power field. Red cell morphology may be a useful indicator as to the source of bleeding. Red cells with a normal outline usually – though not always – arise from the renal collecting system or from a point downstream of that, whereas red cells arising from the glomeruli are often

Table 14.2 Proteinuria

Mild (<500 mg/day)	Moderate (up to 3 g/day)	Heavy (>3 g/day)
Benign hypertensive nephrosclerosis	Chronic pyelonephritis	Acute glomerulonephritis
Obstructive nephropathy	Acute tubular necrosis	Chronic glomerulonephritis
Prerenal uraemia	Acute glomerulonephritis	Diabetic nephropathy
Renal tumour	Chronic glomerulonephritis	Pre-eclampsia
Fever	Obstructive nephropathy	Myeloma
Tubulointerstitial nephropathy	Accelerated phase hypertension	All causes of nephrotic syndrome
Chronic pyelonephritis	Orthostatic proteinuria	
Early diabetic nephropathy	Urinary tract infection	
Orthostatic proteinuria		

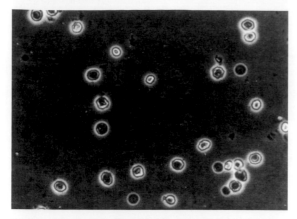

Figure 14.5   Erythrocytes in urinary sediment.

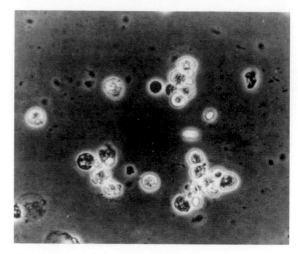

Figure 14.6   Leukocytes in urinary sediment.

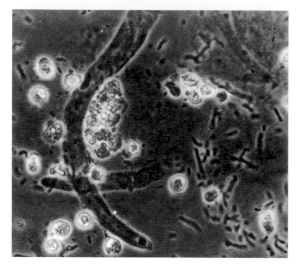

Figure 14.7   Hyaline casts, leukocytes and bacteria in urinary sediment. (Reproduced with permission from Spencer E.S., Petersen I. *Hand atlas of urinary sediment*. Copenhagen: Munksgaard, 1971.)

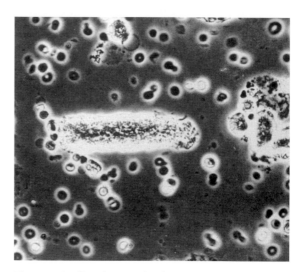

Figure 14.8   Granular casts in urinary sediment.

distorted, probably as a result of movement through the glomeruli or osmotic insults during passage down the renal tubule.

MICROBIOLOGICAL EXAMINATION OF THE URINE

Midstream urine specimens are normally satisfactory, but are always contaminated to a certain extent during passage to the exterior. Extensive studies have shown that the finding of more than 10^5 bacteria per mL in a midstream specimen is usually associated with active urinary infection, especially when accompanied by leukocytes. Occasionally urine is taken directly from the bladder for diagnostic purposes. It should be sterile.

MEASUREMENT OF THE GLOMERULAR FILTRATION RATE

Accurate assessment of the GFR requires measurement in blood and urine of a compound that is

filtered freely at the glomerulus and neither reabsorbed nor secreted by the tubules (Table 14.3). Inulin is the best agent, but involves a continuous infusion of inulin and measurements of inulin concentration in plasma and urine – a laborious and not routinely available investigation that is generally confined to research. A number of surrogates for the inulin clearance method exist, however, and details of these are given in Table 14.3. The most frequently used surrogates, and also the crudest ones, are the plasma urea and plasma creatinine concentrations. Both compounds are produced endogenously (at an inconstant rate in the case of urea) and excreted by glomerular filtration. Neither is particularly accurate when used to establish the absolute level of glomerular filtration in an individual patient, although the plasma creatinine concentration is certainly very useful when used to follow changes in an individual patient's renal function, especially when the GFR is significantly reduced (Fig. 14.9). Creatinine clearance is more precise, but requires a 24-hour urine collection with measurements of plasma creatinine concentration and urine creatinine excretion rate. The clearance is then calculated using the simple formula UV/P, where U equals the urinary concentration of creatinine, V the urinary flow rate (usually expressed in mL/min) and P equals the plasma creatinine concentration. This formula can be applied to urea or to any other compound subject to renal excretion. Only those compounds that are freely filtered at the glomerulus and neither secreted nor reabsorbed by the renal tubules are suitable for GFR measurement. The use of mathematical formulae to calculate GFR has been gaining in popularity, as most of these calculations require simple information such as the age, sex, weight and serum creatinine to derive an estimated GFR (Table 14.4). Precise measures of GFR used in clinical practice depend on measurement of the excretion of radiolabelled compounds. The most commonly used is ^{51}Cr-EDTA, which gives a relatively easy and reproducible measure of GFR. It should be remembered that the GFR peaks at 20–25 years of age and at about 120 mL/min, and declines steadily thereafter at a rate of approximately 1 mL/min/year. Appreciation of this age-related change in GFR is important in clinical practice, particularly when prescribing drugs to the elderly.

MEASUREMENT OF RENAL TUBULAR FUNCTION
The two tests most frequently utilized are:

- Tests of renal concentrating ability when investigating possible causes of polyuria
- Tests of renal acidification in patients with metabolic acidosis and possible underlying renal tubular acidosis.

Renal concentrating ability involves perturbing the patient in a way that should lead to the production of a concentrated urine. Water deprivation is the most common provocation, and after 12 hours the urine osmolality should be at least 750 mmol/kg (specific gravity 1.020). Failure to concentrate the urine in these circumstances indicates either impairment of vasopressin output (pituitary diabetes

Table 14.3 Measurement of the glomerular filtration rate

Method	Comments
Plasma urea	Poor surrogate – variable production rate – variable excretion rate
Plasma creatinine	Better than urea Poor discrimination at near-normal GFR
Calculated GFR	Useful surrogates of creatinine clearance
Creatinine clearance	Reasonable surrogate but depends on accurate timed urine collection (usually 24 hours)
^{51}Cr-EDTA	The best surrogate in clinical practice Expensive
Inulin clearance	Near-perfect measurement of GFR but – Needs continuous infusion – Difficult urine and plasma assays – Research studies only: not suited to clinical practice

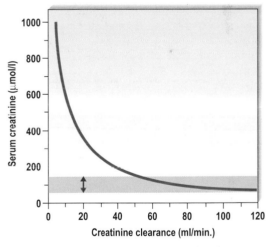

Figure 14.9 Relationship between creatinine clearance and plasma creatinine concentrations. The normal range of serum creatinine concentration can be maintained only when the renal creatinine clearance is greater than about 60 mL/min. The red area represents the normal range of creatinine concentration.

Table 14.4 Estimation of GFR formulae

Cockcroft and Gault	Male GFR = [1.23 × weight (kg) × (140 – age)] / creat Female GFR = [1.03 × weight (kg) × (140 – age)] / creat
MDRD	GFR = 186 × Pcr – 1.154 × age – 0.203 × 1.212 (if black) × 0.742 (if female)

Pcr, plasma creatinine ion mg/dL.

insipidus) or resistance of the renal tubules to the action of vasopressin (nephrogenic diabetes insipidus). These two possibilities may be distinguished by measuring the urine osmolality after an injection of vasopressin or an analogue thereof – again, the urine osmolality should increase to at least 750 mmol/kg.

Renal tubular acidification can be assumed to be adequate if the pH of a random specimen of urine is below 5.5. Urine pH >5.5 in the presence of metabolic acidosis usually indicates renal tubular acidosis. If the patient is only minimally acidotic and the urine pH is >5.5 a provocative test in which ammonium chloride is given at a dose of 0.1 g/kg body weight to provide an acid load and an acute mild metabolic acidosis can be performed. The pH should fall to <5.4 if acidification is normal.

ASSESSMENT OF THE URINE IN THE STONE-FORMING PATIENT

This involves measurement of the important constituents of stone whose outputs may be abnormally increased, and also measurement of at least one of the natural inhibitors of stone formation. Ideally this should be combined with analysis of the stone itself. The tests that should be undertaken in all patients are:

- Plasma calcium, phosphate, alkaline phosphatase, urea, urate, creatinine and electrolytes
- 24-hour urine collection for simultaneous measurement of:
  - calcium
  - uric acid
  - oxalate
  - citrate
  - creatinine
  - sodium
- Nitroprusside test for cystine.

The identification of increased excretion rates of calcium, uric acid, oxalate or cystine indicates a strong predisposition to recurrent stone formation. Conversely, citrate is a natural inhibitor of stone formation, and a low urine citrate is associated with increased stone risk. All patients who make radio-opaque stones should be screened for cystinuria using the nitroprusside test. If hypercalciuria or hypercalcaemia are noted, PTH and serum ACE should also be measured.

KIDNEY BIOPSY

This investigation, in which one or two small cores of renal cortex are removed using a needle biopsy technique, is performed in patients in whom diffuse renal parenchymal disease is suspected. However, not everyone with renal parenchymal disease requires a biopsy. The test is invasive and carries a small but definite risk of serious complications. It is therefore important to define the indications and contraindications carefully. The risk of the procedure can be minimized by the following preconditions:

- A cooperative patient
- Prior knowledge of the position and size of both kidneys (usually provided by ultrasound)
- A solitary functioning kidney should only be biopsied if the diagnostic yield is deemed to be crucial
- Absence of a bleeding disorder
- Availability of blood for transfusion in the event of haemorrhage
- An appropriate indication.

Kidney biopsy is often the only way to distinguish the various forms of glomerulonephritis, both from one another and from tubulointerstitial diseases of the kidney.

IMAGING OF THE URINARY TRACT

PLAIN RADIOGRAPHS

In many people one or both of the kidneys can be seen outlined by perirenal fat on plain abdominal films or nephrotomograms. The information gleaned is limited, although certain types of renal stone or other calcifications may be identified.

ULTRASOUND

Ultrasound provides good images of the renal parenchyma and collecting system, and in nearly all patients gives a reliable estimate of renal size as well as identifying discrete lesions within the parenchyma, hydronephrosis and stone. Doppler studies often permit assessment of blood flow in the main renal arteries and in the larger intrarenal branches. The resistive index, measured by Doppler ultrasound, indicates the degree of chronic intrarenal ischaemic injury. Although the upper ureter can be seen quite well in most patients, the lower ureter is not adequately visualized. Ultrasound examination of the bladder is also extremely useful, allowing calculation of the bladder capacity when full and also after micturition (emptying should be virtually complete), as well as visualization of the bladder wall and lesions projecting into the bladder itself (e.g. tumours). It is sometimes combined with measurement of urinary flow rate.

INTRAVENOUS UROGRAPHY

Intravenous urography involves the injection of organic iodine compounds that are excreted and concentrated radiographically. It is an extremely good technique for examining the renal collecting system, the ureters and the bladder, but gives less information than ultrasound about the renal

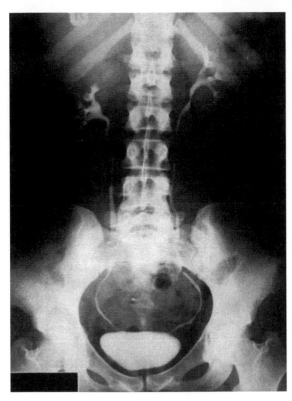

Figure 14.10 Normal excretion urogram. In this film, taken 15 minutes after intravenous injection of the iodine-based contrast medium, the calyces of both kidneys, the ureters and the bladder can be seen.

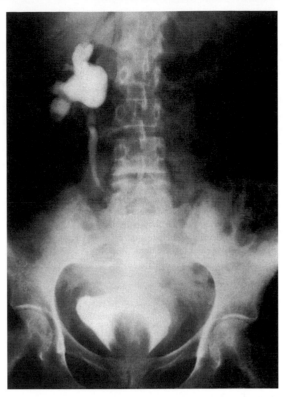

Figure 14.11 Excretion urogram. In this film, made 30 minutes after injection of contrast, the left kidney fails to excrete a detectable concentration of contrast (non-functioning left kidney) and the right kidney shows dilated, hydronephrotic calyces. The right ureter is partially obstructed at the level of the body of the fifth lumbar vertebra. The circular lucency in the bladder is the dilated balloon of a Foley catheter.

parenchyma (Fig. 14.10). Imaging by IVU depends on renal function. This is useful in that it gives a crude measure of the symmetry or otherwise of excretory capacity, but it also means that the image quality is poor in patients with renal insufficiency in whom the GFR is low (Fig. 14.11).

ANTEGRADE AND RETROGRADE UROGRAPHY

Here X-ray contrast material is instilled directly into the urinary tract via a percutaneous needle (*ante-grade*) or a ureteric catheter inserted via a cysto-scope (*retrograde*). These tests are invasive and are most often used in the evaluation of patients with obstruction of the urinary tract.

CYSTOGRAPHY

In cystography the bladder is filled with contrast medium via a urethral catheter and X-rays are taken before, during and after micturition. The test indicates the completeness of bladder emptying, and also whether or not urine refluxes up the ureters during micturition. This also is an invasive test, the principal risk being the introduction of infection. Pressure and flow measurements may be included in more detailed studies of bladder function – uro-dynamics.

RADIONUCLIDE STUDIES

Diethylenetriamine penta-acetic acid (^{99}Tc-DTPA) is used to investigate the excretory function of each kidney selectively (Fig. 14.12). The test is very useful for the assessment of symmetry of function, delayed onset of excretion (as may happen in renal artery stenosis) and retention of excreted isotope (as seen in the presence of obstruction). ^{99}Tc-DMSA (dimercaptosuccinic acid) is a similar technique used to show the gross renal morphology.

COMPUTED TOMOGRAPHY AND MAGNETIC RESONANCE IMAGING

Computed tomography (CT) scanning of the kidneys sometimes complements the information gained from ultrasound and certainly yields important information about the surrounding structures in the retroperitoneum (Fig. 14.13). It is particularly useful in patients with ureteric obstruction from, for

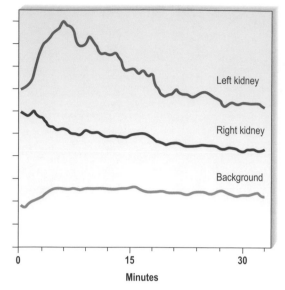

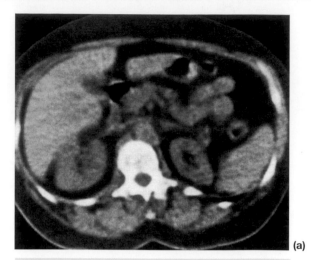

(a)

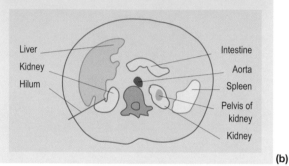

(b)

Figure 14.12 Radioisotope excretion (ordinate) during the 30 minutes after intravenous injection in a patient with right renal artery stenosis and hypertension. The left kidney achieves more rapid excretion of isotope. The malfunctioning right kidney was the cause of the patient's hypertension.

Figure 14.13 **(a)** CT scan with **(b)** Drawing showing normal kidneys.

example, retroperitoneal malignancy or retroperitoneal fibrosis. Spiral CT is becoming the investigation of choice for renal calculi as well. In some cases, more information is obtained using magnetic resonance imaging (MRI).

ARTERIOGRAPHY AND VENOGRAPHY

These are both invasive and are used in selected patients in whom detailed evaluation of the renal blood supply (arterial or venous) is required. The commonest indication is the patient with hypertension and/or renal insufficiency in whom renal artery stenosis is suspected. In the context of renal insufficiency contrast-induced deterioration of function is often seen, but can usually be minimized by adequate prehydration and the use of non-ionic contrast agents. *Magnetic resonance imaging* generates images of the major renal vasculature – *magnetic resonance angiography (MRA)*. Although the images are generally not as good as those from conventional arteriography, the technique has the advantage of avoiding contrast nephropathy and of being non-invasive. CT imaging may also be used in this way.

Gynaecology and obstetrics

T. Beedham

15

GENERAL POINTS

The gathering of relevant information by observation, questioning and examination is crucial to the effectiveness of the diagnostic process in any specialty. In gynaecological practice intimate details must be elicited; therefore, tact, discretion, consideration and the maintenance of proper confidentiality are fundamental. Women have particular expectations of their doctors, and complying with these may not be easy. Gentleness of manner and a genuine interest in the patient helps the development of a good professional relationship. Adequate time should be allowed, but as time is at a premium a sense of direction and purpose is essential, so that the important is quickly separated from the trivial.

PRESENTING PROBLEMS AND BACKGROUND

A detailed account of the patient's problems is best achieved by general open-ended questions. Whatever your own views, avoid questions that imply criticism as they will probably ruin the basis for a constructive interview and may prove unjustified as more information is forthcoming. Sometimes it is important to ask direct questions, such as: 'Which pill are you using?' or 'Do you know the dose of the medicine you were taking?'. Once the interview is progressing satisfactorily, an opportunity must be made to ask about more sensitive issues, e.g. *menstrual disturbance, especially pain or irregularity*, *postcoital bleeding* and *dyspareunia* (pain or difficulty with intercourse). If a woman is too apprehensive to discuss her problems with you, this should be acknowledged as soon as it is recognized and alternatives offered. If you are a man, a female colleague or a colleague with particular skills, for example someone skilled in psychosexual counselling, may be able to help.

Menstruation – 'the natural cyclical loss of sanguineous fluid from the uterus' – is recorded as the days of menstrual loss and the duration of the interval from the first day of one period to the first day of the next, e.g. 5/28. An additional note giving the character of the loss and the daily variation is often more useful than specific labels such as *menorrhagia* (heavy regular periods), *metrorrhagia* (heavy irregular and frequent uterine bleeding) or *polymenorrhoea* (abnormally frequent and less than 21-day intervals), as patterns may not conform exactly to these definitions. Where the problem is infertility, direct questions should be asked about the timing and frequency of intercourse, and whether dyspareunia or other sexual difficulties have occurred. Do not be embarrassed to make these enquiries, as women with these problems will be expecting them. Questions about sexually transmitted disease are equally difficult to pose. They will usually naturally follow those about abnormal discharge in an at-risk person. An accurate diagnosis, contact tracing and treatment are usually best achieved by asking all contacts to attend a sexually transmitted disease clinic. If *prolapse* (where a woman has noticed a bulge at the introitus) is the problem, associated symptoms of bladder or pelvic floor disturbance and backache should be sought.

CURRENT AND PREVIOUS PREGNANCIES

If a woman tells you she is pregnant, remember that some women may not wish to continue with the pregnancy. Therefore, ascertain as gently as possible whether the pregnancy is welcome or not. Remember too that whatever the woman's initial reactions, by the time of their birth most babies are genuinely wanted. In particular, ask the date of the first day of the *last menstrual period (LMP)*, with a note as to its likely accuracy. Record the previous menstrual pattern before conception, and whether this was a natural cycle or due to the use of the contraceptive pill. The *expected date of delivery (EDD)* of the child can be calculated, provided there has been a natural 28-day cycle for some months prior to the conception cycle. The EDD is then 9 months and 7 days from the onset of the last menstrual period (i.e. 280 days or 10 lunar months; alternatively, the date of delivery is 266 days from the date of conception). Clearly, the first is only an approximation, as calendar months are not standard in length, and *term* is regarded as a time stretching from the end of the 37th to the start of the 42nd week from the last menstrual period. Thus although a target date is always given the natural variation should be explained.

Data are usually assembled chronologically in 3-monthly episodes (*the trimesters*) as a healthy normal pregnancy has different characteristics and different problems occur at different stages. The course and outcome of previous pregnancies must be explored and recorded, as these are an essential guide to the progress of the current pregnancy. Where early loss of pregnancy has occurred it must be established whether this was by *spontaneous abortion* ('miscarriage') or *therapeutic termination of pregnancy* ('abortion'), and on how many occasions it occurred. The gestation, symptoms leading to miscarriage, complications and any treatment must be noted. If a termination has taken place, the method used, any complications, and the time taken for the woman to return to a normal menstrual pattern after the event are important

The outcome of each previous pregnancy is recorded as a *live birth*, a *neonatal death* or a *stillbirth*. The birth of a child showing any signs of independent life is recorded as a *live birth*. This occurs beyond 24 weeks' gestation (or 500 g weight), but with improved neonatal care fetal viability may soon be obtained from an even earlier stage. If such a child dies, that event in the UK requires a death certificate. Also in the UK, since the Births and Deaths Registration Act 1953 (as amended by the Still Birth (Definition) Act 1992), Section 41, 'a child which has issued forth from its mother after the 24th week of pregnancy and which did not, at any time after being expelled from its mother, breathe or show any signs of life' is stillborn, 'and the expression *stillbirth* shall be construed accordingly'. Such a birth requires a stillbirth certificate. If the child is born dead at an earlier gestation it is regarded as an *abortion* or *miscarriage* and certification is unnecessary. These are the legal requirements. All parents who lose children under any of these circumstances should receive compassionate consideration and emotional support and, if necessary, professional counselling, e.g. from the Stillbirth and Neonatal Death Society (SANDS). Where possible, they will also need to understand the reasons for their loss.

When a child is born its gestation, weight (to see if this was appropriate for gestational age), and condition at birth should be ascertained (Apgar score if known). Any complications of pregnancy, delivery or the puerperium should be enumerated, as should the developmental milestones of the child. Where events are complex or uncertain an enquiry to the hospital where the delivery occurred may be invaluable.

A woman's *gravidity (the condition of pregnancy regardless of outcome)* is described by the notation *para* (to bring forth or bear) $x + y$: x is the number of babies delivered, whether live births or stillbirths, and y is the number of other pregnancies the woman has had. The latter should include any ectopic pregnancies and abortions prior to 24 weeks' gestation, including both spontaneous abortions and terminations of pregnancy.

MEDICAL BACKGROUND

A broadly based review of the patient's medical background, with particular reference to the problems under investigation, is particularly useful. For example, chronic appendicitis may be related to infertility; or a previous blood transfusion, which has produced blood group antibodies, may be related to subsequent pregnancy loss. Always find out about any current or previous medical disorders, such as diabetes mellitus or systemic lupus erythematosus, particularly when pregnancy is being planned or medical or operative treatment considered. Women with complex or life-threatening medical conditions can also have gynaecological problems and may embark on pregnancy accidentally or deliberately.

MEDICATION OR TREATMENT HISTORY

Any medication taken regularly – or even occasionally – must be noted, as this may be important if other medication is to be prescribed, surgery is to be performed, or an early pregnancy is likely. The effects of alcohol and tobacco are aggravated by a poor diet, and when drug abuse exists (associated with an increased risk of hepatitis and HIV infection) it must be recognized and treatment offered; the risk of vertical transmission of HIV can be reduced if treatment begins early. Allergic reactions should be recorded and clearly displayed, as this information may be required if in an emergency the patient is unable to respond. Be aware that patients report reactions that are not true allergies, and increasingly take supplements of all kinds, which they do not regard as medicines.

FAMILY AND SOCIAL HISTORY

Employment, home conditions and the quality of relationships are of great importance when assessing the prospects for recovery from illness or when planning the support of a child. The ethnic origins and social circumstances of the family may give a clue to the presence of haemoglobinopathy or tuberculosis. One of the underlying anxieties most frequently expressed at interviews is the possibility of familial cancer. When a congenital abnormality is suspected in the offspring of relatives, antenatal screening or diagnosis may be possible (e.g. Tay–Sachs disease, thalassaemia and cystic fibrosis).

GENERAL AND ASSOCIATED SYSTEM ASSESSMENT

Once all the other information has been obtained, ask about changes in appetite, bowel habit, weight, responses to exercise, and variations in sleep patterns. Questions about urological function, estimated by the *frequency* and *volume* of urine passed, with a note about *nocturia* or *dysuria*, should be posed and answers recorded. The presence of *urgency* (an overwhelming desire to micturate), which may or may not result in incontinence, or *stress incontinence* (the involuntary leakage of urine from the full bladder when the intra-abdominal pressure is raised), should be assessed. Short-term mild stress incontinence is very common, particularly after childbirth or in the menopause.

EXAMINATION

GENERAL

Appearance, gait, demeanour and responsiveness can all be observed, and the level of intelligence and education generally assessed as soon as the person is with you. Any abnormality of affect should be noted. Measurements of height and weight (giving the body mass index, BMI) are important. A female chaperone should be present for the physical examination but may inhibit the process of history taking, and so may best assist from the time when the patient needs to undress. However, the maintenance of professional demeanour and behaviour by the doctor, so that there is no possibility of the patient misinterpreting their motives, is more important still.

The examination should be a non-threatening process and should be undertaken by following a predictable sequence, such as the following:

- Hands (to assess the pulse)
- Arms (blood pressure)
- Eyes (conjunctivae)
- Head, chest (heart)

- Breasts (see also page 17)
- Abdomen
- Legs
- Pelvic examination (PV/PR) (also note secondary sexual development, and hair distribution).

ABDOMINAL EXAMINATION

The system of examination described in Chapter 8 should be followed. In addition, in the fertile years, or even later with assisted fertility techniques, the possibility of pregnancy must be considered. When an abdominopelvic mass is present its characteristics and size, either in centimetres measured from the symphysis pubis upwards, or estimated as weeks' gestation of an equivalent-size pregnancy, are recorded. If ascites is suspected check the supraclavicular and inguinal lymph nodes and look for an associated hydrothorax.

ABDOMINAL EXAMINATION IN PREGNANCY

Make sure the light is good, the room comfortably warm, and that there is maximum exposure of the area to be examined (Box 15.1). *Striae gravidarum, linea nigra,* previous *caesarean section or other scars* and any visible *fetal or other movements* should be noted. Ideally the patient is examined flat, but she may be more comfortable semirecumbent. Ask about any tender areas before palpating the abdomen. Using the flat of the hand as well as the examining fingers can enhance comfort and gentleness; this allows the outline of a mass or pregnant uterus to be delineated more readily. In late pregnancy palpation may produce uterine contractions, which can obscure details of the uterine contents. If part of the examination is likely to be painful this should be left to the very end.

The size of the uterus (Fig. 15.1) is traditionally estimated by the *fundal height*, even though this is

---

Box 15.1 Abdominal examination in pregnancy

Inspection
- Striae gravidarum
- Linea nigra
- Scars
- Fetal movements

Palpation
- Fundal height
- Fetal poles and fetal lie
- Presentation: breech, head etc.
- Attitude
- Level of presenting part
- Fetal movements
- Liquor volume

Auscultation
- Fetal heart rate

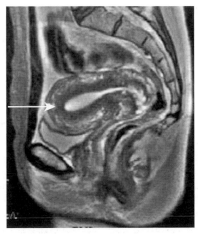

Figure 15.1 Magnetic resonance image of the female pelvis. The uterus is arrowed.

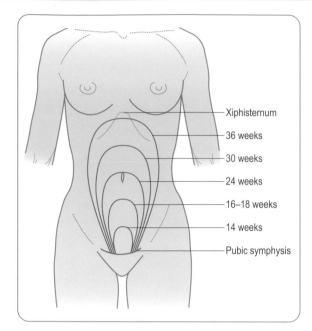

Figure 15.2 Approximate fundal height with changing gestation.

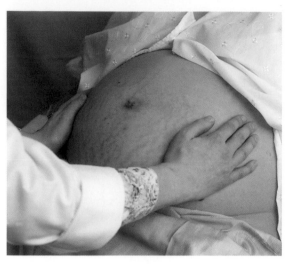

Figure 15.3 Method of abdominal palpation to determine fetal lie and location of back.

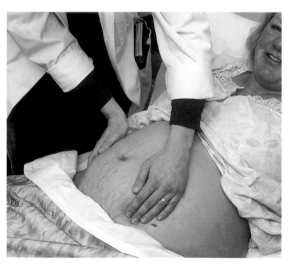

Figure 15.4 Method of abdominal palpation to determine presenting part.

only one dimension of a globular mass. Under normal circumstances the fundal height is just above the symphysis pubis at 12 weeks' gestation, at the umbilicus at 22 weeks and at the xyphisternum at 36 weeks. When the fundus is equidistant from the symphysis pubis and the umbilicus the gestation is 16 weeks, and when equidistant from the xyphi-sternum and umbilicus it is about 30 weeks. From 36 weeks the fundal height is also dependent on the level of the *presenting part*, and will reduce as the presenting part descends into the pelvis (Fig. 15.2). Comparative measurements can be made using either symphysis–fundal height (in centimetres) or the minimal girth measured at the level of the umbilicus (in inches); each of these correlates with gestation.

Next, determination of the number of *fetal poles* will allow assessment of the fetal axis and hence the *fetal lie* (Fig. 15.3). This is the relationship of the long axis of the fetus to the long axis of the uterus. To confirm the lie, the location of the fetal limbs and back should be identified.

At term, over 95% of babies present by the head, but at 30 weeks, because of the greater mobility of the fetus and the relatively larger volume of amniotic fluid, only 70% do so. The breech can usually be distinguished by its size, texture and ability to change shape. However, an ultrasound examination may be necessary for confirmation of *breech presentation*

If the baby is cephalic, the smallest diameters presented to the pelvis occur when the head is well flexed, i.e. a vertex presentation. Flexion of the head is termed the *attitude*, and decreasing amounts of flexion lead to brow or face presentations, which cause difficulty in labour, often requiring delivery by caesarean section. For a breech presentation an equivalent assessment is made to determine whether the breech is *extended* (frank), *flexed* (complete) or *footling* (incomplete). Once the presenting part has a relationship to the pelvis, that relationship can be vertical (the *level*) (Fig. 15.4) or rotational (the *position*). When the flexed head presents, the fetal occiput is termed the *denominator*. When the face presents, the denominator is the mentum (chin), and when the breech presents it is the sacrum. Thus with a vertex presentation the position can now be described as 'left occipitolateral (LOL)' or 'right occipitolateral (ROL)' etc. The common positions of the head before the onset of labour are LOL 50%, ROL 25%. This relationship changes during

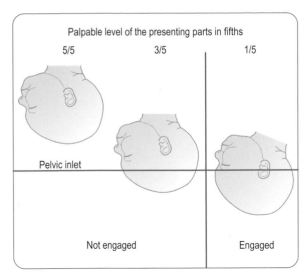

Figure 15.5 The vertical relationship of the presenting part to the pelvic inlet (the level).

Palpable level of the presenting parts in fifths
5/5   3/5   1/5
Pelvic inlet
Not engaged   Engaged

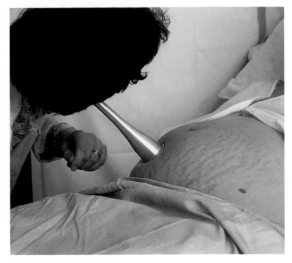

Figure 15.6 Listening over the fetal back to the fetal heart with a Pinard stethoscope. (Historical)

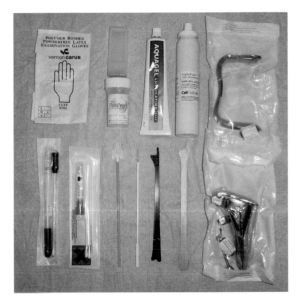

Figure 15.7 Equipment for the gynaecological examination.

the course of labour because of internal rotation, and at the end of labour the common presenting positions are left occipitoanterior (LOA) 60% and right occipitoanterior (ROA) 30%.

Engagement of the presenting part occurs when the largest diameters have passed through the pelvic brim. The number of fifths of the head palpated through the abdominal wall indicates its level (Fig. 15.5). Thus, if there are three or more fifths palpable, the baby's head will be unengaged. If less than three-fifths are palpable, then the baby's head is probably engaged in the pelvis, but this does depend on the overall size of the fetal head and of the pelvis. It must be remembered that the pelvic brim has an angle of approximately 45° to the horizontal when the mother is lying flat. If the abdominal wall is reasonably thin the unengaged head can be palpated by the examiner's fingers passing round its maximum diameter. This means it is above the pelvic brim. When this does not occur the widest diameter must be below the examining fingers, and fixity of the baby's head in the pelvis is also a guide. This means it is engaged. Engagement will usually occur as the leading edge of the baby's head, on vaginal examination, reaches the level of the ischial spines (zero station).

Fetal movements, both as reported by the mother and observed by the examiner during the examination, are noted. A record is made of the *volume of liquor*, which changes throughout pregnancy, and which is estimated by palpation and ballottement. This requires considerable practice. Lastly, the *fetal heart rate (FHR)*, which is normally between 115 and 160 beats/min, is recorded either using a Pinard stethoscope (Fig 15.6) or, more often, with a hand-held audible ultrasonic Doppler with an integrated digital beat rate recorder.

PELVIC EXAMINATION

In gynaecology the pelvic examination is usually undertaken vaginally, but it may also be performed rectally as in general surgery. The instruments used are shown in Figure 15.7.

VAGINAL EXAMINATION

It is most important to explain every step to the patient. Begin by inspecting the perineum in the dorsal or left lateral position (Box 15.2). Women who use tampons or who have borne children should be able to tolerate a gentle vaginal examination. For a digital vaginal examination, disposable gloves are used and the examining fingers are lightly lubricated with a water-based jelly. For others,

Box 15.2 Vaginal examination

Inspection of vulva
Digital palpation
- Locate cervix
- Bimanual palpation
- Pelvic tenderness
- Pelvic masses
- Assessment of uterus (position, mobility)
- Ovaries and fallopian tubes

Speculum examination
- Cervix
- Vaginal walls

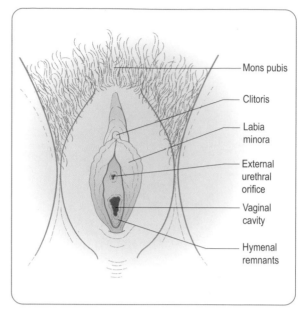

Figure 15.8 The vulva.

pelvic examination may be undertaken per rectum. Inflammation, swelling, soreness, ulceration or neoplasia of the vulva, perineum or anus are noted (Fig. 15.8). Small warts (condylomata acuminata) appearing as papillary growths may occur scattered over the vulva; these are due to infection with the *human papilloma virus* (HPV). The clitoris and urethra are inspected and the patient is asked to strain and then to cough to demonstrate uterovaginal prolapse or stress incontinence (Fig. 15.9). If the latter is the presenting problem it is important that the bladder is reasonably full and that more than one substantial cough is taken, as the first cough frequently fails to demonstrate leakage of urine.

With the patient in the supine position and with her knees drawn up and separated, the labia are gently parted with the index finger and thumb of the left hand while the index finger of the right hand is inserted into the vagina, avoiding the urethral meatus and exerting a sustained pressure on the *perineal body* until the perineal musculature relaxes. Watch for any sign of discomfort. The full length of the finger is then introduced, assessing the vaginal walls in transit until the cervix is located. At this stage a second finger can be inserted to improve the quality of the digital examination, or alternatively a speculum can be used if a cervical smear is required. The examination is continued with the left hand placed on the abdomen above the symphysis pubis and below the umbilicus – the bimanual examination (Fig. 15.10). The hand provides gentle directional pressure to bring the pelvic viscera towards the examiner's fingers in the vagina and serves to assess the size, mobility and regularity of masses. The *cervix* is then identified; it is approximately 3 cm in diameter, with a variably sized and shaped dimple in the middle, the *cervical os*. When the uterus is *anteflexed* and *anteverted*, the os is normally directed posteriorly. The consistency of the cervix is firm and its shape is irregular when scarred. Increased hardness of the cervix may be caused by fibrosis or carcinoma. As a 'soft' cervix

indicates the possibility of pregnancy, even greater caution and gentleness is necessary. The mobility of the cervix is usually 1–2 cm in all directions, and testing this movement should produce only mild discomfort. When attempts are made to move the cervix in the presence of pelvic inflammation, particularly in association with ectopic pregnancy, extreme pain (*cervical excitation*) results.

The size, shape, position, consistency and regularity of the *uterus* and the relationship of the fundus of the uterus to the cervix (flexion) are estimated. Bimanual examination also enables palpation of the *ovaries* and *fallopian tubes*, although these can be difficult to feel in healthy women. The pouch of Douglas is then explored through the posterior *fornix* via the arch formed by the uterosacral ligaments and the cervix.

SPECULUM EXAMINATION

This is an essential part of a gynaecological examination. Several types of vaginal specula are available. These include the *bivalve* type (e.g. Cusco's), used for displaying the cervix (Fig. 15.11), the single- or double-ended *Sims' (duckbill) speculum* (Fig. 15.14), used to retract the vaginal walls, and *Ferguson's speculum*, a tube used to allow the inspection of the cervix when vaginal prolapse is so severe that a bivalve speculum fails to provide a sufficient view. Speculum examination of the vagina can also be undertaken in the dorsal or left lateral position (which is used for examination for pelvic floor prolapse). The speculum should be warmed to body temperature and lubricated with water or a water-based jelly. All the necessary equipment, such as

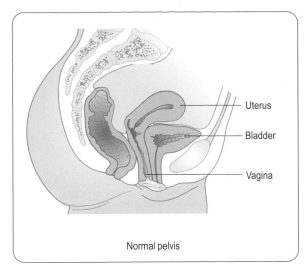
Normal pelvis

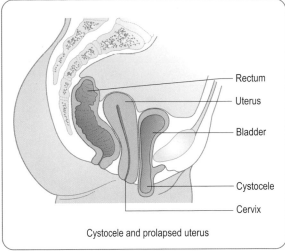
Cystocele and prolapsed uterus

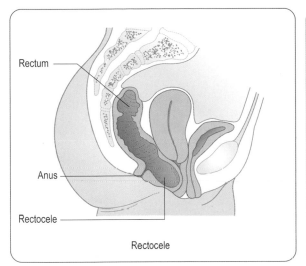
Rectocele

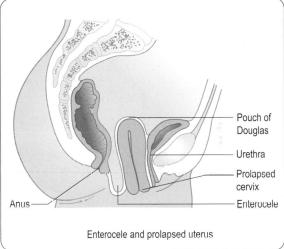
Enterocele and prolapsed uterus

Figure 15.9 In cystocele there is downward prolapse of the anterior part of the pelvic floor, straightening the angulation of the bladder neck and leading to urinary incontinence. In rectocele the posterior part of the pelvic floor is mostly affected, sometimes with associated faecal incontinence. In some patients the whole pelvic floor is weak, with double incontinence or prolapse of the uterus. In enterocele there is a prolapse of viscera from the pouch of Douglas as part of a severe pelvic floor weakness.

spatulas, slides, forceps, culture swabs etc., should be prepared before the examination begins (see Fig. 15.7).

TECHNIQUE FOR TAKING A CERVICAL (PAPANICOLAOU) SMEAR

The procedure is explained to the patient and then she is asked to lie on her back. The labia are separated with the left hand as for the bimanual examination. The lightly lubricated bivalve speculum is held in one hand and the index finger and thumb of the other hand used to separate the introitus; the speculum is then inserted with the handle directly upwards, allowing it to be accommodated by the vagina (which is H-shaped in cross-section). When it has been inserted to its full length, the blades of the speculum are opened and manoeuvred so that

the cervix is fully visualized. The screw adjuster or ratchet on the handle is then locked so that the speculum is maintained in place. Any discharge and the condition of the cervical epithelium, its colour, any ulceration, or scars and retention cysts (*nabothian follicles*) are all recorded.

In the past to detect cervical precancer, an Aylesbury or similar spatula was used with a tip appropriate for the shape of the cervix. The tip of the spatula was placed firmly in the cervical os, so as to allow the removal of surface cells from the whole of the *squamocolumnar junction* when the spatula is rotated through 360°. The use of a brush and liquid-based cytology now allows more accurate diagnosis even in the presence of some bleeding. Computer-aided diagnosis is used with this technique. An example of a stained Papanicolaou slide is

Figure 15.10 Bimanual examination of the pelvis.

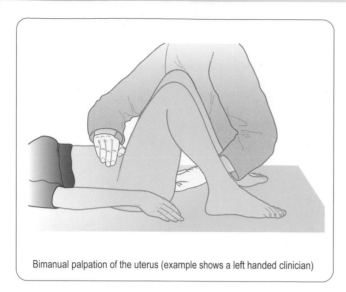

Bimanual palpation of the uterus (example shows a left handed clinician)

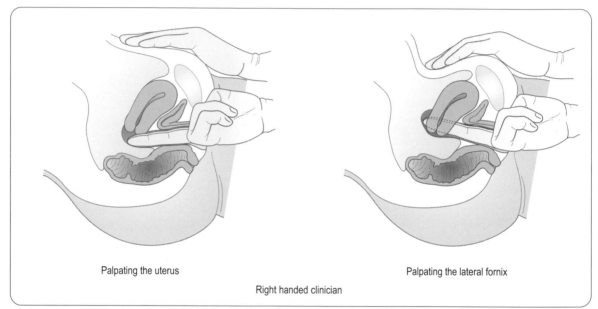

Palpating the uterus

Palpating the lateral fornix

Right handed clinician

shown in Figure 15.12. At the same time, a wet slide for the assessment of *monilia* (*Candida albicans*) or *Trichomonas vaginalis* can be prepared and a culture swab taken from the endocervix or vaginal vault and placed in a bacteriological transport medium. In addition, a Gram-stained smear can be prepared for the detection of *Neisseria gonorrhoeae*, as Gram-negative intracellular diplococci and tests for *Gardnerella*, chlamydia (Fig. 15.13) and herpes should be considered (see Chapter 20). The screw of the speculum is then released and the blades freed from the cervix so that it can be gently removed.

Assessment of the vaginal walls for prolapse or fistula is performed using a Sims' speculum with the patient turned on her left side. The best exposure is given by Sims' position, where the pelvis is rotated by flexing the right thigh more than the left, and by hanging the right arm over the distant edge of the couch. A Sims' speculum is inserted in much the same way as above, using the left hand to elevate the right buttock (Fig. 15.14). The blade then deflects the rectum, exposing the urethral meatus, anterior vaginal wall and bladder base. The patient is then asked to strain and any vaginal wall prolapse is noted. The level of the cervix is recorded as the speculum is withdrawn. The posterior vaginal wall can then be viewed by rotating the speculum through 180°. Uterine prolapse is called *first-degree* when the cervix descends but lies short of the introitus, *second-degree* when it passes to the level of the introitus, and *third-degree* (*complete procidentia*), when the whole of the uterus is prolapsed outside the vulva. Vaginal wall prolapse maybe occurring with, or independent of, uterine prolapse consists of *urethrocele*, *cystocele*, *rectocele* or *ente-*

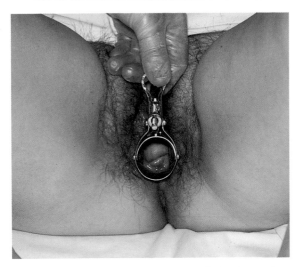

Figure 15.11 Cusco's speculum used to display the cervix.

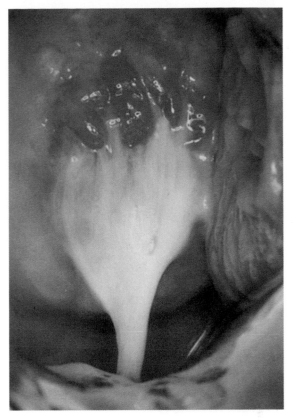

Figure 15.13 *Chlamydia trachomatis.*

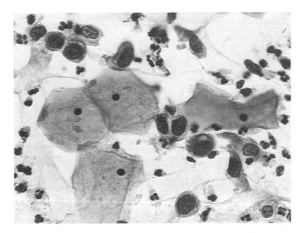

Figure 15.12 Smear from uterine cervix. There are several abnormal squamous cells, indicating in situ carcinoma of the cervix. Large pink-stained normal superficial squamous cells and many inflammatory cells are also included. (Papanicolaou stain, ×160.)

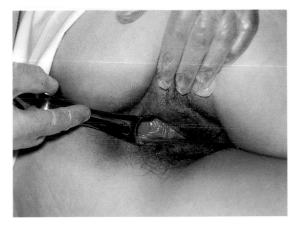

Figure 15.14 Sims' speculum used to display the anterior vaginal wall.

rocele (prolapse of the pouch of Douglas). Several of these anatomical variations usually occur together.

VAGINAL EXAMINATION DURING LABOUR

The examination is made to determine:

- The dilatation and effacement of the cervix
- The presence or absence of amniotic membranes and the state of the liquor
- The level of the presenting part
- The absence of a pulsating umbilical cord, especially if the membranes are ruptured
- The degree of moulding of the fetal head, or the presence of caput succedaneum
- The size and shape of the maternal bony pelvis.

The hands must be washed and sterile surgical gloves worn. The vulva is swabbed clean with an antiseptic such as chlorhexidine in water. An assessment is made of the vulva and then the vagina, which should normally be warm and moist. If it is dry and hot, infection should be suspected. Next the extent of *cervical dilatation* is estimated in centimetres (10 cm is equivalent to full dilatation at term) and the thinness and elasticity of the cervix, which increases with dilatation, is also assessed. The *level* of the presenting part is measured in centimetres from the ischial spines and noted as above (−), below (+) or at (0) '*the station*'. If caput succedaneum (oedema of the fetal scalp) is present there may be difficulty in estimating both the exact level and the position of the presenting part because of the masking of the fontanelles. The *position* can then be assessed by the location and direction of a fetal ear. The method of estimating maternal pelvic dimensions is described in textbooks of obstetrics. If a vaginal delivery is to be achieved safely these measurements must be adequate in relation to the attitude of the presenting part and size of the baby.

RECTAL EXAMINATION

When vaginal examination is not possible or is unacceptable, rectal examination permits bimanual assessment of the pelvic viscera. It is particularly valuable in assessing problems in the pouch of Douglas, the uterosacral ligaments or the rectovaginal septum. Sometimes, disease arising in the rectum (e.g. diverticular disease) can masquerade as a gynaecological problem. (See also Chapter 8)

INVESTIGATIONS

PREGNANCY TESTING

URINE
Most pregnancy tests depend on the detection of *human chorionic gonadotrophin (HCG)* in the urine. The sensitivity of these tests varies, but some detect as little as 25 IU/L HCG in an early-morning urine sample. As the developing placental tissue produces increasing amounts HCG from about 10 days post fertilization, pregnancy diagnosis is now possible even before the first missed period.

BLOOD
Detection of pregnancy earlier still is possible by radioimmunoassay detection of the β subunit of hCG in blood.

BACTERIOLOGICAL AND VIRUS TESTS
Bacteriological and virus tests used in gynaecology and obstetrics include the following:

- Swabs from the throat, endocervix, vagina, urethra and rectum may be needed for sexually transmitted diseases, e.g. direct antigen (DAT) or nucleic acid detection tests for *Chlamydia*
- Culture or DNA detection for herpes virus
- Cervical scrape brush or liquid cytology samples for human papilloma virus
- Midstream urinalysis (MSU) is important in both obstetrics (for bacteriuria) and gynaecology (for frequency and incontinence)
- Serum tests for toxoplasma, rubella, cytomegalovirus and herpes simplex (TORCH)

detect antibodies from previous infections and may be protective of a future pregnancy.

IMAGING TECHNIQUES

HYSTEROSALPINGOGRAPHY   (Fig. 15.15)

The preferred contemporary technique to image the uterine cavity and fallopian tubes is hysterosonography (hysterosalpingo contrast sonography, HyCoSy), rather than X ray hysterosalpingography, in which the flow of saline or galactose microparticles through the tubes and uterus is visualized with a vaginal ultrasound probe, thereby avoiding exposure to radiation.

PELVIMETRY

Pelvimetry is needed less often than in the past, as breech presentations are now always managed with caesarean section. Post delivery MRI is usually used in order to avoid radiation exposure.

ULTRASOUND

Ultrasound scanning (Fig. 15.16) as used over the last 35 years appears safe. Ultrasound waves generated from a piezoelectric crystal transducer are propagated through and reflected from tissue at variable velocities, depending on tissue density. The echo time and signal amplitude give an estimate of the size and consistency of the object scanned. The ultrasonic assessment of gestational age, fetal normality, multiple pregnancy, placental site, blood flow and the expected changes at different gestations are all important parameters of pregnancy monitoring. Two-dimensional imaging by B-mode scanning is the primary modality, and additional information can be obtained by colour and pulsed Doppler, which provide information on blood flow. Transabdominal and transvaginal routes can be used. The former enables a wide field of view,

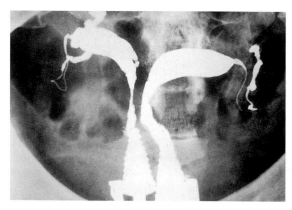

Figure 15.15 An abnormal X ray hysterosalpingogram: uteri didelphys (double uterus).

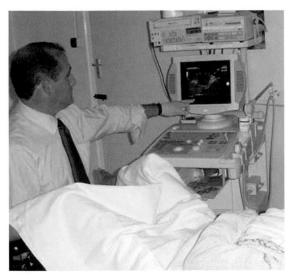

Figure 15.16 This is a picture of a consultant doing a 'one-stop clinic'. This means (a) diagnosis, (b) investigation (in this case by ultrasound), and (c) treatment in one visit rather than the traditional 'come for a check and tests, then return for the results and treatment'.

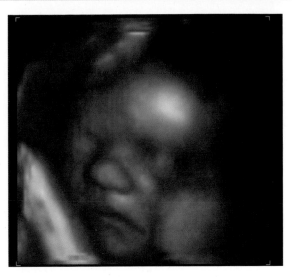

Figure 15.17 This is an ultrasound image with shading which gives an impression of three dimensions. Its use scientifically is not yet determined, but patients love it for the view it gives of their babies.

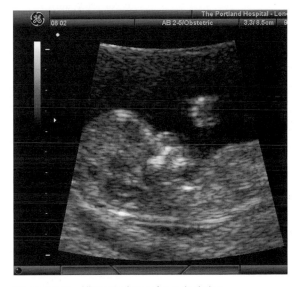

Figure 15.18 Ultrasound scan for early dating.

greater depth of penetration and transducer movement; the latter, with higher-frequency transducers, gives increased resolution and diagnostic power but over a more limited area. More recently 3D scanners have been introduced, and these give improved image quality (Fig. 15.17).

In early pregnancy (5–7 weeks) the integrity, location and the number of gestation sacs can be viewed. At 11–13 weeks mono- or dichorionicity, nuchal translucency, nasal bone development and gross fetal abnormality can be detected (Fig. 15.18). Changes in the cervix can be measured, giving an indication of possible late miscarriage or early premature labour. Anatomical anomaly scanning at 18–20 weeks is performed, particularly of the fetal heart and head and to detect functional activity. By 24 weeks uterine and placental blood flow can be assessed, as can blood flow through fetal arteries.

In gynaecology, ultrasound is useful not only in the assessment of tumours but also to assess bladder function, such as residual volume and bladder neck activity. It is also helpful in the preoperative preparation for repair of anal sphincter damage.

CT AND MRI

CT scanning has proved less useful in gynaecology than was originally anticipated and is now used mainly for staging and follow-up of malignancies. MRI, however, is a better option (Fig. 15.1). It uses no ionizing radiation and no harmful biological effects have been detected in current usage at magnetic field strengths 1.5–2.0 Tesla. Good images are obtained with excellent differentiation of maternal and fetal tissues. Although ultrasound is much cheaper, no artefacts from bone or bowel gas occur. Echo planar imaging is useful to reduce fetal movement artefact and increases the potential for the study of fetal physiology and pathology. In gynaecology MRI has become the standard for assessing carcinoma.

Positron emission tomography (PET) scanning is also useful in gynaecological oncology. It has proved useful in conjunction with fluorodeoxyglucose in the detection of metastatic gestational trophoblastic tumours. Experimentally in animals it has been used successfully to assess placental function.

ENDOMETRIAL SAMPLING (BIOPSY) (Fig. 15.19)

One of the common investigations undertaken in gynaecology is sampling of the endometrium. Formerly, this was performed by a dilatation of the cervix and curettage (D&C) to obtain histological material from the cavity of the uterus. Dilatation of the cervix is very painful and hence an anaesthetic is needed. However, the biopsy is not always representative and may fail to make a diagnosis in up to one-third of cases. Methods of cell sampling have been developed, including surface cytology or from larger quantities of aspirated materials (cell samplers), but the definitive assessment is now usually by hysteroscopy and directed biopsy. With current miniature fibreoptic systems this can also be done under local analgesia in an outpatient setting.

COLPOSCOPY

Colposcopy permits visualization of the cervix, the vaginal vault (vaginoscopy) or vulva (vulvoscopy) with a low-power binocular microscope to detect precancerous abnormalities of the epithelium (Fig. 15.20). Usually an abnormal cervical smear will have alerted the doctor to the need for this investigation. It can be undertaken on an outpatient basis, by accessing the cervix with a speculum, treating it first with acetic acid then with Lugol's iodine. This aqueous solution of iodine and potassium iodide causes the cervix and the normal mucous membrane, which contain glycogen, to stain dark brown. Those areas of abnormality that fail to take up the stain can then be identified (*Schiller's test*). The whole cervix is viewed through a colposcope, which gives low-level binocular magnification, to identify the degree, site and extent of the cervical pathology that has produced the abnormal smear. It also allows examination of the rest of the cervix, including the area most at risk (the transformation zone). Once this has been done, biopsy and appropriate treatment (e.g. large loop electrodiathermy of the transformation zone *LLETZ* or surgical excision) can be undertaken.

HYSTEROSCOPY

This is a technique for viewing the cavity of the uterus using small-diameter fibreoptic telescopes and cameras (Fig. 15.21). Diagnostic hysteroscopy using a 4 mm hysteroscope can be performed as both an inpatient and an outpatient procedure for disorders such as abnormal bleeding, subfertility and recurrent miscarriage. This technique can also be adapted with larger hysteroscopes to be used operatively for the resection of uterine adhesions, polyps, septae, submucous fibroids (Fig. 15.22) and endometrium.

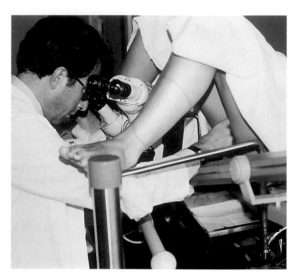

Figure 15.20 Colposcopy.

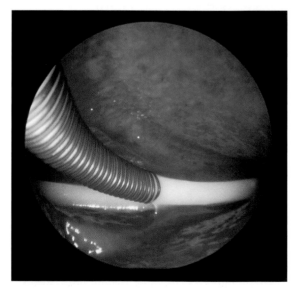

Figure 15.21 Hysteroscopic view of an intrauterine device in situ.

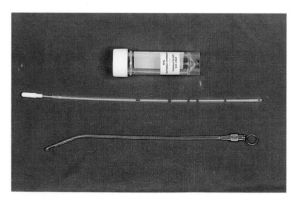

Figure 15.19 An endometrial biopsy curette, a pipette cell sampler and fixing medium.

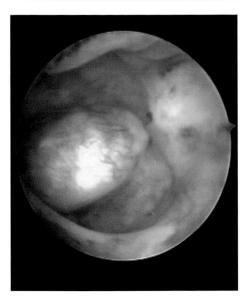

Figure 15.22 Hysteroscopic view of submucosal fibroids.

CYSTOSCOPY AND CYSTOMETRY

The investigation of all voiding difficulties is initiated by checking for urinary tract infection. Following a clinical examination, pelvic/vaginal ultrasound is used to confirm the normality of the pelvis or to assess coincidental pelvic masses. The pressure/volume relationships of bladder filling, detrusor and sphincter activity and urethral flow rate can be assessed with a cystometrogram. The bladder is catheterized and slowly filled with sterile saline. The volume and pressure at which bladder filling is perceived, and at which a desire to micturate is felt, are noted. The urinary flow rate and postmicturition bladder volume are recorded. In developments of this test electromyographic (EMG) activity in the external urethral sphincter can be measured, and the urethral pressure profile established. This is being replaced by real-time ultrasound assessment of bladder neck activity and descent. In *stress incontinence* urinary flow commences at low bladder pressures because of sphincter incompetence; in *urge incontinence* urinary flow develops at low bladder volumes because of uninhibited detrusor activity. Reflux and overflow also show as urethral leakage. Incontinence can also result from a defect in the anatomical integrity of the urinary tract, such as a congenital abnormality or fistula. Viewing the interior of the bladder by cystoscopy gives information about its condition and allows biopsy of the mucosa or the removal of foreign bodies.

LAPAROSCOPY/PELVICOSCOPY

Visualization of the pelvic and abdominal viscera is particularly valuable if it can be done without a major injury to the abdominal wall (Fig. 15.23).

This is achieved by inflating the abdomen with carbon dioxide under general or local anaesthesia, so that the anterior abdominal wall is lifted away from the viscera, allowing inspection of the abdominal and pelvic contents using a fibreoptic telescope illuminated by a light source remote from the patient. The main uses of laparoscopy are diagnostic (e.g. in the investigation of pelvic pain or infertility) and therapeutic (e.g. in sterilization procedures, or in the treatment of a range of pelvic pathologies). Minimal access surgery (MAS) utilizes multiple puncture techniques with high-quality television monitors and video recorders. Treatment for ectopic pregnancy, hysterectomy, lymphadenectomy, cholecystectomy, bladder and bowel surgery are now common place.

TESTS OF FETAL WELL BEING

Besides those tests made to ensure the good general health of the mother, such as haemoglobin, Venereal Disease Reference Laboratory (VDRL), TPHA tests and bacteriuria screening, a number of other investigations of variable complexity can be utilized to check the fetus in utero. These tests are routine in the UK. In addition, anonymous HIV testing is offered to all pregnant women, and particularly to those in known risk groups, in order to obtain an estimate of the community prevalence of this infection. As yet this is *not* carried out routinely.

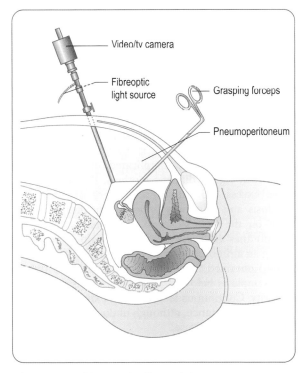

Figure 15.23 Diagram of a diagnostic laparoscopy.

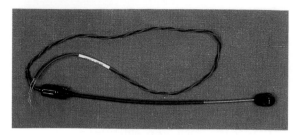

Figure 15.27   Fetal scalp electrode.

Three-dimensional ultrasound images have recently become available. They are beautiful to see but their clinical usefulness is still being established.

DOPPLER BLOOD FLOW

Studies of changes in the uterine circulation may predict the later onset of pregnancy-associated hypertension. Changes in uteroplacental blood flow (absence or reversal of end-diastolic flow) and those in the aortic and cerebral fetal circulation give further clues to the state of the fetus, or even imminent fetal death, especially in already compromised circumstances.

PLACENTAL VOLUME

Ultrasound measurements of placental volume may also help in the prediction of fetal growth retardation.

Children and adolescents

R. Harris

16

INTRODUCTION

'If a child cries when you examine it, then it's probably your fault.' This rather sweeping statement was made by the late John Apley, an eminent paediatrician and teacher in Bristol. The basic philosophy is right. The examiner cannot avoid some discomfort in some parts of the physical examination, but during most of the examination the child should be contented. This is the essence of the art of examining children. A child who struggles and screams is afraid, and the examiner must spend time trying to gain their confidence. The consulting room must have a range of toys suitable for all ages, and the child should be allowed to play with whatever takes his or her fancy. If old enough, the child should be allowed to explore the room, although dissuaded from playing with expensive or potentially dangerous equipment. Younger children will be sitting on their parent's lap, and for some of the time regarding you with suspicion. Do not be afraid to stop what you are doing to pull a face or offer a toy that seems to have caught the child's attention.

As the family enter the room they should be greeted in a friendly manner and introductions made. Ascertain who is with the child. It may not be the mother but another family member, who, in a mixed ethnic population, may be the only one who speaks English. If you can get everyone to relax and laugh in the first few minutes, the child will relax and the subsequent history and examination will be easier. White coats have no part to play in paediatric practice as they frighten and intimidate most children. They should not be worn under any circumstances.

While talking to the mother, an essential part of the examination is to watch the child and assess his/her behaviour. Does the child look unwell? Is he or she interested in the surroundings and exploring them, or apathetic? Watch the child running around: are there any obvious abnormalities in the gait? Is the face normal, or are there features of abnormal development? Are there any obvious physical abnormalities? Is the breathing unusually noisy? Does the child seem well nourished, or wasted?

HISTORY

The history (Box 16.1) will normally be taken from the mother, but when you are seeing an older child, involve him or her by asking relevant points such as the site of a pain etc. Even younger children should be asked simple things in words they can understand. Remember that the mother is giving you her version of the problem, not the child's. Always take notice of what the mother is saying, and listen to her complaints. Do not be tempted to interrupt a mother in full flow to try and ask what you think is a clever question. The mother will know what is worrying her about her child, and any interruptions should be to guide her rather than try and impose your diagnosis on her. Most of all, do not keep looking at your watch or the pile of notes in front of you. A mother and child must be made to feel that they have your whole attention, and that you have all the time in the world for them. Other relatives tend not to be such good historians as the parents, and if well-meaning relatives try to give you the history, make it very clear that it is the parent's view you need, even if this involves the use of an interpreter (but see above). Older children are quite capable of giving a history of their current problems and should be encouraged to do so. All the time you are talking to the parents, keep watching everything that the child is doing and their reactions.

The structure of the history is no different from that of an adult, consisting of the presenting complaint, a history of the present illness, and a history of any previous illness. In children, enquire particularly as to the nature and severity of *previous illnesses*, the age at which they occurred, for example infectious diseases, seizures, bowel disturbances, upper respiratory tract infections, discharging ears and cough. In the case of a cough, always ask when it is worse (for example, asthma sufferers tend to cough at night and when running around), and if vomiting or a 'whoop' is present. Has the child been taking any drugs? Has he or she ever been in hospital, and if so, what was wrong? Have there been any accidents, physical injuries, burns or poisoning incidents?

- Birth
- Milestones
- Mental and physical development
- School
- Specific illnesses, accidents etc.
- Immunizations
- Contacts and travel
- Family history
- Social history
- Consanguinity and genetic risk

Box 16.2   Pregnancy and infancy

- Was the mother well during her pregnancy?
- Did she have any particular illnesses, or was she taking any drugs (including alcohol)?
- Was the baby born at term?
- What were the birthweight and type of delivery?
- Were there any problems in the newborn period?
  - jaundice?
  - breathing problems?
  - fits?
  - feeding difficulties?
- Has the baby had any illnesses?
- How was the baby fed?
- If bottle-fed, which milk formula was used?
- When were solid foods introduced?
- Were vitamin drops given and, if so, how many?
- Was the weight gain satisfactory?
- What immunizations has he/she had?

Next the doctor should pay more specific attention to the *pregnancy, newborn period and developmental progress* (Box 16.2). At this point it is worth asking if the parents have kept any record of child health clinic attendances, such as a 'baby book', containing dates of attendance at hospital or clinic, weights, immunizations etc. It is important to ask about the *'milestones of development'*: When did the child first sit up, smile, crawl, walk and talk? Fuller details will be found in Table 16.2. *General questions* are important (Box 16.3). Ask about *routine immunizations*, and if they have all been given.

FAMILY HISTORY

- How old are the parents?
- How many children are there in the family?
- What are their ages and sex?
- Have there been any stillbirths, miscarriages or other childhood deaths in the family?
- Are there any illnesses in the siblings, parents or any near relatives?
- Is there any background of inherited disease?

SOCIAL HISTORY

Approach the social history with diplomacy; sometimes it is more prudent to leave deeper probing to a later occasion. It is useful to know about living conditions, and whether either or both parents are employed. If the mother is working there is some daily separation from the child. Ask if the child has ever been separated from her for any time in the past, as this may be the basis of a variety of behavioural difficulties. Find out if the child's parents live together, and whether there is any difficulty in the relationship. Is there a supportive family structure involving other relatives, e.g. grandparents? If the family are immigrants, it is important to know how long they have been in their new country. The depth of enquiry in a paediatric social history must always be judged on an individual basis. If the family think that you are prying too much, you may lose the rapport that you have been building up.

Box 16.3   General questions

- What are the child's present habits with regard to eating, sleeping, bowels and micturition?
- What sort of child is he or she?
- Is he or she robust or moody?
- Does he or she cry a lot?
- How does the child compare with siblings or friends of the same age?
- If of school age, what school does the child go to, and how is he or she getting on?
- Does the child miss much time from school and, if so, why? Ask the child if they like school, and one or two questions about it, such as who is their best friend, and the name of their teacher.

Now may be the time to consider talking either to the child or to the parents without the other party being present. This may be particularly valuable in the case of adolescent children, who are often rather resentful of their parents telling you all their problems, and this is the opportunity for them to relax with you. Ask them about the illness, and also a little about themselves and their interests. Parents may also welcome an opportunity to talk in private with you, and it is often during such discussion that the real reason for the consultation emerges. This can be accomplished most easily while the child is undressing or dressing.

By this time you should already have formed an impression of the child, the family and their relationship, and you are now ready to proceed with the examination. By now, a younger child should have found you such a fascinating person that they will be prepared to cooperate with you in most parts of the physical examination. Alternatively, the child may have become so bored that he or she is asleep. In either case physical examination should present no problems. If the child is now crying loudly then you are in for a difficult time, and you should be asking yourself where you went wrong.

EXAMINATION

Older children will usually cooperate sufficiently to be examined lying down, and routine physical examination is no different from an adult examination. A younger child should be examined sitting on his or her mother's lap, as any attempt to get him or her to lie down will result in instant distress. Always talk to children, however young; do not be afraid of looking silly if the result is a cooperative child. Those parts of the examination that are painful or unpleasant should be left until last: if an attempt is made to examine a child's throat at the outset, the immediate response will be crying. Offer the child something to play with – even a stethoscope will be a source of amusement to a young infant. Children often find it amusing if you examine their toy first. Sometimes a small toy clipped onto the stethoscope is interesting enough for a young child to let you examine them without problems. Try to follow the scheme set out in Boxes 16.4 and 16.5.

Start the examination by asking the mother to undress the child. Do not make her hurry. Remember that even very young children may be modest, and prefer to keep their underpants on. Always wash your hands while the child is being undressed. Examination should now proceed by the usual method of inspection, palpation, percussion and auscultation; however, no set routine can be followed, and the examination is by regions rather than by systems. The examination may have to be opportunistic, as each child will dictate the order of the examination by their reactions to various procedures (Box 16.5).

In general, start with the least threatening manoeuvres. Note again the state of *nutrition* now that the child is undressed. If there are bruises on young children, except on the shins, be suspicious of non-accidental injury. Are there any obvious rashes to be seen? Are there any naevi or other skin anomalies?

THE LIMBS

Often the feet are the easiest place to start. There is nothing threatening to the average child about a doctor tickling their feet. This simple trick gives you the first opportunity to touch the child, and will also allow the feet to be checked for a variety of problems, such as minor varus deformities, overriding toes, or such minor plantar abnormalities as flat feet. It is then very easy to run your hands over

---

Box 16.4 Assessments to include in the examination of children

- Observe
- Listen
- Play
- Palpate
- Specific clinical tests
- Other 'background' tests

Box 16.5 Schema for examination of children

- Feet
- Hands and pulse
- Face
- Head
- Neck
- Abdomen
- Chest
- Neurological
- Eyes and funduscopy
- Genitalia, groins, anus
- Other invasive clinical tests

---

the child's legs at the same time, noting any knee or other bony abnormalities. Note any muscle wasting or tenderness, and the movements of the knee and ankle. At the same time an assessment of the muscle tone should be made, as this seems to the child just an extension of the funny game already being played by this strange but interesting doctor. It is easy to notice at the same time whether the skin is dry or moist, and to feel any skin lesions that you may have noticed. All the time the child's reactions should be watched. Is he or she still your friend? Be prepared to stop what you are doing if the child seems to be getting upset, and spend a few minutes trying to re-establish the rapport that you have just built up.

By now there should be no major objections to the rest of the body being felt. The *arms and shoulders* should be examined next, followed by the *hands*. Do the hands have a single palmar crease, as seen in children with Down's syndrome and in a variety of other syndromes, as well as in a small proportion of normal children? Feel the *wrists* for widening of the epiphyses of the radius and ulna – a sign of rickets. Try to feel the pulse and count it, although this will be difficult in a plump, young infant; the rate is best counted at this age when auscultating the chest.

THE HEAD, FACE AND NECK

Look at the child's face and ask yourself the following questions.

- Does it look normal?
- If the baby looks odd, then do not forget to look at the parents. It may then be obvious that what you regard as abnormal may be nothing more than a family trait. If the appearance is still not too clear, ask who the baby looks like.
- Does the child have a large tongue?
- Are the ears in the normal position, or are they low-set and abnormal in any way? There are many hundreds of syndromes diagnosable by the facial appearance, and the salient features should be carefully noted.

Next note the shape of the *head*. It may be abnormally shaped, owing to premature fusion of the sutures, small if the baby is *microcephalic*, or globular if the baby is *hydrocephalic*, sometimes with dilated veins over the skin surface. It is often asymmetrical (*plagiocephalic*) in normal infants who tend to lie with their heads persistently on one side (Fig. 16.1). This is now much more common because babies are placed on their backs to reduce the risk of sudden death in infancy. The parents can be reassured that the head will be normal as the baby grows up.

Assuming that you are still friends, there should be no objection to your feeling the child's head now. Leave the measurement of the head circumference until near the end of the examination, as some babies find this a little threatening and may start crying. Feel the anterior fontanelle. It is normally small at birth, enlarges during the first 2 months, and then gradually reduces until final closure. It is normally closed by 18 months but can close much earlier, and has been reported as staying open in a few normal girls until 4 years of age. Delayed closure may be seen, however, in *rickets*, *hypothyroidism* and *hydrocephalus*. An assessment of the

tension of the anterior fontanelle is important. In health it pulsates and is in the same plane as the rest of the surrounding skull. A tense, bulging fontanelle indicates *raised intracranial pressure*, but it does also become tense with crying. A sunken fontanelle is a feature of dehydration. The posterior fontanelle is located by passing the finger along the sagittal suture to its junction with the lambdoid sutures. It should normally be closed after 2 months of age. Sometimes, when passing the finger along the sagittal suture, a small notch is felt over the vault of the cranium. This is the third fontanelle, and although it can be normal it is seen in some chromosome abnormalities and in congenital infections such as rubella. While feeling the head, any ridging of the sutures should be noticed, suggesting premature fusion (*craniostenosis*), or overriding of the sutures if the head is small (*microcephaly*). In the neonatal period the sutures tend to be separated, and there is sometimes a continuous gap from the forehead to the posterior part of the posterior fontanelle. Sutures close rapidly, and are normally ossified by 6 months of age.

Having assessed the skull, the *neck* can be checked, paying particular attention to the presence of lymph nodes. It is common in childhood to feel small lymph nodes in the anterior and posterior triangles of the neck, as they enlarge rapidly in response to local conditions such as tonsillitis. Enlarged glands in the neck are a common reason for referral to a paediatrician, but parents can generally be reassured that they are of no major significance as they can persist for some years. Examination of other lymphatic areas can be carried out at a later stage of the examination – the inguinal nodes when the napkin area is checked, and the axillary nodes when the chest is examined. In young babies the sternomastoid muscles should be checked for the thickened area known as a sternomastoid tumour, which can lead to difficulties with neck movement and an abnormal head and neck posture.

THE ABDOMEN

The abdomen can be a little difficult to examine if the baby is crying, but most infants will be quite happy sitting on their mother's lap (Fig. 16.2). During the first 3 years of life the abdomen often gives an impression of being protuberant. Causes of true abdominal distension are shown in Box 16.6. It is sometimes possible to quieten a crying infant by placing them over their mother's shoulder and examining them from behind. Small infants can be given a feed to quieten them. Look for any obvious distension or for peristaltic waves suggesting intestinal obstruction. Note the umbilicus, and whether or not there is a hernia. Palpation should be gentle and light. The liver edge can be felt in normal children up to the age of 4 years; it can be anything up

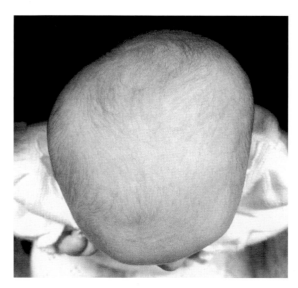

Figure 16.1 Plagiocephalic skull.

to 2 cm below the costal margin. When enlarged, the spleen may be felt below the left costal margin, and in infancy it is more anterior and superficial than in the older child or adult. Slight enlargement of the spleen is common in children with many infections. Faecal masses can be felt in the left iliac fossa in constipated children, and a full or distended bladder presents as a mass arising from the pelvis. Abdominal tenderness is best detected by watching the child's facial expression during palpation. Deep palpation of the kidneys can be carried out last. Although it would be logical to examine the groin area at this time, it is often better to do this at a later stage. If the child has cried persistently, it is still possible to examine the abdomen by the method of *ballottement*: as the baby breathes in, the abdominal muscles relax and the abdominal viscera and other masses, if present, can then be palpated.

THE CHEST

So far, nothing has been done that should cause the child any concern. Examining the chest, however, introduces the stethoscope, which sometimes worries babies. It helps to have let the baby play with the stethoscope at an earlier stage of the examination. Check for any asymmetry, and in girls for any breast development. Minor degrees of pes excavatum are a source of great anxiety to many parents, but are not usually of any importance. Indrawing of the lower ribs (*Harrison's sulcus*) may be seen in obstructive airway disease, due either to asthma or to a nasopharynx blocked by adenoidal hypertrophy. Note any recession when breathing, and count the respiratory rate. In a newborn infant this should be 40 breaths/min; by the second year it has fallen to 30 breaths/min, and by 5 years of age to 20. A child with pneumonia will have a grunting respiration, which is due to reversal of the normal respiratory rhythm. The grunting expiration is followed by inspiration, and then a pause. Thickening of the costochondral junction is felt in rickets (*rachitic rosary*). Palpate the anterior chest wall for the cardiac impulse and for thrills. In children under the age of 5 years the apex is normally in the fourth intercostal space just to the left of the midclavicular line. Vocal fremitus is rarely of any clinical value in children. The axillary nodes may now be felt in the same way as in adults.

Percussion of the chest is useful in older children, but in young children and infants it is only rarely of value. Percuss very lightly, and in babies directly, tapping the chest wall with the percussing finger rather than using another finger as a pleximeter. The chest is more resonant in children than in adults.

A stethoscope with a small bell chest piece is suitable for auscultation of the child's chest. Do not use adult-sized chest pieces, as it is impossible to localize added sounds accurately with a chest piece covering such a wide area in a small child. Often it is less threatening to examine the back of the chest first, and much more information about the lungs can be acquired in this way. Listen for the breath sounds and adventitious sounds. Because of the thin chest wall breath sounds are louder in children than in adults, and their character is more like the bronchial breathing of adults (*puerile breathing*). Upper respiratory tract infections in children often give rise to loud, coarse rhonchi, which are conducted down the trachea and main bronchi (Table 16.1). All is not lost if the child is crying, as this is associated with deep inspiration, and this is the time to listen for the character of the breath sounds.

When you are auscultating the front of the chest, the child's immediate instinct is to push the stethoscope away. Some doctors attach a small toy to the tubing to attract attention, whereas others prefer to distract the child with toys held in the hand (Fig. 16.3). It is a good idea to examine a doll or teddy bear first if the child is playing with one. The normal splitting of the first and second sounds is easier to hear in children than in adults. Venous hums and functional systolic flow murmurs are often heard in normal children. Count the heart rate in young children. The normal rates are as follows:

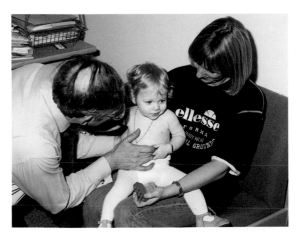

Figure 16.2 Baby sitting on mother's lap while the abdomen is examined.

> **Box 16.6 Causes of abdominal distension**
>
> - Obesity
> - Faeces (constipation, Hirschsprung's disease)
> - Ascites (nephrotic syndrome, cirrhosis)
> - Gas (intestinal obstruction, swallowed air)
> - Pregnancy in adolescent girls
> - Distended bladder (lower abdomen)
> - Pyloric stenosis (upper abdomen)

Table 16.1 Chest signs of some common respiratory disorders of children

Disorder	Chest movement	Percussion (if carried out)	Auscultation
Bronchiolitis	Restricted, with hyperinflation Often tracheal tug and subcostal recession	Hyperresonant	Widespread crepitations, or wheezing
Pneumonia	Rapid, shallow respirations with audible grunt. May be reduced on affected side	Dull or normal	Localized bronchial breathing or crepitations. May have no abnormal signs
Asthma	Restricted with hyperinflation Use of accessory muscles, and subcostal retraction	Hyperresonant	Expiratory wheeze
Croup	Inspiratory stridor, with subcostal recession	Normal	Inspiratory coarse crepitations (crackles)

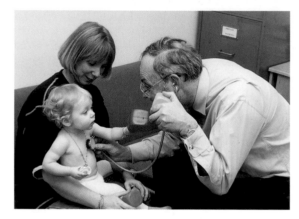

Figure 16.3 Attracting the attention of a 10-month-old baby while examining her heart.

- Newborn infant 140 beats/min (bpm)
- 1-year-old 110 bpm
- 3-year-old 100 bpm
- 8-year-old 90 bpm
- 11-year-old 80 bpm.

Up to this point the baby will have been examined mainly from behind. Take the opportunity to check for spinal abnormalities such as scoliosis or kyphosis, which may otherwise be missed. If there has been no need to stand the baby up at this time, examination of the back can be deferred until the neurological examination, or when the baby is moving around after the examination has been completed.

NEUROLOGICAL EXAMINATION

The neurological examination can usually be carried out in the normal way in older children, but in younger children the extent of the neurological examination will depend on the child's age and willingness to cooperate. A great deal should have been learned already from initial observations. If the child is walking, the gait should have been observed

and muscle tone assessed. Note any abnormal movements:

- Tics or habit spasms are repetitive but not purposeful movements, such as shrugging of the shoulders or facial grimacing.
- Choreiform movements are involuntary, purposeless jerks that follow no particular pattern.
- Athetoid movements are writhing and more pronounced distally.

Cooordination can best be checked by watching a child at play. It is useful to have toys available that require a degree of coordination, such as a toy farm or garage. Otherwise, a modification of the finger–nose test using a toy held in the hand can be used. If the child is old enough, watching them dressing or doing up shoelaces is a good way to assess coordination.

Check *muscle tone* if this has not already been done. Pick the child up if there is still a friendly relationship. This gives a good idea of the feel of a child and of the muscle tone. If the child is hypotonic, it will feel as though he or she is slipping through your hands. Muscle power is difficult to check in young children except by watching playing habits, and assessing power by ability at a variety of lifting games. Always remember to check for neck stiffness. This is detected more readily by resistance to passive neck flexion than by testing for Kernig's sign.

Testing of *sensation* is difficult in young children, and is probably best omitted unless there is a strong suspicion of neurological disease.

Testing the *cranial nerves* takes a little ingenuity. Eye movements are relatively easy using a toy moved in different directions in front of the baby's face; many young infants like poking out their tongue and copying you, which will check the twelfth cranial nerve. If the child can be made to smile, and even if they are crying, any asymmetry of facial movements can be seen.

Getting a child's limbs into the correct position to test *tendon reflexes* may take some time. Often they can be elicited by using a finger rather than a patellar hammer. Tendon reflexes in young infants tend to be brisk, and up to 18 months of age the plantar responses are extensor. The persistence of an extensor response beyond the age of 2 years indicates an upper motor neuron lesion. Primitive responses should have disappeared by 3–4 months of age; their persistence indicates significant neuro-developmental dysfunction. The primitive reflexes will be considered further in the section on examination of the newborn (see p. 338).

THE EYES

The eyes should now be checked. Inspect them for conjunctivitis, cataracts or congenital defects such as colobomata. It is very important to check for *squints*, as immediate ophthalmological referral is necessary, however young the infant. Squints are checked for by shining a light in the eyes from in front of the face; the light reflex should be at the same position in each cornea. A *cover test* should then be used (see Chapter 10), using a doll or some other appropriate toy on which the child can focus his gaze. Pupillary accommodation and light reactions can be noted at the same time. Examination of the *fundus* is particularly difficult in infants, and forcible attempts to keep the eyes open will only make the procedure more difficult. Older children will focus on toys or distant people. In younger children only fleeting glimpses of the fundus are likely. It should be possible to see the red reflex, which if absent is suggestive of a corneal, lens or vitreous opacity, such as cataract or retinoblastoma. Usually enough of the disc can be seen to detect papilloedema.

The testing of vision, hearing, and certain motor functions in young children is included in the section on developmental screening examination (see p. 334).

With the possible exception of the eye examination, nothing so far should have upset a baby unduly. The following examinations should be carried out at the end of the consultation, as they are more likely to upset the child.

THE GENITALIA, GROINS AND ANUS

The nappy or underpants can now be removed if it is necessary to examine the groin or anus. In boys, notice the penis. This is often a source of worry to many parents, especially the lack of retraction of the foreskin. Old wives' tales abound, and few parents realize that the foreskin will only rarely retract under the age of 5 years; they should be informed that forcibly attempting retraction is not only painful but can also result in *balanitis*. Check the hernial orifices and see whether the testes have descended. To feel the testes, make sure that your hand is warm and place a finger in the line of the inguinal canal; advance the finger towards the scrotum. This will stop the cremasteric reflex causing the testes to disappear into the inguinal canal, which tends to happen if the scrotum is approached from below. Having located the testes in the correct place, it is important to demonstrate the normality of the boy to his parents. In young babies it is not unusual to find a testis in the inguinal canal, but it can usually be pushed into the scrotum without too much difficulty. Nothing needs to be done other than to review the boy after a few months, as the testis can be expected to descend into its normal position with increasing maturity.

In girls, check the vulva for soreness or discharge, and for abnormalities such as polyps. Fusion of the labia is not uncommon, so check that they separate normally. Enlargement of the clitoris suggests endocrine disorder.

Check for inguinal lymph nodes at this time, and palpate the femoral artery. If the femoral artery cannot be palpated, this suggests coarctation of the aorta, which requires cardiological assessment.

Examination of the anal margin can best be carried out by gently separating the buttocks with one hand on either side; the anal orifice can then be easily seen and inspected for fissures, which are not uncommon. Rectal examination is rarely necessary in children, and if carried out should be done with a well lubricated, gloved little finger, which should be advanced very slowly. A little time spent talking and waiting will help.

THE NOSE, EARS, MOUTH AND THROAT

The worst parts of the examination as far as the child is concerned are the nose, ears, mouth and throat.

The *nose* need only be examined superficially, looking for nasal patency, any deviation of the septum, or the presence of polyps. Older children are quite good at sniffing, and this will give some idea of nasal patency.

A cooperative child will allow you to look into his or her *ears* but, if not, the child should be held by the mother, as shown in Figure 16.4. Held in such a way, the child can be kept still long enough for the eardrums to be inspected. Look carefully for the light reflex, which can be lost if the child has chronic secretory otitis media ('glue ear'). In acute suppurative otitis media the drum may be bright red and bulging.

The *mouth* and *throat* can be examined by encouraging a cooperative child to 'show me your teeth'; an open mouth will then allow a clear view of the mouth and fauces. If uncooperative, the child will need to be held as shown in Figure 16.5. Sometimes it is not too disastrous if the child cries at this point, as this will give a very clear view of the

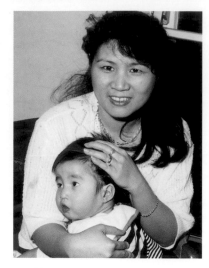

Figure 16.4 How to hold a baby to allow the ears to be examined. The mother faces the baby to one side and holds him firmly, with one arm around the head and the other around the upper arm and shoulder.

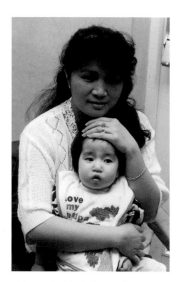

Figure 16.5 How to hold a baby to allow the mouth and throat to be examined. The baby faces the examiner, with the mother holding him firmly with one hand on the forehead and the other holding both arms.

teeth, the tonsils, and sometimes even the epiglottis. A spatula is a terrifying instrument to the average child, causing most to clamp their teeth shut. If this happens, the spatula should be advanced to the back of the tongue to induce a gag reflex. Whatever means are used to open the mouth, the state of the teeth and mucous membranes should be noticed, as well as the tonsils and fauces. Note especially the white patches of *Candida* infection and the Koplik's spots seen in measles.

The child should now be allowed to move freely about the room, allowing a further assessment of gait and of any marked skeletal abnormalities. In younger children and infants the hips must *always* be examined (see page 341).

The general physical examination, with the exception of the special examinations described in the following sections, has now been completed. It is to be hoped that you have retained the friendship of the child. Once the child is dressed, the examiner should sit quietly with the parents and explain what has been found. It is always best for the child to have finished dressing before talking to the parents: they are more likely to consider what you have to say if they are not worrying about buttons or shoelaces. Always involve an older child in the discussion – he or she has every right to know what is wrong. Even young children can be told that they will be all right. Never under any circumstances deceive a child. If they find you out they will never believe you again.

SPECIAL EXAMINATIONS

The following examinations are important.

HEIGHT AND WEIGHT

Measurements of height and weight are essential in the examination of children. In children over the age of 2 years height can be measured against a wall-mounted gauge. Younger children can be measured lying down on special measuring boards. All measurements should be made under standard conditions, and children should be weighed unclothed. If the child keeps any clothes on, this should be noted against the weight so that subsequent weights can be taken with the child wearing the same quantity of clothing. Childhood is a period of growth, the pattern of which may be adversely affected by many disturbances of health, as well as social deprivation. Heights and weights should be compared with those of healthy children of similar sex, age and build, and for this purpose percentile charts are essential (Figs 16.6–16.9). It is also important to have some idea of the height of the parents, as it would be unrealistic to expect small parents to have large children.

Serial measurements over a period are more valuable than single measurements and will give the growth rate – the *growth velocity*. A child who fails to grow at an appropriate velocity needs to be investigated further. However, a child presenting for the first time outside the area between the 10th and 90th percentiles should be regarded with slight suspicion, and those outside the third and 97th percentiles need a very careful history and examination to be carried out. Many of the latter will be normal small children, but it is important to pick up any markers of potential disease such as chronic diarrhoea, recurrent chestiness etc. There are as yet no satisfactory growth charts for children of Asian origin born in the UK, who tend to be smaller than

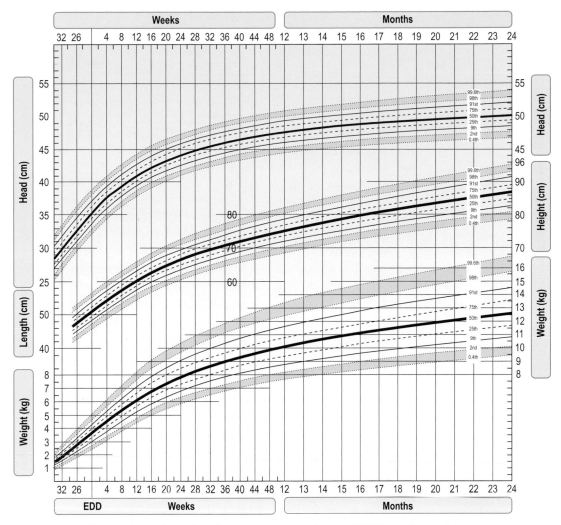

Figure 16.6 Height, weight and head circumference: boys aged 0–2 years. © Child Growth Foundation.

Caucasian children, a least in the first few years of life. As a rough guide, the mean percentile for an Asian child is the 25th percentile on the standard UK charts.

Figures 16.6–16.9 show standard height, weight and head circumference charts for UK boys and girls from birth to 2 years, and standard height and weight charts for UK boys and girls from 0 to 20 years. There are special growth charts for children with Down's syndrome and Turner's syndrome. It will be seen from the percentile charts that there is a wide range above and below the mean. Each chart shows the 0.4th, 2nd, 9th, 25th, 50th, 75th, 91st, 98th and 99.6th percentiles. The meaning of the term '10th percentile' is that 10% of all normal children are respectively lighter or shorter at the age concerned. Slightly different standards are applicable in different races and in different countries.

The term 'failure to thrive' is used to denote children whose weight gain is below that expected (see Figs 16.6 and 16.7).

HEAD CIRCUMFERENCE

In infants under the age of 2 the head circumference should be measured. The standard measurement is the occipitofrontal circumference. Hydrocephalus should be suspected when the rate of growth of the head is greater than normal for the sex, age and size of the infant. Rather than using a chart showing the head circumference alone, it is more useful to use one that combines head circumference, length and weight percentiles, so that the proportions of each individual child can be compared. An additional advantage of these charts is that they allow for prematurity, and so separate charts for preterm babies are not necessary.

BLOOD PRESSURE

Abnormalities of blood pressure are uncommon in childhood, and because the measurement of blood pressure can be frightening it need only be measured when cardiovascular or renal disease is

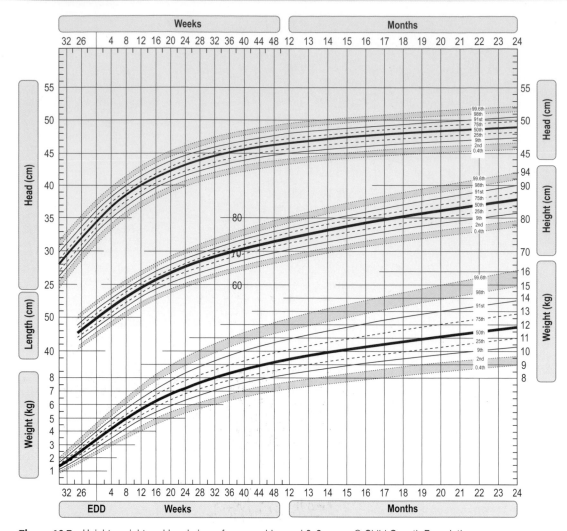

Figure 16.7   Height, weight and head circumference: girls aged 0–2 years. © Child Growth Foundation.

suspected. It should always be carried out at the end of the examination, and preferably when the child is almost dressed. Let the child play with the sphygmomanometer cuff, and talk in simple terms about what is going to happen. The size of the cuff is most important if accurate readings are to be obtained, and a variety of sizes should be available. The inflatable bag should be long enough to encircle the full circumference of the upper arm, and should be of a width roughly equal to one-third of the length of the upper arm and forearm as far as the wrist. Electronic blood pressure monitors are routinely used in most hospitals and are more accurate than most manual methods. In small children and infants the pulse can be palpated to obtain the systolic blood pressure. In babies, the *flush method* may be used. The arm is held up and tightly bandaged to exclude the blood to the level of the cuff, which is then inflated. The bandage is then removed to reveal a white limb. The pressure in the cuff is slowly reduced; the point at which the skin flushes is an approximate indication of the systolic blood pressure. Doppler techniques more accurately measure blood pressure in children, but these are not always available. The blood pressure in the legs must be measured in all suspected cases of coarctation of the aorta.

The blood pressure in the arms is about 65/45 mmHg in the newborn, 75/50 at 1 year, 85/60 at 4 years, 95/65 at 8 years, and 100/70 at 10 years of age.

TEMPERATURE

It is not always necessary to take the temperature as part of the routine examination of children. Fever is a very common finding in children, and may be due to excitement, exercise and minor infections, as well as to severe infections and other serious illnesses. Small infants often respond to infection with low temperatures.

Oral temperature measurements are rarely taken nowadays, and then only in older children. Axillary

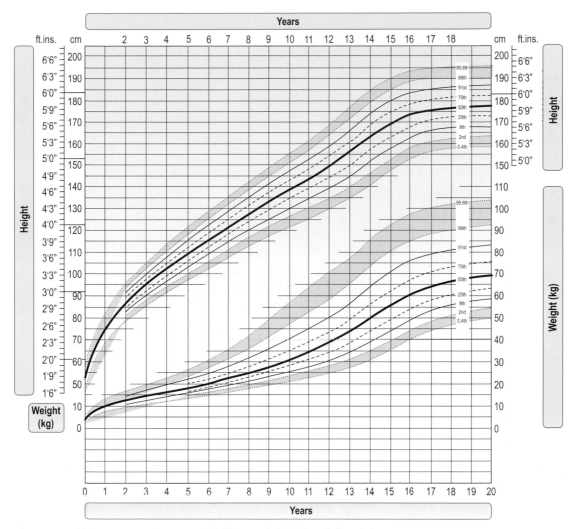

Figure 16.8   Height and weight: boys aged 0–20 years. © Child Growth Foundation.

temperatures are more usually taken, and are 0.5°C lower than oral temperature. Rectal temperature is seldom if ever taken. The more usual way of taking temperature in current use is via the tympanic membrane. This is difficult in a wriggling child, and is probably best used in infants over 3 years of age. The use of chemical dot strips to measure skin temperature is common and easier and safer for parents at home than using glass thermometers. Rapid rises of temperature to 39.5 or 40°C are not uncommon in children under 5, and may be associated with a convulsion.

STOOLS

Never be afraid to see a dirty nappy, or stool. This is part of the examination of a baby, and it is important to know the normal appearance of stools in childhood. The stools of a breastfed infant may be loose and green or pasty and yellow. They have a characteristic odour. Infants fed on cows' milk preparations pass stools that are a paler yellow colour and much firmer in consistency. Babies fed on the newer, modified cows' milk preparations have clay-coloured or greenish stools. The character of the stool in older children is more variable than in adults. Some healthy children pass frequent, loose stools containing undigested vegetable matter – 'toddler's diarrhoea'. The stools of children with coeliac disease or cystic fibrosis are bulky, odoriferous and quite characteristic.

URINE

Collection of urine specimens in infants is difficult, and special techniques are required. Most preferable is a 'clean catch' sample specimen, as many babies pass urine during examination. If you are considering that the child may have a urinary tract infection the parent should be given a sterile bowl or other container to catch the urine as it is passed. Urine can be tested immediately with reagent strips.

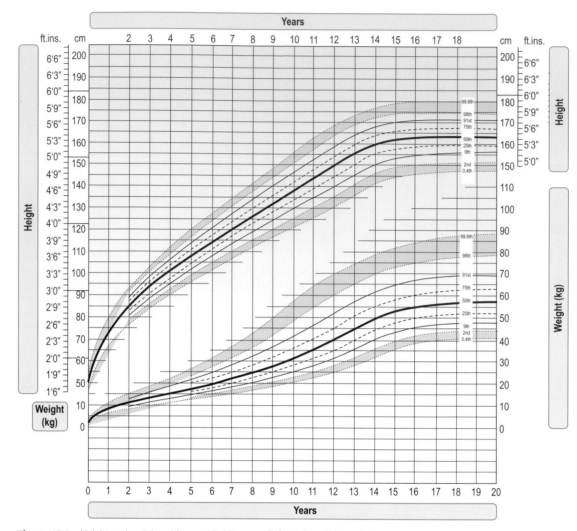

Figure 16.9   Height and weight: girls aged 0–20 years. © Child Growth Foundation.

If it is positive for leukocytes, bacteria or nitrites the specimen should be sent immediately to the laboratory, followed as soon as possible by a second sample. Alternatively, specially made sterile plastic containers with an adhesive opening can be applied to the washed genitalia, but this is liable to be contaminated and the method is unreliable other than as a possible pointer to infection. Unless the child is unwell he or she should not be treated on the strength of a positive reagent strip test, as false positives are common. The results of microscopy and culture should be awaited before treatment is commenced. However, if the child is febrile, there is no other obvious source of infection and the reagent strip is positive, it is reasonable to give an antibiotic such as trimethoprim and review the child after 3 days, by which time the microscopy and culture results should be available. Faecal contamination of urine specimens can be a problem however the urine is collected, and it may be necessary to resort to suprapubic aspiration of bladder urine, a procedure which is not too difficult in infants.

DEVELOPMENTAL SCREENING EXAMINATION

Development is the normal process of maturation of function that takes place in the early years of life. It may be modified by emotional difficulties, environment, and physical defects and illnesses. Lack of intellectual stimulation, and of the normal experiences of childhood, may result in apparent retardation of development. This is commonly seen in children from a neglecting family, which is the commonest variety of child abuse.

All infants should have a simple developmental screening examination at regular intervals. Table 16.2 lists the important milestones. Detailed developmental assessment is a specialist subject, but it is important for all those who examine children to be

Table 16.2 Normal developmental milestones

Age	Movement and posture	Vision and manipulation	Hearing and speech	Social behaviour
6 weeks	When pulled from supine to sitting, head lag is not quite complete (Fig. 16.11) When held prone, head is held in line with body When prone on couch, lifts chin off couch Primitive responses persist	Looks at toy, held in midline Follows a moving person	Vocalizes with gurgles	Smiles briefly when talked to by mother
4 months	Holds head up in sitting position, and is steady Pulls to sitting with only minimal head lag (Fig. 16.12) When prone, with head and chest off couch, makes swimming movements Rolls from prone to supine Primitive responses gone	Watches his or her hands Pulls at his or her clothes Tries to grasp objects	Turns head to sound Vocalizes apparently appropriately Laughs	Recognizes mother Becomes excited by toys
7 months	Sits unsupported Rolls from supine to prone Can support weight when held, and bounces with pleasure When prone, bears weight on hands	Transfers objects from hand to hand Bangs toys on table Watches small moving objects	Says 'Da', 'Ba', 'Ka'	Tries to feed him- or herself Puts objects in mouth Plays with paper
10 months	Crawls Gets to sitting position without help Can pull up to standing Lifts one foot when standing	Reaches for objects with index finger Has developed a finger–thumb grasp Will place objects in the examiner's hands, but not release them	Says one word with meaning	Plays 'peep bo' and 'pat-a-cake' Waves 'bye-bye' Deliberately drops objects so that they can be picked up Puts objects in and out of boxes
13 months	Walks unsupported May shuffle on buttocks and hands	Can hold two cubes in one hand Makes marks with pen	Says two or three words with meaning	Understands simple questions such as 'Where is your shoe?' May kiss on request Tends to be shy
15 months	Can get into standing position without support Climbs upstairs Walks with broad-based gait	Builds a tower of two cubes Takes off shoes	Will say around 12 words, but mostly gobbledegook	Asks for things by pointing Kisses pictures of animals Can use a cup
18 months	Climbs stairs unaided holding rail Runs and jumps Can climb onto a chair and sit down	Builds tower of three cubes Turns pages of a book two or three at a time Scribbles Takes off gloves and socks Unzips fasteners	Is beginning to join two words together	Recognizes animals and cars in a book Points to nose, ear etc. on request Clean and dry but with occasional accidents Carries out simple orders

able to carry out a brief developmental screening examination, and to be aware of all the basic milestones.

It is usual to consider development under four main headings:

- Movement and posture
- Vision and manipulation
- Hearing and speech
- Social behaviour.

Screening for developmental delay involves testing the child's performance of a few skills in each of the four fields of development, and comparing the results with the average for children of the same age. The range of normal developmental progress is wide, and the milestones shown in Table 16.2 are those of an average normal baby. Delay in all fields of development is more significant than delay in one only, and severe delay is more meaningful than slight delay. There are considerable individual variations, and lateness in one particular area should not be taken as evidence of mental handicap or cerebral palsy without other corroborating features.

Allowance must always be made for those infants who were born prematurely, at least until the age of 2 years, by which time they should have caught up.

TECHNIQUES USED

The same rules apply to the techniques used in developmental screening as to those of general physical examination. Time has to be spent gaining the friendship of the child. This time can be profitably utilized by offering, for example, a 10-month-old baby a small toy to see how they grasp it and react to it. Let the baby play with the toys and bricks while sitting on the mother's lap, and if the child remains suspicious, get the mother to offer the various objects. As with all parts of the examination, much more is learned by simply watching a child play and watching his or her reactions to the surroundings.

In the UK, developmental screening is usually carried out by the health visitor. There is always an assessment at 8 months, and usually at 18 months and sometimes at 24 months, but different areas have differing ages of assessment, or are making 18- and 24-month tests more selective by concentrating on 'at-risk' children. The health visitor is trained in developmental skills and will refer to a doctor babies about whom there is any suspicion.

TESTING VISION

Much will be learned about a child's vision by observation. Note whether the child is looking around the room and at particular toys, or staring at nothing in particular, especially if there are random or nystagmoid eye movements: the latter suggest that the child is unable to see. When he or she picks toys up, is accommodation normal? The routine examination of the eye has been dealt with in the first part of this chapter.

Checks of *visual acuity* are not easy in young babies. By 6 weeks of age babies should be following their mother with their eyes and by 6 months they should be able to follow a rolling ball at 3 metres. This is the basis of one method of visual testing at this age. The ability of the child to follow rolling balls of differing diameters gives an accurate assessment of visual acuity. From the age of approximately 2 years, the *Sheridan–Gardiner test* is used. This is a simple comparison test, with the examiner indicating letters or familiar toys on a board, and asking the child to indicate a similar object on a board held by the mother. The acuity is the ability of the child to pick out the smallest objects (see Chapter 18).

TESTING HEARING

In the past, it was usual to check the hearing for the first time between 6 and 8 months of age. Although this is still the case in some areas, there is now a national screening programme for all newborn babies, based on otoacoustic emissions for testing the hearing of neonates and on brainstem auditory evoked potentials for vulnerable babies. Examples of vulnerable babies are where there is a family history of deafness, and in babies who have received ototoxic antibiotics such as aminoglycosides.

Distraction testing is now being phased out in the UK, but details are given as some centres may still need to use it. The test has a large observer error and many children shown subsequently to be deaf pass the distraction test! It does require a quiet room, which can be difficult to find in the average children's unit, and so is now more used as a quick screening test before referring for more specialized testing.

Health visitors use a questionnaire at 8 months of age, concentrating in particular on high-risk factors (Box 16.7), and specifically on the parent's perception of the child's hearing.

To carry out the distraction test, sit the baby on the mother's lap, facing outwards. It helps if an assistant can sit facing them to distract the child with toys etc. (but not funny noises). The examiner then makes a series of soft noises to one side or the other but behind mother and child and out of the child's line of vision (Fig. 16.10). The sounds used are a special high-frequency rattle, a bell, a spoon in a cup, and the rustle of tissue paper or a whisper. At 6 months a baby should turn to the source of the sound when it is about 45 cm from the ear. By 9 months they react more quickly and localize the sound at a distance of 90 cm. If the child fails the test on the first occasion it does not automatically mean that he or she is deaf, but the test should be repeated after a further month. If the child still fails, he or she should be referred for audiological testing.

Box 16.7 Hearing questionnaire for 8-month-old babies

CHILD'S NAME

DATE OF BIRTH

A High-risk factors for deafness
1. FAMILY HISTORY of deafness which required special education or hearing aid fitting in childhood, or an inherited condition known to be associated with childhood deafness, even though there is no known deafness in the family.
    YES   NO
2. CONGENITAL MALFORMATIONS either of chromosomal, syndromic or unknown aetiology, including craniofacial, branchial arch and cervical spine dysmorphologies, cleft palates, and pinna malformations even if unilateral, but excluding isolated ear pits and tags.
    YES   NO
3. CONGENITAL INFECTIONS, including clinically apparent rubella, cytomegalovirus, toxoplasmosis, herpes and syphilis, and also any maternal history of possible infection in pregnancy even in the absence of neonatal stigmata.
    YES   NO
4. PERINATAL ILLNESS requiring admission to the Special Care Baby Unit but only to include those babies with:
    - Gestation of less than 32 weeks
    - Birthweight of 1.25 kg or less
    - An Apgar score of 3 or less at 5 minutes
    - Cerebral illness, e.g. intraventricular haemorrhage, convulsions, meningitis
    - Apnoea requiring ventilation for 4 hours or more
    - Jaundice where exchange transfusion has been considered or undertaken
    - Administration of aminoglycosides at potentially toxic levels.
    YES   NO
5. POSTNATAL ILLNESS of bacterial meningitis, head injury with loss of consciousness or neurological disease.
    YES   NO

B Hearing responses
Go through 'hearing' information leaflet with parents. Try to elicit from them clear examples of the baby's responses to loud and quiet sounds.
    Having done this:
1. Do the parents have any concerns about the baby's hearing?
    YES   NO
2. Do you have any concerns about the baby's hearing?
    YES   NO

C Voice and speech development
The baby should enjoy using his or her voice freely, with variations in pitch and tone.
    The baby should have started making repetitive consonant/vowel sequences, e.g. 'baba', 'mum-mum', i.e. babbling.
1. Do the parents have any concerns about the baby's speech development?
    YES   NO
2. Do you have any concerns about the baby's speech development?
    YES   NO

D Middle ear problems
1. Has the baby had recurrent ear infections requiring treatment?
    YES   NO
2. Has the baby had recurrent upper respiratory tract infections thought to be associated with hearing loss?
    YES   NO
    If YES to any of the above, refer the baby to the secondary audiology clinic (or to the tertiary clinic if a severe loss of hearing is suspected).

E Is there parental consanguinity?
    YES   NO   UNCERTAIN
    Do not make a referral on this factor alone but, if present, take particular care at this and subsequent interviews.

ACTION
F Has a referral been completed?
    YES   NO
If yes, to whom?
Signature of interviewer
Name (please print)
Date of interview

HEAD CONTROL
By 4 months babies can normally keep their head in line with the trunk when pulled from supine to sitting, and when held in the sitting position will keep their head upright. Before this age the head lags behind the trunk (Figs 16.11, 16.12).

Table 16.2 shows the normal development milestones up to the age of 18 months, by which time obvious deviations from normal development will be apparent. Beyond this age developmental testing is more specialized, and is not the concern of this chapter. A baby who appears to have delayed development on screening will need further specialized assessment to establish causation and management.

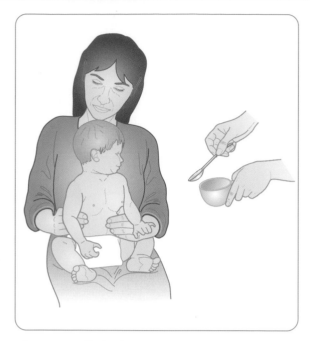

Figure 16.10   Testing hearing at 6 months.

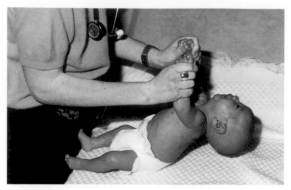

Figure 16.11   Head control at 6 weeks of age.

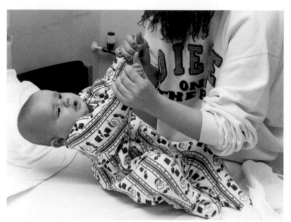

Figure 16.12   Head control at 4 months of age.

EXAMINATION OF THE NEWBORN

The routine examination of the newborn infant (Box 16.8) is designed to assess the general state of health and to detect congenital abnormalities. It is recommended that all babies should be examined within the first 24 hours of life, and again before the end of the first week. Many parts of the examination of the newborn infant are similar to the techniques described above for older babies and children.

The neurological status at birth has implications for the future development of the child, and has been used as an indicator of brain damage sustained during or shortly after birth. The *Apgar Score* (Box 16.9) is in general use as part of this assessment. An Apgar score of 6 or less at 5 minutes after birth is associated with neurological deficit in about 10% of cases, but a low score 1 minute after birth is less predictive of brain damage. A high Apgar score at 5 minutes, on the other hand, may not be sensitive to focal brain injury or infarction.

Weight will usually have been measured by the midwife. Length is not commonly measured nowadays, and the head circumference (occipitofrontal) may not be measured before 48 hours, to allow for moulding to subside. Note the time of passage of the first urine and meconium, which is the dark green, sticky stool of the newborn baby in the first few days of life.

Always examine a newborn baby in front of his or her mother, and involve her at all stages by explaining what you are doing. Have the baby undressed, and in a warm place. Always have warm hands and treat the baby gently, leaving the most unpleasant parts of the examination until last. Talk or even sing to the baby: he or she is as aware of what is going on as an older child, and should be afforded the same courtesy.

Much of the time can be spent just watching the baby, noting the state of awareness. If the baby is awake, seemingly looking around and not crying, examination of the nervous system will yield much information.

THE SKIN

Note the colour of the skin. *Peripheral cyanosis* is a common finding in the normal newborn, but *central cyanosis* indicates cardiac or respiratory disease. So-called '*traumatic cyanosis*' affects the head and neck and is produced by confluent petechial haemorrhages; it is most often seen after prolonged or obstructed labour. Jaundice is common *after* 48 hours in most preterm and some term babies, and is considered physiological. However, jaundice *within* 48 hours of birth has to be considered pathological; the commonest cause is haemolytic disease of the newborn, but any baby jaundiced before 48 hours or after 7 days of age needs to be investigated.

Look for birthmarks, which are either pigmented lesions or haemangiomata. Most babies have a collection of dilated capillaries on the upper eyelids and nape of the neck (sometimes called 'stork bites'), which fade after a few weeks. Some babies develop a crop of small papules on the trunk during the first week (*erythema toxicum* or *urticaria neonatorum*). These are of uncertain cause, of no significance, and usually fade after a few days. Superficial peeling of the skin, especially over the periphery, is common, and is most apparent in post-term and some small-for-gestational-age babies. *Milia* are whitish pinhead spots concentrated mainly around the nose. They are sebaceous retention cysts, and can be felt with the finger. They usually disappear within a month. *Lanugo hair* may cover the body, especially in preterm babies and some dark-haired babies. It usually disappears over the first 2 or 3 weeks. Colour of hair at birth is no guide to subsequent hair colour. *Mongolian blue spot* is the name given to the normal dark blue areas of pigmentation commonly seen over the sacrum and but-tocks or back of the legs in black and Asian babies, as well as some from the Mediterranean region.

THE FACE

Look at the face for obvious abnormalities, such as Down's syndrome and other indications of craniofacial maldevelopment. Check the position of the ears, and whether they are normal and symmetrical. Accessory auricles are small, pedunculated skin tags, usually just in front of the ears, and can be dealt with by tying them off at the base. Make sure that the upper lip is intact.

Once the superficial examination has been completed, more formal examination takes place; again, this should be regional rather than by systems, starting with the head and working down.

THE HEAD

Inspect and palpate the head. The bones of the cranial vault, being relatively soft and connected only by fibrous tissue, change shape readily in response to external pressure. Moulding of the skull takes place during birth, with overriding of the sutures. It usually disappears after a few days. The *caput succedaneum* is an area of oedema of the scalp over the part of the head that presented during labour. It pits on pressure and is not fluctuant. A *cephal-haematoma* is a subperiosteal haematoma which appears a few days after birth as a large, cystic swelling limited to the area of one of the skull bones. It tends to resolve relatively slowly over a few months, and may leave a calcified edge. The anterior fontanelle varies considerably at birth, but should be checked, as described above (p. 326).

THE EYES

The eyes can best be examined when they are open spontaneously. Alternatively, the eyelids can be held open by an assistant, although this tends to make the baby cry. Sometimes a baby will open the eyes if given a feed. The iris gives no indication of its future colour, and is usually greyish-blue in Caucasian infants. A bluish tinge to the sclera is usual. Tears before 3–4 weeks are unusual. Even though newborn infants can see, eye movements tend to be random, often giving the impression of a transient squint. Subconjunctival haemorrhages show as a dark red patch covering the sclera, sometimes ringing the cornea. They commonly follow normal deliveries, and despite their alarming appearance are of no consequence and disappear after a few weeks. Look for evidence of conjunctivitis and check for other abnormalities as described above (p. 329). In particular check for the red reflex, as its absence could indicate a major ophthalmic problem, such as a retinoblastoma or cataract.

THE MOUTH AND TONGUE

Look inside the mouth; this is easy if the baby is crying, and a spatula will not be needed. If the baby is quiet and content, this part of the examination may be left until later. Make sure that there is no cleft of the palate, and note particularly whether the uvula is normal. A bifid uvula indicates a sub-mucous cleft of the palate, which requires surgery. Rounded, thickened areas are often seen on the lips, more especially on the lower lips, and are known as *suckling blisters*. This is a misnomer, as despite their name they do not contain fluid. *Epithelial pearls* are small white areas, best seen on the hard palate. Occasionally teeth are present at birth. They are usually incisors, and can be green in colour. If loose, they are best removed. *Macroglossia* is seen in babies with Down's syndrome, congential hypothyroidism, Beckwith's syndrome, and in some normal children.

THE NECK

The neck of a newborn baby seems rather short, and may be considered abnormal by the inexperienced. Rarely, cystic swellings are seen: *dermoid cysts* and *thyroglossal cysts* in the midline, or *branchial cysts* just in front of the upper third of the sternomastoid muscle.

THE LIMBS

Examine the limbs for abnormalities. Extra digits on the hand are not uncommon and are often familial, but are rarer on the feet. Look for a single transverse palmar crease, which is classically seen in babies with Down's syndrome, but in addition is found in a variety of dysmorphic syndromes, as well as in some normal infants. Common foot abnormalities to look for are syndactyly or talipes equinovarus; the latter requires immediate orthopaedic referral.

THE CHEST

The general appearance and shape of the chest should be noticed. Breast enlargement with exuda-tion of a milky fluid from the nipples is sometimes seen in newborn infants of either sex. This is due to transferred maternal hormones, and disappears in a few days without causing problems. Resist the temptation to squeeze the breasts, as this may result in infection (*mastitis*). Make sure that the clavicles are intact. Note the symmetry of the chest wall, the pattern of respiration, and whether there is any indrawing on inspiration. The remainder of the chest examination is as described earlier for older children; percussion of the chest is of even less value at this age. Transient systolic murmurs are extremely common in the first few days, and may reflect the closing ductus arteriosus or non-specific flow murmurs, as discussed earlier.

THE ABDOMEN

The abdomen of a newborn baby usually seems a little distended and moves with respiration. Slight divarication of the rectus muscles may occur, and this exaggerates this abdominal bulging. The liver edge is palpable 2–4 cm below the costal margin, and the lower poles of both kidneys can be easily felt. The bladder should not be palpable if the baby has just passed urine. Check the umbilical stump: it should contain two arteries and one vein. A single umbilical artery is associated with an increased inci-dence of congenital abnormalities, especially of the renal tract. The umbilical cord should become dry, and then separate between the sixth and tenth days. Some moistness of the stump remains for a further few days. Sometimes excess granulation tissue accu-mulates to form a small granuloma; this can be treated by local application of a silver nitrate stick.

THE PERINEUM AND GENITALIA

Examine the perineum for hypospadias, hydroceles, hernias or undescended testicles. Look for patency of the anus: an imperforate anus is easily over-looked unless it is specifically checked for. While looking at the buttocks and anus, see if there is a sacral dimple, which is usually a blind-ending pit and of no significance. Make sure that the back is straight and that there are no gross spinal lesions, especially spina bifida. Check female external geni-talia for clitoral enlargement – which would suggest a virilizing condition such as congenital adrenal hyperplasia due to 21-hydroxylase deficiency – and for labial fusion. It is not unusual for girls to have a mucous vaginal discharge, and sometimes bleeding. This is the result of transferred maternal hormones and is usually transient. Make sure that the femoral pulses are palpable.

NEUROLOGICAL ASSESSMENT

Combine a formal neurological examination with observation of the baby's behaviour. No two babies react in the same way, but there is a broad, general pattern that applies to most. Spontaneous move-ment normally takes place when the baby is awake and consists of alternating flexion and extension. Any marked difference between the two sides is abnormal. The fingers are more fully flexed than later in childhood, but spontaneous opening and closing of the hands takes place. The thumb may be tucked under the fingers.

The normal position of a newborn baby is one of flexion. When lying prone, the baby's legs are usually drawn up under the abdomen. If the baby is crying, look for any weakness or paralysis in the face, suggesting injury to the facial nerve, or any deficiency of arm movements suggesting injury to the brachial plexus. Note the limb tone, and although tendon jerks are difficult to elicit at this age they should be checked, using a finger rather than a tendon hammer.

PRIMITIVE REFLEXES

Primitive responses are present in the normal newborn infant and disappear at variable times up to 4 months of age. They are responses to specific stimuli, and depend to some extent on the infant's state of wakefulness. The absence of one or more of these reflexes in the newborn infant may indicate some abnormality of the brain, a local abnormality in the affected limb, or a neuromuscular abnormality. Elicitation of these reflexes in front of the mother is often a source of amusement and pleasure to her. Persistence of primitive reflexes beyond the fourth month of life should alert you to the possibility of developmental delay. These reflex responses are as follows:

- Rooting reflexes. In response to a touch on the cheek, a baby will turn his or her head towards the stimulus. Stimulation of the upper lip causes opening of the mouth, pouting of the lips, and tongue movements. Sucking itself is a reflex, and failure of the sucking response beyond the 36th week of gestation suggests significant neurological impairment.
- Palmar and plantar grasp. A finger placed across the child's palm will cause flexion and grasping of the finger. A similar response is seen if a finger is placed on the plantar surface of the foot, but the plantar grasp is not as strong.
- Stepping reflex. The baby is held upright and the feet placed on a firm surface. As the foot presses down, the other leg flexes at the hip and knee in a stepping movement. As this response is alternated from one leg to the other the baby makes a walking movement.
- The Moro reflex. This is the best-known of the primitive reflexes, but it must not be forgotten that because it is a 'startle' reaction it will make the baby cry. It should therefore be left to the end of the examination. Always be gentle in

carrying out the test, and make sure that the baby is well supported. The baby's body is supported with one arm and hand, and the head with the other. The hand holding the head is then lowered a few centimetres, allowing the baby's head to drop back (Fig. 16.13). In a positive response the baby abducts and extends the arms, and then flexes them. A clearly unilateral response suggests some local abnormality, such as a fracture or brachial plexus injury in the arm on the side that does not respond.

ASSESSMENT OF GESTATION

Although a full assessment of gestation is beyond the scope of this chapter, a rough approximation of the baby's gestational age should always be made, especially if the baby is small. This can be made from a combination of maternal menstrual data, and the size and appearance of the baby. The flexed position of the baby at term has already been mentioned, and the more immature the baby, the less flexed he or she will be. Certain physical criteria are the basis of more formal assessments. Among these are the shape and form of the ears: is the pinna flat against the skull and unfolded, or is it folded over with a good development of cartilage? The degree of breast formation, the degree of ossification of the skull, and opacification of the skull to transillumination with a bright light are important specific features.

A neurological assessment, especially of muscle tone and movement, and the development of certain reflexes, will also give a guide to gestation. For example, by 32 weeks the baby will turn his or her head towards a diffuse light; by 34–36 weeks sucking and neck-righting reflexes will have developed.

At the end of the examination of the newborn infant, a comment should always be made on the estimated gestation.

EXAMINATION OF THE HIPS

Examination of the hips is essential but should be left to the end because it is very uncomfortable for the baby. It is illustrated in Figures 16.14 and 16.15. It is usual to differentiate between a tendinous 'click' and the typical 'clunk' of a hip moving in and out of its socket. The latter is more a feeling than an actual noise. Skin creases on the upper posterior thigh may be asymmetrical, but this is not a reliable sign of dislocation; similarly, limitation of abduction is not absolutely reliable. If there is any doubt about the hip, ultrasound examination should be carried out. Routine ultrasound examination of the hips of all at-risk newborn babies should be carried out to screen for congenital dislocation (Box 16.10). At-risk babies are those where there is a breech

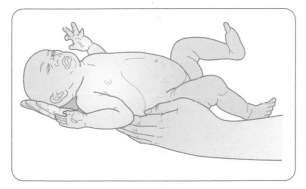

Figure 16.13 Eliciting the Moro reflex.

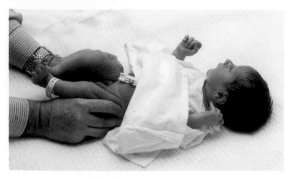

Figure 16.14 Stage 1 of the examination of the hips: the hips are flexed, rotated medially and pushed posteriorly. This will dislocate dislocatable hips.

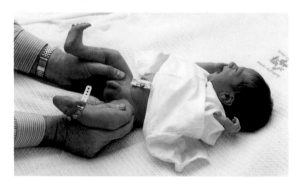

Figure 16.15 Stage 2 of the examination of the hips: the hips are abducted and a 'click' or a 'clunk' is felt for (see text). Note the position of the examiner's hands, with the thumbs on the medial aspect of the thigh and the fingers over the lateral trochanters.

delivery, a family history of congenital dislocation of the hip (especially if female), and any baby in an unusual intrauterine position.

SCREENING FOR GENETIC DISORDERS

There are a number of disorders for which screening is available by testing at birth, and others that may be tested for by measurement of white blood cell enzymes, e.g. gangliosidosis and other lipid storage disorders. In most of these, tests are not carried out routinely, except in genetically isolated populations, or in families known to be at risk. In the UK, all newborn infants are screened for phenylketonuria

Box 16.10   Babies at greater risk of congenital dislocation of the hip

- Breech extraction
- Primipara with extended breech delivery
- Females
- Family history of congenital dislocation

Box 16.11   Inherited conditions screened for at birth

- Phenylketonuria
- Hypothyroidism
- Haemoglobinopathies in vulnerable groups
- Cystic fibrosis in affected families
- Congenital adrenal hyperplasia

and hypothyroidism by a heel-prick blood test at 7 days. Other conditions can be screened for in vulnerable populations (Box 16.11). Direct DNA analysis for genetic disorders is becoming increasingly available for many inherited disorders.

Having now completed the examination, the baby should be dressed and, as in every examination of children, your findings must be conveyed to the parents.

CONCLUSIONS

Throughout this chapter, emphasis has been placed on getting to know the child and treating him or her as gently as possible. Time has to be spent gaining the child's confidence, and indeed building up your own. This can only be acquired by examining or playing with children at each and every opportunity. Students have a natural anxiety when approaching young children, and it is only by play and being with them that confidence in examining them will develop. One of the most rewarding parts of paediatrics is when a child sits on your lap and plays happily with you, and waves good-bye to you as he/she leaves the room. If you can achieve this, you know how to examine children.

Older people

A. Feather

INTRODUCTION

'In the end, it's not the years in your life that count. It's the life in your years.'

Abraham Lincoln

At the turn of the twentieth century there were 65 000 people in the UK aged 85 or older. By 2050 it is projected there will be more than three million. Old age is still associated with frailty, disability and loss of independence. The positive aspects of ageing, such as sagacity, maturity and experience, are too often neglected. One hopes that these commonly held negative beliefs about growing old will gradually disappear, as the period between the average age of onset of disability in the old and the average age of death narrows and the elderly enjoy healthier lives.

Age is traditionally defined in terms of *chronological age*. Older people are considered in three distinct chronological groups: the *young old* (65–74), the *old* (75–84), and the *very old* (85+). However, older people are a very heterogeneous group and each old person should be respected as an individual and not merely classed according to their chronological age. Frailty, disability and dependency are not synonymous with getting old. The accumulation of disability resulting from chronic disease and environmental insults must be separated from the process of merely getting older, i.e. *senescence*. People age at different rates, and it is the interplay of environmental, genetic and acquired pathological processes that determines an individual's *biological age*. *Functional age* takes into account the combination of a person's biological and chronological ages and, although difficult to define, this concept circumvents the negative implications of grouping individuals together because of arbitrary socioeconomic or statutory definitions, such as 'pensioner'. With an increasingly healthy and longer-lived population these concepts will require redefinition according to functional ability.

PRESENTATION OF DISEASE IN OLDER PEOPLE

Two major factors influence the recognition of disease processes in older people:

- Acceptance of ill-health, with delay in seeking help
- Atypical presentation of disease processes.

The acceptance of ill-health and disease as 'ageing', with its resultant disabilities, means that many older people *expect* to be frail, rarely complain, and often seek help late. Coming to terms with some disability or change is necessary at all ages, and acceptance is part of survival. However, the tacit acceptance of inevitable deterioration – for example in vision, hearing, teeth and feet – may lead to treatable conditions being ignored and result in loss of independence. Table 17.1 illustrates what may be regarded as normal ageing and what is pathological.

The range of presentation of disease in old age is an essential element for the student and practitioner to comprehend. The term '*geriatric giants*' (Box 17.1) refers to a set of symptoms and signs that occur in old age which may have as their cause *many* different disease processes. In normal day-to-day circumstances ageing organs are able to maintain normal metabolic function. However, when major stressors are experienced, as in acute illness, functional capacity is exceeded and rapid clinical deterioration may occur. In the elderly patient multiorgan failure may develop rapidly in the context of illness, especially infections. Another important concept is that of *multiple comorbidities*, which may be causally linked, although more typically they are not. *Iatrogenic illness*, most commonly due to *polypharmacy*, often exacerbates disability in the older person.

Recognition of the *social presentation* of disease is of major importance in older patients. The '*social admission*' to hospital and the subsequent failure to cope with this upheaval, often termed '*acopia*' (a made-up word), usually indicates a poor level of information gathering in the process of history taking, examination and investigation. The likelihood of the disease process leading to social decompensation, e.g. relatives leaving a person in the Emergency Department, or the breakdown of the old person's level of physical and mental function during hospitalization or illness at home, can usually be predicted and hence often prevented, thereby avoiding secondary disability.

Table 17.1   Normal ageing and changes in body systems

System	Normal ageing	Pathophysiological changes common in older age
Cardiovascular	Slight increase in heart size Normal stroke volume and left ventricular ejection fraction Exertional oxygen consumption declines 7.5–10% per decade; thus exercise tolerance is reduced	Ischaemic heart disease Heart failure Valvular heart disease Peripheral vascular disease Aneurysms
Respiratory	Vital capacity: 40% reduction by age 70 FEV_1 and FVC: 30% reduction by age 80 Progressive reduction in PEFR after age 30	Haemoptysis Chronic obstructive pulmonary disease (COPD) Lung fibrosis Lung cancers
Alimentary	Reduced and abnormal peristalsis: 'presby-oesophagus' Slower colonic transit Reduced absorption of some nutrients; reduced energy requirements	Weight loss Dysphagia Change in bowel habit Bleeding from the upper or lower GI tract
Hepatobiliary	Reduced hepatic mass and metabolic reserve but maintenance of normal function	Jaundice Deranged liver function tests, including abnormal clotting
Renal	Reduced GFR and numbers of functional tubules and glomeruli Reduced serum creatinine due to loss of muscle mass	Renal impairment with raised serum creatinine Haematuria
Genitourinary	*Men* – Reduced testosterone Normal FSH/LH 50% of men over 70 have 'abundant spermatogenesis' *Women* – postmenopausal low oestradiol; raised FSH and LH Loss of female reproductive capability Atrophic vaginitis due to low oestrogen levels Loss of sexual interest may also occur, but this is complex and multifactorial	Erectile dysfunction Prostatic enlargement Bladder outflow tract symptoms Postmenopausal bleeding (PMB) Urinary incontinence Painful intercourse
Nervous system, including higher senses	High-frequency hearing loss Vision: Close focusing declines from age 40 Distinguishing fine detail (reduced acuity) declines after 70 years. Loss of muscle mass leads to decline in strength Reduced mental agility and minor loss of mental ability	Deafness, tinnitus and vertigo Glaucoma, macular degeneration Cataracts Dementia and delirium Hemiparesis, paraparesis Many other factors, including reduced distal sensation, vascular disease, poor balance
Endocrine	Pituitary dysfunction Abnormal thyroid function Pancreatic function Reduced adrenal response to stress	Hyponatraemia Hypothyroidism Impaired glucose tolerance and frank diabetes mellitus
Musculoskeletal	Increased body fat and loss of muscle mass (although this may be retarded with exercise)	Osteoarthritis and vertebral spondylosis Osteoporosis
Dermatological	Loss of collagen in the skin leads to thin, paparaceous skin Ecchymoses and senile purpura	Basal and squamous cell carcinoma Solar keratoses Malignant melanoma
Haematological and immune system	Loss of T-cell function with age may be associated with late-onset autoimmune disease Possible link between changes in immune system and: (a) Age-related cancers (b) Response to disease	Anaemia Myelodyplasia Haematological malignancies Chronic lymphatic lymphoma and myeloma

Box 17.1 The 'geriatric giants': major clinical syndromes that may result from any disease process

- Immobility, instability/falls
- Incontinence
- Intellectual impairment/confusion
- Pressure sores
- Impaired senses: vision, hearing and speech and language

Box 17.2 History taking: points to note

- The introduction – observation as they enter; greeting
- Cadence and interest
- Position and comfort of patient
- Vision, hearing, cognition
- Environment
- Autonomy and respect
- Use of multiple sources of information
- Interview versus interrogation

Proper diagnosis and management in older people requires the identification and treatment of amenable clinical problems, and recognition of the special needs and the specific clinical presentations of older people. Thus, social aspects of care may be as important as the disease process itself. Understanding this encourages a patient-centred multidisciplinary team approach. Caring for older people requires clinical acumen and much skill. Geriatricians not only recognize diseases and their presentations in older people, but perhaps equally importantly act as their patients' advocate in all areas of healthcare.

HISTORY

Taking a good history is always essential but requires particular sensitivity in the elderly. Respect for autonomy should always be afforded, just as for the young. 'Don't talk about patients, talk with them', especially when dealing with carers. Negotiate how much information the patient would like to share with carers when giving investigation results or trying to obtain corroborative information. Avoid being judgemental and paternalistic. The grey-haired are not necessarily disabled or confused! Even severely physically disabled people, no matter what their age, may have the brightest minds.

There are several universal practical points in the way the history is approached which are particularly important when taking a history from an older patient (Box 17.2). *The first contact* is extremely important (Box 17.3). Eye contact, a greeting, an outstretched hand (expecting a returned handshake), your name and the purpose of the meeting are all that are required to begin with. These relatively simple gestures can provide a wealth of information in the first few minutes. *Depressed* and *very anxious* patients may avoid eye contact. The handshake is often revealing. Some patients with *dementia* may not respond, not recognizing the meaning of the social gesture. *Frightened* older patients may continue to clutch one's hand. Giving your name and purpose puts people at ease and can also be used later to assess short-term memory. Ask the person 'What is your name?'. Be alert for

Box 17.3 Observations during the introduction

- Can the patient see and hear you?
- Is behaviour normal?
- Is language normal?
- Does the patient understand your role as a doctor?
- Is the patient at ease, or in pain?
- Is there evidence of support from family or friends?

hearing impairment. The reply will indicate how a person wishes to be addressed; alternatively, the patient may be specifically asked this.

The environment should be changed to suit the individual patient, particularly if they are in a wheelchair, have multiple carers or are deaf. Ensure the patient puts on any spectacles or hearing aid. If they are hearing impaired, try to sit in a well-lit area to aid lip reading. Hearing impairment is such a common problem that any setting where older people are seen regularly should have a communication aid available. Talking at the bedside in a busy environment is accepted practice, but be sure the patient is really at ease, especially if any delicate or personal issues need to be discussed. Drawing the bed curtains offers some privacy and dignity to the patient but does not ensure privacy.

The cadence of the history may be slower than with younger people. Try to avoid interrupting the patient. There may be multiple medical and social issues, and it is important to let them tell the story in their own way, as they will often prioritize issues. Learning to interrupt politely and redirect the conversation is a necessary but difficult skill to learn. Only when the patient has given consent should you attempt to corroborate information with relatives or carers.

THE SOCIAL HISTORY AND SOCIAL NETWORKS

The social history has extra significance in older people. Routine questions regarding occupation, smoking and alcohol are often forgotten, but should provide a familiar stepping stone to discussing the

---

Box 17.4   Social networks

Informal
- Family, friends and neighbours: available, concerned and committed, familiar, flexible

Formal
- Financial entitlements: pension and other income
- Statutory services: health care and social services
- Voluntary services: church and charity

---

patient's home, how they are managing and what support they have. Find out the kind of home they live in, the number of internal and external stairs, where the toilet and bathroom are situated, and who does their cooking, shopping and cleaning. Remember that most older people, including many of those with severe functional impairment, live in private households. Many are dependent to a greater or lesser extent upon friends and relations who contribute to their social networks, whether informally or formally. No assessment of an older person with even a slight disability is complete without a description of the people who are available to help. The informal network of support consists of both direct and extended family, and friends and neighbours (Box 17.4). This network is usually limited in size but often has a long history of contact. Although perhaps less skilled than a formal network, it has the great advantage of being flexible, familiar and continuous. The formal network consists of any basic financial entitlements, such as pensions, statutory agencies and, in the UK, the NHS, which includes a community multidisciplinary team, and the local social services, e.g. home care, meals-on-wheels and daycare facilities. Local availability of these organizations will vary. Finally, voluntary organizations, religious authorities and other organizations can provide valuable help.

ACTIVITIES OF DAILY LIVING (ADL)

An enquiry about activities of daily living (ADL) provides useful information in patients with multiple disabilities and health problems (see Table 17.2), and informs the planning of treatment and future care. In general, patients who can dress, get about outdoors, are continent, can do their own housework and cooking and manage their own pension do not require much immediate enquiry other than about their presenting problem. Among the old and the very old, such patients are the exception. If a daily living task cannot be carried out, a detailed enquiry focusing on the reason for this must be made.

It is useful to obtain a 'premorbid' picture of the patient's ADLs. This provides a rough goal for the outcome of treatment. A patient who previously had limited functional abilities and needed a lot of help to remain independent is unlikely to return to an independent lifestyle after a serious illness. One cannot assume that an older person was free from disability before the onset of an acute illness, and a corroborative history of premorbid ability is essential in planning future needs.

DRUG HISTORY

Older people are prescribed more medication than any other age group. A treatment history checklist is useful when enquiring about current and past medications (Box 17.5). This is applicable to any patient with chronic illness or multiple comorbidities. Many patients do not take all (or even any) of their prescribed medications. Checking dates on bottles, and a tablet count, is a rough guide to compliance. Medicine cabinets often contain old medications kept for use in the event of future problems – patients will sometimes change a new medication for an older, trusted remedy without telling the doctor. Compliance may be improved by the use of dosset boxes, or by carers giving the patient their medications. The local pharmacist and GP will also be useful contacts when checking adherence to a treatment regimen.

REVIEW OF SYSTEMS

The systems enquiry used for younger patients may produce spurious symptoms, many of which are not immediately relevant. However, do not be too hasty to dismiss them. If they are a concern to the patient they may be important to your diagnostic search. The traditional review of systems may also be used as a 'medical sieve' when there are multiple, seemingly unconnected, symptoms. In patients with cognitive impairment or in the acutely unwell it may be necessary to check key points in the history from collateral sources. Always obtain all the old case notes. After obtaining permission from the patient, if this is possible, talk to a close relative or friend. The telephone can be a vital piece of equipment for history taking with disabled, older patients. Ensure that any information you obtain is based on recent contact with the patient and is not anecdotal and several years out of date. Always try to check with the patient that the information is reliable.

EXAMINATION

GENERAL

Examination starts at the first contact and continues throughout the consultation. Useful information may be gathered at any point in your assessment, particularly with regard to functional abilities and cognition. The examination of an older person should be thorough, appropriate and respectful, but may be limited by the patient's disability or cogni-

Table 17.2 The Barthel ADL Index (total score 20)

Item	Categories
Bowels	0 = incontinent (or needs to be given an enema) 1 = occasional accident (once per week) 2 = continent
Bladder	0 = incontinent/catheterized, unable to manage 1 = occasional accident (max once every 24 h) 2 = continent (for over 7 days)
Grooming	0 = needs help with personal care 1 = independent face/hair/teeth/shaving (implements provided)
Toilet use	0 = dependent 1 = needs some help but can do something alone 2 = independent (on and off, dressing, wiping)
Feeding	0 = unable 1 = needs help cutting, spreading butter etc. 2 = independent (food provided in reach)
Transfer	0 = unable – no sitting balance 1 = major help (one or two people, physical), can sit 2 = minor help (verbal or physical) 3 = independent
Mobility	0 = immobile 1 = wheelchair independent (includes corners) 2 = walks with help of one (verbal/physical) 3 = independent (may use any aid, e.g. stick)
Dressing	0 = dependent 1 = needs help, does about half unaided 2 = independent, includes buttons, zips, shoes
Stairs	0 = unable 1 = needs help (verbal, physical), carrying aid 2 = independent
Bathing	0 = dependent 1 = independent (may use shower)

The Barthel Index should be used as a record of what a patient does, not as a record of what they were able to do previously. The main aim is to establish the degree of independence from any help, physical or verbal, however minor and for whatever reason. The need for supervision means the patient is not independent. Performance over the preceding 24–48 hours is important, but longer periods are relevant. A patient's performance should be established using the best available evidence. Ask the patient or carer, but also observe what the patient can do. Direct testing is not needed. Unconscious patients score 0 throughout. Middle categories imply that the patient supplies over 50% effort. Use of aids to be independent is allowed.

Box 17.5 Areas to cover in a treatment history

- Current medications
- Previous hospital and family doctor medications
- Treatment from 'alternative' practitioners
- Self-medication
- Past bad experiences with medicines
- Other non-drug treatments
- Medicines kept in the home
- Compliance and help: dosset box, nurses; carers

---

tive impairment, or by lack of appropriate privacy. Be guided by the principle of 'appropriateness and need'. For example: a frail, severely disabled or cognitively impaired patient will find it very difficult to cooperate with a formal neurological assessment, and will tire rapidly. The examination thus becomes impossible, invalid and inappropriate. Likewise, a digital rectal examination may normally be considered part of a comprehensive examination but may simply be inappropriate to the patient's needs. The answer to the question 'How will this part of the examination contribute to the mangement of this patient?' should then direct further assessment. However, disability and cognitive impairment should not be used as an excuse for not performing a complete assessment. Older people may present many years after they last visited a doctor. The examination should therefore include screening tests such as body weight, urinalysis, breast examination and digital rectal examination, including assessment of the prostate. Remember, the patient has the right to refuse these seemingly irrelevant examinations, and full explanations are needed.

Where appropriate, ask the patient to undress themselves. Consider whether they can reach their feet and manage buttons. Can they get on to the examination couch unaided? If the patient does have obvious weakness or disability, help them to undress, making sure there are grab rails around the couch or bed, the height of which should be adjustable, or a step provided for the patient to get

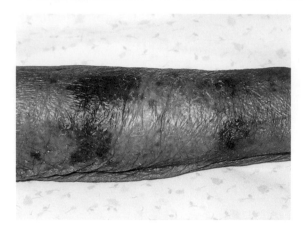

Figure 17.1 Transparent 'paparaceous' skin and senile purpura.

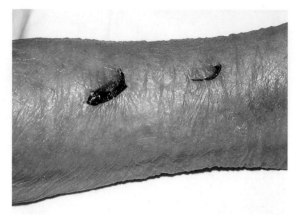

Figure 17.2 Transparent 'paparaceous' skin. The surface has broken with trivial trauma.

on and off. Once the patient is undressed, make sure comfort and dignity are preserved. If the patient is agitated, or if you are intending an invasive examination, a nurse must be present to assist.

SPECIAL CONSIDERATIONS

SKIN

Wrinkles are mainly due to past exposure to ultraviolet light and hence are not usually seen in covered areas. The skin of the elderly bruises easily (*senile purpura*); some people have skin like transparent tissue paper, described as *paparaceous,* especially on the backs of the hands and the forearms (Figs 17.1, 17.2). The skin around the eyes may show yellow plaques – *Dubreuilh's elastoma.* Some solar-induced changes to be aware of include keratoacanthoma, basal cell carcinoma, squamous cell carcinoma and malignant melanoma. The most common skin lesion noted is the small red Campbell de Morgan spot, a benign lesion seen most often on the trunk and abdomen.

Leg ulcers resistant to healing are common in old age; 50% are due to venous stasis (Fig. 17.3), 10% to arterial disease, and 30–40% are of mixed origin. Examination should include sensory (neuropathic ulcers) and vascular (ischaemia and varicose veins) examinations of the lower limbs. Measure the ankle and brachial blood pressures, using a Doppler meter and sphygmomanometer cuff, the Doppler meter being used instead of a stethoscope at the feet. The ankle–brachial pressure index (ABPI) is calculated using the formula:

$$\text{ABPI} = \frac{\text{Ankle systolic pressure}}{\text{Brachial systolic pressure}}$$

An ABPI of 1.0 is normal; an ABPI below 1.0 may indicate arterial disease. An ABPI <0.8 indicates compromised distal circulation, and so pressure bandaging for leg ulceration should be avoided.

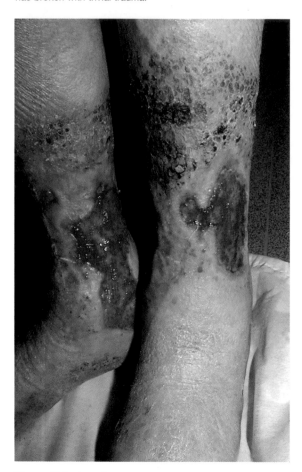

Figure 17.3 Leg ulcers.

Check cutaneous pressure areas, especially the heels, hips and sacrum, for signs of skin breakdown (*pressure or decubitus ulcers*).

CARDIOVASCULAR SYSTEM

Cardiovascular examination in older patients is no different from that in younger adults, but there are a number of important factors to take into account. Bradyarrhythmias and tachyarrhythmias are common in sick, older patients and may lead to cardiovascular collapse despite simlar rates being well tolerated in the young. The increase in heart rate in response to stress (e.g. exercise, illness or pyrexia) is reduced in advanced old age, and this may be exacerbated by medications such as β-blockers and other antiarrhythmics.

A lying and standing (or sitting) *blood pressure* is extremely useful, but may not be obtainable in the more disabled patient. Postural hypotension, defined as a drop in systolic blood pressure on standing of more than 20 mmHg, is a considerable cause of morbidity in old age, often caused or exacerbated by medications. The sitting or standing blood pressue should be measured immediately prior to and then 1, 3 and 5 minutes after changing position. Age-related structural and functional changes in the cardiovascular system account for a slight increase in mean blood pressure with increasing age, although adult hypertensive guidelines should still be applied.

Heart valves, especially the aortic valve, can become less mobile, exacerbated by calcification. This is known as aortic sclerosis and is characterized by a non-radiating ejection systolic murmur, heard loudest in the aortic area. Degeneration and calcification of the mitral valve can result in either apical ejection murmurs or the more common pansystolic mitral regurgitant murmur (see Chapter 7).

Arterial abnormalities auch as an *aortic aneurysm*, arterial bruits and evidence of peripheral vascular disease should be sought. Palpation of the pulses can be difficult because of atheroma or oedema, and in the lower limbs Doppler measurement (see above) may be necessary to assess the peripheral circulation. Assessment of retinal vessels for signs of disease, as in hypertension and diabetes, can prove difficult in old people owing to the frequent presence of cataracts.

RESPIRATORY SYSTEM

Kyphosis, owing to intervertebral disc degeneration and osteoporosis, and calcification of the costal cartilages make the chest wall more rigid and less expansible. A reduction in pulmonary elasticity with age may be responsible for some hyperinflation on a chest radiograph, but this is principally due to pathological hyperexpansion associated with chronic obstructive pulmonary disease (COPD). Generally, the physical signs of respiratory system disease are the same in the old as in the younger patient. Measurements of peak expiratory flow rate (PEFR) and vital capacity (VC) are reduced (see Table 17.1), but despite these changes normal oxygenation is maintained and the normal adult ranges for oxygen saturation should be used.

'All that crackles is not necessarily heart failure or pneumonia.' Coarse basal crackles caused by air trapping owing to loss of pulmonary elasticity can make the interpretation of breath sounds difficult. It is important to note their presence when the patient is well, so that inappropriate therapy is not initiated if and when they become ill. In this situation a chest radiograph is essential, regardless of the presence or absence of other signs and symptoms of cardiopulmonary disease. Common changes on the chest radiograph include calcification from old tuberculosis, calcification in chondral cartilages and major blood vessels, pleural calcification from past pneumonia, and old rib fractures. Pleural effusions, cardiomegaly, areas of collapse and consolidation, interstitial changes and pleural thickening should not be accepted as normal at any age.

GASTROINTESTINAL SYSTEM

The older patient should be weighed at every visit. As in younger patients, nutritional assessment includes estimation of the body mass index (BMI): weight (kg) / height (m^2). Because of osteoporotic vertebral collapse and other age-related changes, height may reduce in the old and so trends in weight are a more useful benchmark. If a true nutritional assessment is required skin folds at the biceps, triceps, waist and thigh should also be measured.

The majority of older people are edentulous. If dentures are used they should be worn during the examination so that problems with fit – for example poor speech or eating difficulties – can be corrected early. Oral candidiasis is common in the unwell older patient and is easily treatable. Leukoplakia appears as small white patches on the oral mucosa. It is associated with repeated mucosal trauma and may become malignant. Varicosities on the underside of the tongue are seen in about 40% of older people; their significance is unknown, but vitamin C deficiency has been implicated.

Abdominal examination may be limited by patients' orthopnoea, kyphoscoliosis or other disabilities. However, always try to perform an appropriate assessment. If abdominal examination is limited by such disabilities, the patient will also find it difficult to lie supine for investigations such as CT scanning or colonoscopy. The indications for digital rectal examination are the same as for younger patients, but this may not be feasible or appropriate, particularly in the very disabled or frail older patient. Constipation severe enough to cause faecal impaction is not uncommon and can have serious consequences (Box 17.6). This is often iatrogenic, but if of recent onset should be investigated appropriately.

Box 17.6 Faecal impaction may cause:

- Faecal incontinence (ball-valve effect, with spurious diarrhoea)
- Intestinal obstruction
- Restlessness and agitation in the confused (but never itself causes confusion)
- Retention of urine
- Rectal bleeding

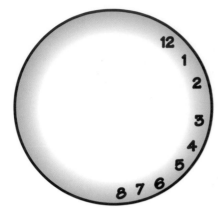

Figure 17.4 Clock-face drawing.

NERVOUS SYSTEM

Central nervous system examination should routinely include an assessment of higher cortical function (language, perception and memory). If cognitive impairment is suspected, assess the mental state early in the interview before the patient tires and record the result in the clinical notes (see below). As well as the AMTS and MMSE (see below) use the 'clock test'. The patient is presented with a drawn circle, about 10–15 cm in diameter, and asked to fill in the numbers of a clock face (Fig. 17.4). Abnormalities may be due to visual impairment, *agnosia* (owing to right parietal lobe lesions) or cognitive impairment. This test is easily reproducible and less influenced by cultural and language problems than the AMTS or MMSE.

It is important to recognize difficulties with communication. Communication is a two-way process that involves understanding and comprehension, as well as the production of appropriate speech. Communication problems can be considered in terms of:

- Disorders of language (dysphasia)
- Disorders of articulation (dyspraxia, dysarthria)
- Disorders of voice (dysphonia) or of fluency (dysfluency).

Dysphasia, i.e. difficulty in encoding and decoding language, is usually associated with a left hemisphere lesion (see Chapter 10). *Dyspraxia* is difficulty initiating and carrying out voluntary movements, for example of the tongue, and hence can affect speech. *Dysarthria* has many causes, including local factors in the mouth and dentition, stroke, Parkinson's disease, and other neurological disorders. *Dysphonia*, an abnormality of the quality of the voice (e.g. hoarseness), can be due to anxiety, vocal abuse, local disease of the larynx and pharynx, or hypothyroidism. It is common after surgery to the throat and intubation. *Dysfluency* (stammer) is found in people of all ages.

The formal assessment of the peripheral nervous system by examining muscle bulk, tone, power, sensation and tendon reflexes is something the inexperienced clinician often finds difficult. In older, disabled patients, where judgements about normality and abnormality may be more subjective, this can be especially difficult. As with all clinical skills such judgement is only acquired with practice. As part of this assessment it is useful to ask the patient to hold their upper limbs fully extended and supinated, at shoulder height, with their eyes closed. Observe for *pronator drift*, which is a sign of pyramidal weakness. The reflexes should be examined in the normal manner. It is not uncommon for the ankle jerks to be diminished or hard to elicit in very old people, but as with all clinical signs this should be viewed in the context of other findings and not in isolation.

It is essential to observe the *walking or gait pattern* wherever possible. This may reveal subtle evidence of hemiparesis, poor balance (Box 17.7), or the furniture-clutching gait of the patient with long-standing mobility problems. When observing the gait always have someone walk alongside the patient to offer a helping hand in case they stumble or fall. Occasionally patients claim that they are capable of carrying out activities when in reality they cannot. Always check the feet for chiropody problems (e.g. onychogryphosis), which cause a 'painful' or antalgic gait.

VISION AND THE EYES

Age-related loss of periorbital fat may give the eyes a sunken appearance; this may be severe enough to cause drooping of the upper lid (*ptosis*) and redundant skin at the lateral borders. The loss of fat can also cause the lower eyelid to curl in (*entropion*) and irritate the cornea, causing redness and watering (*epiphora*), or to fall outwards slightly (*ectropion*). A whitish rim around the iris (*arcus senilis*) is a zone of lipid deposition around the periphery of the cornea.

Visual acuity should be assessed and any loss of vision noted, together with the history of development of the visual disorder. Acute and chronic causes of loss of vision should be considered during the examination (Box 17.8). If the patient wears

Box 17.7   The causes of falls in elderly people

Premonitory
- Forerunner of acute, usually infectious, illness

Medication
- Multiple drug therapy
- Psychotropic drugs
- L-Dopa
- Antihypertensives

Postural hypotension
- Drugs
- Alcohol
- Cardiac disease
- Autonomic failure/dysfunction

Neurological disease
- Neurocardiogenic syncope
- Multiple strokes
- Transient ischaemic attack
- Parkinson's disease
- Cerebellar disease
- Epilepsy
- Age-related loss of postural reflexes
- Spastic paraparesis (usually due to cervical spondylosis)
- Peripheral sensory or motor neuropathy
- Situational and postprandial syncope

Cardiovascular disease
- Carotid sinus syndrome
- Brady- and tachyarrhythmia: second-degree and complete heart block, sick sinus syndrome, atrial and ventricular tachyarrhythmias
- Structural abnormalities: valvular stenosis and regurgitation, hypertrophic obstructive cardiomyopathy
- Myocardial infarction and ischaemia

Musculoskeletal disease
- General muscle weakness (e.g. due to systemic malignancy)
- Muscular wasting due to arthritis
- Unstable knee joints
- Myopathy (e.g. osteomalacia)

Miscellaneous
- Drop attacks
- Hypoglycaemia
- Cervical spondylosis
- Alcohol
- Elder abuse (e.g. physical mistreatment)
- Poor vision
- Multisensory deprivation:
  – deafness
  – poor vision
  – labyrinthine disorder
  – peripheral neuropathy

Box 17.8   Common causes of acute and chronic loss of vision

Acute
- Retinal detachment
- Vascular (central retinal artery/vein thrombosis)
- Angle-closure glaucoma

Chronic
- Cataract
- Macular degeneration
- Open-angle glaucoma
- Diabetic retinopathy

glasses, ask to see them. A state of disrepair may be an indication of cognitive impairment and/or their underuse, thereby explaining falls and misinterpretation of the environment. The visual fields should always be assessed. It is common to see irregular, assymetrical pupils due to previous iridotomy. Pupillary responses are normal in the well, older patient, but stroke and medication may cause abnormal size and responses. Abnormalities such as Horner's syndrome and palsies of the third, fourth and sixth cranial nerves are relatively common in the elderly, related to stroke and neoplastic disease. Funduscopy should be attempted wherever necessary, but may be difficult when there are cataracts.

HEARING

Communication is often compromised in the older patient by hearing impairment. Patients are described as confused when in fact they are simply hearing impaired. If deafness is detected the external ear should be inspected for wax. This should be softened with bicarbonate drops and then removed by gently syringing the external auditory canal. Hearing loss is often due to presbyacusis, an age-related degeneration of the cochlear hair cells. If a hearing aid is being worn, make sure it is switched on. This is easily tested by placing one's hand over the aid. If it is on it will let out a shrill whistle. Communication is aided by raising your voice (but *not* by shouting), obtaining attention, sitting face to face, reducing background noise, and speaking slowly and clearly. When the patient has severe hearing impairment you may need to use written communication, provided their vision is good enough.

THE 'GERIATRIC GIANTS'   (see Box 17.1)

Professor Bernard Isaacs drew attention to the four 'geriatric giants': *immobility, instability (falls), incontinence* and *intellectual impairment* in the mid-1970s. Impaired senses (vision, hearing, speech and language), iatrogenesis and pressure sores are now commonly included. These are important causes of disability and illness, but are not diagnoses in themselves so much as presentations of disease. In any older person presenting with one of the geriatric giants the underlying causes must be considered.

IMMOBILITY

Impaired mobility is one of the most common clinical presentations in the elderly. It is almost invariably multifactorial, and frequently the patient has several other medical problems. A careful history is necessary to elucidate the likely underlying issues and in separating cause from effect. The essential information is the onset of symptoms. Sudden immobility should be straightforward to diagnose, yet stroke and impacted subcapital femoral fractures are easily missed. A steady deterioration in mobility over several years implies a chronic process, e.g. Parkinson's disease or osteoarthrosis. A stepwise decline indicates a disease that has periods of exacerbation and remission, for example recurrent strokes or rheumatoid arthritis. Rapid deterioration from full mobility to total immobility over a few days indicates a serious acute medical problem. The most difficult patients are those in whom the disease process caused immobility a long time ago and the clinical picture has become clouded by the complications of immobility.

Within the bounds of common sense the patient should be asked or helped to stand up and attempt a few steps, during which the gait can also be assessed (see above). Always have someone in close attendance in case of falls. The patient may be able to mobilize but unable to get out of a chair or bed unaided. Look for signs of distress on standing that may not have been mentioned by the patient. Tentative steps, clutching helpers, may indicate loss of confidence or apraxia. Sometimes a diagnostic gait pattern is found (Box 17.9).

INSTABILITY/FALLS

It is said that 'young people trip, but old people fall'. With age, muscle strength is lost and postural reflexes become impaired. Falls are therefore common in old age, especially in the very old. Several causes may coexist (see Box 17.8). Even a single fall should lead to a detailed history and examination, and a corroborative history sought from spouse or friends. In a patient who was previously well, a search should be made for new acute illness. If none is present the fall may be deemed 'accidental' due to environmental or mechanical factors, although this is a diagnosis of exclusion. Information about the pattern of any previous falls can be helpful: frequency, relationship to posture, activity or time of day, pre-warning and residual symptoms following the fall, and any avoiding steps taken by the patient should be ascertained. The absence of any warning implies a sudden event, usually neurological or car-

---

Box 17.9   Abnormalities of gait

- The broad-based, unsteady gait of cerebellar ataxia
- The high-stepping, foot-slapping unsteady gait of sensory ataxia
- The apraxic gait, with rapid small steps like a slipping clutch, or with feet apparently glued to the floor
- The parkinsonian gait, with loss of postural reflexes, festination, a fixed posture, tremor, rigidity, hypokinesia of face and limbs, excess salivation and seborrhoea
- The gait of stroke with dragging of one leg
- The myopathic waddling gait due to weak proximal muscles, e.g. from osteomalacia
- The tentative antalgic or painful gait of patients with acute pain from, e.g., arthritis, injury or ulceration

---

diovascular in nature. Sinister symptoms associated with falling include loss of consciousness (although, notoriously, this is poorly reported), focal neurological deficit, features of seizure, chest pain, palpitations, or other cardiorespiratory symptoms. The most useful clinical investigation in older fallers is to watch them walking. Patients may also require 24-hour ambulatory ECG monitoring, a CT head scan and sometimes tilt table testing.

INCONTINENCE

Incontinence is an involuntary and inappropriate voiding or leakage of urine or faeces. Continence depends on intact sphincter mechanisms and the functional ability to toilet oneself, or at least to acknowledge the need for toileting. Age-associated changes in the lower urinary tract predispose older people to incontinence, but despite these changes most well older people are continent. Incontinence should not be regarded as a normal part of ageing and is more specifically associated with sphincteric damage, loss of neurological control mechanisms, especially in dementia or stroke, and with severe disability, chronic illness and frailty. Among the institutionalized older population as many as 50% may suffer urinary and/or faecal incontinence.

When taking a history of urinary of faecal incontinence, try to differentiate between loss of ability to control voiding and failure to identify or reach an acceptable place. Find out how socially disabling the incontinence has become: many patients become isolated or afraid to go out because of the associated anxiety and potential embarrassment. Clinical examination should include rectal and vaginal examinations, assessment of the prostate gland, evaluation of the pelvic floor muscles, and culture of a midstream specimen of urine. An incontinence chart kept for a few days may suggest a recognizable pattern of urinary and/or faecal incon-

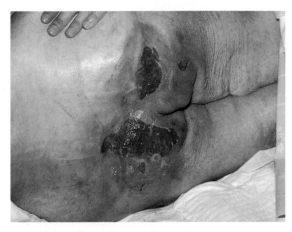

Figure 17.5   Superficial pressure sores.

tinence. The specialist help of a continence adviser is often useful. Causes of urinary incontinence are shown in Box 17.10.

Faecal incontinence is relatively rare in well older men, but is principally associated with severe chronic disability or cognitive impairment. In women it is more frequent relatively, but still rare. It may result from pelvic floor weakness. In both sexes it may occur with carcinoma of the rectum, diverticular disease, laxative abuse and excess, faecal overloading with impaction, and neurogenic bowel.

PRESSURE ULCERS

The mean capillary pressure in the skin of healthy young adults is approximately 25 mmHg. A bedridden patient or a person lying on the floor generates pressures in the skin in excess of 100 mmHg, especially over the sacrum, heels and greater trochanters (96% of 'decubitus' pressure ulcers occur below the level of the waist). Such pressures lead to occlusion of cutaneous blood vessels, causing the surrounding tissues, including the skin, to become hypoxic. In such circumstances necrosis of the skin, adipose tissue and muscle may develop in as little as 4 hours. About 80% of pressure ulcers are superficial (Fig. 17.5). They occur mainly in dehydrated, immobile and incontinent patients exposed to sustained pressure. People with impaired sensation, or with diabetes, are especially vulnerable. Decubitus ulcers are always potentially preventable, but will occur in any setting if skin care is disregarded. Any superficial ulcer will deepen if the pressure is not relieved. Deep ulcers (Fig. 17.6) are formed when localized high pressure applied to the skin cuts off a wedge-shaped area of tissue, usually adjacent to a bony prominence.

All at-risk patients should have active skin care management, including good nursing care and adequate hydration, started immediately a new illness or injury occurs, whether at home or in hospital. All pressure area sites must be inspected at the first clinical assessment, and again at regular intervals during the illness. An alternating-pressure air mattress (APAM) in which horizontal air cells (Fig. 17.7) inflate and deflate over a short cycle,

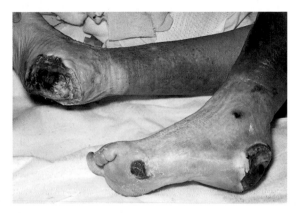

Figure 17.6   Deep pressure sores.

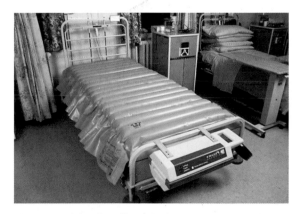

Figure 17.7   An alternating-pressure air mattress (APAM).

constantly supporting the patient, provides periods of low pressure at all pressure sites, and good protection.

CONFUSION

Delirium is an *acute confusional state* that occurs in the context of a depressed level of consciousness. Delirium may occur in patients with underlying brain disease, such as dementia, often termed 'acute or chronic confusion' but more often occurs acutely in the previously unimpaired. Often there are several underlying causes, including pneumonia, toxic states and metabolic abnormalities, e.g. uncontrolled diabetes, or hyponatraemia. Failure to recognize delirium and therefore to diagnose and treat the underlying condition can have fatal consequences. During any hospitalization a person's level of cognitive functioning should be monitored periodically.

Dementia is a *chronic confusional state* associated with loss of higher mental function, e.g. judgemental capacity, memory and language, but unlike delirium it is not associated with altered consciousness. There are, however, reversible causes even of such long-lasting confusion – for example drugs, depression and endocrine abnormalities – and appropriate diagnosis and treatment may produce improvement. Dementia is increasingly common in old age (10% above age 65 years, 20% above age 80 years) but is not a component of normal ageing. Regardless of age, a search for the cause is warranted. The differential diagnoses include benign senescent forgetfulness, amnestic syndromes and depression (*pseudodementia*).

THE CONFUSED OLDER PATIENT

'Patient confused, no history available' is a phrase that should never be used. It is crucial to establish whether the patient is orientated in place, time and person, and whether they are alert. A corroborative history from a friend or relative, and thorough clinical examination, will help decide whether the confusional state is acute or chronic. It is important to use a standard test of mental function (Box 17.11). Explain to the patient that you wish to test their memory. With experience, it is possible to check most of the items in the mental test score by working them into your introductory conversation.

Box 17.11 Abbreviated mental test (AMT): total score 10 (1 point for each item)

A score of 7 or less implies significant cognitive impairment and should be followed up if persistent, with an MMSE and futher investigation

- Age
- Time (to nearest hour)
- Address for recall
- Year
- Where do you live (town or road)?
- Recognition of two people
- Date of birth (day and month)
- Year of start of first or second world war
- Name of present monarch/prime minister
- Count backwards from 20 to 1

Hearing and speech impairments (such as nominal dysphasia) can make people appear very cognitively impaired, but should be easy to recognize. Depressed patients tend to perform poorly on mental test scores. If a problem is detected with a simple test, proceed to a more in-depth assessment using the Mini-Mental State Examination (see Chapter 4). Assessment of mental state is most valuable when applied serially over a period of time.

Management of suspected dementia should aim to confirm the diagnosis, to identify potentially reversible causes, and to determine a management plan with the patient and carers. This is best achieved in a diagnostic memory clinic, where a multidisciplinary approach involving a geriatrician, psychiatrist, psychologist and nurse specialist may be taken. As with any other group of patients, examination and investigation should be appropriate and directed towards helping with the management plan.

OTHER ISSUES

ETHNIC ELDERS

Ethnic minority elders form a small but significant proportion of the older population in many contemporary societies. Older ethnic populations may have a racial predisposition to certain conditions, but often develop similar diseases to the indigenous population within one to two generations. Indeed, environmental excesses, such as the western diet, alcohol and cigarettes, may contribute to an increased incidence and premature death compared to their own indigenous population. The availability of health services for this group is often inadequate and insensitive to their specific needs. Any healthcare professional must always try to understand and respect the cultural background of the patient and their family. Find out about the beliefs and cultural background of your patients – you will find it interesting as well as helpful in your work.

INADEQUATE CARE AND ELDER ABUSE

There are many types of abuse and any older person can be a victim. About 5% of older people suffer abuse. The most vulnerable are female partners, those living with adult children, perhaps because of financial difficulties or unemployment, and older people in poorly run institutional care homes. In the domestic setting abusers are often dependent on their victims for finance. They may themselves have health and financial problems, especially alcohol and psychological difficulties, and frequently their relationship has been dysfunctional for a long time. In institutions, inadequate staffing levels, poor staff training, repeated complaints, and poor client and environmental hygiene are all indicators of potential abuse.

Potential elder abuse should be considered if carers make frequent visits to doctors, preoccupied with their own problems and often seeming to indicate their inability to cope, perhaps using non-verbal cues. Marked changes in a carer's lifestyle (bereavement, unemployment, illness) may also precipitate abuse. Recognition of elder abuse is made more difficult by the physiological and the pathological changes that occur with ageing (e.g. senile purpura). However, abrasions, pressure ulcers and poor nutrition should raise the *possibility* of abuse. Assessment requires a history that includes open questions about *the possibility of violent behaviour*.

Enquiry regarding the full social background is important, including a sympathetic description of the carer's role. A thorough physical examination should be made and the patient's mental state assessed and recorded. If abuse is suspected, expert help from senior colleagues, social services, psychiatrists or clinical psychologists may be necessary for recognition, disclosure and management. It may be necessary to involve the police. Elder abuse is a complex phenomenon which is only beginning to be recognized. We fail the most vulnerable people in our society, however, if we are not sufficiently aware of the problem.

18 Eyes

A. Coombes

HISTORY

Disturbance of vision, the most important ocular symptom, may be sudden or gradual, unilateral or bilateral, causing loss of central vision or partial field loss. Simultaneous bilateral visual symptoms are usually due to disease in optic pathways at or posterior to the optic chiasm. Sudden visual disturbance should be assessed urgently. Visual hallucinations may be formed or unformed. Some visual symptoms have particular significance (Table 18.1). For example, haloes around lights occur in acute angle-closure glaucoma due to corneal oedema. 'Floaters' and flashes (*photopsia*) are indicative of vitreous or retinal disorders, respectively. The latter may also cause objects to appear smaller (*micropsia*), larger (*macropsia*) or distorted (*metamorphopsia*). Disorders of ocular movement may cause double vision (*diplopia*) or visual blurring. Are the visual symptoms binocular or monocular? Are they related to eye movements?

Other common presentations are a *red eye*, abnormal lid position, protrusion of the globe, pupillary or eyelid abnormality. Ocular pain is often associated with a red eye (Table 18.2). Ocular pain due to a *foreign body* may be described as 'a gritty sensation' in the eye, often worsened by blinking. It may be associated with sensitivity to light (*photophobia*) but this, particularly in conjunction with ocular aching, usually indicates serious corneal or intraocular disease. Severe ocular pain with vomiting may indicate *acute glaucoma*. *Migraine* often presents with bilateral visual symptoms and headache. *Raised intracranial pressure* and *giant cell arteritis* should also be considered when headache is associated with visual symptoms. Pain may be referred to the eye because of neighbouring disease, for example sinusitis. Excessive tear production (*lacrimation*) associated with discomfort may indicate ocular surface disease. There may be abnormal secretions from the eye, such as mucus or pus. With insufficient tears the eye typically feels dry, whereas a painless overflow of tears (*epiphora*) typically indicates blockage of the lacrimal drainage system.

Note any previous ophthalmic history, such as a *squint* in childhood, and any pre-existing poor vision, or previous ocular injury or surgery. Note what type of glasses or contact lenses are worn: extended-wear soft contact lenses are associated with an increased risk of corneal infection. The family history may reveal glaucoma, decreased visual acuity, colour blindness, squint, or neurological disease associated with visual loss. In addition to the ocular history the medical, drug and social history is important.

EXAMINATION

Eye examination is part of the cranial nerve examination. It includes ocular movements (cranial nerves III, IV and VI), corneal sensation (ophthalmic division of the trigeminal nerve) and eye closure (VII). Assess the optic nerve by testing visual acuity, colour vision, the visual fields and the pupillary light reaction. Inspect the optic nerve head (the optic disc and cup) with the ophthalmoscope. Detailed examination of the anterior segment of the eye requires use of the slit lamp, which, with additional equipment, can also be used to test the intraocular pressure and examine the retina.

VISUAL ACUITY

Visual acuity is most reliably tested at 6 m (20 ft) using a standard chart such as the Snellen chart (Fig. 18.1). Tests of acuity in near vision are portable but limited by age-related loss of accommodation (presbyopia), which necessitates refractive correction in older patients. These use test types of varying sizes, based on the printers' point system (Fig. 18.2), and the smallest type that can be read comfortably at a distance of 33 cm is recorded (normally N4.5 or N5 type).

SNELLEN DISTANCE VISION

On the Snellen chart each line of letters is designated by a number that corresponds to the distance at which those letters can be read by someone with 'normal' distance vision. For example, the largest letter, at the top of the chart – designated 60 – would be read at 60 m by a person with 'normal' vision.

Table 18.1 Sudden visual disturbance

Diagnosis			History: visual symptoms
Vascular	Ocular	Amaurosis fugax	Transient (minutes), unilateral
		Retinal artery/vein occlusion	Permanent, unilateral, often associated systemic vascular disease, e.g. ischaemic heart disease, hypertension, diabetes
		Non-arteritic ischaemic optic neuropathy (NAION)	Permanent, unilateral, often associated systemic vascular disease, e.g. ischaemic heart disease, hypertension, diabetes
		Arteritic ischaemic optic neuropathy (AAION)	Permanent unilateral, typically associated with symptoms of giant cell arteritis, e.g. temporal headache/tenderness, jaw claudication, features of polymyalgia rheumatica
		Papilloedema/optic disc swelling	Transient (seconds) bilateral visual obscurations, often precipitated by coughing or bending
	Cortical	Transient ischaemic attack (TIA)	Transient (minutes), bilateral, associated with systemic vascular disease, e.g. ischaemic heart disease, hypertension, diabetes etc.
		Migraine	Transient, bilateral, typically followed by nausea and headache
		Cerebrovascular accident (CVA)	Permanent homonymous field defect, may be preceded by TIA symptoms; note central acuity usually preserved except in bilateral occipital lobe infarction
Non-vascular	Vitreous	Posterior vitreous detachment (PVD)	Transient (weeks), unilateral, floaters, occasional photopsia, central vision normal
		Vitreous haemorrhage	Transient (weeks), unilateral, multiple floaters, central vision typically reduced
	Retina	Wet age-related macular degeneration (AMD)	Progressive, unilateral central visual distortion (metamorphopsia). This condition is also known as exudative or neovascular AMD
		Retinal detachment	Progressive, unilateral field loss, central vision reduced if macula involved, often associated with symptoms of PVD
	Optic nerve	Optic neuritis	Transient (months), unilateral, may be associated with features of MS
		Acute compression	Progressive unilateral, bilateral if chiasm involved, e.g. pituitary apoplexy (infarction of a pituitary tumour)
Pseudo		Suddenly noticed	Unilateral gradual visual loss from e.g. dry AMD or cataract
		Functional	Bilateral or unilateral; diagnosis of exclusion

Technique

The patient sits or stands 6 m (20 ft) from the chart. Where space is limited a mirror may be used 3 m from both patient and chart, giving a total of 6 m. Distance glasses should be worn if necessary, and each eye tested separately. The patient should read line by line from the top of the chart. If a patient cannot see the largest letter, designated 60, then the test distance should be reduced. If at 1 m the 60 letter cannot be seen, assess the following:

- Counting fingers held up at about 1 m (CFS)
- Hand movements (HMS)
- Perception of light (PL).

When testing low vision ensure that the eye not being tested is completely covered. If a patient cannot read 6/6 or better in either eye, check the vision again using a *pinhole occluder* (Fig. 18.3). This test distinguishes patients with poor vision due to refractive error from those who have ocular or neurological conditions. In a *myopic* (short-sighted) eye the rays of light are focused in front of the retina. In *hypermetropia* (long-sightedness) light is focused behind the eye, because the eye is abnormally short. In *astigmatism* the cornea is not uniformly curved and light is not focused evenly on the retina. When using a pinhole only the central rays of light pass through to the retina.

Table 18.2   Red eye

Diagnosis	History	Examination
Subconjunctival haemorrhage	Typically asymptomatic, spontaneous. May be associated with trauma	Unilateral (except some trauma), contiguous red area
Viral conjunctivitis	FB sensation, watering, no visual loss or photophobia, ?recent contact with person with red eye or URTI	Bilateral, prominent inflamed conjunctival vessels, follicles, enlarged tender preauricular lymph node
Bacterial conjunctivitis	FB sensation, discharge, no visual loss or photophobia	Bilateral, prominent inflamed conjunctival vessels, mucopus
Allergic conjunctivitis	Itch, watering, no visual loss or photophobia, history of atopy	Bilateral, prominent inflamed conjunctival vessels, follicles
Iritis (anterior uveitis)	Reduced vision, aching sensation, photophobia. PMH or systemic enquiry may elicit underlying disease	Unilateral, prominent pericorneal vessels, small pupil, aqueous cells and protein (at slit lamp), hypopyon
Acute angle-closure glaucoma	Severe pain, haloes/rainbows around lights, reduced vision, hypermetropic, elderly	Unilateral, pericorneal prominent vessels, semidilated (oval) pupil, corneal oedema, shallow anterior chamber (slit lamp)
Episcleritis	Mild discomfort, tenderness, no visual loss or photophobia, young adult, otherwise fit and well	Unilateral, typically sectorial prominent inflamed subconjunctival vessels (may also be nodular or diffuse)
Scleritis	Significant aching pain, tender, photophobia, occasionally reduced vision, systemic enquiry may elicit underlying disease	Unilateral, typically sectorial prominent inflamed deep scleral vessels (may also be nodular or diffuse)
Bacterial keratitis	FB sensation, watering/discharge, visual loss, photophobia, ?pre-existing ocular surface disease, recent trauma or contact lens wear	Unilateral, opacity in cornea (slit lamp) stains with fluorescein
Herpetic viral keratitis	FB sensation, watering/discharge, visual loss, photophobia, ?cold sores or ophthalmic shingles	Unilateral, branching linear dendrite(s) on cornea (slit lamp) stains with fluorescein

FB, foreign body; BP, blood pressure; URTI, upper respiratory tract infection.

Recording visual acuity

The top figure, the numerator, records the distance of the subject from the test chart – usually 6 m. The bottom figure records the line read by the patient. The normal person can read the line designated 6 at 6 m, i.e. 6/6 (20/20) vision.

Record a mistake in one letter as '–1' and a single letter read from the next smaller line as '+1'. Like all ophthalmic findings except visual fields, right eye visual acuity is traditionally written on the left side of the page (as the patient's eye appears to you), and vice versa. Whether the patient was using glasses, pinhole (ph) or was unaided (ua) is recorded in the middle (Fig. 18.4).

COLOUR VISION

Tests of colour vision are important because colour perception, especially for red, is affected in optic nerve disease before changes in visual acuity can be detected. Show the patient a red target one eye at a time (any bright red target can be used) and ask if there is a difference between the eyes. In the affected eye, red appears 'washed out' (*desaturated*). Acquired defects of colour vision may also occur in macular disease. The Ishihara test (Fig. 18.5) was devised to test for congenital colour anomalies (*colour blindness*), but is often used to assess acquired visual disorders. Most inherited colour blindness occurs in males (sex-linked recessive inheritance). It ranges from total colour blindness (*monochromatopsia*) to subtle confusion between colours, typically between red and green. About 8% of men and 0.5% of women in the UK have congenital colour perception defects. Blue/yellow deficiencies and total colour blindness are uncommon.

VISUAL FIELD TESTING

Visual field testing is described in Chapter 10. Field defects may affect one or both eyes. Symmetric bilateral (homonymous) field defects are characteristic of lesions posterior to the optic chiasm, and asymmetric field defects are usually due to lesions

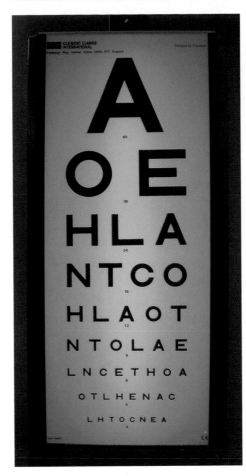

Figure 18.1 Snellen chart for testing distance vision.

anterior to the chiasm, i.e. in the optic nerves or retinae. Characteristic field defects (scotoma) occur in glaucoma, when damage to nerve fibres occurs at the optic disc, typically at the inferior or superior aspect of the optic cup. Funduscopy shows an increase in vertical length of the optic cup and field loss is arc-shaped (*arcuate scotoma*). If both the inferior and superior fields are involved a ring-shaped scotoma develops. Untreated glaucoma results in loss of the peripheral field so that only a small central island of vision remains (*tunnel vision*). Computerized perimetry is useful in identifying early visual field loss. The Humphrey field test analyser, for example, provides statistical information indicating the reliability of the test in comparison with a group of age-matched controls (Fig. 18.6).

PUPILS

Examination of the pupils in neurology is discussed in Chapter 10. In ophthalmic practice there are three key aspects to pupil examination: *size, shape* and *reactions*.

PUPIL SIZE: ANISOCORIA

In 12% of normal individuals the pupils are slightly unequal, particularly in bright light (*anisocoria*), but in these subjects they react normally. Abnormal pupils dilate and constrict abnormally, and the degree of anisocoria varies with the ambient illumination. However, it is often difficult to decide which pupil is abnormal. In the absence of local eye disease a *small pupil* may be due to paralysis of the dilator pupillae muscle (sympathetic innervated), part of *Horner's syndrome* (Fig. 18.7), in which anisocoria is more pronounced in low ambient light. An *enlarged pupil* suggests a *parasympathetic* lesion, which may be preganglionic in oculomotor lesions or postganglionic as in the *tonic pupil* of Adie's syndrome. Adie's tonic pupil tends to be dilated in bright light and is very slow to react. A feature of both parasympathetic and sympathetic lesions is denervation hypersensitivity caused by upregulation of receptors at the neuromuscular junction (adrenergic in sympathetic and cholinergic in parasympathetic). This is the basis of pharmacological pupil testing. In both pre- and postganglionic parasympathetic blockade the pupil is supersensitive to weak cholinergic drops (e.g. pilocarpine 0.1%). In sympathetic block dilute adrenergic agonists such as phenylephrine 1% are unreliable, so the uptake blocker cocaine 4% is used. This dilates normal pupils but has no effect in pre- or postganglionic lesions. Hydroxyamphetamine 1% causes norepinephrine (noradrenaline) release from normal or intact postganglionic neurons and allows pre- and postganglionic lesions to be distinguished (the synapse is located in the superior cervical ganglion). In complex pupil abnormalities, for example bilateral Horner's syndrome, infrared pupil imaging can be valuable. Causes of anisocoria are highlighted in Box 18.1. In congenital Horner's syndrome the affected iris is depigmented and appears blue.

PUPIL REACTIONS: AFFERENT AND CENTRAL DEFECTS

The swinging light test is used to detect an afferent pupillary defect (RAPD) resulting from retinal or optic nerve disease. The test loses sensitivity in symmetrical bilateral optic nerve disease, but this is rare, and in most bilateral cases the defect will be detected on the more abnormal side. RAPD is often associated with reduced vision, but if central vision is retained the acuity will be normal, although severe peripheral field damage may cause RAPD. In neurosyphilis the pupils are small and irregular and show the Argyll Robertson phenomenon (normal pupil constriction to a near target but reduced reaction to light) owing to a midbrain defect. In Parinaud's syndrome the pupils are typically large and poorly reactive to light, with abnormal vertical gaze, convergence retraction nystagmus, and lid retraction on attempted upgaze (Collier's sign).

Figure 18.2 Near vision chart based on the printers' point system.

READING TEST TYPES

as approved by

THE FACULTY OF OPHTHALMOLOGISTS,

LONDON, ENGLAND

N. 5

He moved forward a few steps: the house was so dark behind him, the world so dim and uncertain in front of him, that for a moment his heart failed him. He might have to search the whole garden for the dog. Then he heard a sniff, felt something wet against his leg — he had almost stepped upon the animal. He bent down and stroked its wet coat. The dog stood quite still, then moved forward towards the house, sniffed at the steps, at last walked calmly through the open door as though the house belonged to him. Jeremy followed, closed the door behind them; then there they were in the little dark passage with the boy's heart beating like a drum, his teeth chattering, and a terrible temptation to sneeze hovering around him. Let him reach the nursery and .establish the animal there and all might be well, but let them be discovered, cold and shivering, in the passage, and out the dog would be flung. He knew so exactly what would happen.

(From "Jeremy" by Hugh Walpole).

wire sons vain error unwise cream remove

N. 6

The camp stood where, until quite lately, has been pasture and ploughland; the farm house still stood in a fold of the hill and had served us for battalion offices; ivy still supported part of what had once been the walls of a fruit garden; half an acre of mutilated old trees behind the washhouses survived of an orchard. The place had been marked for destruction before the army came to it. Had there been another year of peace, there would have been no farmhouse, no wall, no apple trees. Already half a mile of concrete road lay between bare clay banks, and on either side a chequer of open ditches showed where the municipal contractors had designed a system of drainage. Another year of peace would have made the place part of the neighbouring suburb. Now the huts where we had wintered waited their turn for destruction.

(From "Brideshead Revisited" by Evelyn Waugh)

nervous manner immune over unanimous wear

N. 8

And another image came to me, of an arctic hut and a trapper alone with his furs and oil lamp and log fire; the remains of supper on the table, a few books, skis in the corner; everything dry and neat and warm inside and outside the last blizzard of winter raging and the snow piling up against the door. Quite silently a great weight forming against the timber; the bolt straining in its socket; minute by minute in the darkness outside the white heap sealing the door, until quite soon when the wind dropped and the sun came out on the ice slopes and the thaw set in a block would move, slide and tumble high above, gather way, gather weight, till the whole hillside seemed to be falling, and the little lighted place would crash open and splinter and disappear, rolling with the avalanche into the ravine. *(From "Brideshead Revisited" by Evelyn Waugh)*

immense snow came near arrow use.

Figure 18.2 Near vision chart based on the printers' point system.

The causes of light–near dissociation are given in Box 18.2.

PUPIL SHAPE

Slit-lamp examination is the best technique to assess intrinsic ocular disease that may affect the shape and position of the pupil (Box 18.3).

DIRECT OPHTHALMOSCOPY

The direct ophthalmoscope is an indispensable clinical instrument that allows direct visualization of the retina – which is part of the CNS – and its cir-culation. It consists of a bright, focused light source that illuminates the retina to allow the observer to see the image, magnified about 15 times.

PREPARATION

1. Decide the objective of the examination.
2. Consider dilating the pupils with 1% cyclopentolate (Mydrilate) or 1% tropicamide (Mydriacyl). This blurs the vision for at least 2 hours, so patients should be forewarned and instructed not to drive. Some patients have a predisposition to closed-angle glaucoma

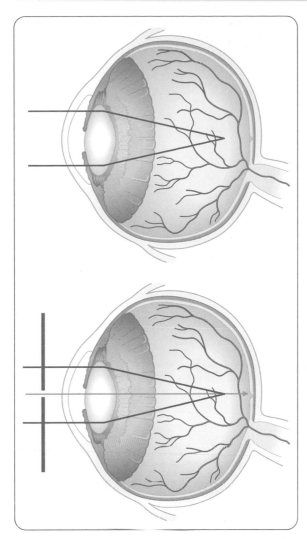

Figure 18.3 Testing vision with a pinhole. Top: light is not focused on the retina owing to refractive error (in this case in front of the retina, as in *myopia*: short-sightedness). Bottom: the use of a pinhole selects rays of light not needing to be focused, giving a better indication of a patient's true best corrected visual acuity despite refractive error.

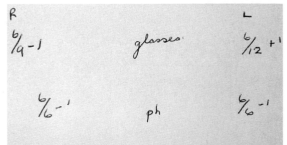

Figure 18.4 Recording visual acuity: the numerator is the test distance. ph, pinhole.

Examining the fundi

Look carefully at the optic disc/cup, the retinal vessels and the retina and macula (Fig. 18.9).

Optic disc

This marks the point where the retinal axons exit the back of the eye to form the optic nerve. It corresponds to the physiological blind spot. The normal disc is round or slightly oval. If there is astigmatism the disc may appear more oval than normal. There are four key questions to consider when viewing the optic disc:

- *Is the colour normal?* The normal disc is yellow-pink and its temporal side is paler. An abnormally pale disc is a sign of optic atrophy (Fig. 18.10). In addition, in optic atrophy there is a reduction in the number of capillaries crossing the edge of the disc, from the normal 10 to seven or fewer (Kestenbaum's sign). The causes of optic atrophy are listed in Box 18.6. In primary optic atrophy due to optic nerve lesions the disc is flat and white, with clear-cut edges. Secondary optic atrophy follows swelling of the optic disc due to papilloedema: the disc is greyish-white, with indistinct edges.
- *Are the margins distinct?* The disc margin should be sharply defined. In optic disc swelling this clear edge is obscured (Fig. 18.11) and venous pulsations are abolished. However, venous pulsations may be difficult to see in some normal subjects. Some important causes of disc swelling are listed in Box 18.7. In *papilloedema*, caused by raised intracranial pressure, the disc is abnormally red and its margins are blurred, especially at the upper and lower margins, and particularly in the upper nasal quadrant. The physiological cup becomes obliterated and the retinal veins are slightly distended. As the condition progresses the disc becomes more definitely swollen (Fig. 18.12). In order to measure the degree of swelling, start with a high plus lens in the ophthalmoscope and reduce the power until the centre of the disc is just in focus. The retina, a short distance from the disc, is then brought into focus by further reduc-

(Box 18.4) and dilatation may precipitate an attack. At-risk individuals must be warned to return if symptoms of acute angle closure occur.

3. Briefly explain the examination so that the patient can cooperate fully. Ask the patient to fixate on a distant target – they should continue to look in this direction even if the examiner's head obscures the target.
4. Dim the room lights.
5. Set the ophthalmoscope lens wheel to zero dioptres (D), unless correcting for your own short- or long-sightedness.
6. Check the ophthalmoscope light is bright. Unless the pupil is small, select a large light spot size (Box 18.5, Fig. 18.8).

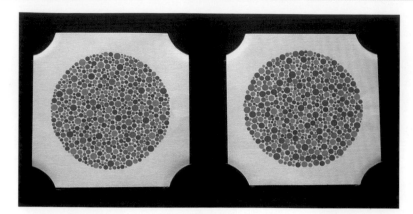

Figure 18.5 Ishihara colour vision test.

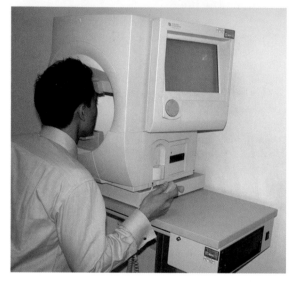

Figure 18.6 Automated static perimetry: the Humphrey field test analyser.

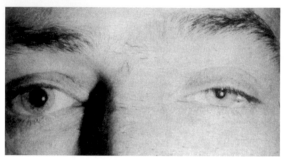

Figure 18.7 Horner's syndrome. On the affected side there is ptosis, which may be very slight, and a small pupil (miosis) that reacts to both light and accommodation.

Box 18.1   Causes of anisocoria

- Idiopathic (12% population)
- Parasympathetic:
  - Third-nerve palsy (external ophthalmoplegia)
  - Tonic pupil (internal ophthalmoplegia, e.g. Holmes–Adie)
- Sympathetic:
  - Horner's syndrome
- Argyll Robertson
- Pharmacological
- Ocular:
  - Iris inflammation, e.g. iritis
  - Iris ischaemia
  - Trauma
  - Iatrogenic

Box 18.2   Light–near dissociation

- Argyll Robertson pupil
- Holmes–Adie pupil
- Parinaud's syndrome
- Aberrant third-nerve regeneration
- Myotonic dystrophy
- Diabetes mellitus

tion of the lens power. This further reduction indicates the degree of swelling of the disc (3 D is equivalent to 1 mm of swelling). If papilloedema develops rapidly, there will be marked engorgement of the retinal veins with haemorrhages and exudates on and around the disc, but with papilloedema of slow onset there may be little or no vascular change, even though the disc may become very swollen. The retinal vessels will, however, bend sharply as they dip down from the swollen disc to the surrounding retina. The oedema may extend to the adjacent retina, producing greyish-white striations near the disc (Paton's lines), and a macular fan of hard exudates temporal to the fovea may develop in some cases.

- *Is the central cup enlarged?* The cup is a physiological central depression formed at the optic disc as nerve fibres leave the retina to form the optic nerve. It marks the point where the retinal vessels enter and leave the eye. It is paler than the surrounding rim of the disc. The optic cup:disc ratio is estimated by comparing their ratios vertically. In chronic open-angle glaucoma the ratio is increased (>0.3) – optic disc cupping. When the cup is deep, in advanced glaucoma, retinal vessels disappear as they climb from the floor to the rim, and reappear as they bend sharply over the edge of the rim (bayonetting); in less advanced cases the cup appears as a vertical oval extending to the edge of the disc (Fig. 18.13). In myopes the disc and cup appear large, and mimic glaucoma. Myopes often have a partial ring of pigmentation or white sclera surrounding the disc, which is easily mistaken for the edge of the cup. In severe myopia degenerative chorioretinal changes may occur in the fundus, which can involve the macula and impair central vision.

- *Are there any other abnormal features?* In proliferative diabetic retinopathy new blood vessels (*neovascularization*) develop at the optic disc. Myelinated nerve fibres have a dramatic white appearance, but they are a unilateral, harmless and non-progressive congenital anomaly (Fig. 18.14). They have a characteristic feathered edge that may obscure the retinal vessels.

Blood vessels

There are four pairs of arterioles and venules, which form the main retinal vascular arcades that

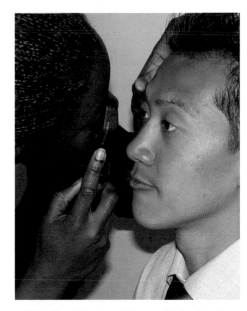

Figure 18.8 Examining the right eye with the direct ophthalmoscope.

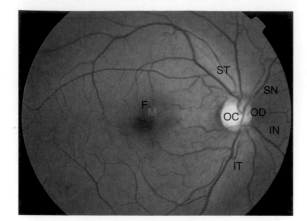

Figure 18.9   Normal fundus anatomy. OD, optic disc; OC, optic cup. Retinal vascular arcades: superotemporal (ST)/inferotemporal (IT)/superonasal (SN)/inferonasal (IN), macula (M), fovea (F).

emerge from the optic disc: superotemporal (above the macula); inferotemporal (below the macula); superonasal; and inferonasal. Study each in turn. Arterioles are thin, bright red in colour, and with a longitudinal streak of light reflection. In branch arteriolar occlusion a bright yellow (*cholesterol*)

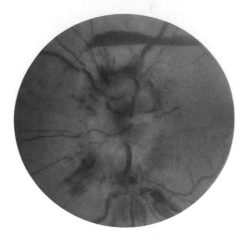

Figure 18.12   Severe papilloedema with retinal haemorrhages.

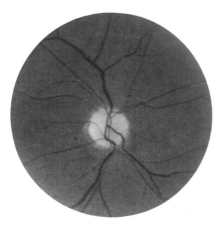

Figure 18.10   Primary optic atrophy. The disc is pale and whiter than normal, and its edges are unusually sharply demarcated from the retina. The retinal vessels are slightly attenuated.

Box 18.6   Causes of optic atrophy

- Congenital
  - Dominant and recessive
- Optic neuritis
- Chronic papilloedema
- Toxic
  - Tobacco, lead, alcohol
- Optic nerve compression
  - Thyroid
  - Tumour
- Post-traumatic (direct optic nerve or indirect vascular damage)

Box 18.7   Causes of the appearance of optic disc swelling

- Raised intracranial pressure (papilloedema)
- Infiltration
  - Lymphoma
  - Sarcoid
- Vascular
  - Hypertension (grade 4)
  - Central retinal vein occlusion
  - Anterior ischaemic optic neuropathy
- Pseudopapilloedema
  - Congenital small discs
  - High hypermetropia
- Optic disc drusen

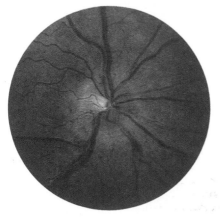

Figure 18.11   Papilloedema: optic disc swelling due to raised intracranial pressure.

embolus may occasionally be seen (Fig. 18.15). In diabetes or venous occlusion the venules are larger, darker, and often dilated or tortuous. Look carefully at arteriolar/venous crossings: compression and localized dilatation of venules (*arteriovenous (AV) nipping*) with arteriolar narrowing (*attenuation*) is a sign of hypertension (Box 18.8, Fig. 18.16). *Spontaneous arteriolar pulsation* is an abnormal finding that may occur if the intraocular pressure is very high or the central retinal artery pressure very low. *Spontaneous venous pulsation* is frequently seen in normal eyes, but is reduced in papilloedema.

Retina and macula

As each main vascular arcade is followed and examined the adjacent and peripheral retina can be systematically assessed. The macula is the central retinal area bounded by temporal vascular arcades. It measures approximately five disc diameters across. The fovea at its centre is one disc diameter in size. The fovea, with its high density of cone photoreceptors, is responsible for fine discriminatory vision. To find the fovea, locate the optic disc and move the ophthalmoscope beam temporally (move

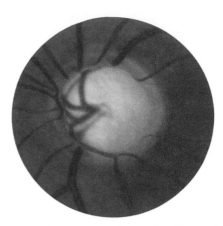

Figure 18.13 Glaucomatous disc cupping. The cup is oval in the vertical plane and appears pale. The retinal vessels are displaced nasally.

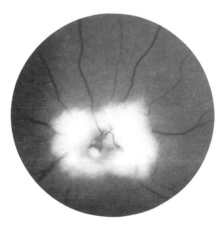

Figure 18.14 Myelinated nerve fibres: the white area obscures the disc; this is a normal variant.

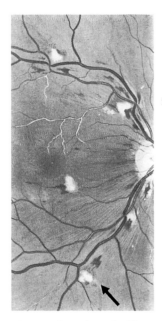

Figure 18.16 Hypertensive retinopathy. The arteries are irregular in calibre and show 'silver wiring'. Arteriovenous nipping is present. Characteristic 'flame-shaped' haemorrhages and 'cottonwool' spots (arrow) can be seen.

Box 18.8   Appearance and classification of hypertensive retinopathy

- Grade 1: arteriolar narrowing and vein concealment
- Grade 2: severe arteriolar attenuation and venous deflections at crossings (AV nipping)
- Grade 3: arteriolar copper wiring, haemorrhages, cottonwool spots and hard exudates
- Grade 4: all of the above, plus silver wiring and optic disc swelling

---

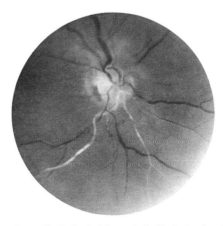

Figure 18.15 Retinal arteriolar emboli. Cholesterol emboli in the retinal arteries of a patient with atheromatous disease of the internal carotid artery in the neck.

Box 18.9   Common retinal abnormalities

White

- *Cottonwool spots:* white fluffy indistinct areas indicative of retinal ischaemia. This is the accumulation of axonal proteins in the nerve fibre layer. Causes include severe hypertension, diabetes and retinal vein occlusion.
- *Chorioretinal atrophy:* well defined 'punched-out' lesions (the white is the sclera). May occur in conjunction with retinal pigment hypertrophy. Associated with previous retinal inflammation or injury (including retinal laser).

Yellow

- *Hard exudates:* bright yellow with well demarcated edges consisting of lipid deposits that have leaked out of abnormal blood vessels. Most commonly associated with microaneurysms in diabetes (Fig. 18.17).
- *Drusen:* small multifocal round yellow features, usually located in the central macula. Generally smaller and less bright yellow than hard exudates. Typically bilateral and relatively symmetrical. Common in elderly people associated with 'dry' age-related macular degeneration.

Red

- *Microaneurysms:* the dots that typify diabetic retinopathy. They may leak to cause exudates or bleed to cause blot haemorrhages (Fig. 18.17).
- *Blot haemorrhages:* rounded localized intraretinal blood, typically due to diabetic retinopathy, but other causes include severe hypertension and retinal vein occlusion.
- *Deep large haemorrhages:* associated with retinal ischaemia when numerous.
- *Flame haemorrhages:* have a characteristic feathery shape as the blood is in the nerve fibre layer; may be present in retinal vein occlusion (Fig. 18.18). Not typically associated with ischaemia.

Black

- *Retinal pigment hypertrophy:* well defined black lesions, often in conjunction with chorioretinal atrophy. May occur with previous retinal inflammation or injury (including retinal laser therapy).

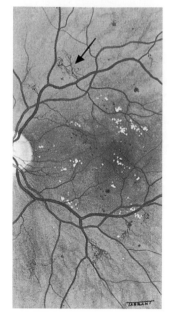

Figure 18.17   Diabetic retinopathy. Microaneurysms (tiny red dots), blot haemorrhages, hard exudates and areas of new vessel formation (arrow) are characteristic of this condition. In many patients hypertensive retinopathy is also present.

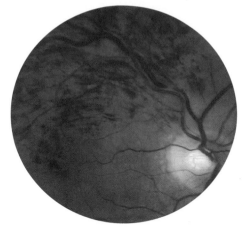

Figure 18.18   Branch retinal vein occlusion. There are flame-shaped retinal haemorrhages, but the disc is normal.

SLIT LAMP AND INTRAOCULAR PRESSURE

The slit lamp (Fig. 18.19) provides a stereoscopic, magnified view of the eye and is the key examination tool for ophthalmologists. Many A&E departments have a slit lamp, and it can be invaluable for assessing suspected foreign bodies and corneal abrasions. Some direct ophthalmoscopes are equipped with a slit-lamp beam, which can be useful. Alternatively, the anterior orbital structures and globe can be examined with a bright torch and basic magnification, and the same principles of systematic examination apply. The slit lamp comprises a

yourself nasally). Alternatively, ask the patient to look directly into the light. However, if the pupil is undilated it tends to constrict at this point, and the patient may recoil because of dazzle (you can dim the light beam to make it more comfortable). In young patients the retina is very reflective and there is often a small yellow dot in the middle of the fovea (macula lutea or fovea centralis). Box 18.9 and Figures 18.17 and 18.18 identify common retinal abnormalities by their colour and appearance.

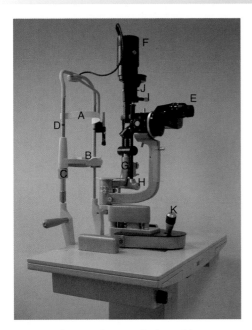

Figure 18.19 Slit lamp (see text for legends).

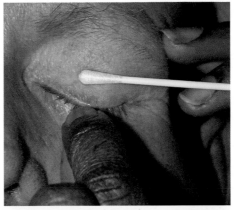

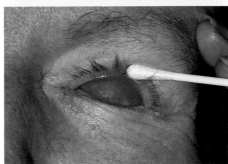

Figure 18.20 Everting the upper eyelid to expose the tarsal conjunctiva.

table-mounted binocular microscope column with an adjustable illumination source that produces a narrow, slit beam of light. The patient is seated with forehead and chin supported. The slit beam illumination and microscope have a common axis of rotation and coincident focal lengths, allowing the angle of illumination to be varied along with its width, length and intensity. Projected on to the globe, the slit beam illuminates an optical cross-section of the eye's transparent structures, and this can be viewed with magnification varying from 10× to 40× power. An attachment allows the intraocular pressure to be measured (*tonometry*). The drainage angle can be seen with a special contact lens (*gonioscopy*) and, with the aid of a handheld lens or a contact lens, the retina can also be viewed.

The following structures can be examined:

- *Lid margins, meibomian gland orifices and lashes.* Inflammation of the lid margins (*blepharitis*) is one of the commonest ophthalmic conditions. It is related to chalazia, blocked meibomian glands and infected lash follicles (styes). The puncta, on the medial aspect of the lids, drain tears into the canalicular tear drainage pathway. Misdirected lashes (*trichiasis*) causing foreign body sensations occur with chronic lid disease.
- *Conjunctival surfaces (tarsal, forniceal and bulbar).* This mucous membrane lines the eyeball (bulbar conjunctiva) and the inner surface of the eyelids (tarsal conjunctiva). The conjunctiva may be pale in anaemia, yellow in jaundice, or red (injected) in conjunctivitis and other inflammatory eye disorders. Directing the patient's gaze up, down, left and right ensures that all the bulbar conjuctiva is viewed. To examine the inferior tarsal conjunctiva of the lower lid, the lower lid should be gently everted and the patient asked to look upwards. To examine the superior tarsal conjunctiva – for example if a foreign body is suspected – ask the patient to look downwards (Fig. 18.20). Grasp the lashes between the forefinger and thumb, gently pull down on them and rotate the eyelid upwards over either the other thumb or a cotton bud.

- *Cornea and tear film.* The transparent cornea can be viewed in cross-section. The addition of a drop of 2% fluorescein reveals defects or foreign bodies in the corneal epithelium and the tear film can be assessed (Fig. 18.21). The tear meniscus on the lower eyelid should be symmetrical and less than 1 mm thick, and the tear break-up time should be more than 10 seconds. Fluorescein also aids the identification of aqueous leakage in a penetrating corneal injury (Seidel's test). Arcus senilis is a common crescentic opacity near the periphery of the cornea. It usually starts at the lower part of the cornea, extending to form a complete circle. It is common in old people, but may occur in the young (arcus juvenilis) in association with type IV hyperlipoproteinaemia. Corneal sensation should be tested.
- *Anterior chamber (filled with aqueous).* In iritis, a cause of red eye, there is inflammation in the aqueous, with flare (protein) and cells (typically

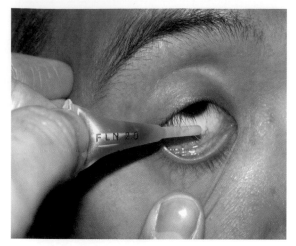

Figure 18.21 Fluorescein used to stain the cornea and tear film.

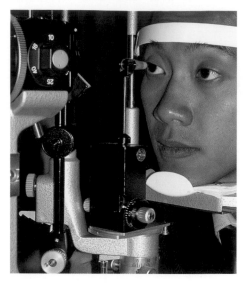

Figure 18.22 Goldman tonometry.

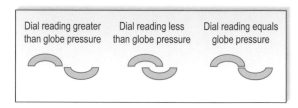

Figure 18.23 Diagrammatic representation of tonometry.

leukocytes). In severe iritis the inflammatory exudate settles inferiorly to create a white fluid level in the anterior chamber (*hypopyon*). Hyphaema has a similar but red appearance caused by bleeding into the anterior chamber, usually due to trauma.

- *Iris*. Note any difference in the colour of the two eyes (*heterochromia*), abnormality in the shape or size of the pupils, or signs of iritis. In iritis the pupil may be constricted (*miosis*) or irregular owing to the formation of adhesions (posterior synechiae) between the edge of the pupil and the anterior surface of the lens. Blunt trauma can cause a dilated (*mydriasis*) unreactive pupil with radial ruptures in the iris. An irregular or teardrop-shaped pupil with a history of a high-velocity foreign body is highly suspicious of a penetrating eye injury where the iris has plugged the leaking wound. Other abnormalities of the pupils are described in Chapter 10.
- *Lens*. Cataracts are usually due to ageing (central nuclear sclerosis), but also occur in diabetes mellitus, after injury, and in certain hereditary diseases, for example myotonic dystrophy. Posterior subcapsular cataract is a common side effect of corticosteroid therapy. Blunt eye injury may cause partial dislocation of the lens (subluxation) or complete dislocation into the vitreous cavity.
- *Anterior vitreous*. This is best examined when the pupil is dilated. Opacities may be observed, most easily using a green light. Cells in the vitreous may be associated with ocular inflammation (*vitritis*), trauma (vitreous haemorrhage) or retinal holes/detachment (retinal pigment).

MEASURING INTRAOCULAR PRESSURE: APPLANATION TONOMETRY

Intraocular pressures (IOP) between 10 and 21 mmHg are considered normal. An increased IOP is a char-

acteristic feature of glaucoma. A diminished IOP occurs in diabetic coma and in severe dehydration from any cause. The IOP may be assessed by palpating the eyeball, although only gross variations from normal can be appreciated. More accurate is applanation tonometry, in which the force required to flatten (applanate) an area of a sphere (the cornea) is proportional to the pressure within the sphere (Fig. 18.22). Topical anaesthetic and fluorescein are applied to the cornea and a bright cobalt blue filter is used to illuminate the sterile tonometer head. Contact between tonometer head and cornea creates a thin green circular outline of fluorescein, and a prism in the head splits this into two semicircles. The tonometer force is adjusted manually until the semicircles just overlap, and is read in millimeters of mercury (mmHg; Fig. 18.23).

EYELID, LACRIMAL AND ORBITAL ASSESSMENT

EYELIDS

People of Asian origin have a long, narrow palpebral aperture with an upward and outward obliquity and a characteristic fold of skin along the upper lid. The highest point of the aperture is typically at the junction of its middle and inner thirds.

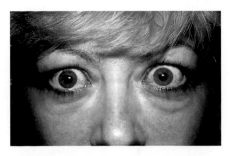

Figure 18.24 Thyroid eye disease with upper eyelid retraction and mild exophthalmos (bilateral proptosis).

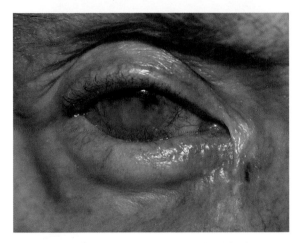

Figure 18.25 Lower eyelid entropion causing infective keratitis and corneal opacification.

In Down's syndrome the palpebral fissure is also oblique. However, it is also short and wide, with its highest point at the centre of the lid.

Normally no sclera is visible above the limbus (the corneoscleral junction). The commonest cause of *scleral show* is eyelid retraction (Fig. 18.24) due to dysthyroid eye disease, accompanied by other signs such as *lid lag*, in which movement of the upper lid seems to lag behind that of the eyeball when the patient looks downwards. In *parkinsonism* there may be reduced blink frequency. Look for reduced eyelid closure (*lagophthalmos*) and levator muscle function. *Ptosis* (drooping of the upper lid) may be congenital or acquired (check old photographs). In age-related ptosis, owing to levator disinsertion, levator function is retained and there is a high upper eyelid skin crease. In ptosis due to myogenic or neurogenic lesions there is reduced levator function (see Chapter 10, Fig. 10.10). In *entropion* there is inversion of the lid margin with associated malpositioning of the lashes, which may rub on the cornea (Fig. 18.25); and in *ectropion* eversion of the eyelid is often associated with watering. The lower lid is prone to skin tumours, particularly basal cell and squamous cell carcinomas (see Fig. 11.25). Xanthelasmas are fatty deposits that develop in the upper and lower eyelids in patients with long-standing hypercholesterolaemia.

LACRIMAL

Examine the lacrimal gland by pulling up the outer part of the upper lid while the patient looks downwards and inwards. Acute inflammation (*dacroadenitis*) causes a tender swollen gland, with oedema of the upper lid and localized conjunctival injection. Chronic dacroadenitis, a painless enlargement of the lacrimal gland which is frequently bilateral, occurs in *sarcoidosis* and *lymphoproliferative disorders*. Tumours of the lacrimal gland produce a hard swelling of the gland associated with displacement of the globe. Involvement of the lacrimal gland by any disease process may cause a dry eye.

Assess the position and size of the puncta (see Slit-lamp examination). Painless watering is a feature of obstruction of the tear drainage pathway, but exclude reflex tearing and overflow from, for example, a dry eye. Schirmer's test uses a standardized strip of filter paper to detect dry eyes by assessing the extent of wetting at 5 minutes (Fig. 18.26). Overt nasolacrimal duct blockage can be excluded if the patient reports fluid at the back of the throat on probing and syringing with normal saline (Fig. 18.27).

ORBIT

The most common cause of forward displacement of the eyeball – *proptosis* when unilateral, or *exophthalmos* when bilateral – is thyroid eye disease (TED) (see Fig. 12.13). This can cause corneal exposure and ulceration. Optic nerve damage may occur despite minimal proptosis. *Axial proptosis*, in the primary direction of the eye in forward gaze, is typical of TED and of tumours in the extraocular muscle cone behind the eye (intraconal mass lesions) (Fig. 18.28). *Non-axial proptosis* occurs in association with space-occupying orbital lesions outside the muscle cone, e.g. lacrimal gland tumours; these displace the globe forward and inferomedially. Apparent ('pseudo') proptosis causes diagnostic confusion: for example in ipsilateral eyelid retraction or myopia (where the eye is longer than normal), or when there is contralateral ptosis or enophthalmos.

Proptosis and enophthalmos can be measured with the Hertel exophthalmometer (Fig. 18.29). A difference of >2 mm between sides is abnormal. A proptosis that increases while the patient performs a Valsalva maneouvre is suggestive of a venous abnormality. Pulsatile proptosis with an orbital bruit is a feature of carotid cavernous fistula.

Blunt trauma to the orbit may cause a blowout fracture of the thin orbital floor. Orbital contents may prolapse through the fracture, restricting the

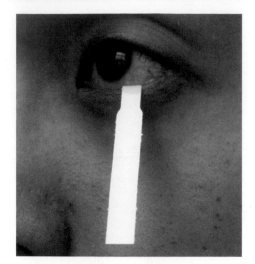

Figure 18.26   Schirmer's test for dry eyes.

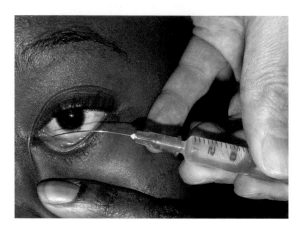

Figure 18.27   Syringe and probing to assess nasolacrimal duct function.

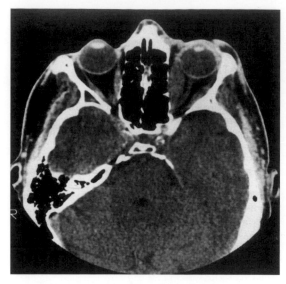

Figure 18.28   Axial CT orbits in TED. Left-sided thyroid eye disease with exophthalmos and marked hypertrophy (inflammation) of the medial and lateral rectus muscles on that side. These muscles in the other eye are also slightly enlarged. The optic nerve can clearly be seen between the enlarged muscles on the left side.

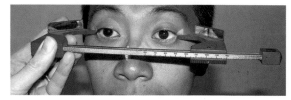

Figure 18.29   Hertel exophthalmometry to quantify proptosis or exophthalmos.

movement of the inferior rectus muscle and limiting upgaze. A full orbital examination should include palpation, eye movement examination, optic nerve assessment, and testing of the trigeminal nerve for altered sensation.

EXAMINATION OF THE EYE IN CHILDREN

The advice given in Chapter 16 on the examination of children in general is also important when examining children's eyes. Children may object strongly to lights and instruments, particularly when they are wielded by white-coated strangers. Allow the child to get used to the surroundings while taking a history from the parent, but do not ignore the child. Constantly observe the child, noting visual behaviour, the position and movements of the eyes, and the general appearance of each eye.

Visual maturation continues until the age of 8. Without a focused retinal image the visual pathways fail to develop properly, a condition known as amblyopia. After this age, sight loss from amblyopia becomes irreversible. It is therefore important to assess visual acuity in preverbal and young children. Babies should rapidly fix a large object – for example the examiner's face – and follow it. After 6 months 'continuous' and 'steady' fixation that is 'maintained' during a blink should be demonstrable ('CSM'). If an infant strongly objects to your covering an eye for even a short time, consider whether the non-covered eye may not be seeing well. A more sophisticated assessment can be made using 'preferential looking'. Cards are presented to the child with a grating drawn at one end and none at the other. The child will prefer to look at the image rather than nothing. Successively smaller spatial gratings are shown until the child does not see them. The grating seen can be converted to an approximate Snellen acuity (the vision of a 1-year-old equates to approximately 6/12), although testing each eye independently in this age group is difficult. From the age of 2 years a more accurate estimate of

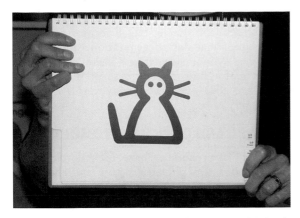

Figure 18.30 Kay picture-matching test to assess the visual acuity of children 2 years and older.

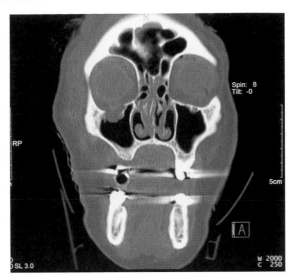

Figure 18.32 Coronal CT orbits in blowout fracture. The right bony orbital floor is fractured and the orbital contents prolapsed.

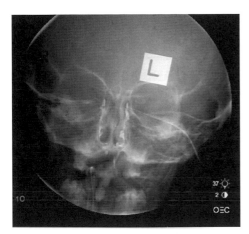

Figure 18.31 Dacryocystogram showing restricted flow of radio-opaque dye in the right nasolacrimal duct.

acuity can be made using the Kay picture-matching test (Fig. 18.30), and from 3 years the Sheridan–Gardiner letter-matching test. In these tests the child, or the child's parent, holds a card with a number of pictures or numbers on it. The examiner holds up an image and asks the child to match this target to one on the card – the targets vary in size.

Next, the position and movements of the eyes should be assessed. The least disturbing method is to observe the corneal light reflex: a light held at about 1 m should produce a reflection in the centre of each pupil. If the reflection in one eye is at a different location from that in the other, there may be a squint (although a wide intercanthal distance may give this appearance). If a squint is suspected, a cover and alternate cover test should be performed. Assess the ocular movements and the pupillary responses to light and accommodation. Examine the media and fundi with the ophthalmoscope through the dilated pupil. Because of limited cooperation refraction testing may be limited to the retinoscopy assessment. In general, only children with refractive errors so severe that there is a risk of amblyopia require treatment.

IMAGING

PLAIN X-RAYS

Plain X-rays have a limited role in the detection of foreign bodies, but have been largely superseded by CT or MRI. Ultrasound is used to assess the globe. A dacrocystogram uses a radio-opaque dye introduced into the lacrimal drainage system to identify sites of lacrimal duct obstruction (Fig. 18.31). It is particularly useful in the watering eye, when carcinoma is suspected, when repeat surgery is planned, or when trauma has occurred.

CT AND MRI

These are used extensively in the diagnosis of orbital disease. CT is often considered superior because it defines the bony orbit, but the X-ray dose to the eye and lens is not inconsiderable. CT is the investigation of choice in blunt orbital trauma and blowout fractures (see Orbital examination above), where fine-cut coronal spiral images are desirable (Fig. 18.32).

A- AND B-MODE ULTRASOUND

The A-mode scan is a one-dimensional time–amplitude study commonly used to assess axial length, which is an essential measurement for lens implant calculation prior to cataract surgery. The B-mode scan gives a two-dimensional cross-sectional view of the eye for the diagnosis of both intraocular and orbital tumours, retinal detachments and intraocular disorders when the fundal

Ear, nose and throat

M. J. Wareing

There is a close functional and anatomical relationship between the ear, the nose and the throat.

THE EAR

ANATOMY

The ear (Fig. 19.1) consists of the external, middle and inner ears. The external ear consists of the pinna and external auditory canal (*meatus*). The cartilaginous *pinna* is covered with perichondrium and skin, forming the helix and antihelix. The *meatus* has an outer cartilaginous and an inner bony component. The skin overlying the external auditory meatus contains modified sebaceous glands, which produce wax (*cerumen*), and hair cells. Desquamated skin debris, mixed with cerumen, migrates outward from the drum and deep canal. The external ear is thus a self-cleaning system.

The opaque or semitranslucent eardrum (*tympanic membrane*) separates the middle and external ears (Fig. 19.2). The *pars tensa*, the lower part of the drum, is formed from an outer layer of skin, a middle layer of fibrous tissue and an inner layer of middle ear mucosa. It is attached to the *annulus*, a fibrous ring that stabilizes the drum to the surrounding bone. The *pars flaccida*, the upper part of the drum, may retract if there is prolonged negative middle ear pressure secondary to Eustachian tube dysfunction. The *malleus, incus* and *stapes* are three small connecting bones (*ossicles*) (Fig. 19.3) that transmit sound across the middle ear from the drum to the *cochlea*. The handle of the malleus lies within the fibrous layer of the pars tensa. Within the middle ear the head of the malleus articulates with the incus in the attic, the upper portion of the middle ear space. The long process of the incus articulates with the stapes. This articulation (the incudostapedial joint) is liable to disruption from trauma or chronic infection. The stapes footplate sits in the *oval window*, and transmits and amplifies sound to the fluid-filled inner ear.

The *inner ear* has two portions. The *cochlea* (Fig. 19.4), the spiral organ of hearing, is a transducer that converts sound energy into digital nerve impulses that are transmitted by the cochlear (eighth cranial) nerve to the brainstem and thence to the auditory cortex. The *organ of Corti* (Fig. 19.5) within the cochlea contains *hair cells* that detect frequency-specific sound energy: low-frequency sounds are detected in the apical region, and high-frequency sounds are detected in the basal region. The inner ear is also concerned with balance. The *semicircular canals* and the *vestibule* contain receptors that detect angular and linear motion in the three cardinal x, y and z planes. The inner ears are only one component of the balance system; *visual input* and *proprioception* from joints and muscles are also important.

The *facial (seventh cranial) nerve* (Fig. 19.6) is important in otological practice. It runs from the brainstem through the *cerebellopontine angle* to the *internal auditory meatus* (IAM) with the cochlear and vestibular (eighth) nerves. The facial nerve passes through the temporal bone and leaves the skull through the stylomastoid foramen near the mastoid process. It may be damaged when there is suppurative middle ear disease. The *chorda tympani* leaves the descending portion of the facial nerve in the temporal bone to provide taste fibre innervation to the anterior two-thirds of the tongue. It supplies the facial muscles through upper and lower divisions that arise as it passes through the parotid gland.

SYMPTOMS OF EAR DISEASE

The five main symptoms of ear disease are:

- Otalgia: earache or pain
- Otorrhoea: discharge
- Hearing loss
- Tinnitus: a perception of sound in the absence of an appropriate auditory stimulus
- Vertigo: an illusion of movement.

OTALGIA

Pain from disease of the external ear, tympanic membrane and middle ear reaches the brain by branches of the fifth, ninth and tenth cranial nerves, together with branches of the greater auricular nerve and the lesser occipital nerve (anterior primary rami C2 and C3). Because branches of these nerves also supply the larynx and pharynx, as well as the temporomandibular joint and teeth, disease

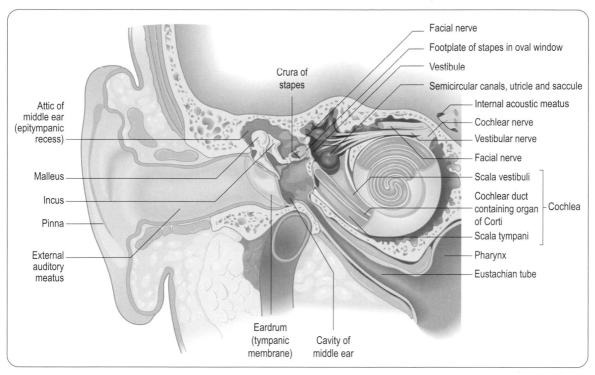

Figure 19.1   Anatomy of the ear.

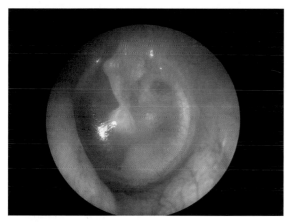

Figure 19.2   A normal left tympanic membrane.

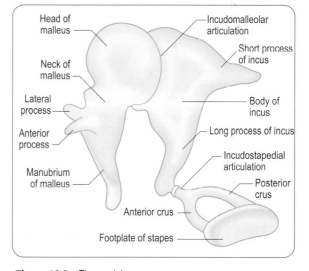

Figure 19.3   The ossicles.

of these structures may give rise to referred pain in the ear. Therefore, if otoscopic examination is normal, examination of these other sites should be considered. In half of affected patients the ear pain is referred.

The main causes of otalgia are listed in Box 19.1. Of the otological causes, acute infection of the cartilage of the pinna (perichondritis) can be very painful. A *subperichondrial haematoma* secondary to trauma requires prompt drainage if a 'cauliflower ear' is to be avoided. Despite its name, *malignant otitis externa* is not neoplastic but is due to infection, usually with *Pseudomonas* species. This can be a serious condition and may spread to the skull base,

especially in diabetic or immunocompromised individuals.

OTORRHOEA

Pus draining from the ear varies in character depending on its origin (Table 19.1) A profuse mucoid discharge with pulsation suggests a tympanic membrane perforation. The length of history is important. Persistent discharge suggests *chronic otitis media*, with perforation (Table 19.2). *Cholesteatoma*

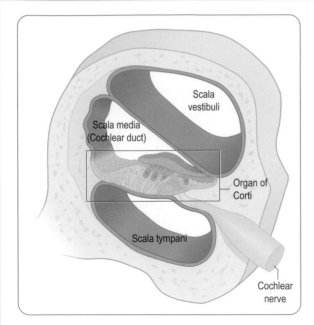

Figure 19.4 Section through the cochlea.

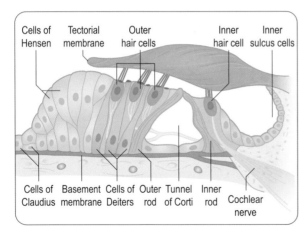

Figure 19.5 The organ of Corti.

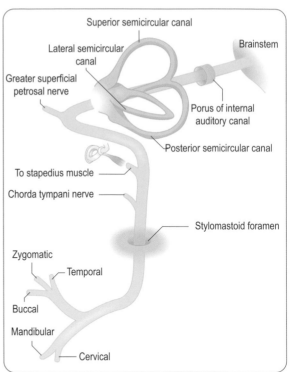

Figure 19.6 The course of the peripheral facial nerve.

usually begins with tympanic membrane retraction and blockage of migrating desquamated skin from the drum and external meatus. The retraction deepens and infection leads to destruction of middle ear structures, sometimes causing damage to the facial nerve or inner ear. The infection may spread outside the temporal bone, even causing meningitis or intracranial abscess. Bleeding from a chronically discharging ear is usually due to infection, but may rarely indicate malignant change. Cranial trauma followed by bleeding and leakage of cerebrospinal fluid suggests fracture of the base of the skull.

HEARING LOSS

Deafness may be gradual or sudden, bilateral or unilateral. There may be an obvious precipitating cause, such as trauma or noise exposure. There are two characteristics of hearing loss: to use the analogy of a radio, a decrease in volume, or a change in the tuning corresponding to impaired speech discrimination, so that words are not clear even with a hearing aid. Hearing loss may be *conductive, sensorineural,* or *mixed* with both conductive and sensorineural components (Box 19.2). *Conductive deafness* is due to disease in the external ear canal, tympanic membrane or middle ear. Characteristically, the patient retains normal speech discrimination. *Sensory deafness* implies pathology in the cochlea, and *neural deafness* implies pathology in the cochlear nerve or the central connections of hearing, but in practice this distinction is difficult to make and rarely useful, and the term *sensorineural deafness* is used instead. Sensorineural deafness causes impairment of speech discrimination with *recruitment;* the latter is an abnormal perception of the increase of intensity of sound with increasing signal volume that results from damage to the hair cells in the cochlea. This leads to a decreased functional dynamic range, so that a small increase in sound intensity is uncomfortable. The patient may also notice an apparent difference in the pitch or frequency of a tone between the two ears (*diplacusis*).

Most hearing loss is gradually progressive and related to ageing. Deafness is often secondary to occupational or social noise exposure, and is often inherited. Many drugs are ototoxic, and there are associations between hereditary hearing loss and neurological and renal disorders. Occasionally, sensorineural hearing loss occurs suddenly. A cause is only rarely identifiable.

TINNITUS

Tinnitus is a ringing, rushing or hissing sound in the absence of an appropriate auditory stimulus. It can be caused by almost any pathology in the auditory pathways. It is strongly associated with hearing loss, although it occasionally occurs with normal hearing. It is common, affecting up to 18% of the population of industrialized countries. In a small proportion (0.5%) daily life is affected. It usually improves with time, but in most cases there is no specific treatment, although correction of any underlying hearing loss may help. Management of tinnitus includes the use of hearing aids or masking devices.

VERTIGO

Vertigo is an illusion of movement such that the patient either feels the world moving or has a sensation of moving in the world. Patients frequently have difficulty describing the symptom. Higher centre dysfunction, as in anxiety states or drug effects, may also cause dizziness. There are therefore many causes for symptomatic 'dizziness' (Box 19.3). A feeling of the room spinning associated with nausea or vomiting suggests an acute labyrinthine cause, especially if there are changes in hearing or tinnitus. Fortunately, most acute vestibular events are self-limiting, because even if one vestibular system is abnormal the central connections can 'reset' the system over a period of a few days. The elderly are less able to compensate. In all age groups

---

Box 19.1   Causes of otalgia

Otological
- Acute suppurative otitis media, mastoiditis
- Acute otitis externa
- Barotrauma
- Furunculosis
- Perichondritis
- Herpes zoster (Ramsay Hunt syndrome – shingles of the facial nerve)
- Myringitis bullosa – viral myringitis
- Necrotizing external otitis (malignant otitis externa)
- Neoplasia

Non-otological
- Tonsillitis or quinsy
- Dental disease
- Temporomandibular joint pathology
- Cervical spine disease
- Carcinoma in the upper air and food passages

Table 19.1   Characteristics of otorrhoea in relation to site and aetiology

Diagnosis	Purulent	Mucopurulent	Mucoid	Serous	Watery
Acute otitis externa	√√	√		√	
Chronic OE	√√	√		√√	
ASOM	√	√√	√		
CSOM	√	√√	√√		
CSF leak				√	√√

Table 19.2   Classification of chronic otitis media (COM)

COM classification (synonym)	Otoscopic abnormalities
Healed COM (Healed perforation with or without tympanosclerosis)	Thinning and/or local or generalized opacification of the pars tensa without perforation or retraction
Inactive mucosal COM (Dry perforation)	Permanent perforation of the pars tensa but the middle ear mucosa is not inflamed
Active mucosal COM (Discharging perforation)	Permanent defect of the pars tensa with an inflamed middle ear mucosa that produces mucopus which may discharge
Inactive squamous epithelial COM (Retraction)	Retraction of the pars flaccida or pars tensa (usually posterosuperior) which has the potential to become active with retained debris
Active squamous epithelial (Cholesteatoma)	Retraction of the pars flaccida or tensa that has retained squamous epithelial debris and is associated with inflammation and the production of pus, often from the adjacent mucosa

---

Box 19.2   Causes of deafness

Conductive
- Occluding wax in the external meatus
- Middle ear effusion
- Acute suppurative otitis media
- Chronic otitis media: perforation, ossicular erosion, cholesteatoma
- Otosclerosis
- Trauma to the drum or ossicular chain
- Otitis externa
- Congenital atresia of the external meatus or congenital ossicular fixation
- Carcinoma of the middle ear

Sensorineural
- Age associated hearing loss: presbyacusis
- Noise-induced hearing loss
- Genetic: syndromal or non-syndromal
- Ménière's disease
- Infective: meningitis, measles, mumps, syphilis
- Sudden sensorineural hearing loss (idiopathic)
- Perinatal: hypoxia, jaundice
- Prenatal: rubella
- Trauma: head injury, surgery
- Ototoxicity: aminoglycosides, diuretics, cytotoxics
- Neoplastic: vestibular schwannoma, other cerebellopontine angle lesions

---

Box 19.3   Causes of vertigo

Of sudden onset
- Acute viral labyrinthitis
- Vestibular neuritis

With focal features
- Brainstem ischaemia (TIA)
- Multiple sclerosis
- Migraine
- Temporal lobe epilepsy

With deafness and tinnitus
- Ménière's disease
- Vestibular schwannoma

With positional change
- Benign paroxysmal positional vertigo
- Cervical vertigo

After trauma
- BPPV
- Perilymph fistula

With motion
- Motion sickness

Drug induced
- Vestibulotoxic drugs, e.g. gentamicin, salicylate, quinine, antihypertensives

With aural discharge
- Middle ear disease

With systemic disorders
- Postural hypotension
- Syncope
- Cardiac dysrhythmia
- Carotid sinus hypersensitivity
- Anxiety and panic attacks
- Hyperventilation syndrome

---

vertigo may cause residual vague imbalance, particularly in association with movement, or after alcohol ingestion. It is important to test for positional changes, as the commonest cause of vestibular vertigo is *benign paroxysmal positional vertigo (BPPV)*, secondary to loose debris floating in the posterior semicircular canal.

CLINICAL EXAMINATION OF THE EAR AND HEARING

PINNA AND POSTAURICULAR AREA

First, inspect the pinna and the surrounding skin. Congenital abnormalities may be associated with accessory skin tags, abnormal cartilaginous fragments in the skin surrounding the ear, or small pits and sinuses. Look also for any lymphadenopathy and for abnormal protrusion of the pinna, often associated with failure of development of the antihelical fold (*bat ear*). Look for surgical scars. A hot, tender postaural swelling, pushing the pinna forward, suggests mastoid infection (Fig. 19.7). Incomplete development of the ear (*microtia*) occurs with narrowing (*atresia*) of the external meatus, but the auricle can also be displaced from its normal position (*melotia*) or pathologically enlarged (*macrotia*). These abnormalities may be associated with cysts or infection in a preauricular sinus. Occa-

sionally, otitis externa is associated with a tender postauricular lymph node. If the external meatus is clear, examine the scalp for signs of cellulitis.

EXTERNAL EAR CANAL

Inspect the external auditory canal using a handheld otoscope (Fig. 19.8). To bring the cartilaginous meatus into line with the bony canal, retract the pinna backwards and upwards. Always use the largest speculum that will comfortably fit the ear canal. Hold the otoscope like a pen between thumb and index finger, with the ulnar border of your hand resting gently against the side of the patient's head. In this way any movement of the patient's head during the examination causes synchronous movement of the speculum, limiting any risk of accidental injury to the ear canal. Wax may be removed with a Jobson Horne probe or wax hook (Fig. 19.9), or

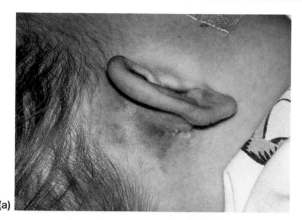

(a)

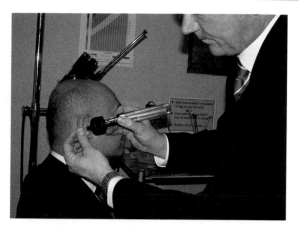

Figure 19.8 Examining the ear.

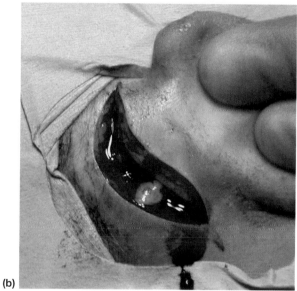

(b)

Figure 19.7 Acute mastoiditis, **(a)** incised and **(b)** drained.

by syringing with water. Never syringe if there is a history of previous perforation, or discharge. It is important to use water at 37°C lest vertigo be induced by caloric stimulation of the labyrinth. Keratin debris, pus or mucopus in the meatus can be removed, and if there is purulent or mucopurulent otorrhoea a swab should be taken for microbiology. Foreign bodies in the ear canal are sometimes found in children; they may be difficult to remove without a general anaesthetic.

THE TYMPANIC MEMBRANE

The handheld otoscope is satisfactory for most examinations, but the outpatient microscope offers the best view. Be familiar with the variability in appearance of the normal drum. The most common abnormality is *tympanosclerosis* (Fig. 19.10), which consists of white chalky patches in the drum caused by hyaline degeneration of the fibrous layer, due to previous infection. Prolonged *negative middle ear pressure* may cause the drum to become thinned and

atelectatic (Fig. 19.11), either diffusely or with a retraction pocket. *Eustachian tube dysfunction* and/or *acute otitis media* may cause a middle ear effusion (Fig. 19.12). Fluid behind the drum is often obvious, but when the drum is opaque increased vascularity or retraction are useful clues. *Perforations* of the pars tensa are either central or marginal (Fig. 19.13). Marginal perforations extend to the annulus and may be associated with *cholesteatoma* (Fig. 19.14), whereas with central perforations there is a rim of retained membrane between the defect and the annulus. Both are described by their position in relation to the handle of the malleus (anterior, posterior or inferior) and by their size (Fig. 19.15). Drum retraction may mimic perforation.

The *fistula test* is indicated if the patient is dizzy with middle ear pathology. Press on the tragus to occlude the meatus and then apply more pressure. If the labyrinth is open then this pressure change will be applied to the inner ear. The patient will be dizzy and nystagmus may be induced.

THE FACIAL NERVE

Test the facial movements. A peripheral facial palsy can be graded using the House–Brackmann scale (Box 19.4). Function of the greater superficial petrosal nerve can be tested with *Schirmer's test*: absorbent paper strips are applied to the inferior margin of the eye to detect tear formation (Page 151). Chorda tympani function can be tested by the sense of taste and by electrogustometry. Stapedius function can be tested with tympanic impedance tests; hyperacusis may occur if the stapedius is paralysed.

CLINICAL ASSESSMENT OF HEARING

Conversational hearing will indicate any possible deafness. The television may be too loud, or varying amounts of background noise make conversation unexpectedly difficult. Establish which is the patient's better-hearing ear. Test using words or

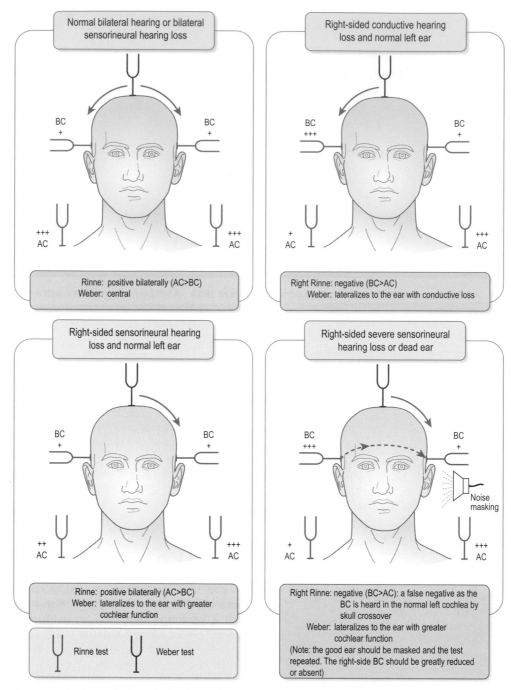

Figure 19.16   Interpretation of tuning fork tests.

a pure sensorineural loss on the other the tuning fork will be louder in the normal ear. Conversely, if there is a purely conductive hearing loss the sound will be louder on the side with the conductive deficit. The Weber test has the merit of simplicity and speed, but there is a high test–retest variability and it adds little to clinical assessment. Because all clinical tests of hearing have limited reliability, accurate formal audiometry in the ENT clinic is essential.

CLINICAL ASSESSMENT OF BALANCE

The unsteady patient requires a full neuro-otological examination. It is also necessary to examine the cardiovascular system (see Chapter 7). The aim is to localize the site of any potential lesion and possibly confirm a diagnosis, although sometimes all that is possible is to differentiate between central (*brainstem*) and peripheral (*labyrinthine*) lesions.

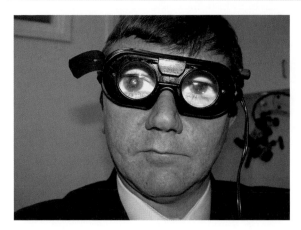

Figure 19.17 Frenzel's glasses.

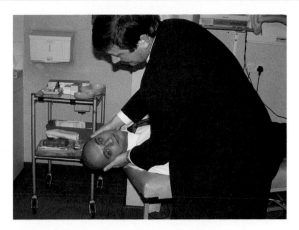

Figure 19.18 The Dix–Hallpike test position.

- *Examine the cranial nerves* (see Chapter 10). Cranial nerve palsies will help localize the site of a lesion. Pay particular attention to *eye movements*. Conjugate eye movements should be tested and any strabismus or nystagmus noted.
- *Nystagmus* (see Chapter 18) is a rhythmic involuntary movement of the eyes defined by the direction of the fast movement. The characteristic saw-toothed nystagmus of vestibular disease has a slow (labyrinthine) and a fast (central) component and is enhanced by movement of the eyes in the direction of the fast phase. The eyes are first observed looking forwards and then to right and left. Eye movements can also be assessed using Frenzel's glasses (Fig. 19.17). These are illuminated and have 20 dioptre lenses that abolish visual fixation for the patient, thereby possibly unmasking nystagmus.
- *Pursuit (slow) movements*, which depend on the fovea and the occipital cortex of the brain, are assessed by asking the patient to track an object moved slowly horizontally and vertically across the visual field about 35 cm away.
- *Saccadic movements* are driven by the frontal lobes and the pontine gaze centres. These are tested by asking the patient to alternate their gaze rapidly between two objects held approximately 30° apart.
- *Romberg's test* involves the patient standing with the feet together, initially with the eyes open and then with them closed. Patients with disorders of the posterior columns in the spinal cord, i.e. with impaired position sense, will sway (or even fall) when the eyes are closed, but will stand normally with the eyes open. Patients with uncompensated unilateral labyrinthine dysfunction are unstable, tending to fall to the side of the lesion. Patients with central dysfunction sway to both sides, whether the eyes are open or shut.
- *Unterberger's stepping test* has the patient standing with their arms outstretched and then taking steps on the spot with the eyes closed. Unilateral vestibular hypofunction leads to rotation to the affected side.
- *Gait assessment.* Ask the patient to walk heel to toe with their eyes first open and then closed. The patient with a cerebellar lesion is unable to do either. The patient with a peripheral vestibular lesion will struggle, particularly with the eyes closed.
- *The Dix–Hallpike test* assesses the effect of positional change. The patient sits on an examination couch. It is wise at this stage to test neck movements, to make sure they are free and painless. The head is then turned 45° to the side of test. The patient is laid back rapidly with their head extended over the end of the bed (Fig. 19.18). The classic response in benign paroxysmal positional nystagmus (BPPV) involves a variable latent period when nothing happens. There is then a torsional nystagmus beating to the lower ear, with a variable feeling of vertigo. This lasts perhaps 5–30 seconds. With repetition the response becomes less or absent. The condition is caused by debris in the posterior semicircular canal. It is frequently self-limiting, but if it persists it may be cured by the *Epley particle repositioning manoeuvre*. Other positive results are possible. Persistent positional nystagmus implies central pathology; the nystagmus appears immediately, is not necessarily associated with vertiginous symptoms, and shows no adaptation.

SPECIAL INVESTIGATIONS OF HEARING

PURE TONE AUDIOMETRY   (Figs 19.19, 19.20)
A single-frequency tone is presented at standardized levels into each ear in turn. This is done in noise-free surroundings, usually in a soundproofed booth. Air conduction is tested first through headphones. A level well above threshold, as predicted by free field testing, is chosen and the patient responds when

they hear the sound. The intensity is then reduced in 10 dB steps until the patient cannot hear it. It is then increased in 5 dB steps to establish the quietest sound that can be heard – the *threshold*. The better ear is tested first at 1, 2, 4 and 8 kHz, then at 500

and 250 Hz. Bone conduction tests are performed using a vibrating headset applied to the mastoid. In conductive loss bone conduction is better than air conduction. The difference is called the air–bone gap. This may be correctible by surgery to the middle ear and tympanic membrane.

SPEECH AUDIOMETRY

A pure tone audiogram does not test discrimination. A speech audiogram measures the patient's ability to recognize words from phonetically balanced lists delivered at different sound levels to the test ear from a tape recording. The percentage of words correctly repeated by the subject is noted at each level. With normal hearing all words are heard (100% optimal speech discrimination – ODS) at a sound intensity of 40 dB. Patients with sensorineural deafness are often unable to achieve 100% ODS, and in particular patients with neural/retrocochlear loss have poor ODS, with a phenomenon called 'rollover': increasing intensities lead to fewer words being understood (Fig. 19.21).

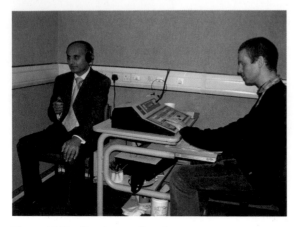

Figure 19.19   Pure tone audiometry.

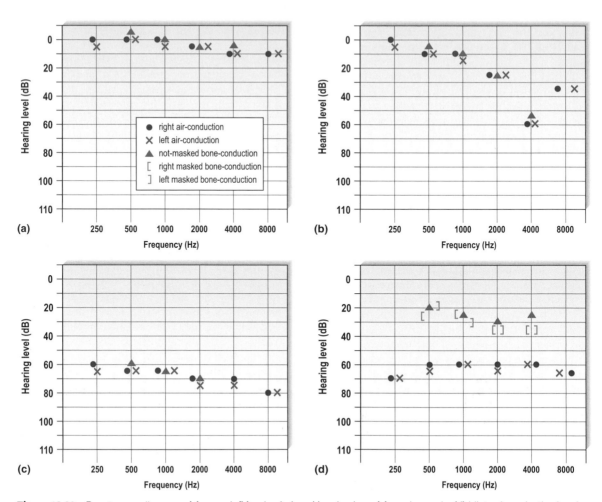

Figure 19.20   Pure tone audiograms: **(a)** normal; **(b)** noise-induced hearing loss; **(c)** presbyacusis; **(d)** bilateral conductive hearing loss.

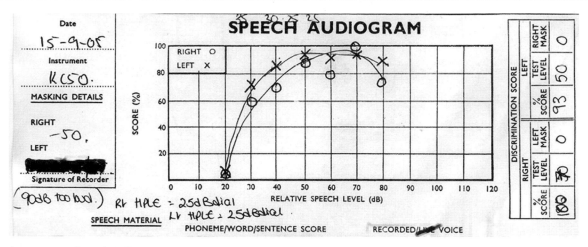

Figure 19.21 Speech audiogram.

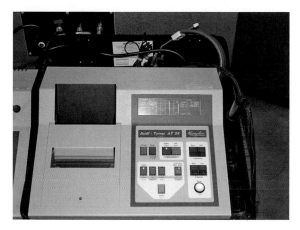

Figure 19.22 The tympanometer.

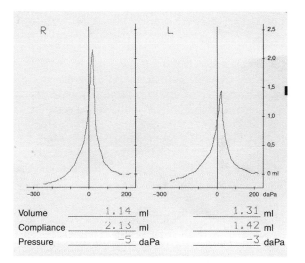

Figure 19.23 A tympanogram.

TYMPANOMETRY

An earpiece is inserted into the external meatus through which pass three channels. The first delivers a continuous tone into the ear canal during the test (probe tone); the second has a microphone to record the sound intensity level within the ear canal; the third channel connects to a manometer so that the pressure within the canal can be altered (Fig. 19.22).

The external meatus is a rigid tube with a compliant end (the drum). Normally the middle ear and ear canal pressures are equal, and most of the sound introduced into the system is transmitted into the ear; only a minimum of sound energy is reflected back and measured by the microphone. Changing the pressure difference between the external and the middle ear causes the tympanic membrane to become less compliant. This increases the sound energy reflected back to the probe. These changes are plotted graphically on a tympanogram (Fig. 19.23), which gives a measure of movement of the eardrum and the compliance of the middle ear. The test also measures the volume of the canal: a large volume indicates a tympanic perforation. Impedance

(the reciprocal of compliance) is increased when the tympanic membrane is thickened or when there is fluid in the middle ear, and is decreased when the drum is hypermobile or atrophic. Tympanometry is an objective test. It has particular value in children in the assessment of glue ear.

OTOACOUSTIC EMISSIONS

When a click or tone-burst is played into the ear a very small noise is emitted in return, probably arising from the outer hair cells. These emissions are particularly prominent in neonates. Testing does not require cooperation. A probe with two channels, a speaker and a microphone is used, and the responses averaged. When there is hearing loss there is no response. The technique is valuable in the screening of neonates, but not in adults.

EVOKED RESPONSE AUDIOMETRY

A click presented to the ear causes a nerve impulse to be sent to the auditory cortex via the brainstem.

Each impulse is very small in the context of background brain activity, but if a large number (2000+) of responses are averaged then evoked responses in brainstem and cortex can be seen and their amplitudes and latencies measured. The *auditory brainstem* response is not affected by sedation and has been used in monitoring neuro-otological surgery. The main indication for auditory cortical evoked response studies is in the establishment of hearing thresholds, especially in infants.

SPECIAL TESTS OF BALANCE

Caloric testing is the most commonly performed routine test of the vestibular end-organ. The patient lies on a couch with the head up 30°, in order to bring the lateral semicircular canals into the vertical plane. They are then instructed to fix upon a point in central gaze and the external ear canal is irrigated with water at 30°C, and then at 44°C for 30–40 seconds. Cold water induces nystagmus away from the ear being irrigated, and warm water induces nystagmus towards the ear under test (COWS: cold opposite, warm same). Each ear is irrigated with water at both temperatures, with a suitable delay between each test. The induced nystagmus is recorded and analysed using electronystagmography (Fig. 19.24). Nystagmus can be enhanced by the abolition of optic fixation, so Fresnel's glasses (see above) are useful in this test. Peripheral lesions tend to cause a diminished response on one side (a canal paresis), although a directional preponderance (where nystagmus in one direction is more prominent than the other) may be observed and may represent incomplete compensation or central disorders, especially in the brainstem.

RADIOLOGICAL EXAMINATION

CT scanning is the investigation of choice, especially for cholesteatoma and cranial trauma (Figs 19.25, 19.26). It also helps in the evaluation of temporal bone neoplasia. *MRI* is useful in identifying retrocochlear pathology, especially vestibular schwannoma (Fig. 19.27) when there is asymmetric sensorineural hearing loss, and tumour spread outside the temporal bone. *Angiography* is useful for embolization of vascular tumours.

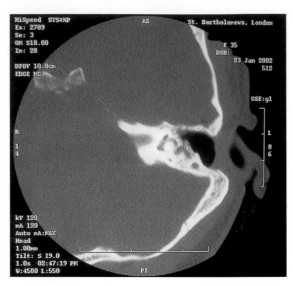

Figure 19.25 CT scan of left ear showing a fistula of the lateral semicircular canal in a patient who had previously undergone a mastoidectomy.

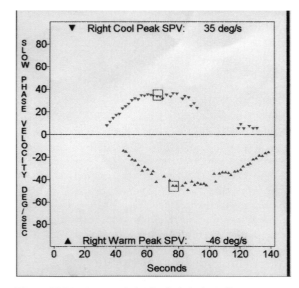

Figure 19.24 A computerized caloric test result.

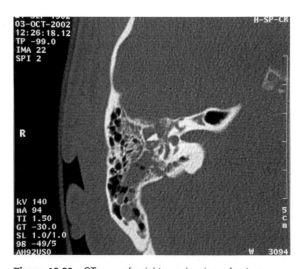

Figure 19.26 CT scan of a right ear showing a fracture across the middle ear. The incus is seen and is lying in a displaced position.

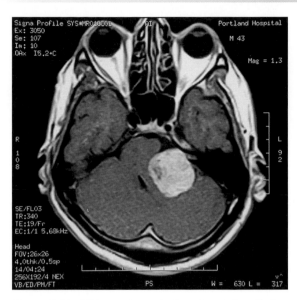

Figure 19.27 MRI scan demonstrating a large left vestibular schwannoma with brainstem compression.

THE NOSE AND PARANASAL SINUSES (Box 19.5)

ANATOMY

The nose is formed by the two nasal bones, which articulate with the nasal process of the maxilla on each side. The lateral cartilages provide support for the nostrils, especially in inspiration (Fig. 19.28). The nasal cavity is divided by the nasal septum, formed of cartilage anteriorly and bone posteriorly (Fig. 19.29). The lateral wall of the nose is formed by the three nasal turbinate bones, inferior, middle and superior (Fig. 19.30). Under each turbinate is a corresponding meatus. The nose constantly produces mucus – a pint a day – which is constantly propelled backwards by the cilia to the posterior choanae, whence it is swallowed, usually unnoticed.

The paranasal sinuses are air-filled spaces in the bones of the facial skeleton (Figs 19.30, 19.31). They comprise the paired maxillary, frontal and ethmoidal sinuses and the unpaired but bisected sphenoid sinus, and form the structure of the adult face. The ethmoidal cells or labyrinth comprises a number of small bony cells. The sinuses open into the nose via small drainage channels (ostia). Their mucus is swept by cilia through the ostia to be mixed with mucus secreted by the nose. The middle meatus is the common pathway for drainage from the maxillary, the anterior ethmoidal and the frontal sinuses. The anterior ethmoids are important because disease in these areas will compromise maxillary and frontal sinus drainage. Blockage of the ostia due to inflammation in the nose, with retention of mucus and secondary infection, is the presumed mechanism for sinus infection (rhino-

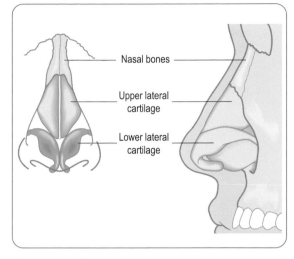

Figure 19.28   The external nose.

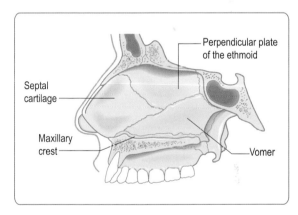

Figure 19.29   The nasal septum.

sinusitis). The upper teeth are closely related to the floor of the maxillary sinus: infection here may lead to sinus problems.

The olfactory neuroepithelium of the nose is located in the roof of the nasal cavity. Neurons run through the cribriform plate to the olfactory bulb lying on the floor of the anterior cranial fossa. The postnasal space contains the adenoids, which are lymphoid tissue, part of Waldeyer's ring, which includes the palatine tonsils. These are largest in childhood and regress from the age of about 8 years onwards, although rarely they may persist into adult life. The inferior opening of the Eustachian tube is on the lateral wall of the postnasal space.

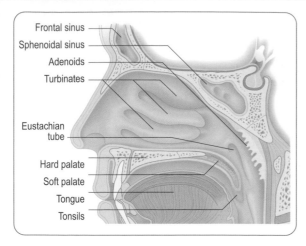

Figure 19.30 The lateral wall of the nose.

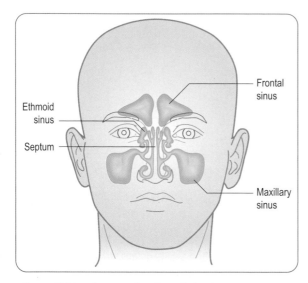

Figure 19.31 Cross-section through the sinuses (semischematic).

SYMPTOMS OF NASAL DISEASE

The important symptoms of nasal and sinus disease are:

- Nasal blockage
- Rhinorrhoea – nasal discharge
- Epistaxis (nasal bleeding)
- Sneezing and itching
- Disturbances of smell
- Facial pain.

GENERAL FEATURES

Orbital and facial pain, proptosis, diplopia, periorbital swelling and conjunctival chemosis may develop if infection or neoplasia spread outside the sinuses. Pathology in the postnasal space may lead to otological symptoms secondary to Eustachian tube involvement.

NASAL BLOCKAGE

Unilateral or bilateral blockage of the nose is common. Maximum resistance to airflow occurs at the front of the nose near the inferior turbinate. In the nasal cycle one side is congested and one side decongested at any one time. This cycle has a normal periodicity of 2–6 hours. The commonest cause of nasal blockage is allergic rhinitis. A constant blockage suggests a structural abnormality, such as a deviated nasal septum or nasal polyposis or, in children, adenoidal hypertrophy.

RHINORRHOEA

Nasal discharge may be mucoid, purulent or watery. It may contain blood. A *purulent discharge* suggests infection, either in the nose or in the sinus. In a child, unilateral discharge may be due to a foreign body retained in the nose. *Mucoid discharge* is more suggestive of allergic rhinitis. *Watery discharge* is indicative of vasomotor rhinitis. CSF leak is a rare but important cause; the discharge is clear, watery and sweet-tasting. *Epistaxis* (a nose bleed) varies in severity from a minor intermittent problem to a life-threatening major haemorrhage that may require cautery. It tends to occur in children and the elderly. The arterial supply of the nose is from branches of the sphenopalatine artery (external carotid), and from the anterior and posterior ethmoidal arteries (internal carotid). These vessels anastomose in the anterior nasal septum, the site of most epistaxes. Epistaxis is associated with hypertension, trauma (including nose-picking), rhinitis and bleeding disorders.

ITCHING AND SNEEZING

Sneezing is a protective expulsive reflex that helps clear the nasal airway of irritants. Paroxysmal sneezing, associated with rhinorrhoea, nasal obstruction and palatal and conjunctival itching, occurs with allergic rhinitis.

DISTURBANCES OF SMELL

Loss of smell (*anosmia*) or impaired sense of smell is most often due to nasal obstruction preventing airborne molecules gaining access to the olfactory cleft, e.g. with nasal polyposis or allergic rhinitis. It also follows damage to nerve fibres passing through the cribriform plate after craniofacial trauma. Rarely, viral infection may cause permanent anosmia. *Cacosmia* is an unpleasant smell, usually unnoticed by the patient, caused by chronic anaerobic sepsis in the nose.

FACIAL PAIN

Pain in the face is very common, but pain limited to the nose is rare. Pain centred over a sinus may indicate infection or, rarely, a malignancy. There are many causes of facial pain. Some, such as trigeminal neuralgia and cluster headache, are functional dis-

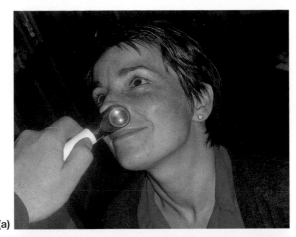

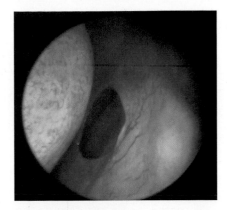

Figure 19.33 A septal perforation.

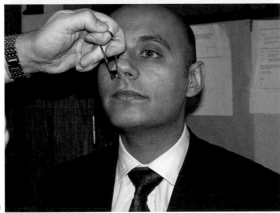

(a)

(b)

Figure 19.32 Examining the nose.

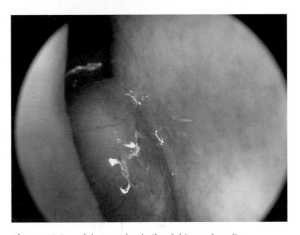

Figure 19.34 A large polyp in the right nasal cavity.

orders, with well defined features. Cluster headache causes transient nasal blockage and rhinorrhoea as part of its symptom complex. Structural disorders, such as infection or tumour involving facial structures, may also present with facial pain. Investigation should usually include imaging by CT or MRI.

OTHER SYMPTOMS
Always enquire about any history of allergy. Most people are aware of hay fever.

EXAMINATION OF THE NOSE

Inspect the nose from the front, side and back in a good light. With age the tip of the nose tends to droop. Deformities of the nasal bone and cartilage, such as saddle deformity, often follow a nasal fracture or other destructive disorders of the bony septum or cartilaginous septum. *Palpate* the nose and facial skeleton, especially the orbital margins, noting tenderness and any swelling, expansion or depression of bone. Facial swelling is unusual in maxillary sinusitis, but occurs with dental root infections and in carcinoma of the maxillary antrum.

Inspect and palpate the palate and alveoli from inside the mouth using a gloved finger.

Examine the *nasal vestibule* and intranasal contents by gently pushing the tip of the nose upwards with a finger, preferably using reflected illumination from a head mirror. The nasal vestibule is lined with skin and contains vibrissae: these become prominent in older men. Inspect the anterior nasal cavity with Thudicum's nasal speculum or an otoscope (Fig. 19.32). The nasal septum is often deviated or thickened. When deviated, hypertrophy of the contralateral inferior turbinate may also develop, causing bilateral nasal blockage. Look for any area of granulation on the nasal septum and for any perforation (Fig. 19.33). Perforations may be secondary to cocaine snorting, nose-picking, surgical trauma, granulomatous conditions, or inhalation of industrial dusts, notably nickel and chrome.

Nasal polyps are usually easily identifiable by their pale colour (Fig. 19.34) and their softness and lack of sensitivity to probing. In a child, an apparent polyp may be seen arising from the roof of the nose: this should not be probed as it may be the intranasal presentation of a meningocele. In children and adults airflow through a patent nostril causes

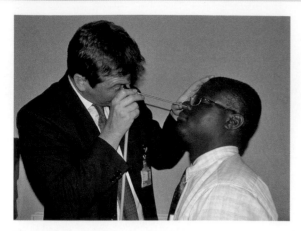

Figure 19.35   Rigid nasal endoscopy.

Box 19.6   Common inhalant allergens

- House dust and house dust mite
- Grasses
- Trees
- Weeds
- Animal dander: cat, dog, rabbit
- Feathers
- Moulds

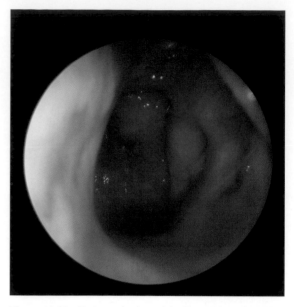

Figure 19.36   Endoscopic view of the Eustachian tube orifice and the postnasal space.

misting on a cold metal tongue depressor or mirror held at the nose. In a neonate nasal patency is best estimated by observing any movement of a wisp of cotton wool held in front of each nostril, after blocking each in turn with the thumb. *Nasal endoscopy* (Fig. 19.35), after applying a topical decongestant such as xylometazoline with topical lignocaine anaesthesia, allows inspection of the middle meatus for oedema, draining pus or polyps. The postnasal space and the opening of the Eustachian tube (Fig. 19.36) can be seen, with the fossa of Rosenmuller, the site of origin of postnasal space carcinomas, lying directly above and behind. In children and young adults, look for adenoidal swelling.

SPECIAL TESTS

ALLERGY TESTING

If allergic symptoms are severe there is merit in confirming extrinsic allergy by skin-prick testing. A solution containing the allergen is introduced into the superficial epidermis of the flexor surface of the forearm using a disposable lance. Any antihistamine therapy should be stopped, as this may cause a false negative response. The common inhalant allergens (Box 19.6), together with any agents that have been suspected from the history, should be tested and compared to positive and negative controls (histamine and saline). A positive response is a wheal and flare. However, a negative response does not definitely exclude atopy. If clinical suspicion is strong, the radioallergosorbent test (RAST), which measures specific IgE in blood, may be considered, although it is expensive. Nasal provocation tests are time-consuming, as only one allergen at a time can be tested.

NASAL PATENCY

Objective assessment is difficult. Rhinomanometry, which measures nasal airflow and resistance, and acoustic rhinometry, which measures nasal volume and cross-sectional area, remain specialized research tools.

MUCOCILIARY CLEARANCE

This is a test of impaired ciliary function used, for example, in Kartagener's syndrome of impaired ciliary motility. Saccharin placed on the anterior end of the inferior turbinate should be tasted in the mouth about 20 minutes later.

RADIOLOGICAL EXAMINATION

Plain X-rays are unreliable in the management of sinus disease. However, a lateral X-ray may be useful in estimating the degree of adenoidal hypertrophy in young children (Fig. 19.37). Endoscopic nasal examination and CT scanning are the investigations of choice for sinus disease (Fig. 19.38). CT is useful in the management of chronic infection, trauma and neoplasia. However, the radiation dosage to the eyes is significant and the investigation should be used only as a presurgical technique, or when the diagnosis is uncertain. Magnetic resonance imaging (MRI) is less useful in sinus disease.

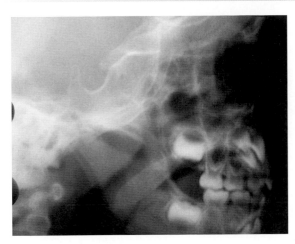

Figure 19.37 Lateral X-ray of the nasopharynx demonstrating adenoidal hypertrophy.

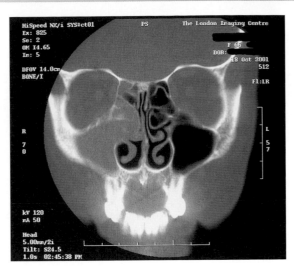

Figure 19.38 Coronal CT scan of the nose showing an opaque right maxillary antrum and anterior ethmoid cells.

THE THROAT

ANATOMY

The throat includes the oral cavity (see Chapter 20), the pharynx (oropharynx, nasopharynx and hypopharynx), the larynx and the major salivary glands. The pharynx extends from the base of the skull to the cricopharyngeal sphincter (Fig. 19.39). The *oropharynx* is bounded above by the soft palate and below by the upper surface of the epiglottis. Its anterior margin is defined laterally by the anterior faucial pillar, containing the palatoglossus muscle, and by the posterior third of the tongue. The posterior pharyngeal wall is its posterior boundary. The palatine tonsils are situated laterally between the anterior and posterior pillars of the fauces. The base of the tongue contains the lingual tonsils. This lymphoid tissue, together with the adenoids and the tubal tonsil (lymphoid tissue around the Eustachian tube opening), makes up Waldeyer's ring, an important line of immunological defence. The *hypopharynx* consists of the posterior pharyngeal wall, the piriform fossae and the postcricoid area. The *piriform fossae*, which comprise the lateral walls of the pharynx adjacent to the larynx, are the routes by which food is passed into the upper oesophagus. The *larynx* is a rigid structure consisting of cartilages, the most prominent of which are the paired thyroid cartilages, which articulate with the cricoid cartilage below. The epiglottis is attached to the inner surface of the thyroid cartilage and aids the separation of air and food passages during swallowing. The larynx consists of three compartments (Fig. 19.40): glottis, supraglottis and subglottis. The *glottis* is formed by the vocal folds. The glottis has poor lymphatic drainage, which may help to delay the spread of malignancy from this area. The *epiglottis* extends from the false cords below to the hyoid bone above. It has a rich lymphatic drainage, and therefore malignancy in this area is more frequently associated with metastatic disease. The *subglottis* is the narrowest part of the upper respiratory tract and extends from the glottis to the lower border of the cricoid.

The prime function of the *larynx* is to separate breathing and swallowing, thereby protecting the airway. Voice production is a secondary function that has arisen with evolution. *Phonation* occurs with movement of the vocal folds into the midline (Fig. 19.41). Changes in volume of the voice are caused by alterations in the subglottic pressure, whereas alterations in pitch are due to modification of the length and tension of the vocal folds. The quality of this basic laryngeal sound is modulated by resonance in the pharynx, air sinuses, mouth and nose.

The *pharynx* is innervated from the pharyngeal plexus (cranial nerves IX, X, XI). Interruption of this nerve supply by lesions at the jugular foramen leads to swallowing problems and severe morbidity. All the muscles of the larynx except the cricothyroid are supplied by the *recurrent laryngeal* branch of the vagus (cranial nerve X). In the chest this nerve loops around the arch of the aorta on the left and the subclavian artery on the right, before running up to enter the larynx. The long course of the left recurrent laryngeal nerve means it is more frequently affected by disease. The cricothyroid is supplied by the external branch of the superior laryngeal nerve (CN X).

The lymph nodes of the head and neck (Fig. 19.42) provide a barrier to the spread of disease, whether inflammatory or neoplastic. Enlargement implies that there is either primary disease within the nodes or that they have become involved secondary to pathology in the areas they drain. Occasionally they may become involved by pathology below the clavicle.

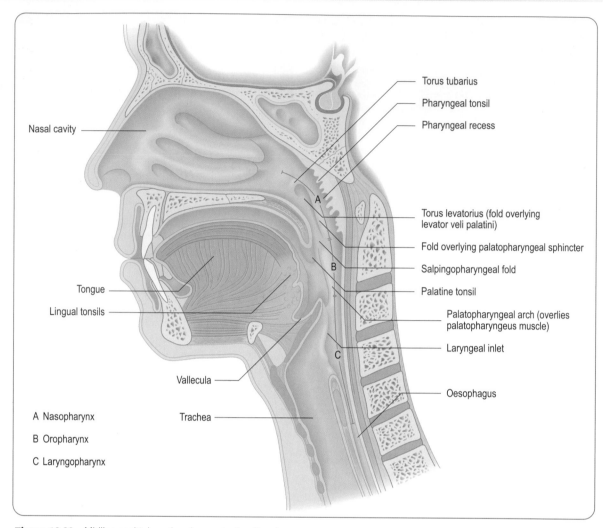

Figure 19.39   Midline sagittal section demonstrating the pharynx.

SYMPTOMS OF THROAT DISEASE

Patients with throat disorders present with:

- Pain
- Stridor, or stertorous (noisy) breathing
- Dysphonia (hoarseness)
- Dysphagia (difficulty in swallowing)
- A mass in the neck.

Occasionally lesions in the upper airway may present with overspill of food and fluids into the upper trachea or nose, or with weight loss. Malignant throat and airway disease is very strongly associated with smoking.

SORE THROAT

A sore throat is one of the commonest of all symptoms. Viral pharyngitis is the most common cause. Tonsillar inflammation is also common. Acute follicular tonsillitis begins with local redness, developing into a punctate or confluent yellow exudate on the tonsils, often due to group A α-haemolytic *Streptococcus* infection. In *glandular fever* (Epstein–Barr virus infection) the tonsils are covered with a white membrane with palatal petechiae. A grey membrane is the classic feature of the now-rare infection with *Corynebacterium diphtheriae*. A throat swab for culture and sensitivity is a useful test. Find out the frequency and severity of attacks of tonsillitis, as estimated by the amount of time lost from schooling or work, and any antibiotic treatment: such considerations help to decide whether tonsillectomy is merited. Generally in children at least four attacks a year for 2 years is the minimum indication for tonsillectomy.

An abscess adjacent to the tonsil (*quinsy*) is very painful, causing dysphagia and *trismus* (spasm in the lower jaw). Surgical drainage is usually required. Squamous cell carcinoma of the tonsil is also often painful. It presents as an *exophytic mass or ulcer*. In the early stages diagnosis is difficult. Ulceration in the oropharynx also occurs in glan-

Labels in figure:
Torus tubarius
Pharyngeal tonsil
Pharyngeal recess
Torus levatorius (fold overlying levator veli palatini)
Fold overlying palatopharyngeal sphincter
Salpingopharyngeal fold
Palatine tonsil
Palatopharyngeal arch (overlies palatopharyngeus muscle)
Laryngeal inlet
Oesophagus
Nasal cavity
Tongue
Lingual tonsils
Vallecula
Trachea
A Nasopharynx
B Oropharynx
C Laryngopharynx

dular fever, rubella and streptococcal tonsillitis, as well as from trauma due to ill-fitting dentures or broken teeth.

STRIDOR AND STERTOR

Stridor is noisy breathing associated with upper airway obstruction at the laryngeal level (Box 19.7). *Stertor* is noisy breathing at the oropharyngeal level and is nearly always caused by adenotonsillar hypertrophy. Epiglottitis is particularly important in infants and small children up to the age of 7 years. It is associated with infection by *Haemophilus influenzae* type B, and may present with rapidly progressive airway obstruction and dyspnoea, fever, pharyngeal pain and drooling. Vaccination has reduced its incidence. Immediate antibiotic therapy may need to be supplemented by intubation or even tracheostomy. In adults laryngeal carcinoma may cause stridor owing to direct blockage of the airway, to fixation of the vocal fold, or with recurrent laryngeal nerve involvement. *Croup* – acute laryngotracheobronchitis – in young children causes less severe airway obstruction. The thick tenacious secretions are relieved by air humidification.

DYSPHONIA

Dysphonia or hoarseness covers a range of symptoms, from subtle changes noticed by professional voice users to *aphonia*, when there is no voice. It may be caused by structural problems affecting the vocal fold, or by neurological disease (Box 19.8). Hoarseness followed by increasing airway obstruction is the typical presentation of a laryngeal neoplasm (Fig. 19.43). Damage to the recurrent

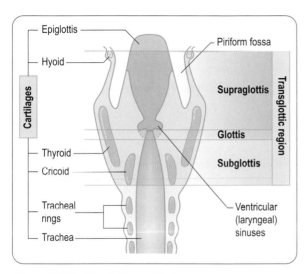

Figure 19.40 The divisions of the larynx.

Box 19.7 Causes of stridor

Neonatal
- Congenital tumours and cysts
- Laryngomalacia
- Subglottic stenosis

Children
- Supraglottitis (epiglottitis)
- Laryngotracheobronchitis
- Acute laryngitis
- Foreign body
- Retropharyngeal abscess
- Papillomatosis

Adults
- Acute laryngitis
- Laryngeal trauma
- Laryngeal carcinoma
- Supraglottitis (epiglottitis)

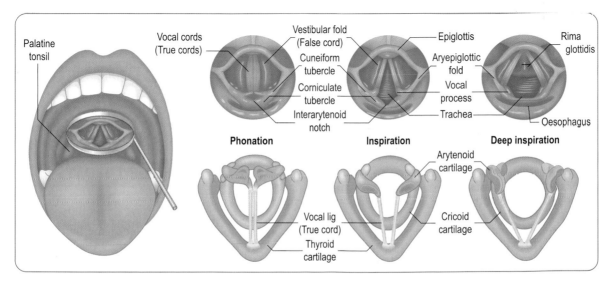

Figure 19.41 The mechanism of phonation.

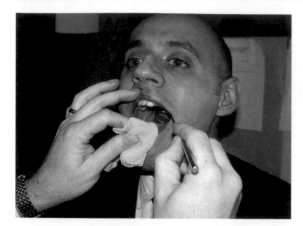

Figure 19.45   Indirect laryngoscopy.

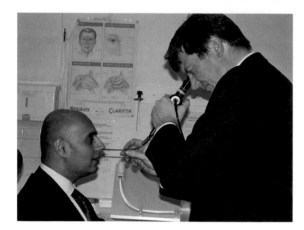

Figure 19.46   Flexible fibreoptic nasendoscopy.

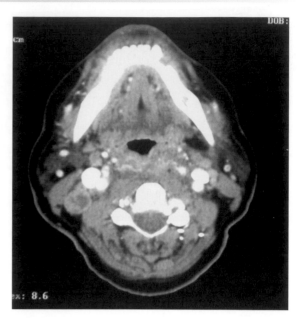

Figure 19.47   CT scan of neck demonstrating a large metastatic lymph node with central necrosis.

parotid and preauricular areas are then examined, followed by submandibular and submental nodes. Finally, the nodes associated with the anterior jugular chain are examined. This brings the fingers to the thyroid gland (Chapter 12). The position and size of the thyroid should be noted: because it lies deep to the small strap muscles of the neck, it is often best examined with the patient's neck partially flexed to relax the overlying structures. Consider whether the gland is enlarged and, if so, decide whether the enlargement is uniform or confined to one or other lobe. Is the gland smooth or nodular, and is it possible to get the fingers below it on palpation? Irregularity, hardness and fixation of the gland to neighbouring structures are features of malignancy.

If there is a midline mass, observe it as the patient swallows a little water. The thyroid gland moves as the patient swallows. Such a manoeuvre may draw a small retrosternal goitre above the examining fingers. Midline lumps should also be assessed with the patient protruding the tongue. Movement suggests attachment to the base of the tongue and implies the presence of a thyroglossal cyst. The larynx should be mobile from side to side, and if

the thyroid cartilage is held between thumb and first finger and gently moved against the cervical spine, should grate. This laryngeal crepitus is a normal phenomenon. It may be reduced or abolished by hypopharyngeal pathology or a mass in the prevertebral space displacing the larynx away from the cervical spine. Finally, auscultate the carotid arteries and, if indicated, the thyroid gland.

SPECIAL TESTS

Fine needle aspiration cytology is described in Chapter 20. If correctly performed, this will diagnose the vast majority of metastatic squamous carcinomas. It is less accurate in distinguishing lymphoma from reactive changes. If doubt remains an excision biopsy should be performed.

RADIOLOGICAL EXAMINATION

A soft tissue lateral neck X-ray is not a sensitive investigation, even for detecting foreign bodies. A barium swallow is a dynamic investigation and can locate obstruction in the oesophagus or demonstrate incoordinate swallowing. It can be combined with video recording (videofluoroscopy). It is less helpful in evaluating the hypopharynx, where endoscopy under a general anaesthetic is the preferred investigation. Endoscopy is helpful in taking biopsies in suspected malignancy. Ultrasound is useful for the evaluation of neck masses and the thyroid gland. Doppler ultrasound assesses the cervical vasculature. CT scanning helps to stage neoplastic disease and may demonstrate metastatic spread that has eluded palpation (Fig. 19.47).

Face, mouth, jaws and neck

J. L. B. Carter

20

INTRODUCTION

The face, head and neck have a special emotional and psychological importance for expression and communication, as well as breathing, chewing and swallowing. Management of disorders of this complex set of functions often requires cooperation between the several medical specialties in a multidisciplinary team.

THE HISTORY

Symptoms are often misleading. For example, dental or jaw disorders may cause earache, facial pain or headache. Neurological disorders, e.g. multiple sclerosis, can present with changes in facial or oral sensation, or with trigeminal pain. Drug-related manifestations are common and dietary habits are important. Sexually transmitted diseases may involve the oral cavity. Swellings of the lymphatic nodes of the neck may precede recognition of a local cause, but careful history taking may suggest the diagnosis. Remember to ask generally about previous dental hygiene and treatment. Previous cosmetic and dental procedures are frequently overlooked in hospital and GP records, and direct questions will be necessary. Diseases that affect facial appearance are often stigmatized; the patient may need time to explain the problem.

The mouth is the entrance to the gastrointestinal tract. Its role in the lubrication of food, mastication, taste, speech and breathing requires sensorimotor integration of mouth, tongue and pharynx. It also has a frequently overlooked role in immune surveillance. Questions about all these functions are important. Cancer of the mouth (Fig. 20.1) is much feared but is not common: about 2000 cases per year occur in the UK. The inside of the lower lip is the commonest site, followed by the tongue, floor of mouth, buccal mucosa (cheek lining) and the area behind the lower back teeth (retromolar area). It presents with a progressively enlarging hard lump, or a persistent ulcer, that may be painful.

THE FACE

EXAMINATION

Inspect the full face in a good light. Note the quality and tone of the skin. A high colour, e.g. flushing of the cheeks, may simply represent embarrassment, but can be a feature of cardiac or dermatological disease. Test facial movements by asking the patient to smile, frown, and bare their teeth together. Examine young children so they can see their mother (Fig. 20.2).

Note any asymmetry of the facial contours, scars, pigmentation or involuntary movements. Are the teeth level and clean, or carious, and do the gum margins look healthy? If dentures are worn are they well fitted, or do they drop when the mouth is opened? Consider the possibility of a congenital anomaly, most commonly Down's syndrome, cleft disorders and other craniofacial syndromes. Does any swelling within the mouth cause facial distortion? Is speech affected? Test facial and oral sensation on both sides using light touch and pinprick. Check sensation in the upper forehead, midface and lower jaw areas corresponding to the three divisions of the trigeminal (fifth cranial) nerve. Check the facial reflexes (see Chapter 10).

FACIAL WEAKNESS

This is not always easy to recognize, especially if it is bilateral. Lower motor neuron facial palsy, due to damage to the facial nerve, as in Bell's palsy, or surgical injury to the facial nerve, causes a dramatic change in facial appearance that is sudden in onset (Fig. 20.3). Infiltration of the nerve by cancer, for example in the parotid gland, causes slowly progressive facial weakness, often partial or localized to one part of the face, which may be painful. Upper motor neuron lesions also cause facial weakness (see Chapter 10) (Box 20.1).

Facial wounds are common. Take particular care to assess facial movement before suturing. If there is abnormality, exploration of the nerve is required. It is also important to search for foreign bodies in such wounds (Fig. 20.4).

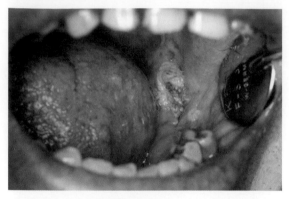

Figure 20.1 Mouth cancer: any mouth ulcer persisting for more than 2 weeks warrants urgent referral.

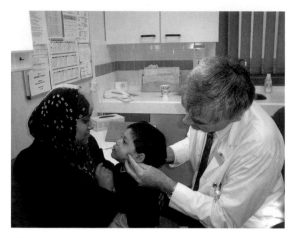

Figure 20.2 Examination of a young child is much easier when he can see his mother.

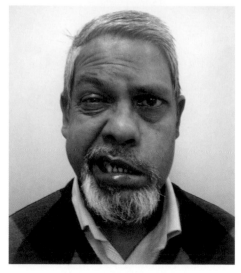

Figure 20.3 Hemifacial weakness, left side, affecting all five branches of the facial nerve (seventh cranial nerve).

Box 20.1   Causes of facial weakness

- Neurological
  - Stroke
  - Bell's palsy
  - Cerebral tumour
  - Moebius syndrome
  - Multiple sclerosis
  - Ramsay Hunt syndrome
- Trauma or surgery
- Middle ear disease
- Skull base malignancy
- Parotid malignancy
- Sarcoidosis
- Myopathies and muscular dystrophies

Glass fragments can often be felt on probing, and they are radio-opaque. An X-ray of the face is therefore very useful. Retained organic material, such as wood, is difficult to identify. Use an ultrasound examination to exclude this.

GENERAL FEATURES

Inspection, palpation, percussion and auscultation all have their place in examination of the head and neck region. An unusual appearance of the facial skin can provide clues to systemic illness or to dermatological disorders. In childhood, 'port wine stains' should be differentiated from more aggressive vascular malformations. Adults are prone to actinic skin changes, especially on the lower lip (Fig. 20.5).

In the elderly, rodent ulcers (basal cell carcinoma) are the commonest malignant lesions of the face and scalp. Pigmented lesions may raise concerns about melanoma.

Minor degrees of facial and jaw asymmetry are common and may raise cosmetic concerns when pointed out by friends or even by clinicians. Look for signs of previous surgical repair of cleft palate or lip. A dental abscess or a blocked salivary duct causes local pain and swelling with signs of inflammation. Parotid gland swelling often causes elevation of the earlobe; it is often best seen from behind the patient, although this may require long hair to be lifted away from the ear (Fig. 20.6).

The eyes should always be included when inspecting the face. Look especially for abnormalities such as iris irregularities, difference in the size of the pupils, redness of the conjunctiva and abnormalities of ocular movement.

THE MOUTH

Examine the mouth with the patient sitting up, head resting comfortably on a pillow or headrest. A good examination light is essential; two dental mirrors and, in the consulting room setting, a chair that

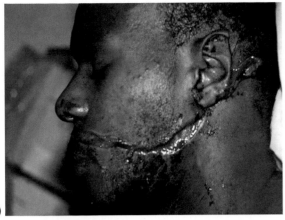

(a)

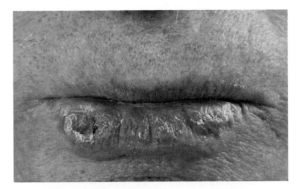

Figure 20.5 Actinic skin changes on the lower lip.

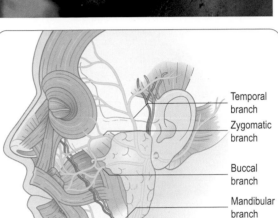

(b)

Figure 20.4 This laceration may involve facial nerve and salivary tissue injury.

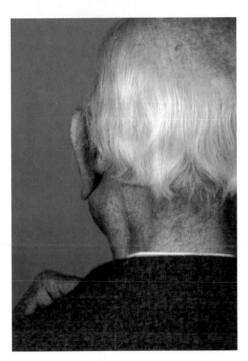

Figure 20.6 Parotid gland swelling elevates the earlobe and is often best seen from behind the patient.

allows positioning of the patient are ideal. The lips, teeth, gums, tongue, palate, fauces, tonsils and oropharynx must be systematically inspected. *Palpation* of the inside of the cheek, sides of the tongue and floor of the mouth is done with gloved fingers to assist retraction of the tongue, to feel for irregularities, and to assess the size and consistency of the tissues (Fig. 20.7). Note the number, type and regularity of the teeth, their state of repair or decay, and any looseness. The gums should be assessed and the patient asked about any tendency for them to bleed when the teeth are brushed (*gingivitis*).

THE LIPS (Fig. 20.8)

Look closely at the philtrum (the shallow depression running from nose to upper lip) for the telltale scar of a repaired cleft lip. In the mouth a submucosal cleft may be difficult to recognize. A bifid uvula is a harmless indicator of minimal failure of fusion. Inspect the corners of the mouth for cracks or fissures (angular stomatitis). In children this is infective, but in the elderly such cracks occur when ill-fitting dentures – or the absence of teeth – result

in overclosure of the corners of the mouth, encouraging candidiasis (thrush). *Cheilosis* may also be seen in severe iron-deficiency anaemia and in vitamin B$_2$ (riboflavin) deficiency. Grouped vesicles on the lips on a red base with crusted lesions are seen in *herpes simplex labialis*. This infection is an acute disorder, and the lack of induration and ulceration serves to distinguish it from malignancy. Recurrent actinic inflammation of the lips (cheilitis) with small blisters and exfoliation, however, is a premalignant condition found in people constantly exposed to the sun and wind (Fig. 20.5) or when there is immune suppression. Any ulcer on the lips should therefore be carefully assessed. *Squamous cell carcinoma* usually occurs on the lower lip away from the midline; it is persistent, indolent, flat and shallow, although in time the edge may become

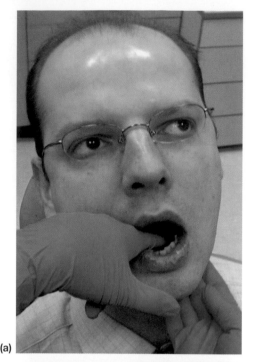

(a)

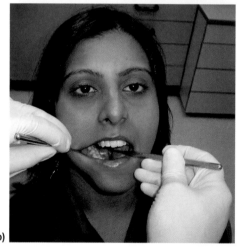

(b)

Figure 20.7   **(a)** Intraoral palpation and **(b)** inspection using two mirrors.

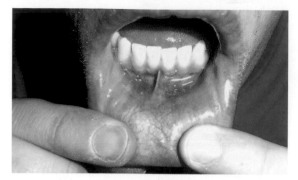

Figure 20.8   Gently grasp the lower lip with the index finger and thumb of both hands to display the mucosal surface of the lip.

painless cervical nodes may often be felt. Oral and perioral light brown pigmentation is a feature of the *Peutz–Jeghers syndrome*, which is associated with small bowel polyposis. On the buccal mucosa this pigmentation resembles that of Addison's disease. Look carefully at the lips and tongue for the fine, red streaks of telangiectasia. Their presence may signal the existence of others elsewhere in the intestine or in other organs, which occasionally bleed. They may also represent a side effect of external beam radiotherapy.

MOUTH ULCERS

An ulcer is the commonest lesion of the mouth. *Aphthous ulcers* are small, painful superficial ulcers of the tongue, buccal mucosa and palate. Although said to be associated with chronic anaemia, this is an unusual cause of mouth ulceration and aphthous ulcers are probably viral in origin. Aphthous ulcers, and ulcers due to trauma from bite errors, usually heal quickly, although they often recur. Chronic ulceration may indicate immune suppression or other chronic conditions, such as Sjögren's syndrome, thrush (an infection with *Candida albicans*) or drug sensitivity. Sharp or decayed teeth, gum infection (periodontal disease) or poor dentures may be the cause of an ulcer, but bleeding gums, dental sinus or foul breath may indicate a more serious underlying disease, such as mouth cancer or leukaemia. Mouth ulcers are sometimes found in inflammatory bowel disease, particularly Crohn's disease. Mouth ulcers in association with genital ulcers may indicate Behçet's syndrome. In general *any mouth ulcer that persists for longer than 2 weeks warrants further investigation* (Fig. 20.1).

FACIAL PAIN

Altered sensation inside the mouth or on the face suggests a lesion in the brain or at the base of the skull (Fig. 20.9). Pain in the mouth or face has many causes. Sharp, shooting pain in the lower third of one side of the face, induced by light contact in

heaped-up and indurated. Squamous cell carcinoma must be differentiated from benign keratoacanthoma, pyogenic granuloma and the chancre of primary syphilis. *Pyogenic granuloma* presents as a soft red raspberry-like nodule on the upper lip. A vertical fissure in the centre of the lower lip is a common, painful problem, but is of no sinister significance.

Primary syphilitic chancre of the upper lip is rare. It appears as a small, round lesion that is firm and indurated. A 'snail-track ulcer', most commonly found on the mucosa in secondary syphilis, has a serpiginous outline with a greyish-white non-purulent exudate. In both carcinoma and chancre, enlarged

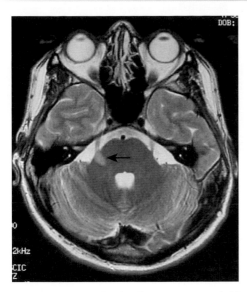

Figure 20.9 MRI scan showing the eyes, nose, periorbita and intracranial base of skull; on the left side (arrow) in this T2 weighted image is a grey lesion suggestive of demyelination (multiple sclerosis).

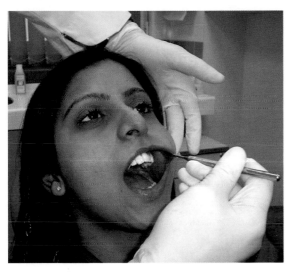

Figure 20.10 To inspect the buccal mucosa, retract the cheek with a dental mirror or a spatula.

the mouth or on the face, suggests trigeminal neuralgia and requires neurological investigation. Sensations of taste, smell, hearing and sight must be assessed in any examination of a patient with facial pain. Always inspect the buccal mucosa, by retracting the cheek with a spatula or dental mirror, to exclude cancer in the mouth (Fig. 20.10).

ORAL MUCOSA

The moist mucosal lining of the mouth can be breached by ulceration or thickened by dysplasia (Box 20.2). Dysplasia may present as discoloration, commonly due to thinning of the tissues causing

---

Box 20.2 Risk factors for mucosal dysplasia

- Smoking
- Chewing tobacco
- Pan (areca/betel nut)
- Alcohol
- Amalgam fillings
- Lichen planus

Box 20.3 Redness of oral mucosa

- Candidosis
- Denture-induced stomatitis
- Irradiation mucositis
- Purpura
- Telangiectasis
- Atrophic lichen planus
- Angioma
- Kaposi's sarcoma

Box 20.4 White patches

- White opalescent patches (rather like white paint) of leukoplakia
  - seen on the inner aspect of the cheek
  - should be differentiated from lichen planus
- Small white points raised somewhat above the surrounding surface
  - thrush (monilial stomatitis), a fungal infection due to *Candida albicans*
- As the infection progresses:
  - lesions coalesce and may form extensive sheets throughout the mouth
  - patches can be removed only with difficulty
  - tend to leave behind a raw surface
  - common in debilitated children, beneath neglected dentures, and in patients on cytotoxic or immunosuppressive drugs
  - seen frequently in ill patients with sepsis
  - with broad-spectrum antibiotics
  - also a feature of cellular immunodeficiency states, including AIDS

---

redness (Box 20.3) or by thickening as keratinization, appearing white (Box 20.4).

When examining the mouth, look for:

- The opening of the parotid duct adjacent to the upper first molar tooth
- Small bluish-white spots, known as Koplik's spots, may be seen opposite the molar teeth (nonpathological)
- Areas of dots of slate-grey or blue pigmentation are seen in Addison's disease

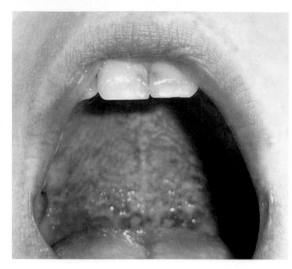

Figure 20.11 Stomatitis in the palate may be triggered by candida or smoking.

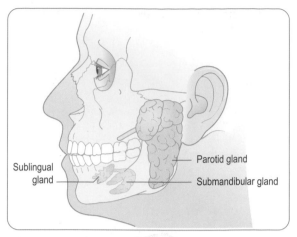

Figure 20.12 The three named major salivary glands are supplemented by hundreds of minor glands.

- Thickening of the buccal mucosa may reduce gape restriction due to hyperkeratosis. In Asian communities this may be due to submucous fibrosis.

White opalescent patches on the oral mucosa, rather like white paint, termed *leukoplakia*, occur on the inner aspect of the cheek. They should be differentiated from lichen planus. Small white points, raised somewhat above the surrounding surface, suggest thrush (monilial stomatitis), a fungal infection due to *Candida albicans* (Fig. 20.11). As the infection spreads the lesions coalesce and may form extensive sheets throughout the mouth. Patches of monilia can be removed only with difficulty and tend to leave behind a raw surface. Candidiasis is common in debilitated children and in immuno-suppressed subjects, e.g. AIDS/HIV infection, or chemotherapy for cancer. It also occurs beneath neglected dentures and when there is poor dental hygiene. It is common during treatment for sepsis and with broad-spectrum antibiotic treatment. In general, *all persistent red and white patches on the oral mucosa warrant urgent specialist consultation.*

SALIVARY GLAND DISEASE

There are three anatomically named major salivary glands on each side of the mouth (Fig. 20.12), but hundreds of tiny accessory salivary glands distributed across the oral mucosa. Many salivary gland problems are more evident at mealtimes. Calculus obstruction is common in the parotid and sub-mandibular ducts, and in the latter the stones are usually radio-opaque. The parotid papilla emerges through the cheek mucosa at a point level with the upper first molar tooth. To confirm free flow of thin, clear parotid saliva, dry this area of the mouth with gauze before gently massaging over the parotid

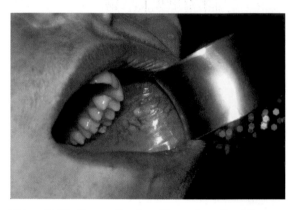

Figure 20.13 Pus exuding from Stensen's papilla at the opening of the parotid duct, which is seen as a tiny swelling adjacent to the upper first molar tooth.

gland in front of the ear, and observing whether there is flow from the duct outlet. Acute bacterial infection may reveal a bead of pus when the gland is massaged (Fig. 20.13).

Blockage of minor salivary glands preventing the secretion of mucus is common, especially around the lips. These *retention cysts* of the mucous glands of the lips and buccal mucosa (mucoceles) appear as round, translucent swellings, elevated from the surface and having a characteristic white or bluish appearance. They also occur on the mucous surface of the lower lip or in the floor of the mouth. A thin-walled blue swelling raising the floor of the mouth under the base of the tongue is called a ranula (Fig. 20.14) and represents a mucus-filled cyst; it usually requires excision.

Causes of salivary gland enlargement are listed in Box 20.5. Mumps usually affects the parotid glands bilaterally and occurs most frequently in children; in men it is sometimes accompanied by painful inflammation of the testicles (orchitis). Non-infective sialoadenitis is seen with dehydration in neonates, in diabetes and in the elderly.

THE TEETH

Look inside the mouth and count the teeth carefully. Counting teeth requires knowledge of the normal: from the usually toothless neonatal mouth to the 20 primary teeth of the 3-year-old, through the mixed dentition stage from 6 years of age, to the final eruption of wisdom teeth (third molars) usually by the age of 21 (Fig. 20.15).

Feel for loose teeth; these are common in children when the primary teeth are ready to exfoliate, but not before then. In adults the commonest cause for loose teeth is chronic periodontal infection. Unexplained mobility of teeth not associated with these factors may relate to damage to the tooth's supporting bone, either by cyst degeneration or by cancer, and must be investigated without delay (Fig. 20.16).

Missing teeth may have never developed or may be located in an ectopic position. Delayed or partial eruption of a tooth may represent impaction against an adjacent tooth, as with impacted wisdom teeth. Ask the patient to grimace so as to show the teeth, and then to open the mouth widely, after removing any dentures. Use a tongue depressor to retract first the lips and then the cheeks, and look for decay (dental caries) on the buccal and lingual aspects of the teeth.

DISCOLORATION

Calculus (tartar) deposition occurs mainly on the lingual aspect of the lower incisor and canine teeth and consists of precipitated calcium salts of saliva, often stained brown in smokers. The chewing of betel nuts may also discolour teeth a reddish-brown or black. 'Pan' is betel-nut chewing quid, flavoured with spices and often with tobacco, commonly used

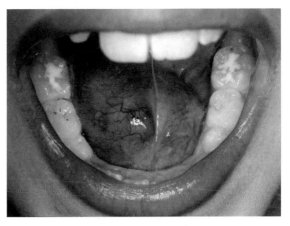

Figure 20.14 Ranula: a mucus-filled thin-walled cyst on the floor of the mouth, arising from a sublingual gland.

Box 20.5 Salivary gland enlargement

- Bacterial infection – acute painful swelling (sialoadenitis)
- Viral infection – mumps; painful swelling and rash
- Obstruction by stone – calculus; variable swelling and pain
- Salivary tumour – gradual increase in size

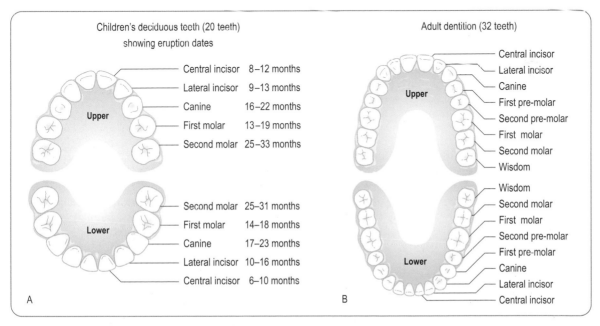

Children's deciduous teeth (20 teeth) showing eruption dates

Upper		
Central incisor	8–12 months
Lateral incisor	9–13 months
Canine	16–22 months
First molar	13–19 months
Second molar	25–33 months

Lower		
Second molar	25–31 months
First molar	14–18 months
Canine	17–23 months
Lateral incisor	10–16 months
Central incisor	6–10 months

A

Adult dentition (32 teeth)

Upper
- Central incisor
- Lateral incisor
- Canine
- First pre-molar
- Second pre-molar
- First molar
- Second molar
- Wisdom

Lower
- Wisdom
- Second molar
- First molar
- Second pre-molar
- First pre-molar
- Canine
- Lateral incisor
- Central incisor

B

Figure 20.15 **(a)** Deciduous teeth in children (20 teeth), showing eruption dates. **(b)** Adult dentition (32 teeth).

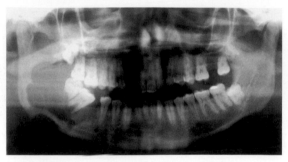

Figure 20.16 Panoral radiograph showing cystic radiolucency in the right ramus, with dental root absorption and, on the left, an impacted lower third molar with apices close to the inferior dental canal.

in Asia and in the Arab countries, which has carcinogenic properties. Children prescribed tetracyclines may develop permanent staining of both the deciduous and the permanent teeth, consisting of horizontal yellowish grey bands. In endemic fluorosis chalk-white patches appear on the teeth, or the teeth appear dull and unglazed.

SHAPE

Malformed hypoplastic teeth may have a broad, concave biting edge, and some notching of the incisors is seen in those who persistently bite cotton threads or hold hairclips between their teeth. Habitual vomiting, e.g. in bulimia, causes acid-induced erosion of the tooth surfaces.

RIDGING

Transverse ridging may follow vitamin C or vitamin D deficiency in infancy. Enlargement of the lower jaw in acromegaly causes alteration of the bite, so that the lower teeth may close outside the upper ones (class III skeletal malocclusion).

THE GUMS   (Fig. 20.17)

The gingivae are keratinized and tough enough to withstand the forces of mastication. Pink, healthy gums adhere closely to the necks of the teeth and have a sharp border. Poor dental hygiene and excess sugar consumption make them vulnerable to infection (Box 20.6). Examine the gums at the same time as the teeth. Gingivitis is the main cause of bleeding within the mouth, and although irregular and poor tooth-brushing technique with inadequate plaque removal is the most likely cause for this common condition, other causes should be considered. These include blood dyscrasias, allergic reactions and chronic debilitating disease, as well as many commonly prescribed drugs.

Acute necrotizing ulcerative gingivitis is a painful and upsetting condition. It occurs with chronic gingivitis when oral hygiene is abandoned completely or there is immune compromise.

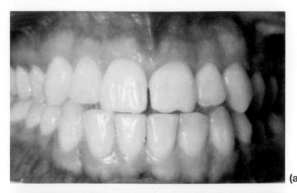

(a)

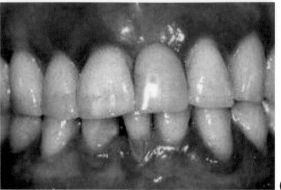

(b)

Figure 20.17   (a) Healthy gingivae. **(b)** Gingivitis.

Box 20.6   Consequences of poor dental hygiene

Poor oral health leads to:
- Gingivitis
- Bleeding of the gums
- Loosening of the gingival attachment
- Weakening the periodontal ligaments
- Infection causes destruction of the alveolar bone support for the teeth

---

BAD BREATH (HALITOSIS)

Carious teeth, periodontal infection or ulceration of the mucosa, stomatitis, and retention and decomposition of secretion in the follicles of enlarged tonsils are the commonest sources of offensive breath (halitosis) (Box 20.7). Obsessive focusing on bad breath may indicate depression. Acute ulcerative gingivitis (Vincent's gingivostomatitis) is an infection due to fusiform spirochaetes that responds swiftly to the prescription of metronidazole, and characteristically destroys the interdental papillae. A thick, felted grey slough is formed and halitosis is present.

PERIODONTAL DISEASE

Gingivitis may progress, leading to breakdown of the gums and destruction of the supportive alveolar bone. Appearing *'long in the tooth'* implies loss of the periodontal and bone support for the teeth, causing the roots to become more exposed and the teeth to loosen. Eventual loss of all the teeth is then inevitable. Shakespeare's '*sans eyes, sans teeth, sans everything*' is greatly accelerated by smoking.

Hypertrophy of the gums and secondary gingivitis are a feature of long periods of treatment with phenytoin (Box 20.8); it may also occur in pregnancy. Haemorrhages can be sometimes be seen in the buccal mucous membrane in thrombocytopenic purpura and acute leukaemia.

DENTAL ABSCESS

Pus forming in a carious tooth causes an alveolar 'dental' abscess (Fig. 20.18). There is local swelling and inflammation, with throbbing pain exacerbated by tapping the affected tooth. A sinus tract may develop, draining pus into the mouth or through the alveolar bone to the skin overlying the upper or lower jaw (Fig. 20.19). This sinus will persist until the underlying infection is treated, usually by extraction of the tooth. *Epulis* is a general term used to describe any soft swelling arising in the gum of the maxilla or mandible. It should be differentiated from a malignant ulcer arising in the gum.

THE TONGUE

Ask the patient to protrude the tongue. Tremor of the tongue may be due to nervousness, thyrotoxicosis,

delirium tremens or parkinsonism. Advanced malignancy of the base of the tongue restricts protrusion. Carcinoma usually involves the side of the tongue (Fig. 20.20). In lesions of the hypoglossal nerve or its nucleus there may be fasciculation of the affected side, followed by weakness and wasting (lingual hemiatrophy). The tongue is large in acromegaly, cretinism, myxoedema, lymphangioma and amyloidosis.

Next examine the dorsum of the tongue. Note in particular Waldeyer's ring of adenoidal and tonsillar tissues and the lingual tonsils, which can become swollen and tender. Systemic conditions, such as amyloid infiltration, can appear dramatic, whereas a papillomatous wart may hardly be noticed (Figs 20.21, 20.22).

COLOUR

Is the tongue pale, red or discoloured? In severe anaemia the tongue is pale. Discoloration is most often due to the ingestion of coloured foods, for example sweets, but can be striking in severe central cyanosis. With the mouth wide and the tongue protruded fully to one side, retract the cheek with a spatula to display the side and undersurface well. Some patients find this impossible to do, so wrap a gauze swab around the tip of the tongue and with index finger and thumb gently pull it out and to one

---

Box 20.7   Halitosis

Characteristic odours that may be recognized
- In ketosis the breath smells of acetone
- In uraemia there is a fishy or ammoniacal odour
- In hepatic failure the odour is 'mousy'
- In lung abscess or bronchiectasis the breath may have a putrid smell
- Paraldehyde and alcohol leave characteristic odours on the breath

---

Box 20.8   Some drugs that cause gum hypertrophy and gingivitis

- Anticoagulants
- Fibrinolytic agents
- Oral contraceptive agents
- Antiepileptic drugs, especially phenytoin
- Protease inhibitors
- Vitamin A and analogues
- Gold compounds
- Calcium channel blockers may cause gingival hyperplasia

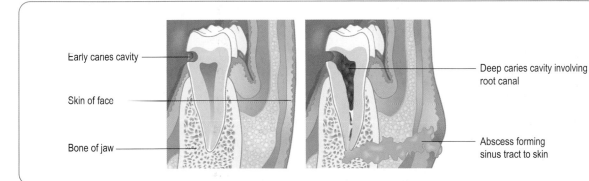

Early caries cavity

Skin of face

Bone of jaw

Deep caries cavity involving root canal

Abscess forming sinus tract to skin

Figure 20.18   Dental caries introduces infection into the pulp chamber, causing a periapical abscess. Pus collects to form an alveolar or dental abscess, with throbbing pain exacerbated by tapping the affected tooth.

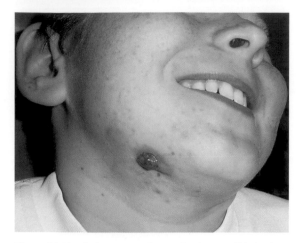

Figure 20.19   A sinus presenting under the mandible is often dental in origin.

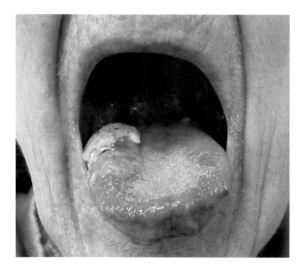

Figure 20.20   Induration in squamous cell carcinoma of the lateral border of the middle third of the right side of the tongue.

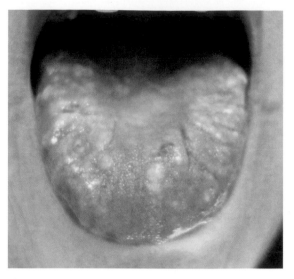

Figure 20.21   Amyloid infiltration in the tongue.

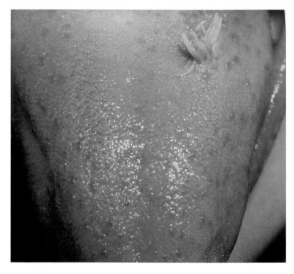

Figure 20.22   A papilloma (viral wart) on the dorsum of the tongue.

side. Benign ulcers in this site are common and may be inflammatory or traumatic in origin, very often due to ill-fitting dentures or broken carious teeth. Unlike malignant ulcers these are painful, superficial, and lack induration.

FURRING
Furring of the tongue is not a sign of disease. It is common in heavy smokers. In scarlet fever the tongue at first shows bright red papillae standing out of a thick white fur. Later the white coat disappears, leaving enlarged papillae on a bright red surface – the 'strawberry tongue'. Hairy leukoplakia may be a feature in patients with HIV infection, but also occurs in immune depression from other causes.

Burning tongue (Box 20.9) is a common complaint but is rarely associated with organic disease.

Box 20.9   Causes of a burning sensation in the mouth

- Deficiency states
  - Iron deficiency
  - Vitamin B$_{12}$ deficiency
  - Folate deficiency
- Infection
  - Candidiasis
- Diabetes mellitus
- Erythema migrans
- Psychogenic
  - Anxiety
  - Depression
  - Cancer phobia

A fissured (scrotal) tongue and atrophic areas (geographic tongue) may respond to dietary change, gentle brushing of the tongue surface and hydrogen peroxide mouthwash.

TONGUE PAPILLAE

Generalized atrophy of the papillae produces a smooth or bald tongue, a characteristic of vitamin B_{12} deficiency, but also found in iron-deficiency anaemia, coeliac disease and other gastrointestinal disorders and deficiency states, especially pellagra (niacin deficiency). In median rhomboid glossitis a lozenge-shaped area of loss of papillae and fissuring is seen in the midline anterior to the foramen caecum.

THE SIDES AND UNDERSURFACE OF THE TONGUE

Now ask the patient to retract and lift the tongue, still with the mouth wide open, to show the under-surface of the tongue and the floor of the mouth. Note the frenulum and the orifice of the sub-mandibular duct on either side of its base. The ampulla of each duct lies just proximal to the orifice and is a common site for calculi, formed in the submandibular salivary gland, to lodge.

Two types of cyst may be found in the floor of the mouth: *ranula* (see above) and *sublingual dermoid cyst*, a round opaque swelling.

THE PALATE, FAUCES, TONSILS AND PHARYNX

With the mouth wide open inspect the hard and soft palates and note the position of the uvula. Get the patient to say 'ah', which raises the soft palate and increases the visibility of the fauces, tonsils and oropharynx. If a good view of these structures has not been obtained, introduce a spatula to depress the base of the tongue and, if necessary, another spatula to retract the anterior pillar of the fauces to view the tonsils properly. Look for ulcers, erythema or vesicles. Herpetic vesicles of the hard palate are unilateral, painful oval ulcers that usually occur in older patients and are accompanied by a similar

rash on the corresponding maxillary dermatome of the face. Herpes zoster infection of the glosso-pharyngeal nerve produces similar lesions in the pharynx.

Malignant ulcers are uncommon on the hard palate: they more commonly present as erosions from the maxillary antrum or as metastases. Ectopic salivary gland tissue may be present in the mouth, and the hard palate is the commonest site. A tumour of this tissue presents as a smooth, hard swelling projecting from the surface of the hard palate, sometimes with central ulceration. The palate is sometimes perforated (Box 20.10).

Petechiae on the palate occur in glandular fever, rubella and streptococcal tonsillitis, and in any form of thrombocytopenia. In glandular fever the tonsils are enlarged and covered with a white exudate, which tends to become confluent. There is oedema of the fauces and soft palate, and erythema of the oropharynx. This contrasts with the yellow punctate follicular exudate seen in streptococcal tonsillitis. A membranous exudate occurs in diphtheria and, as in all cases of mouth infection, a swab should be taken for bacteriological examination. The membrane in diphtheria varies in colour from white to green, and often starts on the tonsil before spreading to the fauces and pharynx.

Finally, look at the pharynx. The presence on its surface of a number of small round or oval swellings, somewhat like sago grains, is so common as to be almost normal. In pharyngitis these are much increased. Note any vesicles or ulcers. In *chickenpox* (herpes varicella) oral lesions may be apparent before the characteristic rash appears. Erythema precedes vesicle formation. In *herpangina* (Coxsackie virus infection), also common in the young, similar lesions may be seen in the oropharynx, soft palate and uvula. In the *common cold (coryza)*, mucopus is seen on the posterior wall of the pharynx running down from the nasopharynx. Less common nowadays are *peritonsillar abscess* (quinsy) and retropharyngeal abscess. The latter forms a smooth, tense, tender swelling that bulges forwards from the posterior wall of the oropharynx.

CLEFT LIP AND PALATE

Cleft lip abnormality can vary from a simple notch in the vermilion of the upper lip to an open gap with discontinuity of all the tissues supporting the lip and the floor of the nose (Fig. 20.23). Cleft palate may be limited to a bifid uvula or a hardly noticeable submucous cleft, or extend forwards unilaterally or bilaterally, resulting in gaping of the palate and the tooth-bearing alveolar bone. The variety of cleft lip and palate deformities makes classification complicated (Fig. 20.24).

The repair of cleft lip and palate requires collaboration between specialists able to manage

---

Box 20.10 Perforations of the hard palate

If a hole is seen in the maxilla it may be due to one of the following:

- Imperfect closure or breakdown after repair of a cleft palate
- Osteoradionecrosis of bone (ORN) following radiotherapy
- Malignant tumour eroding the bone
- Oronasal fistula (after injury)
- Oroantral fistula (after upper tooth extraction)
- Tertiary syphilis with formation of a gumma (rare)

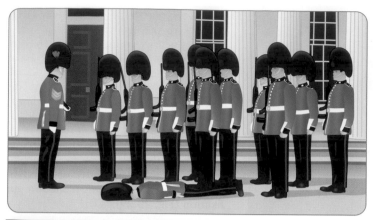

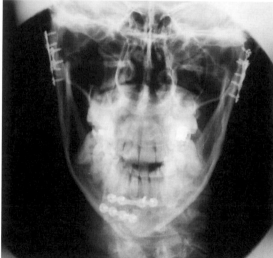

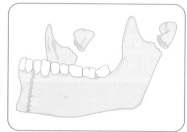

Figure 20.28 The 'guardsman's fracture', where a blow to the point of the chin causes a classic pattern of fracture, involving both mandibular condyles and the symphysis at the point of the chin. X-ray shows open repair with internal fixation using titanium plates and screws.

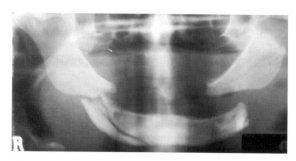

Figure 20.29 Accurate realignment of the broken bone gives the best chance of sensory recovery.

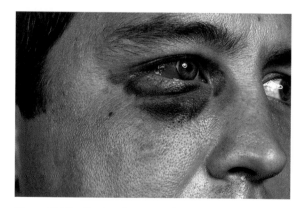

Figure 20.30 Fractured zygoma, showing depressed cheekbone, 'black eye' and 'subconjunctival haemorrhage without posterior limit'.

Box 20.12   Signs of retrobulbar haemorrhage

- Proptosis
- Worsening pain in or around the eye
- Deteriorating vision
- Increasing swelling in or around the eye
- Decreasing pupil response
- Dilated pupil

More complex facial fractures, such as frontonasal ethmoidal fractures, are characterized by collapse of the nasal bridge prominence, splaying of the nasal bridge, and increased width (telecanthus) between the orbits and an upturned nose tip owing to collapse of the support of the nasal root (Fig. 20.33). It is important to recognize the significance of loss of

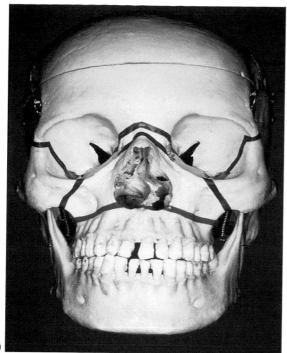

(a)

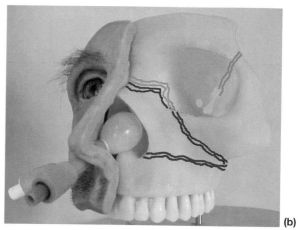

(b)

Figure 20.31 The Le Fort I level of fracture crosses the maxillary sinus and nasal walls horizontally. The Le Fort II has a pyramidal pattern, running obliquely across the anterior walls of the maxillae towards the orbital floors and crossing the thin medial orbital walls to the nasal root. The high Le Fort III level fracture crosses from the lateral orbital (frontozygomatic) sutures to the medial walls, again with fracture of the nasal root. Both Le Fort II and Le Fort III also include fracture across the bridge of the nose. (See Fig. 20.32).

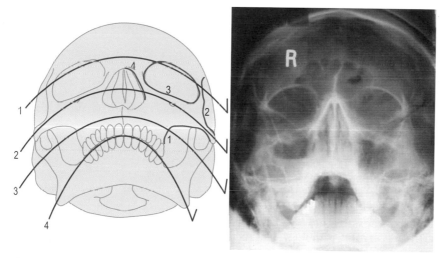

Figure 20.32 Noting asymmetry and visualizing Campbell's lines aids diagnosis in facial radiograph interpretation.

smell and increased orbital separation (telecanthus) in these injuries.

Look for 'panda eyes', swollen periorbital tissues, midface mobility and profuse nasal epistaxis. Disturbance of dental occlusion, resulting in an anterior open bite, may imply posterior impaction of the maxilla but can also be due to mandibular injury. Massive nasal haemorrhage responds well to forward traction on the maxilla and posterior nasal tamponade using tampons or commercially designed epistat (Fig. 20.31).

FRACTURE OF THE SKULL BASE

Bruising over the mastoid (Battle sign) and CSF leakage (otorrhoea) are signs of a fracture involving the skull base (Figs 20.34 and 20.35).

Modern spiral scanners take only moments longer to scan the face and neck than the brain alone; such images are invaluable (Fig. 20.35). Ultrasound may be useful to locate radiolucent foreign bodies.

Pathological fractures (Box 20.13) occur especially when there is malignant invasion of the bony skeleton (Fig. 20.35).

Table 21.1 The Glasgow Coma Scale (GCS)

Eye-opening		Best verbal response		Best motor response	
Spontaneous	4	Oriented	5	Obeys commands	6
To speech	3	Confused	4	Localizes pain	5
To pain	2	Inappropriate	3	Normal withdrawal	4
None	1	Incomprehensible	2	Abnormal flexion	3
		None	1	Abnormal extension	2
				None	1

The three categories of information required in the GCS assessment require no special skills and are thus particularly suited for serial observations by relatively untrained staff. The GCS is much used in the management of head injury. This simple non-linear clinical rating scale enables relatively accurate assessment of improvement or deterioration in a patient's conscious state by physicians, nurses and ambulance staff alike. The best score is 15; the worst is 3, representing 'none' in all three categories assessed. Abnormal extension implies decerebrate posturing.

life and look for reversible causes of the unconscious state (Box 21.2). Airway, breathing and circulation (*ABC*) can be rapidly assessed, and critical interventions made as required. Every patient should be given high-flow oxygen, have an intravenous cannula placed and have early measurement of blood sugar by fingerprick testing. A pulse oximeter should be applied and a brief examination made to establish if the patient is fitting. Patients who are fitting should be treated immediately, before a diagnosis of the cause is made. At this stage consciousness is graded using the AVPU scale (*A*lert, responds to *V*erbal stimulus, responds to *P*ainful stimulus or *U*nresponsive). Protection of the airway by intubation and ventilation should be considered in any patient who does not respond to a verbal stimulus (i.e. is either 'P' or 'U' on the AVPU scale). Before going any further make sure the patient is breathing and is adequately oxygenated, that the pulse and blood pressure are satisfactory, that the blood sugar is normal and the patient is not fitting.

HISTORY

The history is of great importance and attempts should always be made to find witnesses to the onset of the coma. It is essential to discover whether the coma was *gradual, rapid* or *sudden in onset*. Sudden coma is typical of *trauma, fitting* or disorders such as *subarachnoid haemorrhage* or *stroke*. Rapid onset, often preceded by abnormal behavior and confusion, occurs in metabolic disorders such as *hypoglycaemia*, or when there is impairment due to infection, such as *meningitis* or *encephalitis*. A gradual onset suggests a more slowly evolving cause, such as *chronic subdural haematoma* or a *tumour*.

Events preceding the onset of unconsciousness will give clues as to the cause. A history of headache before coma is frequent in patients with intracranial space-occupying lesions of any cause. *Seizures* of recent onset, whether focal or generalized, strongly suggest cerebral disease, which may be due to

tumour, encephalitis, abscess or trauma. Patients with *drug-induced coma* may be known by neighbours, family, medical attendants or the ambulance driver to have abused drugs or medication, or the paramedics may report the presence of drug containers or alcohol in the patient's home. A history of depression or previous episodes of deliberate self-harm may be known. A *search of the patient's clothing* may reveal hospital outpatient attendance cards, unfilled prescriptions, drugs, or even syringes. Diabetic or epileptic patients often carry some form of *identification*, either in their clothing or as a 'medical alert' wristband or necklace. *Hypoglycaemia* is characterized by stupor or coma from which the patient can sometimes be roused to a resentful and aggressive state of partial awareness; there is pallor and sweatiness, a bounding pulse and slurred speech, and an unsteady gait. This state is easy to confuse with drunkenness. If there is *any* suspicion that the patient might be hypoglycaemic, a blood sample should be taken for blood glucose estimation and then 20 g of 50% glucose given intravenously.

Do not be misled by a history of alcohol ingestion. It is a great mistake to assume that a decrease in the level of consciousness is due to alcohol, just because there is evidence the patient has been drinking. An alcoholic patient with a decreased level of consciousness is at risk of intracranial bleeding, Wernicke's encephalopathy and hypoglycaemia – all of these should be actively sought and treated.

A history of trauma with concussion, followed a few days later by fluctuating drowsiness and stupor, suggests *subdural haematoma*, although the injury may be trivial and not recalled by the patient or relatives. Concussion followed by a *brief lucid interval* before rapidly deepening coma suggests *extradural haematoma*. If there is a history of trauma, remember always to consider whether there may be a fracture of the cervical spine; if this is suspected, splinting of the neck and an X-ray are mandatory (Box 21.3). These aspects are described in Chapter 22 in relation to clinical methods in major trauma.

Box 21.1 Outline of causes of coma

A. Functional
Lack of substrate
- Hypoglycaemia
- Hypoxia
- Hypotension
- Stroke

Depression of function
- Hypothermia
- Drugs (including alcohol)

Abnormal function
- Epilepsy
- Metabolic
  - Diabetes mellitus
  - Renal failure
  - Hepatic failure
  - Hypothyroidism

B. Structural
Diffuse
- Meningitis
- Encephalitis
- Other infections (e.g. cerebral malaria)
- Subarachnoid haemorrhage
- Head injury
- Hypertensive encephalopathy

Focal
Supratentorial lesions
- Cerebral haemorrhage
- Cerebral infarction with oedema
- Subdural haematoma
- Extradural haematoma
- Tumour
- Cerebral abscess
- Pituitary apoplexy

Subtentorial lesions
- Cerebellar haemorrhage
- Pontine haemorrhage
- Brainstem infarction
- Tumour
- Cerebellar abscess
- Secondary effects of transtentorial herniation of brain due to cerebral mass lesions

---

Box 21.2 Basic neurological examination in coma

- Assess level of consciousness (Glasgow Coma Scale, see Table 21.1)
- Signs of head injury
  - local bruising, fractures and wounds
  - bleeding from nose or ears
- Splint the neck: head injury may be associated with fracture of the cervical spine
- If no evidence of injury (history and examination) check for neck stiffness
- Check resting pupillary size, and pupillary responses to light
- Ocular movements: spontaneous, following and to 'doll's head' (if no voluntary response)
- Limbs: posture, tone and movement
- Reflexes and plantar responses
- Fundi

Box 21.3 Head injury: basic management

- Control ventilation
- Control circulation
- Exclude intracranial haemorrhage by CT scan
- Obtain neurological/neurosurgical opinion
- Control intracranial pressure

EXAMINATION

Always proceed to examine the patient in a logical order (Box 21.2). The general features of the patient's clinical state are of great importance. Do they appear clean, well-nourished and generally cared for, or are there signs of *social decline*, such as a dishevelled appearance, lack of personal cleanliness, malnutrition or infestation? Is there evidence of trauma or exposure? A rapid search must be made for injuries, and especially for signs of cranial trauma (Box 21.3). Bruising of the scalp is difficult to see, but scalp oedema or haematoma can usually be palpated. Bruising of the skin behind the pinna, – called '*Battle's sign*' – is a useful indicator of middle fossa skull fracture, as is *bleeding from the external auditory meatus* or *haemotympanum* (blood behind the eardrum). Pallor, circulatory failure and other evidence of shock must be recognized and a search made for external or internal haemorrhage, especially if trauma is suspected.

The odours of alcohol, uraemia, diabetic acidosis and hepatic coma may be recognizable in some instances. The rapid, stertorous respiration of *acidotic coma* (air hunger), usually due to diabetes, can be quickly recognized (see below). The presence of jaundice, liver palms or spider naevi, even in the absence of hepatic enlargement, raises the suspicion of hepatic coma.

The ocular fundi must always be examined by *ophthalmoscopy* for signs of papilloedema, retinal haemorrhages or exudates, or intra-arterial emboli, which appear as luminescent, highly refractile yellow or white plaque-like material occluding vessels (see Fig. 18.15). *Coma with neck stiffness* (Box 21.4) implies meningeal irritation, such as *infection* or *subarachnoid haemorrhage*.

After the general examination special attention must also be directed to an assessment of the *level of*

Box 21.4   Causes of coma with neck stiffness (neck stiffness may be relatively inapparent in a deeply comatose patient)

- Subarachnoid haemorrhage
- Meningitis
  - bacterial
  - viral (aseptic)
- Encephalitis
- Intracerebral haemorrhage
- Cerebral malaria

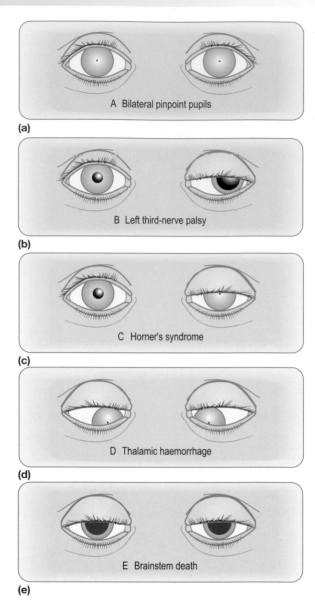

(a)

(b)

(c)

(d)

(e)

Figure 21.1   Pupillary anomalies in coma. **(a)** Bilateral pinpoint pupils occur with brainstem lesions, opiate and other drug intoxications, and with pontine infarction. **(b)** Left third-nerve palsy. There is ptosis, dilatation of the pupil with absence of the light reaction, and slight lateral deviation of the eye. **(c)** Horner's syndrome. There is ptosis and a small reactive pupil. **(d)** In thalamic haemorrhage the eyes tend to 'look towards the tip of the nose' and the pupils are small; later they become large and unreactive as upper brainstem involvement follows. **(e)** When brainstem death occurs the midbrain disturbance is manifest by midposition, fixed (unreactive) pupils with eye closure.

consciousness, pupillary reactions and *ocular movements*, both volitional and reflex, to the *pattern of breathing* and to *limb motor responses*, either spontaneous or reflexly evoked. Localizing responses to painful stimuli are important as they imply preservation of sensation with associated motor responses. If localized responses are absent there may be hemiparesis, or deep coma. Flexion or extension responses of an upper limb to pain signify decortication or decerebration, respectively (see below). Extension of the legs to a painful stimulus applied to the sternum suggests decerebration or decortication.

LEVEL OF CONSCIOUSNESS

Define the state of consciousness by using the Glasgow Coma Scale (Table 21.1). *Change in level of consciousness* is the single most important piece of information: it always indicates the need for reassessment, and perhaps a change of management. The scoring system of the Glasgow Coma Scale is useful in identifying this change. The GCS can readily be assessed by a nurse or by a doctor and is reproducible; it is therefore a highly practical instrument. It is important to note exactly the *degree of responsiveness to external stimuli*, including conversation, calling the patient's first name; painful stimulation (such as placement of an intravenous cannula); and deep noxious stimuli such as squeezing the Achilles tendon, nailbed pressure applied with a pen, or supraorbital pressure from the examiner's thumb.

PUPILS

Pupillary size and responsiveness to a very bright unfocused light beam (not the light of an ophthalmoscope) should be noted (Fig. 21.1). If the pupils are unequal, a decision as to which is abnormal must be made. Usually the larger pupil indicates the presence of an *oculomotor (third) nerve palsy*, whether from damage to the oculomotor nerve by pressure and displacement or from a lesion in the mesencephalon itself. Occasionally the smaller pupil may be the abnormal one, as in *Horner's syndrome*.

If the larger pupil does not react to light it is likely that there is a *partial oculomotor nerve palsy* on that side. If the smaller pupil also fails to react to light this may be the *midposition pupil* of complete sympathetic and parasympathetic lesions, indicating extensive brainstem damage.

In *drug-induced coma and in most patients with metabolic coma* the pupillary responses to light are normal (Box 21.5). Exceptions to this rule are glutethimide poisoning and very deep metabolic coma, in which the pupils may become dilated but only rarely become unreactive to light. In pontine and in thalamic haemorrhage the pupils may be very small (*pinpoint pupils*) and unreactive to light.

OCULAR MOVEMENTS

In comatose patients the eyes become slightly divergent at rest. If there is a pre-existing strabismus deviation of the ocular axes may be pronounced, both at rest and during reflex ocular movements.

DOLL'S HEAD MOVEMENTS

If the patient is too drowsy or stuporous to test voluntary or following eye movements, '*doll's head*' movements should be tested. If possible the patient should be placed supine, although the test can be carried out in any position. The examiner grasps the patient's head with both hands, using the thumbs to hold the eyelids open gently, and firmly rocks the head from side to side through about 70°, and then from passive neck flexion to passive neck extension. The patient's eyes tend to remain in the straight-ahead position despite these passive movements of the head, a phenomenon like that found in some children's dolls, i.e. the eyes tend to deviate in the opposite direction to the induced head movement.

This doll's head ocular movement depends on intact vestibular reflex mechanisms and is thus a test of the peripheral sense organs involved, the labyrinths and otoliths, and their central connections in the brainstem, including the vestibular nuclei, the medial longitudinal fasciculi, and the efferent pathway through oculomotor, trochlear and abducent nerves and their nuclei. Sometimes lesions in these structures can be recognized during the doll's head test by the presence of disturbances in ocular movements consistent, for example, with an abducent or oculomotor nerve palsy. Absence of the reflex on one side indicates an ipsilateral pontine lesion, but complete absence of doll's head movements may be found both in extensive structural lesions in the brainstem and in deep metabolic coma. However, in most patients with drug-induced coma doll's head ocular movements are intact.

CALORIC REFLEXES

Brainstem function can also be assessed by testing caloric reflexes. In the comatose patient, irrigation of the external auditory meatus on one side with at least 20 mL of ice-cold water induces slow conjugate deviation of the eyes towards the irrigated side after a few seconds' delay (the mnemonic COWS – cold, opposite; warm, same – is useful in remembering the

> **Box 21.5   Metabolic and drug-induced coma**
>
> - Coma without localizing signs is characteristic syndrome
> - Full range of ocular movement to 'doll's head' testing
> - Pupils may be small, e.g. opiate poisoning
> - Altered respiratory pattern may signify metabolic acidosis (consider diabetic coma), or respiratory alkalosis (with hypercapnia)
> - Decerebrate extension may occur in extremis
> - Look for signs of metabolic disorder, e.g. jaundice, uraemia, respiratory failure, hypocalcaemia, endocrine disease (especially hypothyroidism or hypopituitarism)
> - Drug-induced coma is associated with access to medication or drugs of abuse, or signs of repeated venous access

direction of the nystagmus that compensates for the deviation, in the patient who is awake).

In the awake or drowsy patient this slow tonic deviation is masked by a fast, coarse nystagmus towards the opposite side. Normal caloric nystagmus is characteristically also found in cases of psychogenic coma. After a few minutes' delay the opposite ear should also be tested. It is important to inspect the tympanic membrane on each side *before* irrigating the external auditory meatus, as it is unwise to perform this test in the presence of a large perforation, or if there is an active otitis media.

SPONTANEOUS OCULAR MOVEMENTS

Occasionally in patients with infarction or other structural lesions in the posterior fossa *spontaneous ocular movements* may be observed. These may be accompanied by marked ocular divergence, sometimes with elevation of one eye and depression of the other. Rarely there may be a spontaneous '*see-saw*' nystagmus, in which one eye rotates up and the other down, the movements alternating at a very slow rate. *Rapid ocular oscillations* may occur, especially after poisoning with tricyclic antidepressant drugs, and a slow – once or twice a second – conjugate downward *bobbing* movement is sometimes a sign of cerebellar haemorrhage or tumour. In *thalamic haemorrhage* the pupils are pinpoint, and the eyes seem to be looking downwards as if at the patient's own nose. *Rapid conjugate lateral movement*, at a rhythm and rate reminiscent of cerebellar nystagmus, occurring in an unconscious patient should suggest focal motor seizures originating in the contralateral frontal lobe. Such seizures are often accompanied by deviation of the head and eyes in the direction of the 'nystagmoid movement', but not necessarily by a fully developed focal seizure involving face and limbs on the same side.

Nystagmus cannot occur in the comatose patient because it requires ocular fixation to develop the fast corrective phase.

PATTERN OF BREATHING

Alterations in the rhythm and pattern of breathing are an important aspect of the assessment of the unconscious patient.

CHEYNE–STOKES (PERIODIC) RESPIRATION

In Cheyne–Stokes respiration, breathing varies in regular cycles. A phase of gradually deepening respiration is followed, after a period of very deep rapid breaths, by a phase of slowly decreasing respiratory excursion and rate. Respiration gradually becomes quieter and may cease for several seconds before the cycle is repeated. Depressed but regular breathing at a normal rate occurs in most drug-induced comas, but *Cheyne–Stokes respiration* can occur in coma of any cause, especially if there is coincidental chronic pulmonary disease. Cheyne–Stokes breathing in a comatose patient is a sign of a large unilateral space-occupying lesion with brainstem distortion, for example subdural haematoma, or of bilateral lesions from other causes, for example cerebral infarction or meningitis.

KUSSMAUL RESPIRATION

Deep, rapid sighing breathing at a regular rate should immediately suggest metabolic acidosis. Metabolic ketoacidosis or uraemia is the commonest cause of this acidotic (Kussmaul) breathing pattern, but a similar pattern may occur in some patients with respiratory failure, and in deep metabolic coma, especially hepatic coma.

CENTRAL PONTINE HYPERVENTILATION

Deep, regular breathing may also occur with rostral brainstem damage, whether due to reticular pontine infarction or to central brainstem dysfunction secondary to transtentorial herniation associated with an intra- or extracerebral space-occupying lesion. This breathing pattern is called *central neurogenic (pontine) hyperventilation*. Interspersed deep sighs or yawns may precede the development of this respiratory pattern.

Rapid shallow breathing occurs if central brainstem dysfunction extends more caudally to the lower pons. When medullary respiratory neurons are damaged, for example by progressive transtentorial herniation, irregular, slow, deep gasping respirations, sometimes associated with hiccups (*ataxic respiration*), may develop. In patients with raised intracranial pressure this sequence of abnormal breathing patterns is often associated with other evidence of brainstem dysfunction, including a rising blood pressure, a slow pulse, flaccid limbs, absence

---

Box 21.6 Coma with hyperventilation (and low $Paco_2$)

- Metabolic acidosis
- Diabetic ketoacidosis
- Brainstem lesion, e.g. stroke
- Rising intracranial pressure
- Bacterial meningitis
- Renal failure
- Liver failure
- Pneumonia complicating brain lesion

Box 21.7 Causes of coma with focal neurological signs

- Epilepsy (postictal state)
- Stroke
- Encephalitis
- Subarachnoid haemorrhage
- Cerebral abscess
- Bacterial meningitis with cortical infarction
- Cerebral venous sinus thrombosis

---

of reflex ocular movements and dilatation of the pupils.

Changing patterns of respiration in an unconscious patient, particularly the development of central neurogenic hyperventilation, provide important and relatively objective evidence of deterioration. These changes in respiratory pattern may occur in structural lesions with raised intracranial pressure, in brainstem infarction, and less commonly in some varieties of metabolic coma, especially hepatic coma. They are indicative of progressive and potentially fatal brainstem dysfunction, but not of its causation (Box 21.6).

MOTOR RESPONSES

It is often difficult to elicit signs of focal cerebral disease in the unconscious patient. The presence of focal neurological signs implies localized dysfunction in the central nervous system, and is important in considering the causes of altered consciousness (Box 21.7). If progressive brainstem dysfunction due to raised intracranial pressure with transtentorial herniation has occurred, focal signs indicative of the causative lesion may no longer be recognizable. However, papilloedema is usually present in such cases.

In the drowsy or stuporous patient it may be possible to recognize a hemianopia by testing the response to *visual menace* or, sometimes, by testing for optokinetic nystagmus (see page 195). Visual threat, or menace, consists of moving a hand rapidly towards the patient's face, first in the left and then

- Fingerprick glucose measurement (always confirm hypoglycaemia by laboratory measurement)
- Check haemoglobin, haematocrit, WBC count, clotting
- Electrolytes and liver function tests
- Blood gases and pH
- CT head scan
- Chest X-ray
- X-ray of suspected fractures/bruised limbs
- Blood for cross-matching
- Drug screen

in the right field. Normally this threat induces rapid eye closure or a flinch. It is necessary to obtain the patient's attention transiently to assess any meaningful response, and the test is, unfortunately, only rarely useful. *Hemiplegia* may be evident either from abnormal flaccidity of the arm and leg on the affected side or, in the stuporous or lightly comatose patient, by the absence of spontaneous movements on that side. In the drowsy or stuporous patient flaccidity can be assessed by picking up each arm in turn and allowing it to drop by the patient's side. A flaccid arm drops 'like a stone', whereas if some tone is preserved the fall of the arm is more gentle. *Noxious stimuli*, for example pinching the skin of the forearms and thighs, deep rubbing pressure with a hard object applied to the sternum or – often most effective – lightly pricking the skin and mucous membranes near the nasal orifices on both sides, will fail to induce movement of the paralysed limbs. Sometimes in a patient with a dense hemiplegia the cheek blows flaccidly in and out with each breath on the hemiplegic side. The *tendon reflexes* may be asymmetrical, but in most comatose patients both plantar responses are extensor. *Asymmetry* of these motor responses is the important feature to assess. In both structural lesions and metabolic disorders coma may be accompanied in its terminal stages by *decorticate* or *decerebrate* postures. These may occur asymmetrically and may at first be apparent only when induced by noxious external stimuli, such as deep sternal pressure or pressure on a nailbed or Achilles tendon. These postural reactions are features of severe upper brainstem dysfunction and are thus usually found in association with pupillary abnormalities, the absence of doll's head and caloric reflexes and a disturbed breathing pattern. Decerebrate and decorticate postures are found much more characteristically in structural than in metabolic coma, and thus do not usually occur in patients with drug-induced coma unless there has been additional hypoxic or ischaemic brain injury.

INVESTIGATION

The initial investigations performed on the comatose patient are outlined in Box 21.8. Immediately treatable structural or metabolic disorders require rapid diagnosis and management. CT head scanning will need to be performed in almost all unconscious patients to look for structural causes, and is mandatory if there is a suspicion of trauma or the patient is at high risk of an intracranial haematoma, especially if they are alcoholic or on warfarin. The early involvement of a radiologist is useful.

Blood tests (U&E, FBC and paracetamol levels) may help (paracetamol overdose will not be the primary cause of coma, but may have been taken with other drugs and may need urgent treatment in its own right). A drugs screen is not usually rapidly available, but may help with the long-term diagnosis. Alcohol level is not helpful, as it may be misleading if a high alcohol level is assumed to be the cause of unconsciousness. Coagulation (the INR) will be abnormal in hepatic coma.

A pattern of change is much more informative than a single data point, so several of the investigations, for example fingerprick blood sugar measurement, blood gas analysis, electrolytes and haemoglobin, may require repeated measurement during management. The GCS should be assessed serially at frequent intervals as long as the patient is thought to be in danger.

SPECIFIC TYPES OF COMA

MENINGITIS

Meningitis can usually be recognized by the rapid onset of drowsiness, lethargy or stupor, with fever and signs of meningeal irritation (see Chapter 10). In pyogenic meningitis the pulse may be unexpectedly slow in relation to the fever, although respiration is usually rapid. Seizures and focal neurological signs may develop and there is usually a history of headache and neck stiffness, perhaps with vomiting. In *meningococcal septicaemia* there may be a characteristic rash (Fig. 21.2). A *primary site of infection*, such as otitis media or sinusitis, may be apparent in other forms of purulent meningitis or *brain abscess*.

METABOLIC COMA

Metabolic coma is common and has many causes (see Box 21.1), the most common being hypoglycaemia. It is characterized by altered consciousness without focal neurological signs or neck stiffness, and with preservation of vestibulogenic ocular movements (doll's head responses) (see Box 21.5). In certain *drug-induced coma* states there may be signs of repeated intravenous injections under conditions of imperfect sterility, causing venous

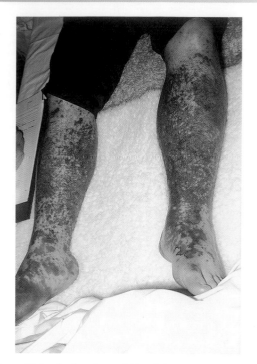

Figure 21.2 Confluent petechial rash in an unconscious patient with overwhelming meningoccocal septicaemia and meningitis.

thrombosis in forearm or antebrachial veins. There may be signs of underlying hepatic or renal disease.

SIMULATED COMA

Psychologically disturbed patients sometimes feign coma. The eyes are actually closed and the patient is usually lying in a resting position, or supine with the arms and legs extended. The eyelids resist attempts to open them and, on forced eye opening, the eyes point upwards exposing the white conjunctiva (Bell's phenomenon) as part of the patient's attempt to maintain eyelid closure. The eyelids close rapidly when released. The slow roving eye movements of organic coma cannot be simulated. Painful stimuli to the limbs may be ignored, but pinprick to the nasal mucosa or to the lips usually elicits volitional grimacing. The pupillary light reflex is normal, as are plantar responses. Cold caloric testing induces nystagmus with the fast phase away from the stimulated side, rather than deviation of the eyes toward the stimulus as would occur in true coma. Examination, especially invasive tests as above, may induce a return of cooperation and consciousness, or uncover a disturbed mental state.

PERSISTENT STATES OF ALTERED CONSCIOUSNESS

Patients with extensive or diffuse injury to the brain do not always die. In some, partial recovery from coma to a *persistent vegetative state (PVS)* occurs (Box 21.9). This term is used to describe patients who appear to be in a state of wakeful unresponsiveness, rather than a state of unresponsive coma. Despite their apparent wakefulness, patients in a persistent vegetative state make no meaningful response to environmental stimuli.

In PVS the patient is immobile, with decerebrate posturing, but appears to be awake, with eyes open but without purposeful or meaningful response to verbal, visual or other communication, or to noxious stimulation. Apparently normal sleep/wake cycles occur through the day and, when awake, the patient's eyes may move slowly and randomly, with preserved spontaneous blinking. Reflex swallowing in response to fluid placed in the mouth, and to salivary secretion, usually occurs and there may be spontaneous chewing movements. The gag reflex is present, and the patient breathes normally. The patient is mute. Relatives often find it difficult to accept that the patient with PVS, who is clearly awake, is not aware. Indeed, it is not possible to assess the state of awareness in such patients, particularly if there are associated focal brain or cervical cord lesions, and when nursing or talking in the vicinity of a patient with PVS it should always be assumed that some awareness may be preserved. In patients in PVS for longer than 6 months there is no prospect of recovery, and only a few patients with PVS of any duration recover. The term '*minimally conscious state*' has been introduced to refer to patients – perhaps in an initial state of PVS – who achieve some evidence of consciousness, judged by the emergence of some partial ability to interact with their environment, while remaining paralysed with decorticate or decerebrate posturing.

In *akinetic mutism*, as in PVS, the patient appears awake. They show no awareness of self or environment, but may follow the examiner or a moving object with the eyes. Communication can sometimes be established, even partially, by sign language or by a code based on eye-blinking, and fragmented

Box 21.10   Diagnostic criteria for brain death. Note that these are clinically determined criteria and do not require special investigative techniques. (Modified from Lancet 1976;2:1069–1070)

A. Conditions in which the diagnosis of brain death should be considered

The diagnosis of a disorder that can lead to brain death must have been firmly established.

The patient is deeply comatose, being incapable of response to any stimulus, other than reflex responses.

(a) There should be no suspicion that this state is due to drugs that may depress brain function, e.g. sedatives, poisons or anaesthetic drugs. No such drugs should have been administered in the previous 24 hours.

(b) Primary hypothermia as a cause of coma must have been excluded.

(c) Metabolic and endocrine disturbances that can be responsible for or can contribute to coma must have been excluded.

The patient is being maintained on a ventilator because spontaneous respiration had previously become inadequate or had ceased altogether.

(a) Muscle relaxants and other drugs should have been excluded as a cause of respiratory failure.

(b) Blood gases, including both oxygen and carbon dioxide levels, MUST be within the normal range at the time the assessment is made; this may require the help of an anaesthetist (see below, B).

There should be no doubt that the patient's condition is due to irremediable structural brain damage.

B. Diagnostic tests for confirmation of brain death

All brainstem reflexes must be absent.

- The pupils are fixed in diameter and do not respond to sharp changes in the intensity of incident light.
- There is no corneal reflex.
- The vestibulo-ocular reflexes are absent.
- No motor responses within the cranial nerve distribution can be elicited by adequate stimulation of a somatic area.
- There is no gag reflex response to bronchial stimulation by a suction catheter passed down the trachea.
- No respiratory movements occur when the patient is disconnected from the mechanical ventilator for long enough to ensure that the arterial carbon dioxide tension rises above the threshold for stimulation of respiration. In practice this is best achieved by ventilating the patient with 5% CO_2 in oxygen for 5 minutes before disconnection. This ensures a $Paco_2$ of 8.0 kPa (60 mmHg). A period of 10 minutes' observation for respiratory movement should then be carried out.

C. Other considerations

Note the following:

- *Repetition of testing.* The interval between tests must depend upon the primary pathology and the clinical course of the disease. In some conditions the outcome is not so clear cut, and in these cases it is recommended that the tests should be repeated. The interval between tests depends upon the progress of the patient and might be as long as 24 hours.
- *Integrity of spinal reflexes.* It is well established that spinal cord function can persist after insults that irretrievably destroy brainstem functions.
- *Confirmatory investigation.* Electroencephalography is not necessary for the diagnosis of brain death. Other investigations such as cerebral angiography or cerebral blood-flow measurements are also not required for the diagnosis of brain death.
- *Body temperature.* The body temperature should not be less than 35°C before the diagnostic tests are carried out.
- *Specialist opinion and the status of the doctors concerned.* Only when the primary diagnosis is in doubt is it necessary to consult a neurologist or neurosurgeon.
- *Decision to withdraw artificial support.* This can be considered after all the criteria presented above have been fulfilled. The decision can be made by any of the following combination of doctors:
  (a) A consultant who is in charge of the case and one other doctor
  (b) In the absence of a consultant, a deputy, who should have been registered for 5 years or more and who should have had adequate experience in the care of such cases, and one other doctor.

voluntary movements of the limbs may be possible. If the akinetic mutism is due to a localized lesion or a tumour in the third ventricular region, recovery may occur, and such patients may have excellent recall of events during the period of illness. It is wise, therefore, to remember that the apparently comatose patient may be able to hear and understand, and may later recall conversations that took place or comments made at the bedside during a phase of apparent coma.

DIAGNOSIS OF BRAINSTEM DEATH

With the advent of improved methods of intensive care it became important to develop criteria for the diagnosis of death, especially for patients undergoing positive-pressure ventilation in whom spontaneous respirations have ceased, yet body temperature and the systemic circulation continue to be maintained spontaneously. A clear definition is crucially important if organ donation is considered. *The diagnosis of brain death must be certain before any decision is made to cease attempts to keep the patient alive.* A conference of the Royal Colleges and Faculties of the United Kingdom considered this problem in 1976, and agreed guidelines (Box 21.10). These were reviewed in 1995, and have not been changed. The criteria concentrate on the recognition of brainstem death, as independent life and consciousness are not possible without intact brainstem function.

The recommendations fall into three groups, A, B and C. The patient must be deeply comatose and on a ventilator, and it must be clearly established that the coma is due to *irremedial structural brain damage* (part A). Drug-induced coma, hypothermia, metabolic causes of coma and relaxant drugs must have been clearly excluded as a cause of ventilatory failure. If these conditions are fulfilled, brain death may be diagnosed if no brainstem reflexes can be demonstrated (part B). Repeated tests – at least two separate evaluations should take place – are necessary, but the interval between such tests depends on the pathology and the course of the disease (part C). Purely spinal reflexes can persist after total brainstem destruction, but it must always be remembered that decorticate and decerebrate postures are far from necessarily irreversible phenomena, and therefore that their presence does not inevitably indicate that brain death has occurred. Indeed, some authorities would doubt a diagnosis of brain death if such reflexes persisted. All these tests should be carried out at a body temperature not less than 35°C.

Major acute traumatic injury

F. W. Cross

INTRODUCTION

Trauma is the most common cause of death and disability in young adults, and is common at all ages. It should therefore receive appropriate immediate treatment and subsequent rehabilitation. Prevention of major trauma is an issue in all societies.

Major trauma is generally defined as when the Injury Severity Score (ISS) is greater than 14. The ISS is a trauma score based on the severity of injury in the three worst-injured systems; to score 15 the patient usually has multisystem injuries. The highest possible score is 75, and this is incompatible with life (Box 22.1).

The approach to the examination of a patient with major trauma is somewhat different from a routine outpatient or ward examination in that it must be carried out quickly in order to identify and correct life-threatening injuries as they are found. No physical examination, however, should ever be hurried, and it is especially important that the trauma patient should be thoroughly examined. However, the order in which the examination is carried out is fundamentally different from that used in routine practice. This is a major departure from the 'history, examination, investigation' structure adhered to in the rest of this book. *Triage* is a term used to describe the process of assessment, diagnosis and management at first contact with the injured person. If there are several injured patients the order in which they are treated is determined by triage.

ASSESSMENT OF MAJOR TRAUMA

First, make a rapid but thorough primary survey so that any life-threatening abnormalities can be corrected as they are found. This is followed by essential imaging (see below). A slower secondary survey – nothing less than a complete head-to-toe examination, including examination of the back and a rectal examination – should follow. The order in which systems are examined in the primary survey is dictated by the speed with which an injury to a system can kill the patient. Thus, airway obstruction can kill more rapidly than tension pneumothorax, so it is sought and corrected first. If there is severe haemorrhage, say from an open fracture of

the femur, then the airway is still attended to first; a second attendant can apply pressure to the bleeding point while the airway is being secured.

In a large hospital with a well-organized Accident and Emergency department the management of multiple trauma is a team affair (Fig. 22.1). The team leader directs a group of three other doctors, each backed up by a nurse. The team leader should be a consultant, and the three medical members of the team should be an anaesthetist, a general surgeon, and someone from another specialty such as neurosurgery or orthopaedics. Such a team approach has been shown to improve the speed and efficacy of resuscitation. There is a 'golden hour' immediately after injury during which the patient should be resuscitated and definitive systematic management commenced, and this has a bearing on the eventual outcome. *The golden hour runs from the time of injury, not from the time of arrival in hospital.*

If a seriously injured patient is taken to a small hospital without a trauma team, and indeed without facilities for major surgery, the 'ABC' approach (see below), if necessary applied by a single doctor working with nursing assistance, can be seen as a holding measure until the patient can be transferred to a larger unit. This is not ideal but, nevertheless, the application of a rigorous trauma management scheme will save lives if it is carefully applied.

HISTORY AND MECHANISM OF INJURY

It is important to get an accurate history of the accident. The patient may be in no condition to provide this, and information from relatives, ambulance personnel, police or other eyewitnesses to the accident is essential. Much may be deduced from the mechanism of injury. In addition, it is important to learn the previous medical history when possible, especially in older patients, because the presence of intercurrent illness has a bearing on survival. The presence of prescription medicines, hospital appointment cards and other information in the patient's pockets and other belongings may be helpful.

There are three peak risk periods for death following injury (Fig. 22.2). The first and greatest,

Box 22.1 The Injury Severity Score

The Injury Severity Score (ISS) is an anatomical scoring system that provides an overall score for patients with multiple injuries. Each injury is assigned an Abbreviated Injury Scale (AIS) score and is allocated to one of six body regions (head, face, chest, abdomen, extremities (including pelvis) and external). Only the highest AIS score in each body region is used. The three most severely injured body regions have their scores squared and added together to produce the ISS.

An example of the ISS calculation is shown below.

Region	Injury description	AIS	Square top three
Head/neck	Cerebral contusion	3	9
Face	No injury	0	
Chest	Flail chest	4	16
Abdomen	Minor contusion of liver	2	
	Complex rupture of spleen	5	25
Extremity	Fractured femur	3	
External	No injury	0	
	Injury Severity Score:		**50**

The maximum ISS is 75 (where high is severe injury). If an injury is assigned an AIS of 6 (unsurvivable injury) the ISS is automatically 75. The ISS is virtually the only anatomical scoring system in use and correlates linearly with mortality, morbidity, hospital stay and other measures of severity.

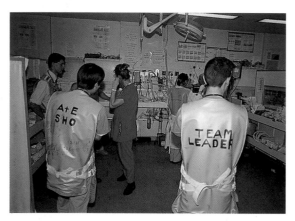

Figure 22.1 Members of the trauma team waiting for the patient to arrive in the resuscitation room. Each member is clearly identified in order to prevent confusion during the resuscitation.

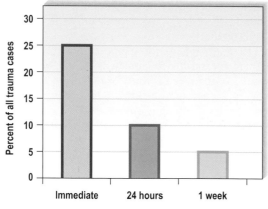

Figure 22.2 Trimodal distribution of trauma deaths.

accounting for over 10% of all traumatic deaths, occurs at the scene of the accident and is due to severe injury to the central nervous system or mediastinal structures. The second, smaller, peak occurs around 24 hours later, usually if major surgery for extensive injury fails to arrest haemorrhage. The third peak is the smallest and occurs about a week after injury; this is due to death from sepsis and multiorgan failure.

There are two basic mechanisms of injury, *blunt* and *penetrating*. The ratio of blunt to penetrating injuries is related to the nature and degree of violence in the society in which such injuries occur. In the UK the ratio is 4:1. In the United States, where firearms are more readily available to the general public, this ratio is reversed.

BLUNT INJURY

The most common causes of blunt injury are falls and motor vehicle accidents. The degree of injury is related to the energy released in the collision between the patient and the solid object concerned. In all cases a sudden deceleration causes brain, bone and soft tissue injury; direct blows in which the velocity of injury is comparatively less are responsible for isolated bony injury. In general terms young people are more resistant to deceleration than older people; the speed at which a car crash will kill half of constrained car occupants is about 65 kph, and the height from which half those falling will die is about 12 m. Occasionally people survive deceleration forces much greater than this, but there are usually mitigating factors such as something to break the fall, or vehicular deceleration occurring in stages. The use of seatbelts has dramatically reduced

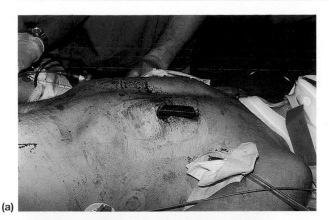

(a)

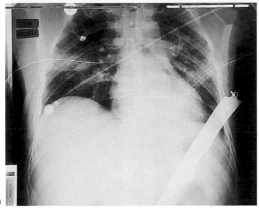

(b)

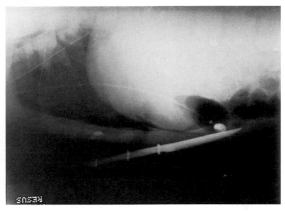

(c)

Figure 22.3 **(a)** The patient has been stabbed in the chest with a very large knife. The AP chest X-ray **(b)** confirms this, but the lateral view **(c)** shows that the blade has not penetrated the chest cavity. The knife was removed and the patient made an uneventful recovery, being discharged from hospital the next day.

road mortality and morbidity among car occupants in traffic accidents, whereas the use of airbags is not so obviously beneficial. Properly designed crash helmets and protective clothing similarly increase safety among motorcyclists and pedal cyclists involved in accidents.

Other causes of blunt injury include fights and, more rarely, blast injury from antipersonnel mines, industrial explosions and terrorist or military bombs.

PENETRATING INJURY

These are usually deliberately inflicted rather than accidental. They are classified as follows:

- **Blade** Stabbings are common injuries. The overall mortality for stab wounds is only 2%, but this is because the majority of them involve the hands, arms and subcutaneous tissues of the trunk (Fig. 22.3). A deep stab wound to the chest or abdomen can cause rapid death by bleeding, either from mediastinal structures or intercostal vessels, or from the abdominal aorta or its main visceral branches. It is even possible to exsanguinate from a stab wound to a vessel as small as the facial artery in the neck or the inferior epigastric artery inside the rectus sheath, and swift attention to such wounds is essential. The size of the entry wound is no indication of its depth, direction or severity.

- **Bullet** The extent of the injury is dependent on the amount of energy transferred from the speeding bullet to surrounding tissue. For example, a high-velocity bullet from an AK47 assault rifle entering the chest between the ribs at the front, passing through the lung tissue and then leaving between the ribs at the back causes very little damage because there is little energy transfer; the same round, perhaps travelling much more slowly at the limits of its trajectory, may cause serious damage by striking mediastinal structures, the vertebral column, or a solid organ such as the liver. Slower bullets do tend to cause less damage because they possess less kinetic energy, but even a very small bullet fired from a short-barrelled weapon can kill instantly if it lodges in the heart or brain, or somewhat more slowly if a major artery is involved. Under these circumstances survival is often a matter of luck (Fig. 22.4). Shotgun injuries are rather different. At short range the damage is caused by blast injury from the cartridge discharge as well as tissue destruction from a large mass of small lead pellets. At longer range the pellets travel much more slowly and tend to cause more superficial injuries, but can still cause blindness at a distance of 40 m (Fig. 22.5).

- **Blast** Explosions often carry the risk of penetrating injury from flying fragments (Fig. 22.6). These can lodge anywhere in the body and cause

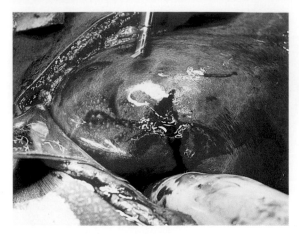

Figure 22.4 A through-and-through gunshot wound of the liver. The patient was shot at point-blank range by an armed policeman (whom he was trying to strangle at the time) using a long-barrelled Colt .44 calibre Magnum weapon, possibly the most powerful handgun available. The round traversed the liver and was found loose in the peritoneal cavity. Only minimal bleeding from the liver wound was found.

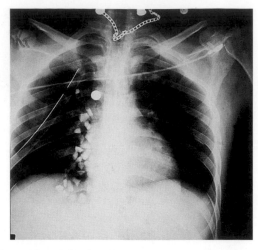

Figure 22.5 A PA chest X-ray showing large-calibre shotgun pellets in the anterior mediastinum. The weapon had been discharged at medium range and none of the pellets had punctured the myocardium.

trivial superficial wounds or serious, fatal, deep wounds. Such fragments often travel at high speed and their irregular shape and aerodynamic instability lead to much more energy transfer in the body than would be expected from a slower streamlined bullet following a stable trajectory.

PRIMARY SURVEY AND TRIAGE

AIRWAY WITH CERVICAL SPINE CONTROL

Resuscitate the trauma patient supine. The so-called 'recovery position' with the patient lying on the left side is not used because it makes it difficult to protect the cervical spine. The airway can be managed perfectly well with the patient supine.

BASIC MANAGEMENT OF AIRWAY OBSTRUCTION

Airway obstruction, if complete, causes death within 3 minutes and must be relieved at once. Even sweeping the index finger around the mouth to remove obstructions such as false teeth, followed by the chin lift or jaw thrust to move the tongue forwards and clear the oropharynx, can be life-saving in the unconscious patient (Box 22.2). The airway can then be protected by a nasopharyngeal or oropharyngeal airway. If the patient has ceased to breathe then a cuffed orotracheal or nasotracheal tube should be inserted immediately; this makes ventilation with a bag and oxygen a lot easier, and the inflated cuff protects the airway against vomit (Fig. 22.7). If necessary, a general anaesthetic can be used when inserting an airway.

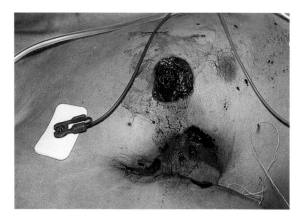

Figure 22.6 A penetrating wound through the right anterior axillary fold caused by a flying bomb fragment. Note the ragged entry and exit wounds caused both by the irregular shape of the fragment and its tumbling flight.

Physical signs of upper airway obstruction are not always easy to recognize, but it is vital to do so.

- *Noisy breathing*, particularly on inspiration, should alert one to the possibility of partial obstruction.
- *Silence*. If there are a number of injured people at the scene of an accident the silent ones should always be attended to before those crying out in pain, as they may have airway obstruction that can be easily relieved. They may, however, already be dead.
- *Suprasternal recession*. Inspiratory effort against a closed upper airway sucks the tissue inwards above the suprasternal notch and the clavicles. This sign indicates an urgent need for airway relief.

• *Deepening cyanosis*. This is an advanced sign of dangerous airway obstruction.

ADVANCED MANAGEMENT OF AIRWAY OBSTRUCTION

If the airway is blocked above the larynx by the inhalation of a foreign body or by direct trauma to the neck, a surgical airway is needed (Box 22.3). Cricothyroidotomy is the safest technique. A stab incision is made into the larynx *below the vocal cords* through the cricothyroid membrane, which lies subcutaneously between the thyroid and cricoid cartilages (Fig. 22.8). The exact surgical technique

---

Box 22.2 Airway 1

Basic management
• Chin lift
• Jaw thrust
• Nasopharyngeal airway
• Oropharyngeal airway

Advanced management
• Nasotracheal intubation
• Orotracheal intubation

Box 22.3 Airway 2

Surgical management
• Cricothyroidotomy
• Tracheostomy

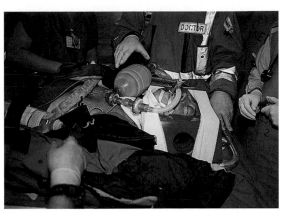

Figure 22.7 Airway with cervical spine control. The airway has been secured with an endotracheal tube. The cervical spine is controlled by means of a hard cervical collar to prevent rotation, with wedges on either side of the head to prevent lateral flexion and a tape across the forehead to prevent forward flexion. All of these measures must be used to provide complete control.

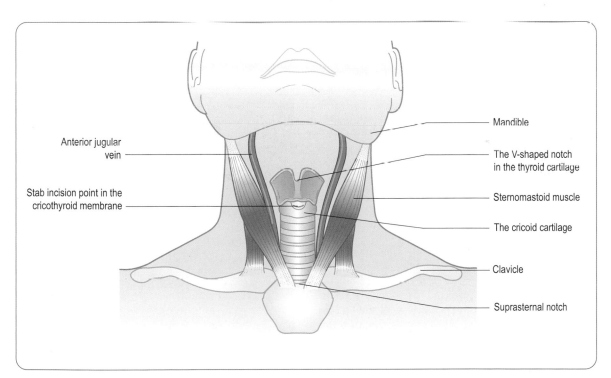

Figure 22.8 Surface markings for cricothyroidotomy. The cricothyroid membrane is located as a depression felt between the 'V' of the thyroid cartilage and the prominent ring of the cricoid cartilage some 2 cm below this. Caudally, the trachea can be felt disappearing into the thorax at the suprasternal notch. The transverse incision should be confined to a length of 2 cm in order to avoid damage to the lateral structures of the neck, the most prominent of which is the anterior jugular vein, which bleeds profusely if damaged.

for this procedure should be carefully learned (see the ATLS manual of the American College of Surgeons). Cricothyroidotomy is done under a local anaesthetic, or under no anaesthetic at all if the patient is unconscious. It is much safer and quicker than tracheostomy.

PROTECTING THE CERVICAL SPINE

Control of the cervical spine is essential at all times during resuscitation. Any injury involving deceleration may lead to a *cervical spine fracture, which may be unstable*. The cervical spine must be immobilized:

- in an inline position
- using both hands

until a *rigid* (not soft) cervical collar can be applied. It is essential to avoid damaging the spinal cord. Full immobilization requires:

- sandbags on either side of the head
- a piece of wide sticky plaster across the forehead attached to the sandbags.

If the airway problem is urgent and no collar is available then an assistant should hold the head steady while the airway is secured (see Fig. 22.7).

BREATHING

In the absence of airway obstruction, failure of breathing is caused either by severe head injury leading to cessation of central control of breathing, or by direct damage to the thoracic wall (Box 22.4). Thoracic injury may result in fractured ribs, a collapsed lung or bleeding into the chest, all of which restrict breathing. Several local problems in the chest can restrict breathing. All need immediate treatment from the moment they are diagnosed during the primary survey.

TENSION PNEUMOTHORAX

Air may enter the pleural cavity as a result of damage to the lung surface by a fractured rib. If there is a pleural flap air may enter the cavity with each breath but not leave between breaths, so that it accumulates under pressure. This increasing intrapleural pressure prevents lung inflation and may displace the mediastinum (Fig. 22.9). Reduced air exchange in the affected lung may lead to cyanosis. Observation of the chest wall shows that the affected side is fixed (does not move with respiration) and hyperinflated. Palpation confirms lack of movement on the side of the lesion, and there is deviation of the trachea *away* from the side of the pneumothorax. Percussion reveals hyperresonance all over the chest wall on the affected side, and there is resonance outside the normal surface markings of the lung in inspiration. Breath sounds are diminished or absent. The diagnosis is clinical and should be obvious without the use of a chest X-ray; indeed, waiting for an X-ray to confirm the suspected diagnosis is a mistake that wastes precious time.

Treatment of a *tension pneumothorax* is by the immediate insertion of a large-bore needle into the second interspace on the side of the lesion. This relieves the tension but does not treat the underlying lesion. A chest drain must be inserted (Fig. 22.10). There is usually a brisk gush of air as the pleural cavity is opened which confirms the diagnosis and is the first step towards successful treatment. The life-saving step is to relieve the tension; the needle does this, but only converts the lesion into a *simple pneumothorax*. A negative-pressure underwater seal drain allows the collapsed lung to reflate (Fig. 22.11).

HAEMOTHORAX

The signs are similar to those of tension pneumothorax, except that the affected side is dull to percussion. The patient is nearly always shocked, with a low blood pressure, elevated pulse rate, sweating, and short of breath (see Circulation below). The

---

Box 22.4 Causes of breathing difficulties

- Tension pneumothorax
- Haemothorax
- Haemopneumothorax
- Simple pneumothorax
- Flail chest
- Open chest wound

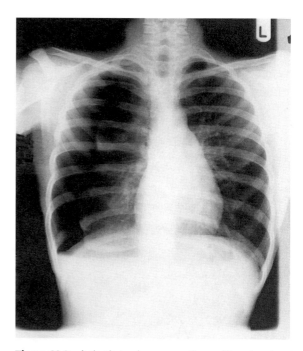

Figure 22.9 A simple tension pneumothorax. There is only slight collapse of the lung and minimal tracheal shift.

insertion of a chest drain confirms the presence of blood, which may be arterial or venous in origin, but which most commonly comes from a torn intercostal artery; massive haemorrhage from the mediastinum is rarely seen in hospital as this usually causes death before a chest drain can be inserted. If more than 750 mL are drained or the bleeding continues at a rate of more than 250 mL/hr, with no signs of slowing, then the patient needs urgent thoracotomy in order to secure haemostasis.

HAEMOPNEUMOTHORAX

Here there is both blood and air in the pleural cavity; it can occur with a simple or tension pneumothorax. Physical signs are similar to those of pneumothorax, except that there is often a fluid level on percussion; dullness to percussion over the lower zone gives way to a sudden increase in resonance as the pneumothorax is encountered. This sign is easier to elucidate with the patient sitting up. A chest drain must be inserted and thoracotomy may be necessary.

SIMPLE PNEUMOTHORAX (Fig. 22.9)

This occurs when a fixed amount of air has escaped into the pleural cavity causing partial collapse of the lung, the leak then sealing itself off. There is seldom any tracheal deviation and the affected side moves normally, or with only slight restriction. The patient is unlikely to be short of breath, distressed or cyanosed unless there is underlying chronic obstructive pulmonary disease. Palpation may reveal some loss of movement on the affected side. The percussion note is more resonant than usual, but not as resonant as that found in tension pneumothorax, and breath sounds may be reduced or muffled but

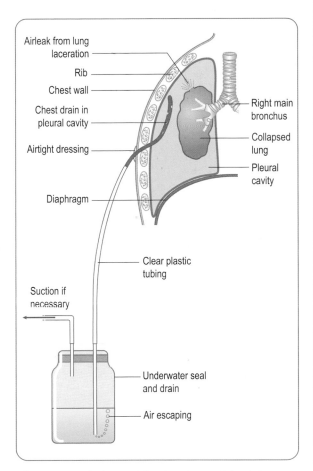

Figure 22.11 An intercostal underwater seal tube drain. The fenestrated drain is introduced into the pleural cavity and, once secured to the chest wall, is connected to an underwater seal. As the pressure in the pleural cavity rises air is forced down the tube and bubbles out through the water. This is particularly evident on coughing. Gentle breathing usually causes the water in the drainage tube to swing up and down. If the patient breathes in sharply the water is drawn up the tube until the hydrostatic pressure equals the pressure inside the pleural cavity. The water thus acts as a one-way valve which prevents air entering the pleural cavity via the chest drain but allows it to escape to the atmosphere. Graduations on the side of the bottle allow the amount of any blood or other fluid leaking from the pleural cavity to be measured.

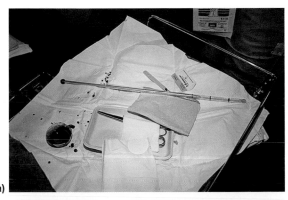

(a)

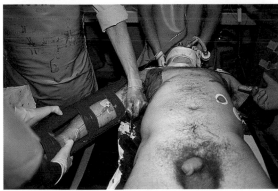

(b)

Figure 22.10 The instrument requirements for insertion of a chest drain (a) are minimal. Antiseptic solution, a knife for making the incision in the chest wall, a pair of artery forceps to deepen the incision through the intercostal muscles, an intercostal tube drain with the sharp trocar removed, and a stitch to secure the drain are all that are required. The drain is placed (b) in the fifth intercostal space in the anterior axillary line. The drain is shown pinched shut by the surgeon while the underwater seal drainage tube is prepared for connection.

seldom absent. Diagnosis without a chest X-ray may be difficult. A chest drain may be required, but this is less urgent than with a tension pneumothorax.

FLAIL CHEST

A flail chest is present when there is more than one fracture in more than one rib (Fig. 22.12). The loose segment of the chest wall takes no part in breathing: it is sucked in during inspiration and bulges out during expiration. If the segment is large the disorder may compromise gas exchange and the patient may need to be ventilated until some healing takes place – normally about a fortnight. The underlying lung injury is usually much more serious: for a flail chest to develop the chest wall has to be forced inwards against the lung, leading to lung contusion, ventilation/perfusion (V/P) mismatch, infection, oedema, and eventually adult respiratory distress syndrome (ARDS), a serious condition where all the above problems are compounded by the accumulation of fluid in the lungs, which makes the V/P mismatch even worse. This can be difficult to manage despite aggressive ventilation, physiotherapy and antibiotic therapy.

OPEN CHEST WOUND

If there is a large hole in the chest wall this should either be covered with an airtight dressing taped down on three of its four sides, or be completely sealed and a separate chest drain with a flutter valve or underwater seal placed in the normal position.

An open chest wound causes collapse of the lung and may be rapidly fatal.

CIRCULATION WITH CONTROL OF HAEMORRHAGE

Circulatory collapse in the absence of airway obstruction or tension pneumothorax is due to haemorrhage (Box 22.5). This may be confined to the body cavities (see Haemothorax above) or due to exsanguination from an open wound. In other words, the blood is either in the chest, in the abdomen, in the pelvis, in the long bones, or visible at the scene of the trauma or in the resuscitation room (Fig. 22.13).

The diagnosis of circulatory collapse may be made by observing the pulse, blood pressure, urine output and skin temperature. The signs of shock are:

- Elevation of pulse rate
- Fall in blood pressure
- Fall in urine output
- Central cyanosis due to circulatory failure
- Sweatiness
- Fall in peripheral temperature.

SOURCES OF BLEEDING

A rare but major cause of shock in the absence of obvious bleeding, either into the body cavities or elsewhere, is acute cardiac tamponade. The accumulation of blood inside the pericardium puts pressure

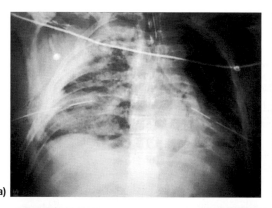
(a)

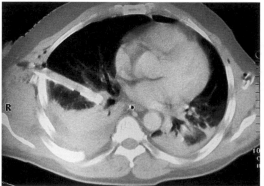
(b)

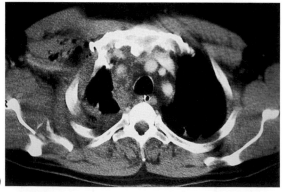
(c)

Figure 22.12 **(a)** Typical X-ray findings in a flail chest. There are obvious multiple fractures on the right side of the chest that include the first rib. There are severe underlying lung contusions. Bilateral chest drains are in place. **(b)** A CT scan through the lower part of the chest shows a collection of blood in both pleural cavities, more on the right, with a chest drain in situ. **(c)** A CT scan through the upper part of the chest shows crushing of the chest wall over the apex of the lung, with heavy extravasation of blood into the chest wall musculature. A ruptured right subclavian vein was subsequently repaired.

on the cardiac atria, impeding venous return and reducing cardiac output. Eventually the pressure difference between the atria and the pericardial space disappears and the circulation comes to a halt. The clinical diagnosis is made by the presence of Beck's triad, which consists of

- Distended neck veins
- Reduced heart sounds
- Reduced blood pressure.

Examination often reveals a penetrating injury in the region of the mediastinum, at the front or the back of the chest. Tamponade is one of the causes of pulsus paradoxus. Treatment is by relief of the intrapericardial pressure, i.e. by removing blood from the space, either by needle pericardiocentesis or, more reliably, by thoracotomy. Thoracotomy is preferred because the bleeding point can be secured (Fig. 22.14).

Long bone fractures may lead to the loss of large volumes of blood into the soft tissues without obvious external signs of bleeding. Bilateral femoral shaft fractures with a fractured pelvis can lead to major exsanguination.

Bleeding into the abdominal cavity is often difficult to diagnose (Box 22.6). It should be suspected if the patient is obviously shocked but there is no pelvic or long bone fracture and the chest is clear. Blood in the peritoneal cavity is irritant and causes abdominal pain, distension and absent bowel sounds. If the diagnosis is unclear then a diagnostic peritoneal lavage (DPL, see below), ultrasound scan or CT scan should be carried out.

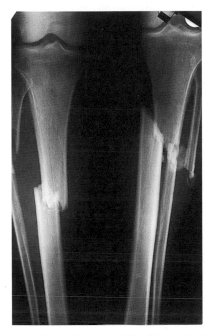

Figure 22.13 Bilateral fractures of the tibia and fibula can cause three to four units of blood loss into the tissues, and even more than this if the fractures are open.

Box 22.5 Sites of haemorrhage

- Intrathoracic
- Intra-abdominal
- Pelvic fracture
- Multiple long bone fractures
- Exsanguination

Box 22.6 Signs of intra-abdominal bleeding

- Pain
- Distension
- Guarding, rebound, rigidity
- Absent bowel sounds

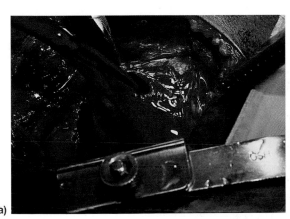 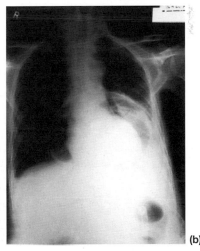

(a)   (b)

Figure 22.14 **(a)** The surgical treatment of pericardial tamponade. The figure shows a gush of blood under pressure leaving the pericardial cavity via a stab incision that has just been made by the surgeon. **(b)** Pneumopericardium may produce similar symptoms to haemopericardium.

Box 22.7   Blood tests in the resuscitation room

- Full blood count
- Urea and electrolytes
- Amylase
- Cross-matching
- Alcohol and toxicology if indicated

Table 22.1   The Glasgow Coma Scale (GCS)

Assessment area	Score
Eye-opening	
Spontaneous	4
To speech	3
To pain	2
None	1
Verbal response	
Orientated	5
Confused conversation	4
Inappropriate words	3
Incomprehensible sounds	2
None	1
Best motor response	
Obeys commands	6
Localizes pain	5
Normal flexion (withdrawal)	4
Abnormal flexion (decorticate)	3
Extension (decerebrate)	2
None (flaccid)	1

Note that a motor response in any limb is acceptable. Ocular movements and pupillary responses do not form part of the assessment. The GCS is suitable for use not only by physicians but also by nurses, ambulance personnel and other paramedical staff.

Treatment of circulatory collapse is by the immediate insertion of two wide-bore cannulae (16 gauge or larger) into the antecubital veins. Blood samples should be taken at this point; a full blood count, urea and electrolyte and amylase estimation and cross-matching should be carried out (Box 22.7). Initial resuscitation is by quick intravenous infusion of crystalloid (low molecular weight solutions of dextrose or saline) or colloid (high molecular weight solutions of starch and other blood substitutes) solution to bring the blood pressure back up. The trauma patient almost always needs blood, especially if arterial blood gases show an acidosis, and if the need is urgent O-Rhesus negative blood may be given until type-specific un-crossmatched or properly cross-matched blood becomes available.

Any obvious bleeding, for example from an open wound, is controlled by direct pressure on the bleeding point until surgical repair can be arranged. Most patients who have bled and whose bleeding has ceased will respond to a 2 L fluid infusion, but if it is not possible to keep the blood pressure up then it must be assumed that internal bleeding is continuing. The source of the bleeding should be found and controlled immediately. Whole blood is the best transfusion fluid; there is much debate as to whether crystalloid or colloid should be given in the initial stages of resuscitation, and it probably does not matter very much which is used. In penetrating trauma in younger, fitter patients it is probably best not to resuscitate too vigorously and restore the blood pressure to normal, as this may provoke further bleeding and worsen the outcome. It is better to conserve the patient's own blood than to replace it with stored blood products. A central venous line may be useful in later management for reading the central venous pressure (CVP). The CVP line should not be used for volume replacement or fluid resuscitation because it is narrow and long. In addition, remember that it is wise always to warm fluids given intravenously.

DISABILITY

The diagnosis of central nervous system injury is made initially by a simple assessment of the level of consciousness. The patient may be alert, responsive to voice, responsive to pain, or unresponsive (AVPU). A rudimentary assessment of limb movement may be made at the same time, but it is seldom necessary to go beyond this level until later in the examination. The assessment can be formalized by using the Glasgow Coma Scale during the secondary survey (Table 22.1).

EXPOSURE

It is important to undress the patient completely in order to carry out a full examination. At the same time, and paradoxically, it is important to keep the patient warm, because trauma and blood loss invariably lead to a reduction in core temperature, even in warm climates. Once the patient is undressed a cellular blanket or a warm-air warming device should be used to maintain body warmth (Fig. 22.15).

RADIOLOGY

Three X-ray films are of most immediate use in the trauma victim:

- Cervical spine
- Chest
- Pelvis.

These augment the physical findings made during the primary survey. Note that a skull X-ray is of little use: brain injury is much more reliably assessed by CT scanning.

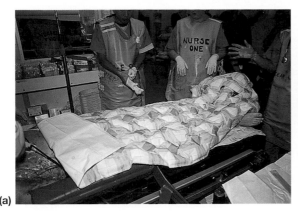

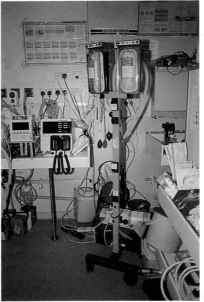

Figure 22.15 Keeping the patient warm by means of **(a)** a warm air blanket and **(b)** a blood warmer.

CERVICAL SPINE

A cross-table lateral view of the cervical spine is important for excluding spinal cord injury or potential injury due to an unstable fracture of the neck. The film must show all seven cervical vertebrae and the top half of the first thoracic vertebra in order to be reliable, and many films have to be repeated, either with traction on the arms or as oblique views. If there is doubt, and particularly if there is neck tenderness on examination, the rigid cervical collar that was fitted when the patient was first seen should be left in place. Do not be distracted from other more urgent injuries by the need to get a good view of the cervical vertebrae. CT scanning or MRI of the neck may be required to 'clear' the cervical spine (Fig. 22.16).

CHEST

A plain chest radiograph is useful for identifying:

- Lung contusions or mediastinal injury not suspected clinically
- Bony injury, such as fractured ribs or flail chest
- Simple pneumothorax and/or haemothorax
- Diaphragmatic injury
- Correct placement of chest drains and CVP lines.

Interpretation is difficult because this is an anteroposterior film taken with the patient lying flat and the normal appearances are quite different from the standard chest X-ray, taken posteroanteriorly with the patient standing. The diagnosis of a ruptured diaphragm may be quite difficult to make; if the rupture is on the left, placing a nasogastric tube may help as it often appears in the chest on a subsequent chest film.

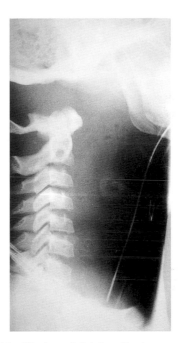

Figure 22.16 Atlanto-occipital disruption is rare and generally fatal, caused by severe traction injury to the neck.

PELVIS

The diagnosis of a pelvic fracture is very important because this may be life-threatening. A large amount of blood may become sequestered in the soft tissues of the pelvis and the injury may be exacerbated by damage to the bladder, uterus, rectum, iliac arteries and veins, and ureters. The extent of the bony injury is usually related to the extent of the soft tissue injury; the main exception to this is where an iliac artery or even the aorta has been breached.

OTHER DIAGNOSTIC X-RAYS

These are carried out as indicated when specific injuries are diagnosed during the secondary survey.

SECONDARY SURVEY

The secondary survey is nothing more or less than a full physical examination of the patient from head to toe.

FACE, HEAD AND NECK

Careful digital examination of the cranium, the facial skeleton, the cervical vertebrae and associated soft tissues is important to exclude fractures. The cervical collar may be removed for this examination, but inline traction of the neck must be maintained by an assistant and the collar replaced afterwards unless a fracture has been clearly excluded. Be particularly alert for the boggy swelling over the cranium that suggests a depressed fracture, and the tenderness in the neck that suggests a fractured cervical vertebra. An open wound over such an injury suggests a compound fracture. Look for penetrating injuries: a tiny stab wound to the neck may hide extensive damage to the carotid arteries, pharynx and other deep neck structures. Facial bruising is a clue to underlying injuries. In particular it is important to exclude an orbital floor blowout fracture, associated with periorbital haematoma, which may lead to loss of sight. Serious maxillary fractures are nearly always associated with bleeding from the nose or mouth, as is a fractured base of skull. Search for broken teeth and a step in the mandible, which suggests a fractured jaw. Finally, fundoscopy can provide important information about ocular injuries, and otoscopy will reveal bleeding from the ear with blood behind the tympanic membrane. A fractured skull base is often associated with a cerebrospinal fluid leak from the nose or ears. Battle's sign – bruising over the mastoid bone – is an important clue to this injury.

CENTRAL NERVOUS SYSTEM

The state of the pupils is important. Bilateral fixed dilated pupils indicate brainstem injury and imply a poor prognosis. A unilateral constricted pupil is caused by stretching of the third nerve across the edge of the tentorium cerebelli as a result of brain displacement, usually due to extradural or subdural haematoma with raised intracranial pressure. If this situation worsens the pupil will become fixed and dilated, and there is a risk of irremediable brainstem damage and death. Immediate CT scanning of the brain is indicated. This situation is usually associated with a very poor GCS score (see below).

The Glasgow Coma Scale (GCS) is an invaluable measure of the level of coma in a patient. It is measured by clinical examination of the conscious state by assessing three domains of function:

- Eye-opening
- Best motor response
- Verbal response.

The detailed scoring system is outlined in Table 22.1. The best possible score is 15 and the worst is 3. The scale is precisely what it says it is, a measure of coma; it does not give information regarding the CNS as a whole. A patient can come into the A&E department with a dense left-sided stroke but still have a GCS of 15, as a moment's thought will show, as the best motor response will be on the unaffected side and therefore normal. The prognosis becomes increasingly grave with a lower score, and full coma is defined as a score of 8 or less.

CHEST

Because of the importance of managing severe chest injuries to maximize the chances of survival, much of the thoracic examination is carried out during the primary survey. During the secondary survey the chest is examined in more detail together with the thoracic spine. The patient is log-rolled on to the left side by four people, maintaining inline traction on the cervical spine and avoiding any twisting of the thoracic and lumbar spine. It is at this point that the back is searched for stab wounds or other open wounds not hitherto suspected, tenderness associated with fractured ribs, and the thoracic and lumbar spine gently probed for tender areas or a palpable step that might suggest a spinal fracture (Fig. 22.17).

ABDOMEN AND PELVIS

Abdominal injuries can be difficult to diagnose. Attention to abdominal signs and symptoms is essential (Fig. 22.18(a)). This is easier if the patient is conscious. The presence of bruising from seatbelt injuries or other direct blunt trauma should be regarded with suspicion and, of course, the presence of penetrating injury very often means damage to internal structures. If the abdomen is soft and pain free, major injury is unlikely. The classic signs of peritonitis – guarding, rebound tenderness and rigidity – can only be elucidated in the conscious patient. A distended, rigid abdomen with absent bowel sounds almost certainly contains major pathology whether the patient is awake or unconscious (Box 22.8).

Haematemesis suggests upper gastrointestinal injury. Pancreatic injury is serious, and in most cases a raised amylase alerts the surgeon to its presence. CT scanning will locate a pancreatic injury.

A nasogastric (NG) tube should always be placed in the trauma patient; if there is bleeding from the nose or mouth the tube is best placed orally in order

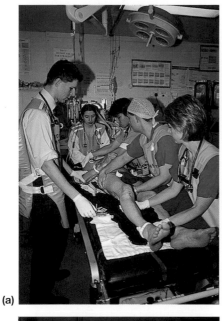

(a)

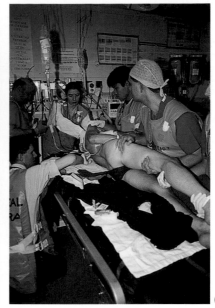

(b)

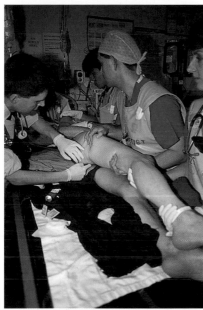

(c)

Figure 22.17 **(a)** Preparing to log-roll a patient. Four people are needed to do this: three to roll the patient while keeping the thoracolumbar spine stable and in line, and the fourth to secure the cervical spine from the top of the table. **(b)** Once the patient is rolled the thoracolumbar spine is examined for evidence of fracture and the back of the thorax and abdomen are searched for penetrating trauma. **(c)** The opportunity is taken to carry out a rectal examination.

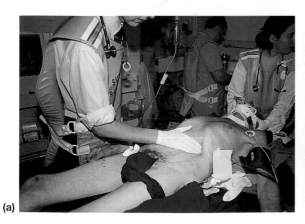

(a)

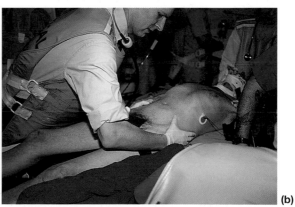

(b)

Figure 22.18 **(a)** Palpating the abdomen for signs of injury and **(b)** examining the pelvis for signs of instability.

ischaemia (Box 22.10). In a young, fit patient pulses may still be present even if a major blood vessel has been disrupted. An open arterial injury is controlled by direct pressure on the wound; this is safer than the application of a tourniquet, which is too easily forgotten. Venous bleeding, such as that seen after disruption of a superficial varicose vein, can be controlled either by local pressure or by elevation of the limb.

SPECIAL TESTS

Additional diagnostic tests may be carried out after the secondary survey. There are probably as many tests as there are injuries.

The mainstay of trauma investigation is the CT scan. Highly sensitive and specific, especially with injected contrast medium, the test will identify most intrathoracic, intra-abdominal and pelvic injuries, including firm and soft organ rupture, retroperitoneal injury to the urinary tract and pancreas, and ruptured thoracic aorta. A modern spiral or multi-slice CT scanner will perform a total body scan in less than 3 minutes, although the dose of ionizing radiation is very high (equivalent to more than 500 chest X-rays). The most important thing to remember about this type of diagnostic imaging is that the patient must have a stable airway and circulation before starting, otherwise they may collapse halfway through the scan. The CT scanner is no place for an unstable patient.

Of less value, but still useful in the early stages of resuscitation or if access to a CT scanner is not available, is diagnostic ultrasound, which will identify fluid in the peritoneal cavity and delineate injury to firm organs, including the kidneys, but not soft ones such as the gut.

Intravenous urography will help diagnose renal tract injury – this is normally done as a one-film procedure 1–2 minutes after the intravenous injection of contrast medium; this film will show whether the kidneys are working. The assessment of ureteric, bladder or urethral injury relies on more complex radiological procedures.

Finally, diagnostic peritoneal lavage (DPL) is useful in some circumstances, usually when ultra-

to avoid the remote risk of passing it through a fractured skull base and into the cranial cavity.

A *rectal examination* is essential, and this should be done during the log-roll described above. Rectal wall damage should be sought, and if such injury is present the jagged edges of fractured pelvic bones may be felt. Blood on the glove is a sign of rectal or other large bowel injury. The presence of bruising in the perineum, haematuria, or a high-riding prostate, suggesting urethral injury, is a contraindication to catheterization, and under such circumstances a suprapubic catheter should be placed. Blood coming from the urethra is usually fresh and undiluted, whereas haematuria from the kidneys and bladder is diluted by the urine. Renal or bladder damage should always be suspected under these circumstances. Otherwise, diagnosis in the unconscious patient relies on the special tests outlined below. Pelvic fracture can be diagnosed clinically by the elucidation of pain on gentle suprapubic pressure (Box 22.9).

EXTREMITIES

The arms and legs should be carefully examined for fractures. Radiography is indicated if there is bruising or obvious deformity. Skin wounds over a fractured bone mean that a compound fracture is present. The presence of a large haematoma, especially when there is a penetrating injury, suggests vessel damage, and the presence of a bruit found on auscultation over the area suggests traumatic arteriovenous fistula. Peripheral pulses should be sought. The absence of pulses usually means that there is major vessel injury, unless the patient is elderly and has pre-existing vascular disease. The presence of pain, pallor, pulselessness, coldness and poor capillary return are diagnostic of acute sound or CT are unavailable. The procedure diagnoses the presence of blood or bowel contents inside the peritoneal cavity but cannot indicate its source. A small vertical incision is made below the umbilicus and a litre of warmed saline instilled, left for 15 minutes, and then drained out. The procedure is positive, indicating the need for laparotomy, if the red cell count exceeds 100 000/mL, the white cell count exceeds 5000/mL, or there are bowel contents in the fluid.

CASE STUDY

A 27-year-old male motorcyclist is admitted to the emergency department after falling from his motorcycle on a bend and hitting a tree. No other vehicle was involved. His helmet was removed at the scene by the emergency medicine technicians and he arrives in the department strapped to a long spinal board with full cervical spine restraint, including a hard collar, a tape and sandbags. He is awake and alert but complains of pain in the right side of the chest, and the right tibia and fibula are clearly broken, with an open wound just behind the knee from which arterial blood is pouring through the bandage. The GCS is 15. The pulse is 140, the blood pressure is 90/40 and the respiratory rate is 40.

Questions
1. What must you attend to first?
2. What comes second?
3. What comes third?
4. What investigations would you like to carry out?

Answers
1. Check the *airway* by examining the patient and asking him some questions. Check the cervical spine restraint. Give oxygen via a facemask.
2. *Breathing.* You expose the chest and find a right tension haemopneumothorax. You insert a chest drain and 500 mL of blood comes out, mixed with air.
3. *Circulation.* If you are by yourself you will have carried out the above two manoeuvres first; if you have an assistant you should already have arranged for pressure to be put on the wound. Put up two large drips in the antecubital fossae and start some fluid. Do a quick neurological examination.
4. Send blood for grouping and order six units of type-specific blood followed by six cross-matched units. If the patient fails to respond well to the initial fluid challenge you can give O-negative blood. Send blood for arterial blood gases. Then order a trauma series of X-rays, but only when the patient is more stable. The main purpose of the chest X-ray is to check the position of the chest drain and exclude mediastinal injury. Then move on to the secondary survey.

In a modern well-equipped hospital expert help will already be on its way, but the following personnel may all be needed: a consultant anaesthetist, a consultant orthopaedic surgeon, a consultant vascular surgeon, and possibly a consultant thoracic surgeon if the bleeding from the chest drain does not stop. The ISS is above 30, and this patient requires rapid expert assistance.

23 Intensive care

J. H. Coakley

INTRODUCTION

The critically ill patient on the ITU presents a bewildering sight to the uninitiated (Fig. 23.1), and it is important to focus on the patient and not be too distracted by the vast array of equipment surrounding them. There are features of the ITU situation that require specific clinical skills.

GENERAL PRINCIPLES

Severe illness, trauma, and planned or emergency surgical interventions may produce life-threatening problems. The role of the ITU is to keep patients alive by providing treatment to support organs or systems, in addition to specific therapy of the precipitating condition. It is therefore important to diagnose the cause of organ failures and physiological disturbances, although it should be recognized that some acute conditions resolve without specific treatment. The absence of a diagnosis is not in itself a barrier to the continuation of supportive care.

One of the fundamental differences between intensive care medicine and other medical and surgical disciplines is that it is often necessary to bypass the normal clinical evaluation processes. For most diseases, a well-defined pathway is followed that encompasses history, examination, investigation, diagnosis, prognosis and treatment. In critical illness, particularly in medical and surgical emergencies, it is often necessary to proceed directly to treatment with no clear idea of the history or diagnosis. This can be challenging, and it is important to learn to recognize the signs of impending death in a patient, either on the ward or in the emergency department, so that the emphasis can be rapidly changed to the urgent provision of life support.

The generally accepted criteria for admission to an ITU are shown in Box 23.1. The more criteria in Box 23.1 that are present, the greater the indication for admission to the ITU.

BEFORE ITU ADMISSION – ASSESSMENT

SIGNS OF IMPENDING DEATH

These would have been familiar to Florence Nightingale and Hippocrates. They are based on clinical observations made at the bedside and recorded in the patient's charts, and on findings elicited on rapid examination. The sequence of clinical evaluation follows the same principles as for major trauma. The difference with the critically ill patient is that the evolution of changes may be slower and more subtle than in the trauma victim. A number of methods have been recommended to aid the early identification of the need for ITU intervention. Figure 23.2 illustrates a system used in many hospitals to highlight important abnormal observations, colour coded to show the severity of the variation from normal. It also gives details of how to contact the critical care team.

HISTORY

It is often difficult to obtain a satisfactory history from a critically ill patient. Of course, if the patient is capable of talking, the history should be taken from him or her. Even in the face of catastrophic illness, there is nothing more irritating to a patient than being ignored. If the patient cannot give a coherent account of their illness, they should at least be acknowledged and asked if they mind someone else being interviewed on their behalf. It is important to be discreet in taking a history from others, even if they are the next of kin. This is particularly important in HIV infection, alcohol or substance abuse. It is, as always, important to obtain an occupational, social and travel history. There may be no time to take a history, and keeping the patient alive long enough to obtain one may need to take precedence.

When taking the history, in addition to standard questions about the illness, it is particularly important to obtain some idea of the stage of disease and

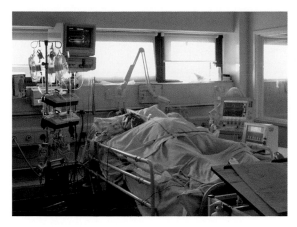

Figure 23.1 A critically ill patient surrounded by (from left to right) several infusion pumps, monitoring screen, mechanical ventilator, oesophageal Doppler probe and ITU chart. Note also the gloves near infusion pumps and the alcohol gel hand rub dispenser at the bottom of the picture attached to the chart holder. Infection control is vital in the ITU.

Box 23.1   Criteria for ITU referral

Airway
- Actual or potential airway obstruction
- Impaired ability to protect airway

Breathing
- Respiratory rate <8 or >30
- Respiratory arrest
- Oxygen saturation <90% on 50% oxygen
- Respiratory acidosis

Circulation
- Heart rate <50 or >140 bpm
- Systolic blood pressure <90 mmHg
- Cardiac arrest
- Metabolic acidosis (pH <7.2)
- Urine output <0.5 mL/kg/h

Neurological
- Repeated seizures without return of consciousness between episodes
- Prolonged seizures
- Deteriorating level of consciousness of any aetiology
- GCS <8 whatever the cause

Other
- Gross metabolic disturbances
- Increased nursing dependency
- After major elective surgery, emergency surgery or any surgery with major comorbidities

---

the physiological reserve. Patients in the terminal stages of a chronic disease process are unlikely to survive intensive care. Likewise, patients with limited cardiac or respiratory reserve will probably not tolerate organ support, as this makes considerable demands on their physiological reserve. For example, the circulatory and respiratory systems may be stressed by mechanical ventilation. It is of little benefit to someone already severely disabled with a chronic disease to be subjected to treatment that might in itself be life-threatening. Furthermore, critical illness induces a severe catabolic state, often leading to rapid muscle wasting and weakness. This severely hampers even previously healthy individuals, who may take several months to recover fitness; those with previous limitations take much longer and may die before rehabilitation is complete, or survive only in a very disabled state. Patients should therefore be asked about their ability to perform such tasks as climbing stairs, doing their shopping and cleaning, and other activities of daily living. People who have been housebound because of limited cardiac or respiratory function will probably not benefit from prolonged intensive care support.

AIRWAY

Airway obstruction may be partial (stridor) or complete. Do not confuse stridulous breathing with wheezing. Stridor is an inspiratory noise and is best heard by listening over the trachea with a stethoscope, although it is usually obvious to the unaided ear. It is due to mechanical obstruction (such as a foreign body, tumour or laryngeal oedema). The degree of physiological impairment should be gauged by the ability to speak in full sentences, respiratory

effort, and the presence of obviously uncoordinated breathing (seesaw breathing). The patient with upper airway obstruction who is struggling to breathe, or who cannot speak or swallow, is threatened and airway patency must be restored immediately. A silent airway is either completely clear or completely obstructed.

A patient with impaired consciousness may obstruct their airway with their tongue, a foreign body or vomitus. Patients with a Glasgow Coma Score (GCS; see Chapter 21) of 8 or less (whatever the cause) are at severe risk of airway obstruction, and constant attention to the airway is necessary.

BREATHING

This should be assessed rapidly. The important features in the deteriorating patient are shown in Box 23.2, and may occur singly or in combination.

Breathing may become unduly rapid in many disease states with or without lung involvement. An abnormal respiratory rate is a highly sensitive but very non-specific indicator of life-threatening illness. Patients who exhibit the signs in Box 23.2 are at risk of respiratory failure and should be closely monitored.

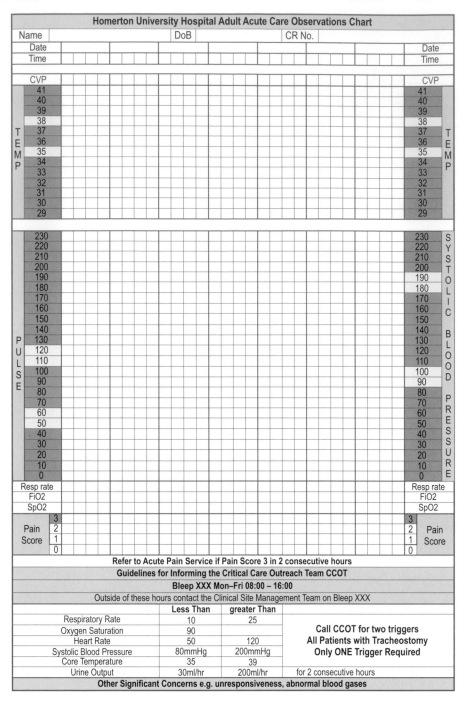

Figure 23.2 Chart for recording of patient observations, with colour coding to emphasize variations from normality.

CIRCULATION

Shock (hypotension, reduced cardiac output) has a number of causes, which are sometimes difficult to distinguish by simple clinical observation. Some clinical methods for differentiating types of shock are outlined below. Evidence of underperfusion of organs can be obtained by estimation of capillary refill. This is defined as the time taken to restore perfusion to the skin following a brief period of applied pressure. In health this is usually less than 2 seconds, and if normal represents a reasonable estimate of skin and, by implication, internal organ, perfusion.

DISABILITY

A brief neurological examination should be carried out. The GCS should be estimated, as should pupillary size and reaction. *Blood glucose* should be measured

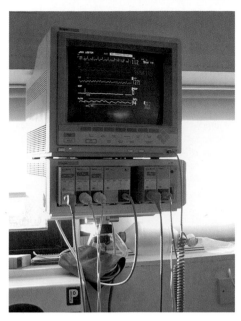

Figure 23.3   A typical ITU monitor showing, from the top, electrocardiograph, arterial blood pressure trace, central venous pressure trace, respiratory rate (the zero is an artefact) and oxygen saturation trace. The number 30.1 in the bottom right corner is the peripheral temperature. This patient has a sinus tachycardia and is hypotensive, with increased filling pressures and poor peripheral perfusion. Work out why.

in all cases of impaired consciousness. The major causes of impaired consciousness for which ITU assessment may be required are shown in Box 23.3.

EXPOSURE

A full physical examination should be carried out as soon as possible after assessing the ABC (airway, breathing and circulation) as above and instituting any life support measures required. Always keep the patient warm, and remember their dignity.

AFTER ITU ADMISSION – ASSESSMENT

RECORDING OF OBSERVATIONS

Several physiological variables are recorded continuously in each patient on the ITU. These are usually displayed on a monitor situated close to the patient (Fig. 23.3), and duplicated at a central nursing console. They are important. A typical chart will have haemodynamic, respiratory and neurological observations, intravenous and enteral fluid input, urine and other fluid output, and drug infusions. Systematic scrutiny of these charts can yield much information about the physiological state of the patient.

EXAMINATION

It is important to examine critically ill patients on at least a daily basis according to the principles laid out in the chapters on specific areas and systems of the body (respiratory, cardiovascular etc.). Remember that many of the techniques used to support the critically ill patient may themselves have serious adverse effects, and careful monitoring is required. It is therefore mandatory to examine carefully all indwelling tubes and cannulae, in addition to all organ support devices. The noise made by equipment in the ITU may render auscultation difficult, particularly when examining heart and lungs. Subtle changes may be missed, and it is important to maximize the use of collateral sources of information, such as radiographs and portable ultrasound devices.

RESPIRATORY SYSTEM

The patient's chest should be inspected to ensure adequate, symmetrical expansion with good air entry to both sides. The chest should be palpated for tracheal shift, surgical emphysema, and adequacy and symmetry of expansion; then auscultated for stridor, adequacy of air entry, wheeze, crackles and bronchial breathing.

An expiratory wheeze indicates impaired expiratory airflow. Inspiratory crackles may indicate pulmonary oedema, infection or fibrosis. Bronchial breathing suggests pulmonary consolidation. These findings may be due to the disease that precipitated ITU admission, but may be due to the development

Box 23.4   Features of ARDS

- A recognized underlying cause (e.g. sepsis, trauma, pancreatitis)
- Increased radiological lung shadowing
- Stiff lungs – increased airway pressure in the ventilated patient, or tachypnoea in the patient breathing spontaneously
- Impaired gas exchange – worsening hypoxia
- Increased physiological dead space – increased arterial Paco$_2$

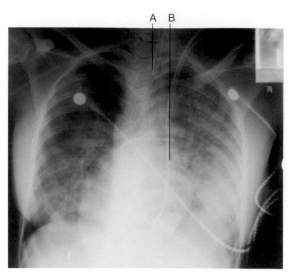

Figure 23.4   Chest radiograph of a patient with severe ARDS. There is diffuse shadowing throughout both lung fields. Note the position of the endotracheal tube A and the presence of a pulmonary artery catheter B, which allows determination of pulmonary artery pressure and cardiac output (both likely to be elevated in this patient).

of one of the most serious complications of critical illness – the *acute respiratory distress syndrome (ARDS)*. This condition usually arises in patients on the ITU, although subtler forms may occur on the general wards. It is characterized by increased extravascular lung water (non-cardiogenic pulmonary oedema), which causes a number of clinical and radiological features (Box 23.4). ARDS may occur in association with primary respiratory disease such as pneumonia or chest trauma, or secondary to an extrapulmonary cause. A wide range of conditions may precipitate ARDS, but the most common causes are severe sepsis, trauma, burns and pancreatitis.

The excess lung water results in an increased work of breathing, leading to tachypnoea, and ultimately exhaustion and respiratory arrest in the non-ventilated patient. More commonly it arises in patients already receiving ventilatory support. A typical radiograph of a patient with ARDS is shown in Figure 23.4.

It is important to check the position of endotracheal or tracheostomy tubes, both clinically and radiologically. The depth from the lips or teeth to which the tube is inserted originally should be marked on the ITU chart. Tubes may be displaced down one of the bronchi (usually the right) or upwards out of the trachea. Either may prove fatal if not diagnosed rapidly. Downward displacement is readily diagnosed by noting any difference from the original depth of insertion, and secondly by auscultation. Air entry to one lung is highly suggestive of a downwardly misplaced tube. Upward migration is diagnosed by observing a gush of air from the mouth on inspiration. *Always* take a chest radiograph to confirm endotracheal tube placement: the tip of the tube should be approximately 2 cm above the carina. The correct position is shown in Figure 23.4.

The integrity of the defence mechanisms against aspiration of pharyngeal contents is reduced for the reasons shown in Box 23.5.

In the ventilated patient, oxygenation is monitored continuously with a pulse oximeter, and a regular check kept on the arterial blood gases. The pressure with which the oximeter probe is applied is not great, but in patients whose blood flow is jeopardized even this may lead to pressure necrosis. It is therefore important to check the skin under the probe on a regular basis.

Patients should have a daily chest radiograph. This should be examined for the presence of new infiltrates suggestive of infection or oedema. It is also valuable in ensuring that lines and tubes remain correctly placed. These devices may easily become displaced, for instance when the patient is turned or moved, and these displacements may become life-threatening.

It is also important to check that ventilator equipment used to support respiration is functioning. Most ventilators display essential respiratory information such as respiratory rate, inspired and expired tidal volume, inhaled oxygen concentration, peak airway pressure and so on. A typical modern ventilator is shown in Figure 23.5.

Mechanical ventilation is associated with a number of adverse effects, which should be sought on clinical examination. In spontaneous respiration the pressure within the thoracic cavity during inspiration is subatmospheric, whereas in mechanical ventilation the pressure is above atmospheric. This leads to impaired venous return to the right side of the heart. The consequences of this are first, hypotension and second, venous engorgement leading to peripheral oedema.

Expiratory airflow limitation, usually manifest as expiratory wheeze, may occur if the endotracheal tube has kinked or become partially obstructed with

- Presence of endotracheal tube
- Sedative and analgesic drugs
- Muscle relaxants
- Paralytic ileus
- Recumbent posture
- Presence of nasogastric tube
- Reduction in gastric exocrine function leading to loss of gastric acidity and hence colonization of gastric contents with Gram-negative organisms

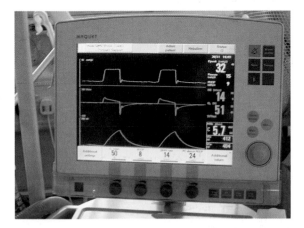

Figure 23.5 A typical modern ventilator. The screen shows three traces. From the top: airway pressure (yellow), inspiratory and expiratory flows (green) and tidal volume (blue). The figures along the bottom of the screen show, from left to right, inspired oxygen, applied end-expiratory pressure, set respiratory rate and applied end-inspiratory pressure. The blue figures at bottom right show minute ventilation, inspired and expired tidal volumes.

secretions, and if the patient has developed bronchospasm. This is dangerous in the ventilated patient, as one ventilator breath may occur before exhalation from the previous one is complete. In such circumstances there is progressive hyper-inflation of the lungs, and if overdistension occurs, cardiovascular collapse may follow as venous return to the right side of the heart is impaired by raised intrathoracic pressure. Such air trapping may be detected by briefly disconnecting the ventilator tubing and timing exhalation.

CARDIOVASCULAR SYSTEM

In the critically ill patient, circulatory failure presents clinically as reduced tissue perfusion. This may be assessed rapidly prior to ITU admission as outlined above, but after admission much more information should be obtained by clinical examination and scrutiny of the monitors and observation charts. The consequence is a metabolic (usually lactic) acidosis that occurs as a result of tissue hypoxia.

Observe the state of the peripheral pulses and also the temperature of the peripheries. Warm peripheries suggest that the cardiac output is adequate; cold, that it is not. This is not an infallible clinical tool. The blood pressure should be noted, bearing in mind the patient's normal reading.

In general, *shock* is manifest by a rapid heart rate and low blood pressure, with evidence of reduced cardiac output leading to underperfusion of tissues or organs. There is a large variation in blood pressure in a population of healthy individuals. Caution should therefore be exercised in interpreting isolated low blood pressure as shock, or in assuming that an apparently normal blood pressure is evidence of the absence of shock. It is important to judge a patient's blood pressure in the context of previous readings, either in hospital or by contacting the GP. A low diastolic blood pressure suggests either the hyper-dynamic circulation of sepsis or inflammation (common), or aortic regurgitation (rare).

Ensure that the circulation is monitored to a level appropriate for each patient. The patient with a normal heart rate and blood pressure, with no evidence of organ underperfusion or metabolic acidosis, is unlikely to benefit from invasive monitoring, but in the ITU such patients are rare. Most patients on the ITU will have a line inserted into an artery and a central vein to measure simple haemodynamic variables such as arterial and central venous blood pressure. It is important to check the insertion sites of these regularly to ensure that there is no evidence of infection. It is important to check the arterial cannula site for complications (Box 23.6).

Cardiac output is monitored either clinically (evidence of reduced tissue perfusion or metabolic acidosis) or by *thermodilution* using a pulmonary artery catheter (Fig. 23.4), or non-invasively using a *Doppler* oesophageal probe. The latter two techniques give reasonably accurate estimates of cardiac output. Figure 23.6 shows a chest radiograph with the oesophageal probe and the waveform obtained from it, allowing estimation of cardiac output, stroke volume, systemic vascular resistance, and a rough guide to the 'fullness' of the circulation.

Hypovolaemic shock is manifest by a falling central venous pressure, hypotension and reduced cardiac output. *Cardiogenic shock* is also a low cardiac output state, but also often associated with high central venous or pulmonary artery wedge pressures. In *septic shock* there is an increased cardiac output. It is not uncommon for these three types of shock to coexist – the patient with septic shock will inevitably lose fluid because of fever, tachypnoea and reduced oral intake, and may therefore become hypovolaemic. Cardiogenic shock may

---

Box 23.6 Complications of intravascular cannulae

General

- Infection (initially manifesting as a slight reddish discolouration around the insertion site, progressing to pus oozing from insertion site if not dealt with)
- Bleeding
- Damage to vessel wall
- Thrombosis

Arterial lines

- Vasospasm
- Embolization distal to cannula
- Damage to vessel wall – pseudoaneurysm

Central venous lines

- Pneumothorax or haemothorax
- Subclavian or carotid artery puncture

Pulmonary artery catheter

- As for central venous line, plus
  - Arrhythmias
  - Damage to tricuspid valve

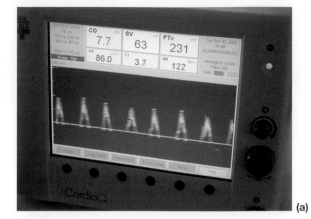

(a)

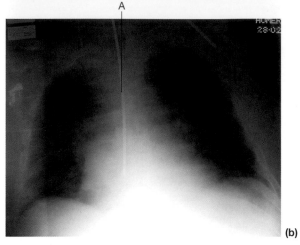

(b)

Figure 23.6 (a) Haemodynamic measurements from an oesophageal Doppler probe. The numbers at the top of the screen from left to right indicate cardiac output, stroke volume and corrected flow time, an indicator of circulating volume. The Doppler probe A is shown on the chest radiograph (b).

occur simultaneously if the patient also has ischaemic heart disease. The other major category of shock is that associated with obstruction to blood flow, or obstructive shock. This occurs when venous return to the heart is impaired or there is obstruction to the flow of blood out of the heart. The most common causes are pulmonary embolism, aortic stenosis, pericardial tamponade and tension pneumothorax. The features of the different causes of shock are shown in Box 23.7.

GASTROINTESTINAL SYSTEM

The abdomen is often difficult to assess in the ITU patient, but it should be inspected for evidence of distension (girth measurements are useless in the critically ill) and palpated for evidence of new masses.

Gross abdominal distension with elevated intra-abdominal pressure has two important effects: compression of the renal vasculature leads to renal underperfusion and hence oliguria or anuria; and upward pressure on the diaphragm may lead to difficulty in securing adequate lung ventilation.

It is not uncommon for critically ill patients to develop a *paralytic ileus*, as a result of either their underlying diseases or the use of narcotic agents, or of the many other drugs used in the critically ill which may reduce gut motility. The gut is roughly assessed by the ability to tolerate enteral feeding. It is important to recognize that the nature of the bowel sounds provides almost no useful information in the ITU patient, and that patients may tolerate feed satisfactorily with absent bowel sounds, and conversely may fail to tolerate feed with apparently normal bowel sounds.

Acalculous cholecystitis is a potentially life-threatening complication of severe illness, and it is therefore essential to look for evidence of jaundice, and in particular to be aware of the possibility of a distended gallbladder. In extreme cases it is possible to palpate this, but more often it is diagnosed by ultrasound scanning.

RENAL SYSTEM

The patient should be examined for evidence of dehydration (such as reduced tissue turgor) or overload (oedema, high CVP), bearing in mind that the state of hydration may not necessarily reflect the circulating volume in the body. Very oedematous patients may have intravascular fluid depletion.

The most common and simple method of assessing renal function in the critically ill is to record urine output and cumulative fluid balance

- Cardiogenic – cold peripheries, acidosis, oliguria,
  low cardiac output
- Hypovolaemic – as above, with low central venous
  pressure
- Obstructive – as above, with high central venous
  pressure
- Septic – warm peripheries, bounding pulse, elevated
  cardiac output, acidosis

on an hourly basis. A urine output of >0.5 mL/kg/h
is generally enough to maintain normal renal biochemistry, but not enough to clear fluid administered to the critically ill (intravenous or enteral feed,
drugs), which may amount to 4 L or more per day.
If the patient is anuric, an ultrasound scan of the
kidneys should be obtained in order to exclude
postrenal causes of renal failure, which may require
urological intervention.

Patients developing renal failure may need to be
treated with haemodialysis or haemofiltration – a
machine typical of those used in the ITU is shown in
Figure 23.7. The use of these machines requires the
insertion of a very large cannula with two lumina
into a large vein under strict asepsis. These cannulae
are subject to the same complications as central
venous cannulae (see Box 23.6). The cannula is connected to the dialysis machine and blood is pumped
from the vein, through the machine and then
returned to the patient. The blood will inevitably
cool on its extracorporeal journey, and thus as it is
returned to the patient, the patient will cool by as
much as 2 or 3°C. It is important to understand that
this happens, because patients may appear to be
apyrexial when they are not. This adverse effect is
sometimes used to cool patients who are hyper-
pyrexial, particularly if the fever is associated with
haemodynamic instability.

The indications for haemodialysis in the ITU are
shown in Box 23.8.

CENTRAL NERVOUS SYSTEM

Given the widespread use of sedatives, narcotic
agents and muscle relaxants it is difficult to assess
the central nervous system in the critically ill. Most
units operate a scoring system for sedation, with the
aim that patients should be just rousable on stimulation while remaining pain and anxiety free. The
finer points of neurological examination are thus
difficult, but it is important to look for evidence of
gross limb movement abnormality.

Epileptic seizures may occur in the critically ill
and may be difficult to diagnose. A high index of

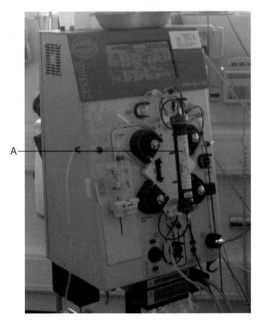

Figure 23.7   A blood purification device. Blood is pumped
through the filtration device A and returned to the patient.

suspicion is required, particularly in those who have
presented to the ITU with epilepsy. In the heavily
sedated patient the only signs may be rigidity, hypertension, and barely detectable shaking. In such cases
continuous recording of the EEG may be required.

Patients with multiple organ failure will inevitably
develop severe muscle wasting and weakness as part
of the catabolic response to injury. This wasting
may initially be masked by the presence of tissue
oedema, but as the patient recovers the magnitude
of the wasting will become obvious. Many patients
will also develop a *peripheral neuropathy*, which
usually reveals itself as attempts are made to wean
the patient from mechanical ventilation. Typically
there is severe weakness with absent or reduced
reflexes, often with relative sparing of the cranial
nerve reflexes.

THE ITU WARD ROUND

The array of information gathered for each critically
ill patient is bewildering, and if it is not considered
and presented systematically it becomes uninter-
pretable. On a ward round, the patient's name, age
and diagnosis should be presented, together with
relevant recent history and the events of the previous 24 hours or so. There should follow a description of each organ system in turn, with problems,
current levels of support and recent results. The
order of presentation is not critical – neurosurgical
units will tend to start with the head for instance –
but it is important to cover each system logically
and completely.

Box 23.8   Indications for haemodialysis

- Fluid overload (peripheral or pulmonary oedema, rising central venous pressure, positive fluid balance)
- Biochemical derangement
  - Rapidly rising creatinine and urea
  - Metabolic acidosis
  - Hyperkalaemia
- Anuria or oliguria

INVESTIGATIONS

HAEMATOLOGY

DAILY FULL BLOOD COUNT

- Patients will tend to have haemoglobin concentrations between 8 and 10 g/dL. This generally requires no action.
- An elevated white cell count is generally an indicator of sepsis, but is not specific.
- In severe sepsis immature white cells appear in the peripheral blood.
- In very severe sepsis there may be neutropenia.
- Thrombocytopenia is common in severe sepsis, but may also be an adverse drug effect or an indicator of disseminated intravascular coagulopathy.
- Prothrombin and activated partial thromboplastin time are routinely monitored as an indicator of liver synthetic function and the integrity of the clotting cascade.

BIOCHEMISTRY

DAILY BIOCHEMICAL PROFILE

- Hyponatraemia is relatively common – nearly always iatrogenic.
- Hypernatraemia is relatively common – nearly always iatrogenic.
- Urea and creatinine – not the best guide to renal function in the critically ill, but gives a crude estimate and is easy to perform.
- Hypoalbuminaemia is nearly universal, reflecting the severity of illness. Rarely if ever requires treatment (hypocholesterolaemia also almost universal).
- Abnormal plasma transaminases may reflect hepatocellular dysfunction (often drug induced), but they are also released from cardiac and skeletal muscle, so look for evidence of myocardial infarction (levels not very high) or muscle necrosis (levels usually very high).
- Elevated bilirubin and alkaline phosphatase levels suggest cholestasis, which may be functional or structural – suggests the need for an ultrasound scan of biliary tree to exclude acalculous cholecystitis.
- An elevation of bilirubin out of proportion to the liver enzymes is quite common, probably owing to a mixture of drugs and sepsis.
- Elevated C-reactive protein may suggest infection or inflammation.

MICROBIOLOGY

- Infection in the critically ill is complex, often with organisms resistant to conventional antimicrobials. The advice of the microbiology department should be sought before using antibiotics, and daily visits from the microbiology team are extremely helpful
- Frequent samples of blood, sputum and urine should be sent for microbiological examination. The presence of organisms does not always mean infection: very ill patients become colonized with microorganisms.
- Meticulous application of the basic principles of infection control is vital.

RADIOLOGY

Imaging on the ITU can only be performed with portable equipment, and the images are often not optimal because it is difficult to place the patient correctly. Plain films of limbs, chest and abdomen can be obtained, as can ultrasound images of chest and abdominal contents. Ultrasound is particularly useful in the diagnosis of pleural effusions (which may not be obvious on plain chest films) and ascites. It is also used to exclude postrenal obstruction in the anuric patient, to examine the liver and gallbladder, and to identify abscesses. Some of these conditions may also be treated by ultrasound-guided drainage.

The other imaging modalities (CT and MRI scanning, angiography and contrast studies) can only be obtained by moving the patient to the radiology department. Because this is potentially highly dangerous and may prove fatal to a critically ill patient, it is vital to ensure that the benefit of any information obtained by such imaging outweighs the risks of obtaining it. A CT scan of a patient with ARDS is shown in Figure 23.8.

ETHICS AND PROGNOSIS

Critically ill patients present challenging ethical dilemmas, principally the issue of whether to withhold or withdraw treatment. It is often possible to restore a semblance of life to a dying patient (for instance by mechanical ventilation and inotropic support) even when there is no prospect of recovery. In such cases, ITU has merely served to prolong the process of dying rather than restored meaningful life. Decisions about not instituting therapy are difficult, and should be made at a senior level. Discus-

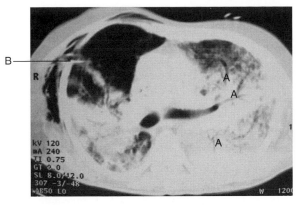

Figure 23.8 The thoracic CT scan of a patient with severe ARDS. There is an increase in lung water as evidenced by the white areas, with obvious air bronchograms A indicating pulmonary consolidation. There is also a chest drain B inserted to treat a pneumothorax.

sions will often have to involve senior members of the referring team, the patient and their family. Any patient has an absolute right not to consent to any treatment, including intensive care, and such decisions must be respected. Relatives cannot overrule the wishes of the patient. These judgements are often difficult to make because acute illness is often associated with confusion or delirium, and the patient's wishes may thus not be clear.

It is important not to be judgemental about the illnesses patients suffer from or their lifestyles when deciding about the advisability of offering intensive care. Decisions must be objective, evidence based (as far as is possible in a relatively evidence-free environment), capable of standing up to scrutiny, and carefully documented.

It is also particularly important to remember that the duty of confidentiality applies to patients at all times, even when they are desperately ill. This has to be tempered by the need to keep family and friends apprised of the situation. Great care should be taken in discussing specific diagnoses that the patient might not wish the family to know. Most critically ill patients are incapable of giving consent, either for therapeutic interventions or for participation in research projects.

The prognosis of a critical illness depends to some extent on the prognosis of the disease that led to ITU admission. Outcomes are also dependent on the degree of physiological derangement present at the time of admission, and the extent to which such derangements change in response to treatment. A number of scoring systems are used to provide some idea of the risk of death, but as they are based on population data they cannot and must not be used to try to predict outcome for individual patients.

Approximately 80% of patients admitted to the ITU survive, and will leave the unit shortly after they have become independent of life-supporting technology. It is important to review patients after discharge to ensure that satisfactory progress is being made.

SUMMARY

The intensive care unit is a high-technology environment, and there is a danger that this may distract attention from the need to concentrate on simple clinical observation. This is as vital in the critically ill patient on the ITU receiving multiple organ support as it is in the general wards, outpatient clinics or surgery.

24 Pain

W. J. Gallagher, S. Nikolic

INTRODUCTION

Pain is a phenomenon with which we are all familiar. It is a part of everyday life and is a feature of various diseases. It most commonly accompanies an injury, where it serves its most important purpose, namely, to protect us, alert us, and to make us remove ourselves from danger. The severity of pain, and its impact on an individual, ranges from a trivial occurrence such as a needle-prick injury to a sensation of such intensity that it induces thoughts of suicide.

Pain is common. In a review of GP practice notes over 45% of patients had a painful condition listed. According to another UK study, pain leads to 12 million GP consultations a year, 900 000 hospital bed days and 119 million days of certified incapacity annually, amounting to an approximate annual cost of £6 billion. It is obvious that pain has enormous impact, not just on individuals, but also on society as a whole.

DEFINITION

Is it possible to define pain? The International Association for the Study of Pain has proposed the following definition (1979): 'Pain is an unpleasant sensory and emotional experience associated with actual or potential tissue damage or described in terms of damage'. It follows from this that pain is always a subjective sensation and is always unpleasant. This definition has two important implications: pain is not necessarily or always associated with ongoing tissue damage; it is a subjective experience and has an emotional as well as a sensory component.

Pain is notoriously difficult to describe. It is difficult to assess despite many efforts to establish ways to qualify and quantify it. None the less, pain assessment is crucial in order to evaluate its impact on the sufferer, plan a treatment strategy and assess its results.

CLASSIFICATION

There are many ways in which pain can be classified in order to formulate an optimal treatment strategy.

Despite this, classifying a particular pain state can be challenging because often the pain syndrome does not fall into a single category. The main reason for this is that the aetiology and pathogenesis of many pain syndromes is multifactorial.

Pain may be classified according to:

- Aetiology and pathogenesis
- Duration
- Site.

AETIOLOGY AND PATHOGENESIS

- **Physiological** – an acute response to an injury.
- **Inflammatory** – when the pain is generated and maintained mainly by inflammatory mediators.
- **Cancer-related pain** – aetiology is usually multifactorial. It may be predominantly physiological, inflammatory, neuropathic or ischaemic, or any combination of the above.
- **Neuropathic** – pain arising from injury or dysfunction of the central or peripheral nervous system.
- **Central** – pain caused by a lesion or dysfunction of the central nervous system. It can affect the brain or the spinal cord, or both.
- **Ischaemic** – related to reduction in blood supply to organs or nerves that supply the organs, or both. It may or may not be associated with cancer.
- **Psychogenic** – pain, especially chronic pain, has almost invariably a strong and important emotional and behavioural component. Purely psychogenic pain is rare.

DURATION

- **Acute** – most commonly a physiological response to an injury. It resolves with the disappearance of a noxious stimulus or within the time frame of a normal healing process.
- **Chronic** – it can either be associated with an ongoing pathological process, such as rheumatoid arthritis or malignancy, or be present for longer than is consistent with a normal healing time. Pain is arbitrarily described as chronic if it persists for longer than 3 months. Chronic pain is often associated with disability and a significant behavioural response.

SITE

- **Somatic** – usually well localized: for example, it may follow a dermatomal distribution.
- **Visceral** – poorly localized. Does not follow a dermatomal distribution.
- **Referred** – pain that originates in one site but is perceived as being present in a closely related or distant site.

TERMINOLOGY

- **Nociceptors** – receptors that are responsible for initiating the generation of pain. They are most commonly free nerve endings found in the small fibre sensory system. There is another class of receptor, termed silent receptors – these are only active after tissue damage.
- **Nociception** is defined as a noxious stimulus, or a stimulus that would become noxious if prolonged, hence **nociceptive** pain.
- **Allodynia** – pain that is produced by a stimulus that is not normally painful. The stimulus that is commonly used is a light touch or light pressure. Allodynia is present to a greater or lesser degree in various pain states, but it is especially a feature of chronic neuropathic pain.
- **Hyperalgesia** – increased sensitivity to painful stimuli. Like allodynia, this is commonly seen in chronic pain states but is also common in acute pain in an area that surrounds the actual area of tissue damage.
- **Hypoaesthesia and anaesthesia** – reduced or absent sensation in response to a stimulus.
- **Disability** – WHO (1980) definition: 'The restriction or lack (resulting from an *impairment*) of ability to perform an activity in the manner or within the range considered normal for a human being'. It may accompany acute pain states, but usually resolves as the healing progresses. It is usually present to a varying degree in chronic pain states.

AETIOLOGY AND PATHOGENESIS

Broadly speaking, pain is generated by a stimulus that excites the central nervous system. Such stimuli may or may not be noxious. This was proposed centuries ago by Descartes, and conceptually still holds true, but it is crucial to appreciate that the final subjective perception of pain is shaped by various factors (Fig. 24.1).

A stimulus (which can be thermal, pressure, cold or chemical) excites nociceptors and is then transmitted to the spinal cord by two different classes of nerve fibre. Faster, myelinated Aδ fibres and smaller, slower, unmyelinated C fibres transmit the sensation to the dorsal horn of the spinal cord, where these primary afferents synapse in lamina I, lamina II (substantia gelatinosa), lamina IV, and some in lamina V. All these afferent sensory fibres are excitatory. Second-order fibres are then carried in the spinothalamic and spinoreticular tracts to the thalamus, where they synapse. From the thalamus, third-order neurons project to the somatosensory cortex, anterior cingulate gyrus and the insular cortex, where they terminate. It is at this cortical level that a stimulus is perceived as pain. Thus, sensory input is modulated at spinal cord level by several different mechanisms, as well as by modulation in higher centres in the brain. Much remains to be understood about the psychophysiology of pain.

The *gate theory* proposed by Melzack and Wall in 1965 states that non-noxious stimulation of the large Aβ fibres inhibit the response to painful stimuli of neurons with wide dynamic range (WDR neurons, located primarily in lamina V), reducing the input of small fibres mediating the sensation of pain. A good example of this effect is 'rubbing it better'. Descending input from higher centres also modulate neural activity in the spinal cord, reducing or enhancing pain sensation. Such descending input is one of the mechanisms by which emotional and cognitive factors modulate pain perception. It is also important to recognize that some pain may be mediated by the sympathetic nervous system. This is more commonly observed in neuropathic pain states, but remains poorly understood.

In recent years a *biopsychosocial model* of pain, implying that no single dimension is adequate to fully understand and explain pain, has highlighted the need to take into account interactions between biological, psychological and social factors in understanding an individual's reaction to pain (Fig. 24.1).

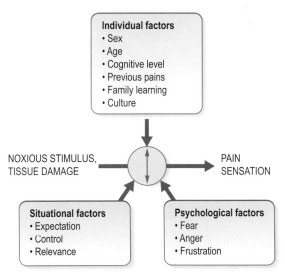

Figure 24.1 Biopsychosocial model of pain.

THE PATIENT IN PAIN

As with any other branch of medicine, careful and meticulous assessment of a patient in pain is important. Two questions should be considered when dealing with a patient in pain:

- Is the pain a symptom of ongoing tissue damage, or of another condition that needs to be dealt with by another medical professional?
- What is the optimal treatment strategy: to either abolish the pain altogether or reduce it to a more bearable level?

Unfortunately, no single standardized approach will allow assessment of pain in every situation. Pain is essentially a subjective experience. Therefore, what the patient describes as their experience is of paramount importance. As in most areas of medicine the history is the most useful tool in assessment and diagnosis.

HISTORY

Taking a history from a patient in pain is more complex than recording the history of the symptoms that provide diagnostic clues. Even in acute pain states, where pain represents a protective function and is a symptom of an injury, taking the patient as a whole and bearing in mind emotional, cognitive and behavioural aspects is crucial in arriving at a treatment strategy.

The first step is to evaluate the complaint of pain, trying to understand its pathophysiology, including the mechanisms that sustain it.

- **The site of pain** – this may give a clue to the underlying pathology.
- **Distribution** – pain may follow a dermatomal or peripheral nerve distribution, or have no relation to anatomical patterns.
- **Character of pain** – nociceptive (somatic or visceral) versus neuropathic (Table 24.1).

- **Duration of pain** – this may have a bearing on the level of disability and psychosocial cost of the pain.
- **Rapidity of onset and any precipitating factors** – a rapid or relatively recent-onset pain syndrome is more likely to follow a conventional medical model, whereby it is appropriate to search for an underlying cause. Chronic pain requires a more biopsychosocial approach.
- **Severity of pain and its change over time** – this requires some method for measuring pain (see below).
- **Alleviating and exacerbating/aggravating factors** – these may lead to a better understanding of mechanisms that sustain the pain.
- **Exclusion of more sinister pathology** – 'red flags'. Two most important conditions are not to be missed. One is pain related to cancer and the other is pain related to inflammation.
- **Evaluation of psychosocial elements** – 'yellow flags'. These are not life-threatening symptoms, but their presence means that the psychosocial history has special relevance.
- **Impact of pain** – consider the effect of pain on the patient's activity, work, mood, sleep, relationships etc.

The next step is to evaluate current and past treatments for pain.

- **Past medical history** – with an emphasis on the relevant system. Taking the full medical history must not be overlooked. It may give invaluable clues as to the aetiology and genesis of pain.
- **Psychosocial history and assessment** – see below.

EXAMINATION

The purpose of examination is as follows:

- To exclude pathology that needs to be dealt with urgently or electively by another medical professional

Table 24.1 Nociceptive versus neuropathic pain

	Nociceptive	Neuropathic
Description of pain	Aching, localized, toothache-like, sharp, squeezing	Shooting, radiating, stabbing, burning, electric shock-like
Movement impact	Associated with movement	Independent
Physical examination	Normal response	Allodynia, hyperalgesia, vasomotor changes
Examples	Injury, postoperative pain	Peripheral neuropathies, shingles, cancer pain
Treatment strategies	More classic approach, conventional analgesics	More biopsychosocial approach, conventional analgesics ± non-conventional (antidepressants, anticonvulsants etc.)

- To understand the mechanisms that sustain the pain
- To elucidate and evaluate any physical signs associated with a particular pain condition
- To reassure the patient that pain does not imply any ongoing damage
- To define baseline parameters and monitor their change over time.

Detailed examination will focus on different systems according to a particular pain condition. It may involve basic orthopaedic, neurological or surgical examination. Regardless of the approach, it should follow conventional basic methods: *inspection*, *palpation*, and *range of movement* where appropriate. For example, a patient who presents with back pain will require at least *inspection* to check for muscle spasm, posture and deformity, and evidence of previous surgery; *palpation* of paravertebral and bony areas; *range of movement* to evaluate any restriction. The examination will also need to include a neurological examination focusing on the signs of nerve root irritation, muscle power, sensation and reflexes.

INVESTIGATION

Investigation of a patient in pain is individually structured. It serves three important goals:

- To exclude more sinister pathology
- To provide diagnostic clues
- To arrive at an optimal management strategy.

The commonest investigation employed by pain specialists is imaging, e.g. using simple X-rays to exclude a pathological fracture, MRI to demonstrate changes within the central nervous system, or an ultrasound examination of the abdomen. Neurophysiological (EMG) studies are helpful to determine the presence and extent of any nerve damage, and various blood tests may be used to determine, for example, the activity of rheumatoid arthritis. Any test used must be considered only as a part of a more global approach, never in isolation.

PSYCHOSOCIAL ASPECTS OF PAIN

The psychosocial assessment of pain should be directed at finding out what is particularly bothering the patient about their pain. Generally speaking this is more relevant in chronic pain states, because acute pain usually resolves quickly.

Pain is described as having at least five dimensions, each of which should be addressed:

- The *sensation* of pain – the subjective experience
- *Suffering* and *distress* – the emotional component
- *Expectations* and *beliefs* – the cognitive component

- *Verbal* (complaints) or *non-verbal communication* – the behavioural component (illness behaviour) is the way in which a patient responds to and expresses the sensation of pain. It is influenced by various cultural and social factors
- *Impact* of the *social environment*.

MEASURING PAIN

Pain is a subjective experience and therefore difficult to quantify. Various measures are in use that consist of *single-dimensional* and *multidimensional* scales (simple and complex).

SINGLE-DIMENSIONAL SCALES
These are very commonly used. They are simple, sensitive, reproducible and quickly applied, and give a numerical value to the pain severity. They can be either *analogue* or *discrete*. The latter may be numerical or verbal. The most common of these scales is the Visual Analogue Scale (VAS). The patient is given a horizontal line 10 cm long with 'no pain' on the left-hand side and 'worst possible pain' on the right, and is asked to mark the line according to the severity of the pain.

The numerical scale is similar to the VAS. The patient is asked to assign a number from 0 to 10 to their pain, 0 being no pain at all and 10 being the worst imaginable pain. In the verbal rating scale the patient rates their pain into one of the following categories: none, mild, moderate or severe.

MULTIDIMENSIONAL (COMPLEX) SCALES
The development of multidimensional scales acknowledges the multidimensional impact of pain on a sufferer's life. The commonest scale in use is the *McGill Questionnaire*. There are two forms of this: the original McGill Questionnaire assesses various aspects of pain, including sensory qualities of pain, affective qualities (tension, fear etc.), and evaluative words that describe the subjective intensity of the total pain experienced. There are various measurements derived from the data, but a short-form of the McGill Questionnaire is most used (Fig. 24.2). It is easy to apply and reproducible.

TREATMENT STRATEGIES

As indicated above, all treatment strategies start from the same question: is there ongoing tissue damage or a condition amenable to treatment by other medical professionals? For example, it is clearly inappropriate to treat a patient who suffers from a lower limb compartment syndrome with analgesics alone. The same would apply to increasing the dose of opioids in a cancer sufferer who has raised serum calcium levels due to a tumour.

Generally speaking, treatment strategies are directed at *symptom control* – this can be pharmacological,

Short-Form McGill Pain Questionnaire:

I. Pain Rating Index (PRI):

The words below describe average pain. Place a check mark (✓) in the column that represents the degree to which you feel that type of pain. Please limit yourself to a description of the pain in your pelvic area only:

		None		Mild		Moderate		Severe
Throbbing	0		1		2		3	
Shooting	0		1		2		3	
Stabbing	0		1		2		3	
Sharp	0		1		2		3	
Cramping	0		1		2		3	
Gnawing	0		1		2		3	
Hot-Burning	0		1		2		3	
Aching	0		1		2		3	
Heavy	0		1		2		3	
Tender	0		1		2		3	
Splitting	0		1		2		3	
Tiring-Exhausting	0		1		2		3	
Sickening	0		1		2		3	
Fearful	0		1		2		3	
Punishing-Cruel	0		1		2		3	

(a = Throbbing through Splitting; b = Tiring-Exhausting through Punishing-Cruel)

II. Present Pain Intensity (PPI)–Visual Analog Scale (VAS). Tick along scale below for pelvic pain:

No Pain   Worst possible pain

III. Evaluative overall intensity of total pain experience. Please limit yourself to a description of the pain in your pelvic area only. Place a check mark (✓) in the appropriate column:

Evaluation		
0	No pain	
1	Mild	
2	Discomforting	
3	Distressing	
4	Horrible	
5	Excruciating	

IV. Scoring

		Score
I-a	S-PRI (Sensory Pain Rating Index)	
I-b	A-PRI (Affective Pain Rating Index)	
I-a+b	T-PRI (Total Pain Rating Index)	
II	PPI-VAS (Present Pain Intensity-Visual Analog Scale)	
III	Evaluative overall intensity of total pain experience	

Figure 24.2   Short McGill Questionnaire.

non-pharmacological, or varying combinations of the two. Pharmacological options include simple analgesics, non-steroidal anti-inflammatory drugs, opioids and non-conventional analgesics. The most commonly used drugs are antidepressants and anti-convulsants. Non-pharmacological options include physiotherapy, occupational therapy, acupuncture, and transcutaneous nerve stimulation. Symptom control can also be achieved by peripheral or central neural blockade. *Physical rehabilitation* aims to improve disability and hence the quality of a patient's life. *Psychological support* aims to improve the quality of a sufferer's life by addressing the emotional, cognitive and behavioural aspects of pain.

DIFFICULT CASES

- **Non-English speakers** – assessment of pain can be extremely difficult even in the presence of an advocate. Cultural differences in behaviour are also often important.
- **Patients with learning difficulties** – in this case the help of a carer or relative who knows the patient well may be very useful.
- **Very sick and confused patients** – it is often necessary to make assumptions in this situation, and a compassionate approach should always be taken.
- **Children** – there is a commonly held misconception that infants have an immature

nervous system and therefore do not feel pain in the same way adults do. Another is that health professionals cannot measure pain in children. Both of these are false. Pain must be assessed and treated as in any other patient. Some assessment tools have been modified for use in children; for example, a pictorial facial expression scale is also used.

CONCLUSIONS

Pain is complex and essentially a subjective phenomenon. The patient should always be believed. Pain assessment includes its social and psychological consequences as well as its sensory characteristics. Perhaps more than with any other symptom, management must be individualized to the patient.

25 People with cancer

P. N. Plowman

INTRODUCTION

Cancer is the term used to refer to the random overgrowth/continued proliferation (or proliferative potential) of cells in the body, resistant to the physiological and homoeostatic mechanisms that normally govern their orderly behaviour. Cancers arising from epithelial tissues, mesenchyme and embryonal tissues are called carcinomas, sarcomas and germ cells tumours respectively. Cancers of the bone marrow/reticuloendothelial system are called leukaemias and lymphomas. A secure, pathologically confirmed diagnosis is the bedrock of good clinical oncology.

Advances in cancer management over the last few decades are dependent not only on improved treatment techniques but also on the earlier detection of tumours, hence improved curability. Here, clinician input is vital. Cancer screening programmes, e.g. mammography and cervical cytology, have proved effective, and new methods such as prostate-specific antigen (PSA) blood testing and CT thorax screening are under investigation.

Clinical genetics allows better prediction for people at high genetic risk of cancer and this may allow 'pre-emptive' cures, e.g. total colectomy in familial polyposis, prophylactic mastectomy in *BRCA* gene carriers, total thyroidectomy in MEN-2 patients, thereby preventing 'near-certain' colon, breast and thyroid (medullary) cancers, respectively. Increased awareness of cancer in the population has also allowed earlier diagnosis of disease, e.g. skin tumours such as melanoma, breast lumps or oral cancers. The clinician should be aware of the need for early detection, alert to risk factors in the clinical history – whether this be daily habits such as smoking or a strong family history of disease – and comprehensive in clinical assessment.

The principal modalities of cancer therapy have, until recently, been regional, such as surgery and radiotherapy, or systemic, such as chemotherapy and hormonal therapy. Immunotherapy and molecularly targeted therapies are now adding a new dimension to systemic therapy for many malignant diseases.

SYMPTOMS, SIGNS AND ANCILLARY TESTS

The symptoms of many early cancers are few. Thus an early breast cancer may present as a lump in the breast with no other symptom (Box 25.1); the oncologist is familiar with the statement: 'I didn't think it was anything serious because I feel so well'. Symptoms specific to the site of origin of a cancer often facilitate diagnosis: e.g. altered bowel habit in colorectal cancer, or haemoptysis in carcinoma of the lung. Weight loss, lethargy, anorexia and cachexia attend advanced or metastatic cancer. Metastatic cancer may present with symptoms referable to the site of secondary deposits: e.g. fits or focal neurological signs with metastatic spread to the brain. Secondary phenomena may be the presenting feature, e.g. bleeding diathesis due to bone marrow failure in acute leukaemia, obstructive jaundice due to compression/infiltration of the common bile duct by a carcinoma of the head of the pancreas. Less easily explicable associated features of cancer are important for the alert clinician, e.g. finger clubbing in carcinoma of the lung, and acanthosis nigricans in stomach carcinoma. Observation of these clinical symptoms or signs will naturally lead to investigation.

As in all clinical methods, the carefully taken clinical history and examination precede ancillary tests, the clinician being alert to all possibilities, 'running down' each symptom to completion before exploring each physical sign to its full extent, e.g. if a lump is felt, then questioning as to whether it is neoplastic or inflammatory by exploring other corroborative signs of inflammation (heat, redness, pain) or neoplasm (slow progressive growth) to assist in furthering the path to the correct diagnosis. The history will have revealed any changes in health, predisposing factors and information in the family history (Boxes 25.2, 25.3).

SYMPTOMS

CHEST   (Box 25.4)
- **Cough** – irrepressible cough may be a feature of a mass obstructing a major airway

---

Box 25.1   Breast cancer

Symptom	Signs
Mass	Skin discoloration and tethering
Nipple discharge	Inflammation
Ulceration	Lymphadenopathy

Box 25.2   Environmental factors leading to cancer

- Tobacco and lung cancer
- Alcohol and gastrointestinal cancer
- Ultraviolet light and skin cancer
- Dietary habits, such as the chewing of betel nut in oral cancers
- Exposure to industrial carcinogens: asbestos exposure leads to mesothelioma, and heavy metals, leather tanning and coal tar products to bladder cancer
- Occupational hazards, e.g. radiation exposure in lung and prostate cancer
- Radon exposure in lung cancer

Box 25.3   Some hereditary cancer syndromes

- Familial adenomatous polyposis
- Hereditary non-polyposis colon cancer
- Breast/ovarian cancers and BRCA1, BRCA2
- von Hippel–Lindau syndrome
- Li–Fraumeni syndrome
- Multiple endocrine neoplasia
- Retinoblastoma
- Ataxia telangiectasia
- Xeroderma pigmentosa

Box 25.4   Lung cancer

Symptom	Signs
Cough	Clubbing
Breathlessness	Nicotine staining
Haemoptysis	Cyanosis
Pain in the chest	Lower brachial root signs, Horner's syndrome

---

Box 25.5   Gastrointestinal malignancy

Symptom	Signs
Dysphagia	Glossitis
Indigestion	Anaemia
Abdominal pain	Guarding
Nausea and vomiting	Jaundice and ascites
Haematemesis	Epigastric mass and tenderness
Melaena	Palpable colonic mass
Rectal bleeding	Hepatomegaly and hepatic failure

Box 25.6   CNS malignancy

Symptom	Signs
Headache and vomiting	Mental function
Convulsions	Focal neurological signs
Loss of function	

BREAST

- *Lump, pain, nipple discharge*, relationship of symptom to *menstrual cycle* and previous *breast history*.

GASTROINTESTINAL TRACT   (Box 25.5)

- **Appetite**
- **Dysphagia** – solids versus liquids, at what level does the food stick?
- **Vomiting** – when? e.g. relationship to foods
- **Abdominal distension and pain** – *colicky* or *waxing and waning*, with loud bowel sounds, or *constant*? Where in the abdomen does the pain occur? Loud bowel sounds
- **Altered bowel habit**
- **Indigestion** – and what the patient means by this
- **Bleeding** – haematemesis, melaena, fresh bleeding per rectum.

CENTRAL NERVOUS SYSTEM   (Box 25.6)

- **Late-onset epilepsy**
- **Progressive focal neurology** – particularly suggestive of a single focus in the brain
- **Headache, vomiting and obtundation** – suggesting raised intracranial pressure.

In all the above it is the nature of the progression (or not) of symptoms (fast or slow, waxing and waning, intermittent or inexorable) that may be important in the differential diagnosis:

- Stroke – fast onset
- Multiple sclerosis – waxing and waning
- Tumour – inexorable progression.

- **Sputum** – may be productive or non-productive
- **Haemoptysis, breathlessness/dyspnoea, wheeze** – in lung cancer a persistent wheeze develops, rather than an episodic one as in asthma
- **Pain** is a cardinal chest symptom.

These should all be described as to their onset, timing, severity etc.

GENITOURINARY   (Box 25.7)
- Haematuria, dysuria
- Obstructive urinary symptoms – males: hesitancy, slow flow, frequency, *pelvic pain*.

GYNAECOLOGICAL   (Box 25.8)
- Bleeding, vaginal discharge – timing: intermenstrual, postmenopausal etc.
- Pelvic pain.

EAR/NOSE/THROAT   (Box 25.9)
- Lump or ulcer
- Pain, difficulty or pain on swallowing (odynophagia)
- Deafness (conductive versus neuronal – distinguished by Weber and Rinne tests)
- Hoarse voice/dysphonia
- Blocked nose, nasal discharge (?bloody), sputum (?bloody) – these are all symptoms that need to be 'run down' to their origin and lead to further investigation.

SIGNS

General signs of advanced cancer include asthenia, cachexia, and a general appearance of fatigue and ill health. General signs of early cancer may be very subtle. Site-specific signs include the following.

Box 25.7 Urological malignancy	
Symptom	**Signs**
Dysuria	Abdominal and pelvic mass
Frequency	Rectal prostatic mass
Incontinence	Penile or vulval ulceration
Haematuria	Testicular mass
Prostatism	Hard prostatic mass

Box 25.8 Gynaecological malignancy	
Symptom	**Signs**
Vulval pruritus	Vulval ulceration
Vaginal discharge	Cervical mass
Vaginal bleeding	Pelvic mass
Pelvic pain	Mass, discharge
Bleeding	

Box 25.9 Head and neck malignancy	
Symptom	**Signs**
Taste and swallowing disturbed	Ulceration
Hearing and voice abnormal	Discharge
Bleeding	Cranial nerve palsies
Persistent cough	Lymphadenopathy
Sinusitis	

CHEST

Epiphenomena such as finger clubbing, then specific signs such as cough productive of sputum. Remember that bloodstained sputum is more likely to be cytologically positive in patients with haemoptysis. A fixed rhonchus rather than the episodic wheeze of asthma, or restricted air entry into one lung, is suggestive of an obstruction in the airway, such as by tumour (eventually leading to the signs of atelectasis); signs of a pleural effusion – not an infrequent accompaniment of a locally advanced lung cancer. Left recurrent laryngeal nerve palsy, due to involvement of this nerve by tumour in its intrathoracic course, leads to a hoarse voice and a 'bovine' cough. Lymphadenopathy and signs of metastatic disease are often found even at presentation.

In *superior vena cava obstruction* (SVCO) dilated jugular veins are visible in the neck, with suffused head/face and neck and arms, particularly the right arm, together with dilated anastomotic veins visible on the anterior chest wall, owing to obstruction of venous flow by a mass at the level of the thoracic outlet. There is no pulse/wave to the fluid level in the engorged neck veins, which are fixed and, on lifting the right arm above the horizontal, the suffused arm veins do not rapidly empty. Horner's syndrome due to sympathetic chain involvement by tumour may also occur. *Superior sulcus syndrome* is the whole symptom complex of SVCO and Horner's syndrome.

Hypertrophic pulmonary osteoarthropathy
HPOA is a syndrome with pain in the wrists and ankles, sometimes spreading up to the knees and forearms, together with clubbing of the fingers; sometimes it is only the finger clubbing that is observed. This syndrome is a distant epiphenomenon of non-small cell lung cancer, particularly squamous cell lung cancer, but also occurs in other, non-neoplastic conditions (e.g. chronic empyema).

BREAST
A lump should be defined as single or multiple – as dominant with satellite others, or generally within a lumpy breast; by its site in the breast; size; mobility or fixity to skin or pectoralis; tenderness; involvement of the skin (satellite nodules of tumour, *'cancer en cuirasse'* or *'peau d'orange'*) (Fig. 25.1); by nipple discharge – spontaneous or expressible, with or without blood; and by axillary and/or supraclavicular or infraclavicular lymphadenopathy. Careful palpation of the contralateral breast (Fig. 25.2) is essential.

GASTROINTESTINAL TRACT
Look for epiphenomena such as jaundice, anaemia or acanthosis (Fig. 25.3), then specific signs: a distended abdomen (Fig. 25.4), tenderness, lump

(define by site in abdomen, size, mobility, texture – hard, soft, edged, ballotable etc.), all in an attempt to define the site of origin of a mass. Seek signs of bowel obstruction, ascites (dullness in flanks, shifting dullness), inferior vena cava obstruction (oedematous legs/lower abdomen and distended veins over abdomen filling from below – or radially, periumbilically: 'caput medusae'). There may be a rectal mass on digital rectal examination (DRE), and observation of the stools may be appropriate. Signs of distant spread of cancer are:

- **Sign of Troisier** – in the late stages of pancreatic or stomach cancer, lymphadenopathy may be palpable in the left supraclavicular fossa, an observation made first by Charles Troisier (Paris, 1844–1919).
- **Thrombophlebitis migrans** – particularly in the later stages of pancreatic cancer there is a generalized tendency to thrombosis, most commonly manifest in the deep veins of the leg.
- **Courvoisier's law.** This states that if, in a jaundiced patient, the gallbladder is palpably

enlarged, the diagnosis is not impacted stone in the common bile duct; the commonest alternative in an obstructively jaundiced patient is obstruction of the duct by a carcinoma of the head of the pancreas. This aphorism was formulated by Ludwig Courvoisier (1843–1918), Professor of Surgery in Basel, and is worthy of note not only because of its practical usefulness, but also as an illustration of good clinical acumen and deductive power. The rationale is that a gallstone usually occurs in a patient with chronic cholecystitis who, because of the chronicity of the inflammatory condition, has a fibrotic gallbladder that will not easily dilate in an episode of acute biliary obstruction. In carcinoma of the head of the pancreas, there is prompt dilatation of the gallbladder when the obstruction of the bile duct causes back-pressure on the normal gallbladder.

CENTRAL NERVOUS SYSTEM (CNS)

Signs of raised intracranial pressure (headache, vomiting and the cardinal sign: *papilloedema*), focal neurological signs suggestive of a mass developing at one site in the CNS (although metastatic disease and occasional others may be multifocal), and signs of a spinal block (upper motor signs below the level, and lower motor signs and a sensory level at the level of the block) are all sought (Fig. 25.5).

GENITOURINARY

A ballottable flank mass (common presenting sign in childhood Wilms' tumour, unusual in adult renal cancer), tenderness on deep palpation over the hypogastrium and/or a palpable pelvic mass (unusual presenting feature of bladder cancer), prostate mass on digital rectal examination (define overall size of prostate, whether one lobe is larger than the other, and whether it contains a harder area

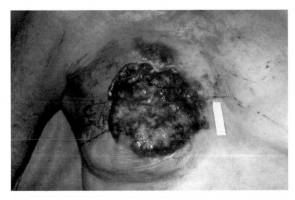

Figure 25.1 Fungating breast cancer fixed to the chest wall.

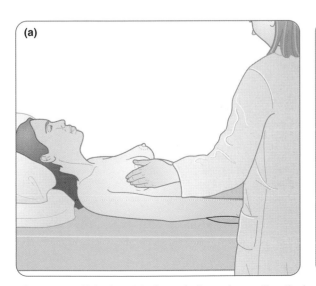 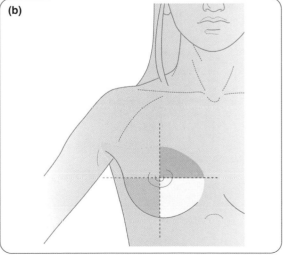

Figure 25.2 Palpation of the breast in the supine position; the four quadrants should be carefully and systematically palpated.

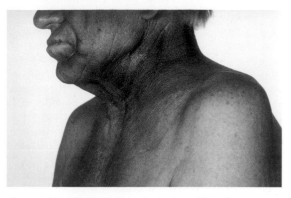

Figure 25.3   The neck of a patient who exhibits the thickened and pigmented skin of acanthosis nigricans associated with a 'distant' stomach cancer.

which is asymmetrically nodular or hard-edged); the observation of haematuria.

A hard testicular mass requires further investigation. The features are explored (hard and solid or cystic and transilluminable, this last being a diagnostic feature of hydrocele), and the ability to 'get above' the mass (hernias have a neck passing up to the inguinal ring) must all be considered. A scar from a previous orchidopexy in youth is a useful adjunctive sign, as patients with maldescent are predisposed to testicular cancer.

A rare distant event in testicular teratomas secreting HCG is the development of mild gynaecomastia. Varicoceles disappear when the patient lies down, and epididymal cysts are palpably separate from the testis. Right-sided varicoceles may also be

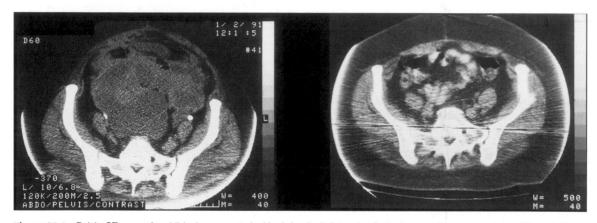

Figure 25.4   Pelvic CT scan of a child who presented with abdominal distension (note the grossly convex nature of the anterior abdominal wall on the left panel) due to a very large malignant ovarian germ cell tumour. On palpation the mass was easily palpable as a large, hard mass filling the lower abdomen. Right panel shows excellent regression after chemotherapy.

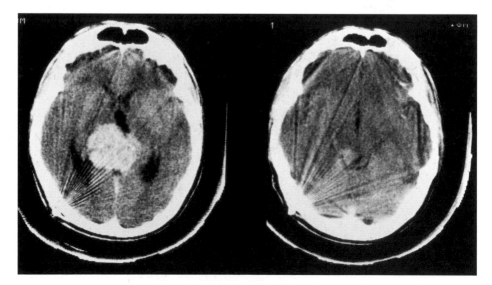

Figure 25.5   CT scan of brain. Left panel demonstrates an enhancing mass (a germ cell tumour) in the region of the pineal gland. The patient had presented with the symptoms and signs of raised intracranial pressure and been treated with a ventriculoperitoneal shunt, which created the artefactual lines seen radially across the scan. After chemoradiotherapy (right panel) the disease has remitted.

a feature of right-sided renal cancer that is invading the inferior vena cava (a back-pressure event via the obstructed renal vein).

GYNAECOLOGICAL

Inspection of the vulva and Cusco's examination of the vagina and cervix by direct inspection are important. Is the cervix smooth, symmetrical and non-ulcerated? Palpation includes a digital vaginal examination of the cervix for palpable irregularities, ballotting the uterus – often bimanually to assist in feeling any masses – and then exploring the adnexae via the fornices; once again this is often best done using a bimanual technique. Digital rectal examination (DRE), alone and in conjunction with vaginal examination, can be useful to define masses and their fixity. Any masses felt must be described by their site, size, texture, regularity of outline, fixity and tenderness. Blood on the examining glove is noted. Lymphadenopathy (groin nodes drain the vulva) and more distant evidence of disease are sought (e.g. ascites is a not infrequent presenting sign in ovarian cancer).

EAR/NOSE/THROAT

Facial asymmetry, lumps or ulcers may be externally visible or on endoscopy (direct or indirect via mirror/endoscope). Biopsy of any suspicious lesion follows, as in any of the above systems. Lymphadenopathy in the neck is a sign that requires ENT review, as it may well be the first sign of a cancer in the head and neck region (e.g. nasopharyngeal carcinoma). Thyroid lumps rise up on swallowing and are more suspicious of a neoplasm if single (demanding further investigation) (Fig. 25.7).

Trotter's triad, described by the English surgeon of that name in 1911, is a trio of signs that suggest a nasopharyngeal cancer (NPC): (1) hearing loss, (2) trigeminal pain, and (3) partial paralysis of the palate. These are features of a laterally extending NPC, all three being ipsilateral to the extending growth. The addition of basal cranial nerve signs, e.g. abducent nerve palsy, suggests that the NPC is invading through the skull base, most frequently via the foramen lacerum.

Certain tumours have typical presenting features, such as a persistently hoarse voice in laryngeal cancer, and a sore persistent ulcer with hard craggy edges on the side of the tongue in carcinoma of the tongue (Fig. 25.6). Tonsillar cancer often presents with pain on swallowing on the affected side, and advanced oral or pharyngeal cancer is often associated with pain and foetor.

ANCILLARY TESTS   (Box 25.10)

The diagnosis of cancer almost always relies on the histopathological examination of the tumour – either biopsy or resection specimen; this is called the

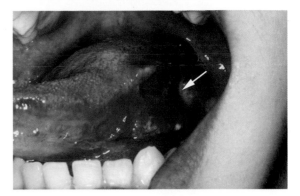

Figure 25.6   Malignant ulcer (arrowed) on the lateral border of the tongue – the commonest site for carcinoma.

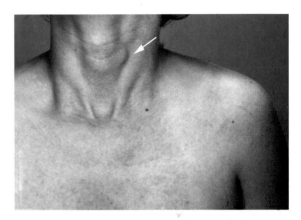

Figure 25.7   Neck of a young woman demonstrating an enlarged lymph node that was histologically (metastatic) papillary thyroid cancer (arrow). The histology may so closely resemble the normal thyroid architecture that early clinicians described this event wrongly as a 'lateral aberrant thyroid'.

tissue diagnosis. Occasionally, the detection of an oversecreted serum 'marker' product from the tumour (e.g. HCG in teratoma, catecholamines in phaeochromocytoma or neuroblastoma, α-fetoprotein in hepatoma/hepatoblastoma) may allow clinical diagnosis without recourse to biopsy, and occasionally a biopsy may be associated with risks that are not considered sufficient to merit this tool, given a near-certain diagnosis by other diagnostic means (e.g. brainstem glioma confidently diagnosed on MRI scanning) – but these are exceptions.

Following tissue diagnosis, the patient is staged, i.e. the extent of the disease in the body is assessed. For decades, staging has been performed to divide localized (non-metastatic) from metastatic disease, as there may be no point in performing a mastectomy for breast cancer, pneumonectomy for lung cancer or gastrectomy for stomach cancer in the presence of established metastatic disease, although there are exceptions, e.g. a colonic tumour that is imminently obstructing the bowel might well be primarily resected, notwithstanding the presence of

Box 25.10   Diagnostic imaging at various cancer sites

Head and neck
- Nasal endoscopy
- MRI or CT scan staging
- PET scan

Lung
- Bronchoscopy
- Chest X-ray and CT scan staging

Gastro-oesophageal
- Endoscopy
- Endoscopic ultrasound
- CT scan staging
- Barium swallow

Pancreatic and biliary
- Endoscopic ultrasound
- CT scan staging
- Endoscopic and MR cholangiopancreatography

Colorectal
- CT scan diagnosis and staging
- Colonoscopy
- Barium enema

Breast
- Mammography
- Ultrasound
- MRI scan
- CT body and bone scan

Gynaecological
- Abdominal and transvaginal ultrasound
- Colposcopy and hysteroscopy
- MRI and CT scan staging

Urological
- IVU
- Cystoscopy
- Transrectal ultrasound
- MRI and CT scan staging

CNS
- MRI scanning

Endocrine
- MRI and CT scanning

Bone, thyroid and carcinoid
- Radionuclide scan

Cancer staging

Cancers are commonly staged using the TNM (Tumour, Nodes, Metastases) system, which is a clinically-based method that can be applied to most cancers.

Clinical staging definitions
T = Size of the tumour and its spread to the skin and chest wall:
0   No primary tumour
1   Tumour no more than 2 cm
2   Tumour 2–5 cm
3   Tumour greater than 5 cm
4   Tumour with direct extension to the skin or chest wall

N = extent of tumour spread to lymph nodes:
0   No growth present in axillary lymph nodes same side as primary tumour
1   Growth present in axillary lymph nodes same side as primary tumour, with axillary lymph nodes still moveable
2   Growth present in axillary lymph nodes same side as primary tumour, with axillary lymph nodes fixed to another, or to other structures
3   Growth present in supraclavicular or infraclavicular nodes same side as primary tumour, or oedema of the arm

M = Metastases
0   No metastases
1   Metastases demonstrable

(a)

Breast cancer staging; how the two systems compare (the TNM system is explained in Fig. 25.89(a))

	Clinical stage			
	1	2	3	4
T1N0M0	□			
T2N0M0	□			
T4N0M0*			□	
	1	2	3	4
T1N1M0		□		
T2N1M0		□		
T3N1M0			□	
T4N1M0			□	
	1	2	3	4
T1N2M0*			□	
T2N2M0			□	
T3N2M0*			□	
T4N2M0			□	
	1	2	3	4
T1N3M0*			□	
T2N3M0*			□	
T3N3M0*			□	
T4N3M0*			□	
T0–4, N0–3, M1				□

* Less common

(b)

Figure 25.8   Breast cancer staging: how the two systems compare. **(a)** TNM; **(b)** Site-specific staging.

---

liver metastatic disease, although stenting has reduced the need for this practice.

Nowadays, staging is more sophisticated and refined, depending on histopathology and many other tests, and there is an important supplementary reason: modern adjunctive oncological therapy is tailored to the risk characteristics for tumour recurrence – 'risk-adapted therapy'. For many tumours a TNM (tumour/nodal/metastasis) staging system is utilized, and this is exemplified in Figure 25.8.

Certain staging tests are performed in the work-up of many tumours before the patient is referred for surgery, whereas other staging data only become available after a definitive surgical procedure, or further staging tests are prompted by the findings at operation.

CHEST
Chest X-ray (PA and lateral, with oblique views being particularly useful to demonstrate some ribs,

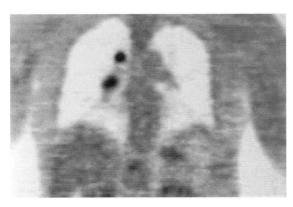

Figure 25.9 Coronal PET scan of chest, demonstrating a hypermetabolic right lung carcinoma with hilar lymph nodal metastases.

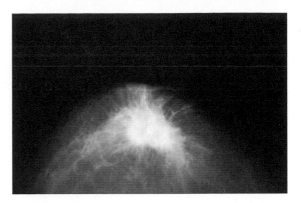

Figure 25.10 Mammogram demonstrating a large solid (white) mass under the nipple that proved to be a carcinoma.

and special views for the sternum) lead on to CT scanning which, with thin-slice spiral CT well delineates any primary lung tumour, small metastases, and hilar and/or mediastinal nodal disease. Bronchoscopy, usually fibreoptic, is used to visualize an endobronchial primary lung cancer and provides the tissue diagnosis by biopsy. Primary lung tumours are divided by the histologist into non-small cell and small cell tumours.

The whole-body PET scan has nowadays replaced some staging tests, e.g. bone and liver scans, and brain scans where appropriate, to exclude as far as possible distant metastatic spread (Fig. 25.9). Non-small cell lung cancer that is not metastatic beyond the hilar nodes is considered for definitive resection. A single pulmonary nodule that is avidly metabolizing glucose on fluorodeoxy glucose PET scan is likely to be neoplastic in origin, and a similar uptake in mediastinal nodes suggests that these nodes are involved by the disease – this is important in considering operability. The chest surgeon may still advise mediastinoscopy with node biopsy prior to definitive resection (but much more selectively in the PET era), and will certainly want to see lung function tests to be reassured that the patient will survive the extent of any planned lung resection.

Postoperatively, pathological staging influences the subsequent recommended treatment plan, as there is increasing evidence that postoperative chemo- and radiotherapy may improve the outlook of those patients with higher risk features such as node-positive disease – this is pathological staging (pTNM). Indeed, trials of preoperative (primary) chemotherapy are in progress.

BREAST
Mammography (Fig. 25.10), often supplemented by ultrasound (and increasingly often by MRI), forms the main tool for breast imaging. Fine needle aspiration cytological biopsy (FNAC) of suspicious lesions or (guidewire) excision biopsy follows. Systemic

staging of breast cancer occurs before definitive therapy: abdominal ultrasound with a chest X-ray or whole-body CT scan and isotope bone scan (nowadays selectively replaced by PET scanning), forms the staging procedure.

GASTROINTESTINAL TRACT
Endoscopy via the oro-oesophageal route for upper gastrointestinal lesions, supplemented by endoscopic ultrasound or ERCP (endoscopic retrograde cholangiopancreatography) and biopsy of suspicious lesions, and colonoscopy (selectively replaced by virtual CT colonography) with biopsy of suspicious lesions, has in the majority of instances superseded barium studies for endoluminal diagnosis. CT or ultrasound scanning of the abdomen and pelvis, selectively replaced by MRI for mainly pelvic disease, forms the main imaging modality for extraluminal disease.

CENTRAL NERVOUS SYSTEM
MR scanning has replaced other imaging of the brain in most instances, although CT maintains an important role in skull base imaging. Angiography, visual field testing, pituitary endocrine testing and other ancillary tests are used on a selective basis.

GENITOURINARY SYSTEM
Ultrasound is extremely useful in the diagnosis of both renal and testicular disease, and transrectal ultrasound is important for imaging the prostate. Ultrasound is also important in the diagnosis of the site of obstruction in postrenal failure. CT scanning complements these tests for renal (and adrenal) disease (Fig. 25.11). Cystoscopy (often now fibreoptic) is the cardinal investigation for exploring bladder disease, with biopsy of any suspicious lesions. Intravenous pyelography maintains a place for imaging the whole genitourinary tract, and nuclear medicine tests such as renography (for obstructive disease) and GFR, DMSA and MAG-3

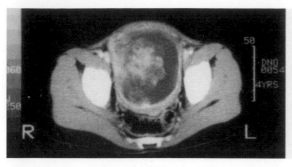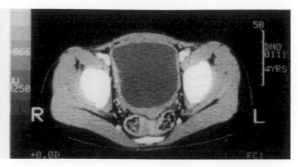

Figure 25.11   CT scan of a child's bladder demonstrating (left panel) a large mass (rhabdomyosarcoma) successfully treated (right panel) by surgery, chemotherapy and radiotherapy.

scans help to define overall and divided (i.e. left versus right) renal function.

GYNAECOLOGICAL
Colposcopy and hysteroscopy are important investigative tools for direct visualization of the cervix and endometrial cavity, and laparoscopy for visualization of the ovaries and adnexae. Transabdominal and transvaginal ultrasound have their place, but MRI of the pelvis is currently the most sensitive non-invasive modality for assessing the extent of gynaecological disease in the pelvis; CT has advantages in the abdomen. Cervical cytology is undoubtedly the most successful type of cancer screening.

EAR/NOSE/THROAT
MRI/CT scanning and biopsy of lumps or ulcers and lymph nodes are common procedures. Cytological analysis of thyroid lumps is difficult, but often precedes thyroidectomy. PET scanning is playing an increasingly important role in the diagnosis and staging of head and neck cancer.

METABOLIC AND ENDOCRINE CANCER SYNDROMES   (Boxes 25.11, 25.12)

- **Hypoglycaemia** associated with *IGF-2-secreting fibrosarcoma*: dizziness, obtundation and sweating, and often hypotension, lead to unconsciousness.
- **Hypertensive crises associated with catecholamine secretion from *phaeochromocytoma*.** 'Anguor animi' (feeling of impending doom) is associated with languor and the excessive 'flight and fright' symptoms.
- **Carcinoid syndrome** due to the oversecretion of *5-hydroxytryptamine* and other vasoactive peptides from neuroendocrine tumours. Episodic flushing is the most common feature, which can become a fixed facial erythema after some time. Diarrhoea and abdominal colic are also part of the syndrome, as may be bronchospasm. Right heart failure with the murmur of tricuspid regurgitation, due to endocardial fibrosis, also occurs with

Box 25.11   Cancer-related metabolic and endocrine syndromes

- Carcinoid syndrome
- Cushing's syndrome
- Cytokine-related hypercalcaemia
- Syndrome of inappropriate antidiuretic hormone (ADH) secretion
- Gynaecomastia

Box 25.12   Primary endocrine cancer

Symptom	Signs
Hoarseness	Thyroid mass
Headache, sweats	Hypertension, oedema
Palpitations, nausea	Adrenal mass, pallor, hypertension, phaeochromocytoma
Hypoglycaemic coma and history of dyspepsia	Pancreatic mass, insulinoma/gastrinoma
Polyuria, polydipsia	Pituitary mass
Visual field loss	Hypopituitarism
Fatigue	Buccal pigmentation of hypoadrenalism

time. There are variations on carcinoid syndrome that occur when other specific neuroendocrine or gut peptide hormones are oversecreted by a carcinoid-like tumour: for example the Verner–Morrison syndrome is associated with watery diarrhoea, Zollinger–Ellison syndrome is associated with symptoms of a severe peptic ulcer, insulinoma with hypoglycaemic symptoms, Cushing's syndrome with excessive ACTH secretion etc.

- **Hypercalcaemia.** This occurs with and without widespread metastatic bone disease. Oversecretion of a PTH-like peptide is one mechanism. The symptoms are thirst and dehydration (as hypercalcaemia causes a nephrogenic diabetes insipidus), constipation, obtundation, and eventually renal failure.

Box 25.13   Paraneoplastic syndromes

Metabolic and endocrine syndromes
- See Box 25.11

Autoimmune syndromes
- Lambert–Eaton myasthenic syndrome
- Cerebellar degeneration with ovarian cancer
- Peripheral neuropathy with various cancers

Immunosuppression
- Reactivation of herpes zoster infection, especially with lymphomas

Coagulopathy
- Thrombophlebitis and pulmonary emboli associated with cancers of the pancreas, stomach, breast and ovary

Pel–Ebstein fever
- An alternating daily fever associated with malignancy

- **Ectopic gonadotrophin secretion.** Precocious puberty in children and gynaecomastia in adult men is recognized in association with human chorionic gonadotrophin (HCG) secretion by germ cell tumours.
- **Syndrome of inappropriate antidiuretic hormone (ADH) secretion.** Excessive ADH secretion is not uncommonly associated with small cell lung cancer in particular, and presents with languor and drowsiness, leading to confusion and coma. A low serum sodium is the diagnostic clue, and a high urine osmolality in the face of a low serum osmolality clinches the diagnosis.

PARANEOPLASTIC SYNDROMES (Box 25.13)

These clinical entities are associated with cancers and often overlap with metabolic and endocrine syndromes – the more so now that the mechanisms are becoming clearer. Fever associated with cancer (e.g. *Pel–Ebstein fever* associated with advanced Hodgkin's disease) is at least partly mediated by IL-2, and the cachexia of advanced cancer (often disproportionate to the extent of cancer) may be partly humorally mediated also. In other paraneoplastic syndromes – for example the glomerulonephritis that occasionally accompanies lung cancer and Hodgkin's disease – a metabolic or immunological humoral link is suspected, although often not known.

Neurological paraneoplastic syndromes are well recognized. *Polymyositis* and *dermatomyositis* may be associated with overt or occult malignancy. Thus, dermatomyositis may be the alerting presenting sign of a deep-seated cancer that has yet to declare

itself. An interesting *myasthenic syndrome* is a rare accompaniment of lung cancer: the *Lambert–Eaton syndrome*. This differs from true myasthenia (which, of course, may be an accompanying event in thymoma) in several respects, but primarily in the lack of response to the edrophonium test. These paraneoplastic syndromes of the muscle and neuromuscular junction may remit when the cancer enters remission, and are thought to have a humoral basis.

Encephalomyelopathies occur as paraneoplastic syndromes often presenting as dementia, less commonly with myelitis – lung cancer is the commonest underlying cancer. However, it should be stressed that the diagnosis is one of exclusion (i.e. it is mandatory for the clinician to first exclude organic pathology – almost always symptomatic metastatic disease). *Paraneoplastic cerebellar degeneration* is most commonly found in association with ovarian cancer. *Myelopathies* may also occur with lymphomas as paraneoplastic events, but some neurological syndromes associated with lymphomas may also have an aetiological contribution from the therapy or infection, e.g. *progressive multifocal leukoencephalopathy*. Visual paraneoplastic events (e.g. cancer-associated retinopathy, optic neuritis) occur but are rare, being best documented in lung cancer and lymphoma: the remarks about 'always ruling out metastatic causes' still apply. The clinically dramatic oscillating eye movements of *opsiclonus–myoclonus*, best associated with advanced *neuroblastoma*, can also occur to some degree with other tumours, e.g. lung cancer. *Peripheral neuropathy* is an unusual paraneoplastic event.

Coagulopathies may be paraneoplastic events, disseminated intravascular coagulopathy (DIC) – e.g. in association with acute promyeloblastic leukaemia and mucin-secreting adenocarcinoma – being one extreme of the spectrum, and excessive bleeding and thrombophlebitis migrans (e.g. in pancreatic carcinoma) being the other.

The *paraneoplastic syndromes of the skin* are protean. *Pruritus* is the most common and best linked to advanced Hodgkin's disease. *Acanthosis nigricans* (see Fig. 25.3) – itchy brown hyperkeratotic skin, most commonly in the flexures and axillae – is rare in association with deep-seated malignancy (e.g. stomach cancer), and other ichthyoses occur. *Bullous conditions* (paraneoplastic pemphigus and dermatitis herpetiformis) may occur. The bullae of shingles remind us that this particular infection not infrequently becomes reactivated in cancer (e.g. Hodgkin's disease).

WORK-UP OF THE UNKNOWN PRIMARY CANCER

This is an interesting topic and relevant to a text such as this. It is not uncommon in medicine that the patient arrives with symptoms/signs/ancillary tests suggestive of cancer and yet no certain primary is apparent. Thus a patient arrives with back pain (the presenting symptom), is found to have tenderness over the spine at a certain level (the sign), and is found on imaging (the ancillary test) to have partial collapse of a vertebral body with destruction of the pedicles on plain X-ray, and destruction highly suggestive of cancerous destruction on subsequent MR imaging of the spine; the MR may well show other foci of disease. Of course, a differential diagnosis may exist, as tuberculous involvement of the spine may also present thus. The alert clinician will search for other corroborative signs: the pattern of destruction of the vertebrae on the imaging may help (e.g. the disc spaces are usually preserved in malignant involvement of the spine, whereas they are often involved in TB of the spine) and the presence of other disease – e.g. a large mass on a chest X-ray suggesting a bronchial primary, versus hazy, extensive upper lobe shadowing with cavitation and calcification – is suggestive of TB.

For spinal disease presentations of malignancy, the clinician needs to consider the primary tumours (e.g. myeloma, osteogenic or chondrosarcoma, Ewing's or other sarcoma, and rarely chordoma and lymphoma) or, more commonly, metastatic disease. Before biopsying the disease in the spine the clinician will be alert to the primary cancers that frequently metastasize to the bones, namely bronchial, breast, prostate, renal and adrenal carcinomas and melanoma, although others may do so late in their natural history. The clinician may well want to exclude myeloma by measuring the immunoglobulins (paraprotein) in the serum and checking for light chain excretion in the urine (Bence Jones test). If screening for all these proves negative, then a biopsy of the affected vertebra will be performed.

If the tissue diagnosis indicates carcinoma, then the histologist is pressed to help further define the possible primary; thus a squamous carcinoma is likely to have an origin in the bronchus, head and neck, cervix uteri or other sites with squamous epithelium that give rise to squamous cancers. An adenocarcinoma may be more difficult to categorize as to its tissue of origin, but with immunohistochemical techniques the short list may be narrowed. Thus, the presence of oestrogen receptors on adenocarcinoma cells strongly suggests a primary breast cancer. Intracellular mucin suggests a gastrointestinal tract origin, and clear cell carcinoma suggests the kidneys or lungs. The presence of thyroglobulin staining points strongly to the thyroid as the site of origin. Melanoma is famous for the black melanin pigment in the cells ('the black cancer') and is diagnostic, and the S100 stain is corroborative; amelanotic melanoma exists. Lymphomas can be diagnosed and typed using special immunohistochemical stains – necessary for modern risk-adapted therapies. The

work-up of bony disease at sites other than the spine is similar, including an assessment of other bony sites of involvement by skeletal 'survey' (a plain X-ray series of most of the skeleton) or isotope bone scanning, the former being most useful in myeloma and the latter in most other types of cancer. Another relatively common presentation of the 'mystery' primary is a node in the neck, biopsy of which yields cancer cells. The histologist can usually tell straight away if this is infiltration by lymphoma, melanoma or thyroid cancer, but a poorly differentiated carcinoma is more difficult. Thus a patient presenting with neck node enlargement and proven carcinoma on biopsy should have full ENT assessment with endoscopy and chest imaging (chest X-ray in the first instance). It is not unusual for nasopharyngeal, tongue base or tonsillar carcinoma to present in this manner before the primary tumour becomes symptomatic. Lung cancer and even breast cancer may also present in this way. If all these are negative then other, rarer, tumours, such as medullary carcinoma of the thyroid, suggested by amyloid in the tumour and a very high serum calcitonin, should be considered. Carcinoma in a residual branchial cyst is a very rare but localized cancer that may well be curable by surgery and radiotherapy, and is therefore an important unusual diagnosis to be considered in the patient presenting with neck nodal disease that is negative on standard work-up.

Patients presenting with liver metastases are usually those presenting with ill-health and weight loss, anorexia, and other symptoms that lead the enquiring clinician to scan the abdomen. Not infrequently, multiple solid liver masses almost diagnostic of metastases are found, with no evidence of the primary. Of course, hepatocellular carcinoma (HCC), a primary liver tumour, may be the cause, and more likely in those with cirrhosis or a background of hepatitis, but overall much less likely than metastatic disease in the liver. Note that hepatocellular carcinoma may be multifocal. A raised serum α-fetoprotein occurs in many cases of HCC.

Certain cancers often present with liver metastases from an occult primary neoplasm; in women breast cancer is particularly likely to do this. Careful examination of the whole patient may well bring to light clues as to the site of the primary cancer, and a breast lump would be a sign that should be actively sought. Obviously, the other sites from which liver metastases commonly arise are those in the gastrointestinal tract, including the pancreas, and a full gastrointestinal endoscopic examination is part of the work-up. Liver preference for metastatic disease is a curious feature of some cancers, e.g. melanoma, particularly ocular primaries. Where cancer is not obvious except in the liver then biopsy of the lesions within the liver, under image guidance, is indicated, and the onus then falls again on the histopathologist to assist in the unravelling of the diagnosis.

The work-up of multiple brain masses discovered following presentation with neurological symptoms/ signs or epilepsy, leading to brain MR scanning, can be surmised from the foregoing. Obviously, the surgeon will not wish to subject the patient to open craniotomy if the diagnosis of metastatic disease, suggested by a multiplicity of lesions in different areas of the brain, can be ascertained from a chest X-ray, breast lump, renal mass, ovarian mass etc. – detected by whole-body screening. Such a body screen should therefore precede the neurosurgical procedure. If a primary is still not obvious after such measures, then biopsy will bring the histologist once again to the fore. Gliomas, and particularly primary brain lymphomas, may be multifocal.

Abdominal lymphadenopathy as a presenting problem – usually brought to light by abdominal symptoms leading to a scan – may be *regional adenopathy* relating to a primary in the area or the initial presentation of a lymphoma. A biopsy may be needed, but if lymphoma is a possibility it is essential to search elsewhere to see if there is a more superficial nodal mass to biopsy for diagnosis, as biopsy of a retroperitoneal node mass, although frequently performed and reasonably safe, nevertheless has a small risk attached. The point here, as so often the case, is to think beyond the presenting problem, paying regard to the bigger picture. Lastly, a malignant midline carcinoma presenting as a retroperitoneal mass may be a germ cell tumour, and serum markers such as HCG and AFP are relevant screening tests.

TREATMENT

Despite its complexity the treatment of cancer follows certain general principles. The diagnosis having been proved, usually by tissue diagnosis, the patient is staged to ascertain whether the disease is localized or metastatic. If localized, then there is often a chance of cure. Surgery and radiotherapy are the two regional therapies for localized cancer. Thus radical gastrectomy and radical prostatectomy are two examples where a gross total removal of the organ bearing the cancer gives the patient a chance of cure. Similarly, radical radiotherapy stands a good chance of curing laryngeal cancer. Sometimes both surgery or radiotherapy carry an equal chance of cure, and, as in prostate cancer, the patient may choose from the available options, bearing in mind the risks and sequelae, in relation to the substaging characteristics or other medical problems of the individual patient. Postoperative radiotherapy is based on the principle of 'mopping up' cancer cells wide of the surgical margin.

Chemotherapy and hormonal therapy (Fig. 25.12) (and in the future perhaps molecular therapy) are more often employed for multisite disease – lymphoma or metastatic cancer. However, in the field of cancer treatment, and where regional control may be followed by late systemic relapse, there is increasingly a role for additional or initial chemotherapy or hormonal therapy. Thus an ostensibly early breast cancer patient treated by surgery, and whose axillary sentinel staging lymph node is positive for microscopic cancer, is at greater risk of later systemic relapse of breast cancer and of dying from this disease. Therefore, even though staging scans (performed prior to surgery) have not demonstrated metastatic disease, the clinician is mindful that the patient is at high risk of later fatal relapse. It has now been unequivocally demonstrated that, by giving such a patient early postoperative chemotherapy (adjuvant chemotherapy), the chance of that late relapse is reduced. The logic is clear: in this day and age, where chemotherapy is imperfect and incapable

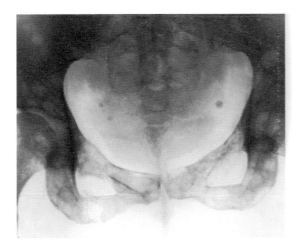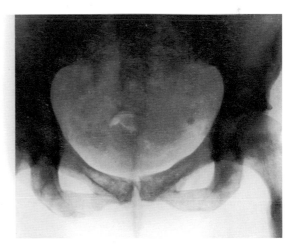

Figure 25.12 Hormone therapy for cancer. Plain X-rays of pelvis demonstrating (left panel) severe metastatic destruction of the pubic rami by metastatic breast cancer. The right panel shows an excellent response, of interest in that not only is there regression of the tumour but the destroyed bone has remodelled. The tumour was a strongly oestrogen receptor-positive cancer and the only therapy that the patient had received between the two pictures was bilateral oophorectomy.

of sterilizing millions of cells (the burden at the time of established metastatic disease), such chemotherapy is capable of sterilizing thousands of cells (the perceived systemic tumour burden at the time of staging negative disease in the above example). Thus adjuvant chemotherapy (and hormonal therapy in oestrogen-positive breast cancer and in prostate cancer) has become established oncological practice for an increasing number of diseases. The subject has been taken further, and in a patient with a locally advanced breast cancer where it would be difficult to obtain clear microscopic borders at the surgical resection margin, it is now often the case that primary chemotherapy is recommended (neoadjuvant chemotherapy). After shrinkage of the tumour within the breast definitive surgery then proceeds. In T3 prostate cancer (stage T3 denoting extracapsular spread), it is now usual to start treatment with endocrine therapy to attempt to shrink the disease within the prostate capsule prior to definitive local therapy. This concept is widening and is almost 'de rigeur' in the oncological therapy of paediatric solid tumours.

SCREENING

The emphasis of modern oncology is very much turning towards the early detection and therapy of cancers. The introduction of cervical screening programmes in middle-aged women has had a profound effect on the death statistics from this disease worldwide. This test relies on the cytological analysis of smears taken from the cervix with a simple wooden spatula, every 2–3 years. This programme has been successful because the test is cheap and relatively easy to perform, and applicable worldwide; it has also fuelled the enthusiasm of the profession to find equally successful programmes for other diseases.

Mammographic screening for breast cancer is now well established and undoubtedly detects breast cancers earlier and in a more curable form. When the programme was introduced there was some controversy as to whether any increased detection would translate into improved survival because of biases that may creep into such a programme; these are worth citing here as they pertain to other programmes. For example, suppose 100 early breast cancers were discovered in a screening programme and it was shown that the life expectancy of these patients was better than that of 100 patients presenting to a symptomatic early breast cancer clinic (i.e. with a breast lump); is it really true that this survival benefit is due to the screening programme, or is it possible that the disease was detected earlier in its natural history, and therefore the base time for survival was shifted backwards in the programme (lead time bias)? Alternatively, could it be that naturally slow-growing (non-aggressive) cancers would be more likely to be detected in a screening programme (as they would have been indolent in the breast for longer), thus biasing the perceived improved survival in the screened group? Although these issues have been resolved for mammographic breast screening, which is now proved to be unequivocally useful, they remain valid for other programmes. Routine colonoscopies or virtual colonography (for the detection of colon cancer), PSA (prostate-specific antigen) serum testing (for the detection of early prostate cancer), thin-cut spiral CT scanning of the chest (for lung cancer screening), ovarian screening ultrasonography, and many other screening programmes need to pass these rigorous tests to be embraced as truly useful to the population as a whole.

In patients with a positive family history of the cancer under scrutiny, or with a syndrome predisposing to cancer in certain sites, the clinician has a lower threshold for screening tests – indeed, pre-emptive surgery may be advised (total colectomy in familial polyposis coli, prophylactic mastectomies in *BRCA* gene carriers etc.).

PALLIATIVE CARE

Once a patient has been deemed incurable of cancer, then the management plan changes to the relief of their symptoms. Of course this may still involve surgery (e.g. for bowel obstruction, tracheostomy for laryngeal obstruction etc.), radiotherapy (e.g. for bone pain from metastatic disease) or chemotherapy/hormonal therapy (e.g. breast, bowel or lung cancer) aimed at prolonging life, but the patient has a right to expect less toxicity from the therapy than they might accept had the treatment been for cure.

Once the disease is beyond any life-prolonging hope, then the judicious use of pain-killing drugs and supportive care is arranged around the patient's home or hospice. The emphasis is that no patient should die in pain or distress, and the patient and family must be supported both physically and psychologically through to a dignified and peaceful death.

Blood disorders

D. Provan

26

INTRODUCTION

Blood is a circulating tissue that is in contact with most other tissue systems. As a result, disorders affecting the blood may cause symptoms or signs at any site in the body. In broad terms, blood diseases may be *malignant* (e.g. leukaemias, lymphomas and others), *potentially malignant/premalignant* (e.g. myeloproliferative diseases, myelodysplasia) or *non-malignant* (anaemias, cytopenias such as thrombocytopenia or neutropenia, coagulation disorders, and others).

The first section of this chapter concentrates on anaemia, which results from a reduction in the number of red cells or of the haemoglobin concentration within red cells. Because the bone marrow manufactures all three cellular components of the blood, anaemia may be associated with abnormalities of white cells and platelets, for example when there is a primary bone marrow disorder such as aplastic anaemia. However, anaemia is more commonly found as an isolated abnormality and is then usually secondary to disorders affecting the gastrointestinal tract or other organs. Thus, the clinical approach to the anaemic patient must be wide ranging, as underlying disease processes may involve any organ system. In both the developing and the developed worlds the most important cause of anaemia is gastrointestinal (GI) blood loss. Appropriate GI investigation should be considered in all cases of unexplained anaemia.

The second section discusses symptoms and signs associated with haematological malignancies, both acute and chronic, highlighting the features of each.

The third section is concerned with coagulation disorders, which result from abnormalities of platelet function or number, or of the plasma proteins involved in haemostasis. These abnormalities can result in either an increased risk of bleeding or, conversely, an increased risk of thrombosis.

ANAEMIA

The term anaemia simply means a reduced haemoglobin concentration (adjusted for age and sex), with no specific cause implied (Table 26.1). There is always an underlying cause and the physician must determine what this is, by obtaining a full history and physical examination before moving to laboratory and other tests. It is worth remembering that immediately after acute massive blood loss the haemoglobin concentration will initially be normal. This clinical situation is dominated by hypovolaemic shock and is not further discussed here.

The causes of anaemia are numerous but can be broadly classified on the basis of the major pathophysiological mechanism. Anaemia results either from increased blood loss (bleeding or haemolysis) or from decreased red cell production. However, in the clinical situation it is often unclear which process is dominant, and a more practical classification is based simply on red cell size (microcytic, normocytic and macrocytic) (Tables 26.2, 26.3 and Box 26.1). Although this classification is extremely valuable practically, it is not exhaustive and non-specific anaemias do occur. For example, the 'anaemia of chronic disease', which can be associated with any infective, inflammatory or neoplastic process, usually results in a normocytic anaemia, but in extreme cases causes a microcytic anaemia. Similarly, most haemolytic anaemias are normocytic, but macrocytosis may develop when haemolysis is particularly brisk, as reticulocytes are larger than mature red cells.

Certain symptoms and signs can be associated with anaemia, whatever its cause (Box 26.2). Several of these will be strongly influenced by the coexistence of cardiovascular disease. For instance, heart failure is most likely to occur in patients with underlying coronary heart disease. Once a clinical or laboratory diagnosis of anaemia has been made, then attention should be paid to features in the history and examination that might suggest a particular underlying aetiology.

HISTORY

Patients with anaemia from any cause are likely to present with the non-specific symptoms of anaemia (Box 26.2). The age and sex of the patient are highly relevant, as inherited disorders of the blood such as thalassaemia are most likely to present in childhood, whereas in women of childbearing age, by far the most common cause of anaemia is iron deficiency consequent on menstrual blood loss and pregnancy. In contrast, older women and males of any age with iron deficiency should undergo investigation aimed at detecting gastrointestinal blood loss.

The patient may describe symptoms that suggest certain underlying pathologies. For instance, drenching night sweats might indicate lymphoma, whereas bone pain points towards myeloma or metastatic cancer. The past medical history may reveal important clues, such as a history of peptic ulcer disease, malignancy or autoimmune disease.

Aspirin or other non-steroidal anti-inflammatory drugs may cause occult blood loss from gastritis. Similarly, steroid therapy can result in peptic ulceration. Excess alcohol consumption is associated with gastritis, macrocytosis, folate deficiency and liver disease, with consequent variceal bleeding and red cell pooling in an enlarged spleen.

The dietary history is particularly relevant in the assessment of anaemia, as nutritional deficiencies of folic acid (and less frequently of iron and vitamin B_{12}) result in anaemia. Dietary folate deficiency occurs in 'skid-row' alcoholics, or when the diet is deficient in green vegetables. As there is usually adequate iron in the diet, iron deficiency is rarely due to poor diet alone. As all the vitamin B_{12} present in the human diet is ultimately animal in origin, dietary B_{12} deficiency is only likely to occur in vegetarians, and is inevitable in strict vegans unless appropriate supplementation is taken.

A family history of blood disorders (e.g. sickle cell disease, thalassaemia) or autoimmune disorders is relevant, as is the ethnic origin of the patient. Sickle cell disease is found in Afro-Caribbeans whereas β-thalassaemia is commonest in the Mediterranean littoral and in the Indian subcontinent. Prolonged residence in or travel to tropical countries may suggest that malaria or other parasitic infestation is present.

Systematic questioning may reveal symptoms suggestive of an underlying disease that is causing the anaemia. Thus, a history of weight loss, dysphagia, dyspepsia, chronic diarrhoea, change in bowel habit or rectal bleeding should instigate appropriate investigations directed at the GI tract, looking for malignancies, peptic ulcer disease, malabsorption states, colitis, haemorrhoids and other causes of GI blood loss. Similarly, a detailed genitourinary his-

Table 26.1   Normal red cell values in adults

	Males	Females
Hb (g/dL)	13.3–16.7	11.8–14.8
RBC ($\times 10^{12}$/L)	4.32–5.66	3.88–4.99
PCV or Hct (L/L)	0.39–0.5	0.36–0.44
MCV (fL)	76–96	76–96

Hb, haemoglobin; RBC, red blood cells; PCV, packed cell volume; Hct, haematocrit.

Table 26.2   The microcytic anaemias (MCV <76 fL)

Impaired haem synthesis	Impaired globin synthesis
Iron deficiency	Thalassaemia
Anaemia of chronic disease	
Sideroblastic anaemia	
Lead poisoning	

Table 26.3   The normocytic anaemias (MCV 76–96 fL)

With increased reticulocytes	With decreased reticulocytes
Bleeding	Aplastic anaemia
Haemolysis	Pure red cell aplasia
	Anaemia of chronic renal failure
	Anaemia of chronic disease
	Myelodysplasia
	Haematological malignancies
	Bone marrow metastases

Box 26.1   The macrocytic anaemias (MCV >96 fL)

- Megaloblastic anaemia (B_{12} or folate deficiency – identical features on blood film)
- Hypothyroidism
- Liver disease
- Alcohol
- Myelodysplasia
- Anaemias with extreme reticulocytosis

Box 26.2   The non-specific symptoms and signs of anaemia

Decreased oxygen transport	Fatigue, syncope, dyspnoea, angina
Reduced blood volume	Pallor, postural hypotension
Increased cardiac output	Pounding in ears, palpitations
Congestive cardiac failure	Orthopnoea, paroxysmal nocturnal dyspnoea; tachycardia, raised central venous pressure, displaced apex beat, gallop rhythm, basal crackles, bilateral ankle oedema

tory should be taken in women, with particular emphasis on the extent of menstrual blood loss. Many women of childbearing age are teetering on the brink of iron deficiency, and the added iron losses of menstruation or pregnancy frequently precipitate anaemia. When haematuria is heavy enough to cause anaemia, it is normally the presenting problem itself.

EXAMINATION

Certain physical signs are likely to be found in patients suffering from anaemia irrespective of the cause (Box 26.2). Pallor is best detected by examination of the mucosae (conjunctival or intraoral), although this is a very unreliable guide to an individual's haemoglobin concentration. In addition, specific causes of anaemia are often associated with characteristic physical findings (Table 26.4). Some specific points are important: B$_{12}$ deficiency is one of

the few causes of both pyramidal tract damage and peripheral neuropathy, and so can present with brisk knee reflexes and absent ankle jerks (neuropathy). The typical facial appearance of inadequately treated thalassaemic patients results from the massive expansion of bone marrow that occurs in an attempt to compensate for the anaemia. Expansion of the facial bones results in so-called 'chipmunk facies', and similar changes result in typical radiological features (Fig. 26.1). Leukaemia and lymphoma can result in protean physical findings. Some specific features include the florid overgrowth of gingival mucosa that occurs in monocytic leukaemias, and the features of meningism (photophobia, headache, stiff neck) that result from meningeal infiltration by malignant cells.

Certain other aspects of the physical examination may also be helpful. For example, anaemia associated with jaundice may well indicate haemolysis. Many haemolytic anaemias are associated with skin

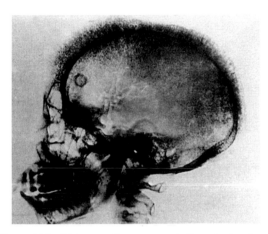

Figure 26.1 'Hair-on-end' appearance in the calvarium in thalassaemia.

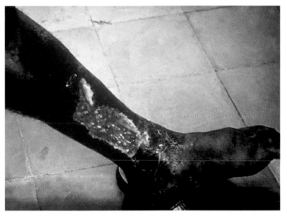

Figure 26.2 Haemolytic anaemia (sickle haemoglobin disease); leg ulcer.

Table 26.4 Specific features of different types of anaemia

Cause of anaemia	Specific clinical findings
Iron deficiency	Angular stomatitis, painless glossitis, dysphagia due to pharyngeal web (Plummer–Vinson syndrome), koilonychia (spoon-shaped nails – very rare nowadays), pica (craving for strange foods, e.g. ice, soil)
Megaloblastic anaemia	Painful glossitis ('beefy' red tongue)
B$_{12}$ deficiency	Peripheral neuropathy, subacute combined degeneration of the cord (damage to the corticospinal tracts and dorsal columns) in severe B$_{12}$ deficiency
Haemolytic anaemias	Jaundice, gallstones, splenomegaly, skin ulceration
Sickle cell disease	Bony tenderness, osteomyelitis
Thalassaemia	Skull bone expansion with characteristic facial abnormalities, e.g. 'chipmunk facies', poor growth and development
Malignancies • Leukaemia and lymphoma • Myeloma • Metastatic cancer	Lymphadenopathy, hepatosplenomegaly, skin nodules, gum hypertrophy, meningism Bone pain and fractures Bone pain and signs of primary malignancy

ulceration (Fig. 26.2). Signs of arthropathy indicate connective tissue disease. Examination of the breasts, chest or prostate may suggest carcinoma, which can sometimes present with anaemia. Epigastric tenderness, abdominal masses, haemorrhoids or a rectal mucosal lesion indicate GI pathology. The presence of telangiectases on the face, lips, or within the mouth suggests a diagnosis of hereditary haemorrhagic telangiectasia, which can cause iron deficiency due to chronic GI blood loss from lesions scattered throughout the length of the bowel. Enlargement of the liver, spleen and lymph nodes commonly occurs in haematological diseases and is discussed in detail below.

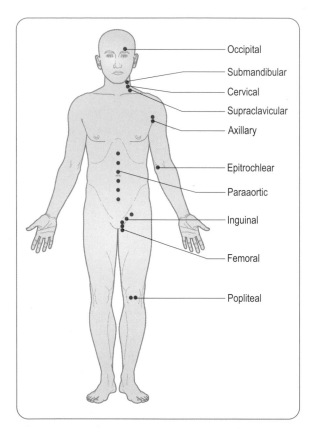

Figure 26.3   The lymph nodes: clinical examination.

EXAMINATION OF THE LYMPH NODES

The distribution of the major lymph node groups that can be felt is shown in Figure 26.3. Although the para-aortic nodes are retroperitoneal, they can occasionally be palpated when markedly enlarged. If lymph nodes are palpated, then the following points should be considered:

- How many nodes are palpable?
- What is the diameter of the nodes?
- What is their consistency?
- Are they discrete or confluent?
- Are they mobile or fixed?
- Is the skin in the vicinity of the nodes abnormal?

Infections tend to result in tender lymphadenopathy (Table 26.5), whereas neoplastic lymph nodes are generally painless. Of course, there are exceptions to this rule, and both TB and HIV infection can cause painless lymph node enlargement. Generalized lymphadenopathy occurs in systemic infections and as a reactive process in skin diseases such as psoriasis or eczema (*dermatopathic lymphadenopathy*). Inguinal lymphadenopathy commonly occurs in normal people owing to current or past infections affecting the lower limb. Marked, asymmetric or generalized enlargement of lymph nodes suggests lymphoma; this should be confirmed by excision biopsy. Lymph nodes involved by lymphoma tend to be 'rubbery' in consistency, whereas nodes infiltrated by metastatic carcinoma tend to be firm or 'craggy'. The finding of regional lymphadenopathy should always prompt examination of the areas drained by those nodes (e.g. breasts, chest), searching for evidence of malignancy. Occasionally, enlargement of nodes which are themselves impalpable will result in specific clinical findings. For instance, enlargement of mediastinal nodes can cause superior vena caval obstruction, manifest by venous engorgement of the neck veins, headache and papilloedema.

EXAMINATION OF THE LIVER AND SPLEEN

Haematological disorders frequently cause enlargement of liver and spleen, although the differential diagnosis is wide-ranging (Table 26.6 and Box 26.3). Palpation should begin in the iliac fossae so that

Table 26.5 Infections that cause enlarged lymph nodes	
Site of lymph node enlargement	**Infections**
Submandibular	Dental infections, aphthous ulceration
Cervical	Tonsillitis (upper cervical, 'tonsillar node'), TB
Generalized lymphadenopathy (often predominantly cervical and occipital)	Epstein–Barr virus infection (glandular fever), cytomegalovirus, HIV, toxoplasmosis
Axillary	Upper limb infections (e.g. paronychia), breast infections (e.g. mastitis, abscess)
Inguinal	Lower limb infections (e.g. leg ulcers), genital infection (e.g. lymphogranuloma venereum, genital herpes)

Table 26.6 Common causes of hepatosplenomegaly and their associated features

Disorder	Associated clinical findings
Myeloproliferative disorders	Usually relatively few findings
Lymphoproliferative disorders	Lymphadenopathy
Congestive cardiac failure	Tachycardia, raised JVP, displaced apex, gallop rhythm, basal crackles, dependent oedema
Chronic liver disease	Stigmata of chronic liver disease (jaundice, palmar erythema, spider naevi, ascites)

Box 26.3 Causes of splenomegaly

Mild/moderate splenomegaly	*Autoimmune disease*	Autoimmune haemolytic anaemia
		SLE
		Sjögren's syndrome
	Globin disorders	Thalassaemia
	Infections	TB
		EBV
		Brucellosis
	Malignant disease	Leukaemias
		Lymphomas (Hodgkin's and non-Hodgkin's)
	Miscellaneous	Felty's syndrome
Massive splenomegaly	*Infections*	Visceral leishmaniasis (kala-azar)
		Malaria (tropical splenomegaly syndrome)
	Malignant disease	Chronic myeloid leukaemia
		Splenic lymphoma
	Myeloproliferative disease	Myelofibrosis
	Storage disorders	Gaucher's disease

massive hepatosplenomegaly is not missed. If palpable, these organs should be measured at rest in centimetres from the costal margin at the midclavicular line to the point of furthest extent. Sometimes, they are palpable only on inspiration, and this should also be noted (see Chapter 8). Some disorders are associated with modest splenic enlargement, whereas others typically result in massive enlargement (Box 26.3).

INVESTIGATION OF THE ANAEMIC PATIENT

Investigations should first be directed towards determining the type of anaemia, and then at identifying an underlying pathology. A patient with significant anaemia for which the cause is not obvious should have initial investigations as in Box 26.4. Examples of normal and abnormal blood and bone marrow appearances are shown in Figures 26.4–26.15. If there is any evidence to suggest a haemolytic process (jaundice, splenomegaly, gallstones, or suggestive features on the blood film), then a haemolysis screen should be included. In the majority of cases the type of anaemia will then be apparent and further investigation can be initiated (Table 26.7). Most primary

haematological disorders (e.g. leukaemia) will have an abnormal blood film and, if so, appropriate referral is indicated.

If the cause of anaemia is not apparent at this stage, then proceed as in Table 26.8. Haemoglobin electrophoresis should be performed at the initial screening if the patient comes from an appropriate ethnic group. Obviously, investigation need not proceed precisely along these lines, and cases should be approached on an individual basis. If the cause of the anaemia is not evident at this stage, or if a haematological disorder has been diagnosed, then referral to a haematologist is indicated.

HAEMATOLOGICAL MALIGNANCIES

There are many types of malignant disease that affect the blood. The broad features associated with haematological disease, which should prompt the clinician to carry out investigations to confirm the diagnosis, will be discussed here.

ACUTE OR CHRONIC

Diseases such as leukaemia and lymphoma are broadly split into two major types: acute and chronic. The acute forms are generally abrupt in onset, often with marked physical signs and laboratory features. These diseases are aggressive in character and rapidly fatal unless treated promptly. By contrast, chronic malignancies have often been present for many months before diagnosis, with relatively few symptoms and signs; these disorders are more indolent (less aggressive) and patients do not require treatment immediately. Although it might not be suspected from the terminology used, a large proportion of the acute haematological malignancies can be cured with treatment, whereas most of the chronic forms cannot – they can usually be controlled with treatment, but not eliminated completely.

Box 26.4   Initial investigations of anaemia

- Full blood count
- Examination of the blood film
- Serum ferritin
- Serum B$_{12}$
- Red cell folate
- Haemolysis screen (if indicated): reticulocyte count, serum bilirubin, serum lactate dehydrogenase, haptoglobins, urinary urobilinogen

---

PRESENTATION OF PATIENTS WITH ACUTE HAEMATOLOGICAL MALIGNANCIES

Patients often consult their GP after a short period of ill health. They may complain of sweats (often severe, drenching, occurring at night, requiring a change of night clothes; Table 26.9). Anorexia is common and weight loss is often prominent. The patient may have suffered with more infections than

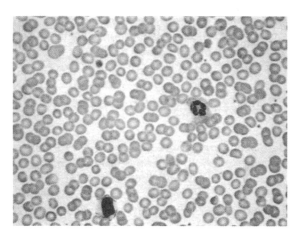

Figure 26.4   Normal peripheral blood. The red cells show little variation in size or shape. A neutrophil granulocyte and a lymphocyte are visible, and platelets are scattered through the film.

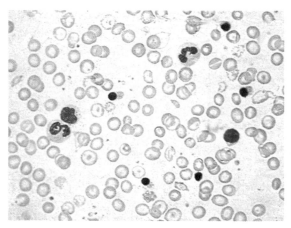

Figure 26.6   β-Thalassaemia major (peripheral blood). There is hypochromia, microcytosis and anisocytosis. Target cells and nucleated red cells are numerous. In β-thalassaemia minor the peripheral blood looks like that in iron deficiency.

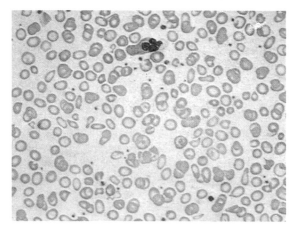

Figure 26.5   Iron deficiency anaemia (peripheral blood). Hypochromia, microcytosis, anisocytosis and target cells are shown.

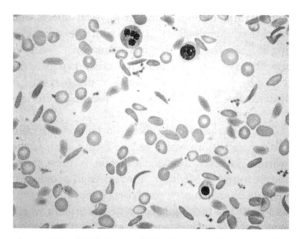

Figure 26.7   Sickle haemoglobin disease (peripheral blood). In homozygous disease (HbSS), sickle cells and target cells are present together with occasional nucleated red cells. Heterozygotes (HbAS) have a normal peripheral blood.

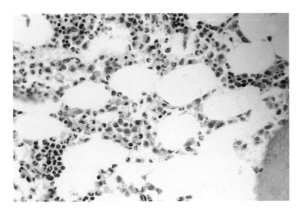

Figure 26.8 Trephine bone marrow biopsy showing a normally cellular marrow.

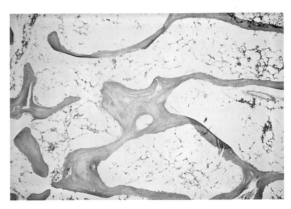

Figure 26.9 Trephine bone marrow biopsy. The marrow is acellular and there is bone resorption in this patient with aplastic anaemia.

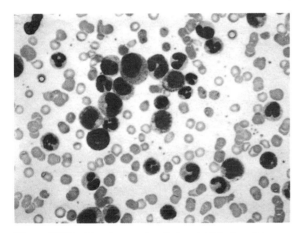

Figure 26.10 Chronic granulocytic (myeloid) leukaemia (peripheral blood). There is an increased number of granulocytes, most of which are mature neutrophils. A few more primitive cells are also present.

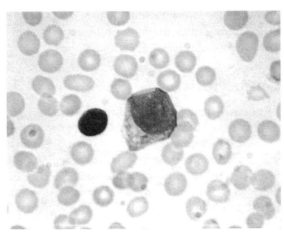

Figure 26.11 Acute myeloblastic leukaemia (peripheral blood). The myeloblast in the centre of the field contains a cytoplasmic Auer rod.

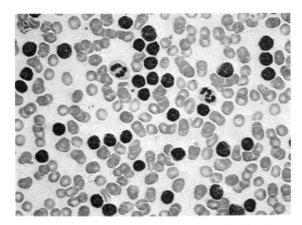

Figure 26.12 Chronic lymphocytic leukaemia (peripheral blood). The white cell count is increased and most of the white cells are small lymphocytes.

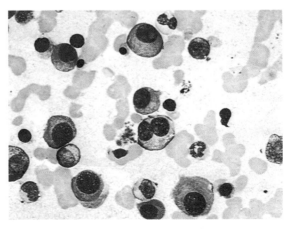

Figure 26.13 Myelomatosis (bone marrow). The marrow is infiltrated with plasma cells and one binucleate form is present. The red cells show rouleau formation.

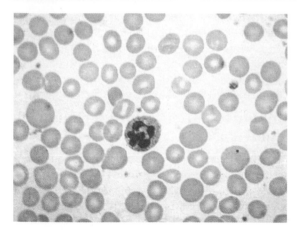

Figure 26.14 Macrocytic anaemia (peripheral blood). Macrocytosis, anisocytosis, poikilocytosis and a hypersegmented neutrophil granulocyte are shown.

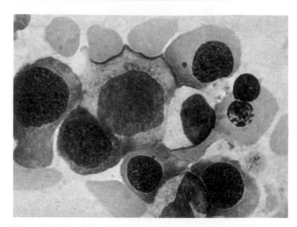

Figure 26.15 Megaloblastic bone marrow. The majority of cells are megaloblastic erythroblasts showing failure of nuclear development and abnormal nuclear morphology.

Table 26.7 Second-line investigations of anaemia

Cause of anaemia	Appropriate investigations
Iron deficiency	Oesophagogastroduodenoscopy (OGD), colonoscopy, gynaecological examination, coeliac antibodies (anti-tissue transglutaminase)
Low serum B_{12}	Gastric parietal cell antibodies (not specific), intrinsic factor antibody (specific for pernicious anaemia), Schilling test (B_{12} absorption test)
Low red cell folate	Coeliac antibodies and/or duodenal biopsy – if small bowel malabsorption, refer to gastroenterologist
Evidence of haemolysis	Direct antiglobulin test (DAT) – if DAT neg: G6PD screen, refer to haematologist

Table 26.8 Third-line investigations of anaemia

Type	Investigations
Microcytic anaemias	Haemoglobin electrophoresis Search for evidence of underlying infective, inflammatory or neoplastic disorder (blood cultures, ESR, C-reactive protein, ANA, CXR etc.)
Normocytic anaemias	Renal function Haemolysis screen (if not already performed) Immunoglobulins and paraprotein screen Search for evidence of underlying infective, inflammatory or neoplastic disorder (see above)
Macrocytic anaemias	Thyroid function tests Liver function tests Haemolysis screen (if not already performed)

are usual for them, owing to the profound immuno-suppression that occurs in any cancer, especially those of the haematopoietic system. A low platelet count is often present in acute leukaemia, and this may cause unexplained bruising or bleeding, including nose or gum bleeding. Anaemia, as discussed earlier, is common in all types of cancer, and especially leukaemias, because the normal bone marrow cells are replaced by leukaemic cells. Patients are often pale and tired on presentation.

Older patients who have coexisting lung or heart problems may have worsening shortness of breath or angina as the haemoglobin concentration falls. Acute haematological malignancies generally involve the reticuloendothelial system, resulting in lymph node enlargement and hepatosplenomegaly. Because white blood cells are in contact with most tissues, acute leukaemias may present with swelling at unusual sites, such as the gums, central nervous system, testes and other sites.

Table 26.9 History and features of acute and chronic leukaemias

	Acute leukaemias	Chronic leukaemias
History	Short history	Long history, often few symptoms, may be detected by chance
	Anorexia	Anorexia
	Sweats	Sweats
	Weight loss	Weight loss
	Infection	Infection
	Gum bleeding	Skin rashes if involvement by e.g. chronic lymphoid malignancy
	Nose bleeds	
	Bruising	
	Bone pain	
	Mucositis, e.g. oral discomfort	
Signs	Pale	Pale
	Bruising	Occasionally bruising
	Oral bleeding	Lymphadenopathy
	± Lymphadenopathy	Hepatosplenomegaly
	± Hepatosplenomegaly	Shingles common in chronic lymphocytic leukaemia
	± Gum swelling	
	± Testicular swelling	
	Candidiasis (oral thrush)	

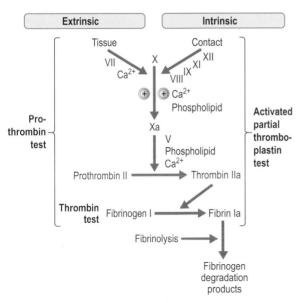

Figure 26.16 The coagulation and fibrinolytic mechanisms.

Overall, when an individual develops acute leukaemia there is a rapid development of the disease, with associated physical signs and marked deterioration in wellbeing.

CHRONIC HAEMATOLOGICAL MALIGNANCIES

Chronic leukaemias and lymphomas affect older individuals (not exclusively, but predominantly). Because of the very slow growth of these disorders patients may not notice any change in their general health. Weight loss, sweating and other constitutional symptoms may occur, but are often less severe than in the acute disorders (Table 26.9). Similarly, infection and anaemia occur but are generally less florid than in the acute diseases. Marked lymphadenopathy occurs, and enlargement of the liver and spleen is quite common. Because patients have few symptoms related to their chronic condition, the disease is often diagnosed by chance. For example, an older patient admitted to hospital for an unrelated reason will usually have a full blood count carried out, and this may show increased numbers of white cells and a reduction in haemoglobin, platelets, or other cells in the peripheral blood.

COAGULATION DISORDERS

The term 'haemostasis' refers to the coordinated physiological processes that prevent excess blood loss following vascular injury, and which can limit and localize the thrombotic process and initiate thrombolysis. The essential components of the haemostatic system are the integrity of the vessel wall, 'primary haemostasis' (the formation of a platelet plug) and 'secondary haemostasis' (the formation of a fibrin clot through the activation of the coagulation cascade) (Fig. 26.16). Disorders of primary haemostasis, which generally result from defects in platelet function or number, result in petechiae and bleeding from mucosal surfaces. Conversely, disorders of secondary haemostasis (as exemplified by haemophilia) usually result in haemorrhage into deeper structures such as muscles and joints (Figs 26.17, 26.18).

HISTORY

Because bleeding after injury is a universal experience it is sometimes difficult to determine whether an

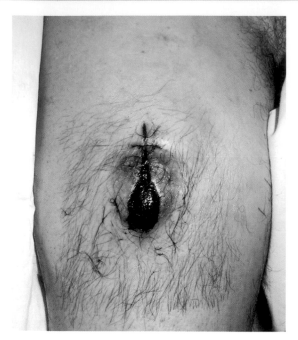

Figure 26.17   Haematoma following an intramuscular injection in a patient with mild haemophilia.

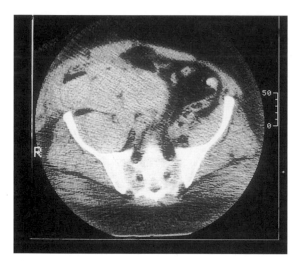

Figure 26.18   CT scan of the abdomen (haemophilia). There is a large haematoma in the right psoas region causing right-sided abdominal pain and swelling.

individual has a significant bleeding disorder or not. Approximately 20% of the population consider themselves to be 'easy bruisers', so it is important to take a 'bleeding history' that will discriminate easy bruising from a potentially important haemorrhagic disorder. An important aspect of the history will be the duration of any bleeding tendency. A lifelong tendency suggests an inherited disorder, whereas a later onset suggests an acquired disorder.

The presence of a haemostatic defect is suggested by frequent and persistent blood loss, often after minimal injury. Blood loss is often overestimated by

a third party (e.g. the concerned mother of a child who has bled after dental extraction), so it is useful to try to obtain some objective evidence of excessive blood loss. Any history of prior dental extraction, surgery or vaginal delivery should be obtained, as these are all significant challenges to the haemostatic system, and if excess bleeding did not occur then a major haemorrhagic disorder is *unlikely*. Features suggestive of a haemostatic defect include the requirement for blood transfusion or for surgical intervention to stop the bleeding. Heavy menstrual blood loss is a common complaint which, unless recent, is unlikely to indicate a haemostatic defect. Certain problems are highly suggestive of specific disorders. For instance, a history of spontaneous bleeding, or of bleeding into muscles or joints after only minimal trauma, is highly suggestive of haemophilia. Excessive bleeding from the umbilical stump after separation of the cord is characteristic of factor XIII deficiency.

Certain drugs affect the haemostatic system, most obviously the anticoagulants warfarin and heparin. Sometimes patients will not spontaneously report drug ingestion because the preparation was bought 'over the counter'. Aspirin is the most important example of this: platelet function is deranged for up to 3 weeks after a single dose of the drug.

EXAMINATION

The first element of the examination is to observe the character of any bruising or haematomata. Bruising due to abnormal platelet function or number most often results in purpura – tiny pinprick bruises due to haemorrhage from small cutaneous vessels. When compressed, purpura does not blanch, unlike similar cutaneous lesions resulting from small vessel inflammation, which will blanch on pressure. This distinction is best made by applying pressure with a glass slide and observing whether there is any blanching or not. However, the distinction is not absolute and some types of vasculitis, such as Henoch–Schönlein purpura, also result in extravasation of blood from tiny vessels. Another common type of cutaneous bruising occurs when the supporting structures of the vessel wall are weakened by age ('senile purpura') or drug therapy (e.g. steroids). When severe, platelet abnormalities may result in retinal haemorrhage. Ophthalmoscopic examination is mandatory in anyone with evidence of widespread purpura and mucosal haemorrhage.

If thrombocytopenia is suspected from the clinical findings, then consideration should be given to possible underlying causes (Table 26.10). In the paediatric setting, many of the congenital thrombocytopenic syndromes also have associated physical abnormalities, for example absent radii and absent radial pulses in the rare Fanconi's anaemia. Be alert to the relevant physical findings of leukaemia and

Table 26.10   The causes of thrombocytopenia

Mechanism		Examples
Reduced production	Congenital Acquired	Fanconi's anaemia Leukaemia Aplastic anaemia HIV infection
Redistribution		Chronic liver disease
Increased destruction	Immunological Non-immunological	ITP Drugs Septicaemia (DIC)

Table 26.11   Initial investigation of the haemostatic system

Test	Purpose
Full blood count	Platelet number
Blood film	To confirm genuine thrombocytopenia Platelet structure, size, colour Other abnormalities (e.g. leukaemic cells)
Prothrombin test (PT)	Tests extrinsic pathway
Activated partial thromboplastin test (APTT)	Tests intrinsic pathway
Thrombin test (TT)	Tests fibrin formation

Table 26.12   The clinical consequences of thrombocytopenia

Platelet count ($\times 10^9$/L)	Clinical features
100–150	Nil
50–100	Possible excess bleeding after major surgery or trauma
20–50	Possible excess bleeding after minor surgery or trauma
<10	Significant risk of major bleeding; cerebral haemorrhage

lymphoma, such as lymphadenopathy and hepatosplenomegaly. Similarly, stigmata of chronic liver disease (see Table 26.6) may be present. Thrombocytopenia has a wide-ranging differential diagnosis that overlaps with that of anaemia. A detailed general physical examination may well provide diagnostic clues.

INVESTIGATION OF THE HAEMOSTATIC SYSTEM

If a haemostatic disorder is suspected certain screening tests are essential (Table 26.11).

FULL BLOOD COUNT
A full blood count includes the platelet count (normal range $150–400 \times 10^9$/L). When abnormal, this should always be correlated with examination of the blood smear. A non-exhaustive list of the potential causes of thrombocytopenia is given in Table 26.10. The clinical consequences of thrombocytopenia are detailed in Table 26.12. Myeloproliferative disorders are commonly associated with a high platelet count, and because platelet dysfunction

Box 26.5   Causes of an abnormal PT/INR

- Warfarin or heparin therapy
- Liver disease
- Malabsorption of vitamin K
- Haemorrhagic disease of the newborn
- Disseminated intravascular coagulation

frequently accompanies these diseases, with an increased risk also of both thrombosis and bleeding.

PROTHROMBIN TIME (PT)
The prothrombin time measures the extrinsic coagulation pathway and final common pathway for haemostasis (factors VII, X, V, II and I) (Fig. 26.16 and Box 26.5). The test sample is compared with a normal control and the result expressed as a ratio. The reagents are standardized, and this ratio is given as the International Normalized Ratio (INR). Common situations in which the PT/INR is abnormal are shown in Table 26.13. For example, a patient with liver disease may have a PT of

Table 26.13   Tests of the coagulation system

Test	Normal range	Comments
Prothrombin time (PT)	11–15 s	Tests the extrinsic and final common pathways
Activated partial thromboplastin time (APTT)	33–47 s	Tests the intrinsic and final common pathways
Thrombin time (TT)	11–15 s	Tests the ability of exogenous thrombin to form a clot

Box 26.6   Causes of an abnormal APTT

- Haemophilia A or B (factor VIII or IX deficiency, respectively)
- von Willebrand's disease
- Warfarin or heparin therapy
- Liver disease
- Disseminated intravascular coagulation

Box 26.7   Causes of an abnormal TT

- Low fibrinogen levels
- Abnormal fibrinogen (dysfibrinogenaemia)
- Heparin
- Elevated fibrinogen degradation products

24 seconds (long). The normal PT is 12 seconds, and so the ratio (INR) = 24 ÷ 12 = 2.0 (normal INR is 1.0). In practice, the test is most commonly used to monitor warfarin anticoagulant therapy and the usual therapeutic aim is an INR within the range.

ACTIVATED PARTIAL THROMBOPLASTIN TIME (APTT)

The activated partial thromboplastin time measures the intrinsic coagulation pathway and final common pathway for haemostasis (factors XII, XI, IX, VIII, X, V, II, I) (Fig. 26.16). The result is not usually expressed as a ratio. Common causes of a prolonged APTT are given in Box 26.6. The APTT is usually used for monitoring heparin therapy.

Deficiencies of factors VIII and IX (haemophilias A and B, respectively), as well as von Willebrand's disease, cause a prolonged APTT. Therefore, an isolated prolonged APTT should be interpreted as indicative of a significant inherited bleeding disorder until proved otherwise by specialized factor assays.

THROMBIN TIME (TT)

In this test, thrombin is added directly to plasma. The thrombin test therefore assesses only the very last stage of coagulation, namely the conversion of fibrinogen to fibrin. The test is abnormal when there is insufficient fibrinogen present, or if there are substances present that inhibit thrombin, classically heparin (Box 26.7). When there is prolongation of the PT, APTT or TT for which the cause is not apparent, then further specialized investigation under the direction of a haematologist is required to elucidate the cause.

Sexually transmitted infections

B. T. Goh

INTRODUCTION

Stigma and shame are often attached to sexually transmitted infections. Remember that two aspects of sexually transmitted diseases are ever present. First, an infected patient implies that at least one other person is also infected. Thus treating a patient in isolation will not control the spread of these diseases. Second, a patient may harbour more than one sexually transmitted infection (Box 27.1). Many infections are asymptomatic, acquired months or even years previously. Remember that babies, monogamous partners and victims of rape and sexual abuse can also be infected.

The interview and examination must be carried out in private, in strict confidence, with sympathy, and avoiding any disapproving or moralistic attitude. As with other clinical problems, diagnosis is achieved by history (Box 27.2), examination and relevant laboratory tests. Following diagnosis, effective treatment and contact tracing should be instituted promptly. Sexually transmitted infections in children should suggest the possibility of sexual abuse, although non-sexual transmission can occur.

HISTORY

PRESENTING SYMPTOMS

URETHRAL DISCHARGE

This is nearly always a complaint of men. Ensure that the discharge is from the urethra and not from under the foreskin. Ascertain the colour and duration of the discharge. A purulent discharge suggests gonorrhoea, whereas 'non-specific' urethritis and *Trichomonas vaginalis* are more likely to give rise to a scanty mucoid or mucopurulent discharge. Sometimes the patient only notices the discharge in the morning, or by staining of his underwear. Prostatic secretions, which are physiological, may present as urethral discharge.

DYSURIA

Urethral pain on passing urine may be described as burning or stinging. False dysuria may occur if urine comes into contact with inflamed areas on the prepuce or vulva (ulcerated).

URINARY FREQUENCY

The frequent passage of urine, usually in small quantities, suggests bladder infection or involvement of the trigone of the bladder from ascending urethritis. It also occurs physiologically in irritable bladder syndrome and in anxiety.

VAGINAL DISCHARGE

Ask if the discharge is itchy or offensive. An itchy vaginal discharge is suggestive of thrush or, occasionally, trichomoniasis. Smelly discharges are usually due to trichomoniasis, bacterial vaginosis, or retained foreign bodies such as tampons. Physiological discharge can occur after sexual stimulation or during pregnancy, but is not itchy or offensive. Vaginal discharge may also arise from gonococcal, chlamydial or herpetic infections of the cervix.

DYSPAREUNIA

This is pain on sexual intercourse. In women, superficial dyspareunia is pain in the vulvovaginal area and can be due to vulvitis or lichen sclerosus. This must be differentiated from vulvodynia, which is chronic localized burning and soreness in the vulva and may be associated with vestibulitis, vestibular papillomatosis or subclinical warts, or may be idiopathic. However, vulvodynia can be aggravated by intercourse or tampon insertion. Deep dyspareunia is pain deep in the vagina and may result from pelvic inflammatory disease, endometritis and other gynaecological diseases, particularly endometriosis.

GENITAL ULCER

This is usually described as a 'sore'. Ask if it is painful or recurrent. *Painful ulcers* are usually due to herpes, chancroid, Stevens–Johnson syndrome, Behçet's disease or trauma, whereas a *painless ulcer* may be due to syphilis or lymphogranuloma venereum. However, syphilitic ulcers can be painful. The evolution of the ulcer is important. Genital herpes may start with local irritation followed by erythema, a group of papules, then blisters which ulcerate and crust before healing, but may present as a genital fissure. If the infection was acquired in a tropical country, chancroid, lymphogranuloma venereum and donovanosis should also be considered.

age of 40 from bacterial urinary tract infection, such as that due to *Escherichia coli*. Testicular cancer may sometimes present as a painful swelling.

PUBIC AND GENITAL ITCH

This is usually due to pediculosis pubis, scabies, or other inflammatory genital conditions, such as allergic dermatitis, but may be psychological or be due to lichen simplex. Ask if sexual or household contacts also complain of itching. In pediculosis pubis, patients may notice 'crabs' and nits on the hair shaft. Itching at night is suggestive of scabies and is likely to be generalized except for the face.

GENITAL RASH

An *itchy rash* on the vulva, glans penis or prepuce is seen in thrush, scabies and inflammatory dermatological conditions such as lichen sclerosus or contact dermatitis. *Non-itchy rash* may be seen in secondary syphilis, circinate balanitis, which is a manifestation of Reiter's disease, and in other genital dermatosis. Fixed drug eruptions, Stevens–Johnson syndrome, lichen planus, and penile or vulval intraepithelial neoplasia may present as a genital rash.

ANORECTAL SYMPTOMS

Anal soreness, pain or itching, rectal discharge, pain on defecation, a feeling of incomplete defecation (*tenesmus*) and constipation may occur in infective proctitis resulting from herpes simplex, gonococcal or chlamydial infection or lymphogranuloma venereum. *Anal itch (pruritus ani)* may be secondary to rectal discharge or due to thrush, anal warts, dermatitis and poor anal hygiene. If the itch is worse at night, threadworm infestation should be considered. *Pruritus ani* is frequently psychological in origin. *Sexually transmitted enteric infections* such as giardiasis, shigellosis and salmonellosis in homosexual men may present with diarrhoea. *Diarrhoea* is also a common problem in HIV infection.

Ask whether the patient has applied any medicament that might interfere with microbiological tests. An acute anogenital ulcer is syphilitic or herpetic unless proved otherwise; herpetic ulceration persisting more than 1 month is an AIDS-defining illness.

PAINFUL SCROTAL SWELLING

Acute epididymo-orchitis may complicate a sexually transmitted infection. Painful scrotal swelling is also a feature of acute surgical emergencies such as torsion of the testis and strangulated inguinal hernia. Other causes include trauma and recent vasectomy. Acute epididymo-orchitis in sexually active men below the age of 35 is likely to result from gonococcal or chlamydial infection, and in those over the

SYSTEMIC REVIEW

The skin, mouth, eyes and joints are commonly associated with sexually transmitted infections.

Rashes may be seen in acute HIV infection, secondary syphilis, gonococcal septicaemia and Reiter's disease. *Conjunctivitis* may be seen in chlamydial and gonococcal infection and is usually unilateral, whereas in Reiter's disease it is usually bilateral. *Anterior uveitis* may be seen in Reiter's disease, syphilis and HIV infection. *Joints* may be involved in gonococcal arthritis, Reiter's disease, and congenital (Clutton's joints) and late syphilis (Charcot's joints). *Lower abdominal pain* may indicate pelvic inflammatory disease, and right hypochondrial pain may indicate perihepatitis or FitzHugh–Curtis syndrome, which are all related to chlamydial or gonococcal infections.

OTHER ASPECTS OF THE HISTORY

A *past history* of genitourinary problems, sexually transmitted infections, gynaecological diseases, e.g. pelvic inflammatory disease and cervical dysplasia, and obstetric problems, such as stillbirths, miscarriages or babies with ophthalmia, is important. A delayed menstrual period with unilateral lower abdominal pain may be due to salpingitis (or ectopic pregnancy). A change in the menstrual cycle may be due to pelvic inflammatory disease. Chlamydial cervicitis may cause postcoital bleeding, but other causes, including carcinoma of the cervix, must be excluded. Ask whether the patient is using contraception, including intrauterine contraceptive devices, which may predispose to pelvic inflammatory disease, or has taken any drugs recently, especially antibiotics. Enquire about drug abuse. Antibiotics, diabetes mellitus, pregnancy and immunosuppression may predispose to thrush.

SEXUAL HISTORY

Enquiry into the less embarrassing aspects of the medical history fosters the patient's confidence, so start with this before moving on to more intimate matters, such as (in the case of women) contraception and the menstrual history. Details of the sexual history should be obtained by simple questions. Ascertain the date of exposure: 'When did you last have intercourse/'sex'?', and particulars of sexual contacts over recent months. If married: 'When did you last have intercourse/'sex' with your wife/husband?' followed by 'When did you last have intercourse/'sex' with someone else?' and whether with regular partners, casual contacts or commercial sex workers. Are sexual partners traceable, e.g. place of intercourse: 'which town?' and 'whether abroad?'. If there are several contacts, it is useful to identify them by first names. Heterosexual, homosexual or bisexual contact should be ascertained: 'Do you have intercourse/'sex' with men, women or both?'.

The incubation period of infection may be assessed from the date of exposure to the onset of symptoms, and hence the probable cause. Tropical sexually transmitted infections should also be considered in patients presenting with genital problems acquired in the tropics. A history of intercourse with homosexual or bisexual men, injecting drug users, or persons in or from an area of high *human immunodeficiency virus* (HIV) endemicity suggest acquired immune deficiency syndrome (AIDS) as the cause of multisystemic symptoms and signs.

The type of sexual practice will dictate the sites from which to take tests (see below). It is also helpful to understand some of the common or unfamiliar terms that may be used in relation to sexual practices. 'Straight sex' indicates heterosexual (penovaginal) intercourse. Ask whether the person also practises insertive or receptive oropenile intercourse: 'Do you receive or give 'oral sex'?'. Certain practices in homosexual or bisexual men ('gay sex') may predispose to particular infections; for example, if there is oroanal contact the possibility of intestinal pathogens should be considered. Hepatitis B and HIV infections are more common in those practising receptive penoanal intercourse. Ask whether the patient practises insertive (*'active'*) or receptive (*'passive'*) penoanal intercourse: 'When did you last have 'anal sex'?', or simply, 'Are you 'active', 'passive' or both?'. Some patients practise oroanal intercourse ('rimming'), insertive or receptive brachioanal intercourse ('fisting') and, rarely, urinating on to each other ('watersports') or using faeces during intercourse ('scat'). 'Barebacking' is unprotected anal intercourse; 'cottaging' is sexual intercourse in public places.

Heterosexual couples may also practise penoanal intercourse. This should be enquired for if rectal infection is found in women, although this commonly occurs in association with infection at other genital sites without having 'anal sex'. Sex 'toys' or 'dildoes' (artificial penises) are objects inserted into the rectum or vagina. 'Fisting' and 'toys' may cause injury presenting as an acute abdomen. 'Bondage', in which the person is tied up during sex, may be associated with masochism (sexual gratification through the infliction of pain on another). This should be considered if superficial injuries are present without an obvious cause.

Enquire about the use of condoms whether or not the patient is using other methods of contraception. Condom use should be advised if the person is at risk of acquiring or transmitting sexually transmitted infections, or if the efficacy of an oral contraceptive is affected by the concomitant use of other drugs. Many infections that may initially be acquired through non-sexual means, for example hepatitis B and HIV infection among injecting drug users and haemophiliacs, may be secondarily transmitted through sexual intercourse. Advice on non-penetrative 'safer sex' practices, such as body rubbing, dry kissing and masturbating each other, can be given to infected individuals who do not wish to have penetrative intercourse.

Sexual dysfunction, including erectile problems and premature ejaculation, often presents to a sexually transmitted disease clinic. Impotence is likely to be psychogenic if it is sudden in onset, related to life events, situational or intermittent, or if nocturnal or early morning erections are unaffected, and organic causes often have a psychogenic component. Curvature of the penis on erection may result from Peyronie's penile fibrosis.

GENITAL EXAMINATION

The patient should be examined in a well-lit room and gloves should always be worn.

MALE GENITALIA

THE PENIS
Note the appearance and size of the penis, the presence or absence of the prepuce, and the position of the external urethral orifice. Examine the penile shaft for warts, molluscum, ulcers, burrows and excoriated papules of scabies, and rashes. In Peyronie's disease there may be induration or a fibrotic lump inside the penile shaft. In the uncircumcised, establish that the prepuce can be readily retracted by gently withdrawing it over the glans penis. This allows inspection of the undersurface of the prepuce, the glans, the coronal sulcus and the external urethral orifice (meatus) for warts (Fig. 27.1), inflammation, ulcers and other rash. Always carefully draw the prepuce forwards after examination, otherwise *paraphimosis* – painful oedema of the foreskin due to constriction by a retracted prepuce – may ensue.

Phimosis is narrowing of the preputial orifice, thereby preventing retraction of the foreskin; it may be due to lichen sclerosus. This predisposes to recurrent episodes of infection of the glans (*balanitis*), the prepuce (*posthitis*) or both (*balanoposthitis*). *Circinate balanitis* in Reiter's disease appears as erythematous eroded lesions which coalesce with a slightly raised and polycyclic edge. Multiple small yellow or white submucous deposits (*Fordyce's spots*) may be seen on the inner prepuce. These are ectopic sebaceous glands and do not require treatment. *Smegma*, which is greyish-white cheesy material arising from Tyson's glands, may accumulate under the prepuce if unwashed.

Hypospadias is a congenital abnormality in which the external urethral orifice is not at the tip of the glans penis but opens at its ventral surface in the midline, anywhere from the glans to the shaft, or even in the perineum. *Epispadias*, a similar opening situated on the dorsal surface of the penis, is rare.

Tiny regular papules arranged in rows around the coronal sulcus are *coronal papillae* and may be mistaken for warts. The coronal sulcus is the commonest site for a chancre. Inspect the meatus for inflammation, urethral discharge, narrowing (stricture) and warts. Retract the lips of the meatus to look for meatal chancre and intrameatal warts. Tyson's gland is on the frenum of the penis and is not normally palpable, whereas the median raphe leads from the frenum to the inferior aspect of the penile shaft; both can be infected by gonococcal or chlamydial infection, leading to tysonitis and median raphe abscess, respectively.

Look at the scrotal skin for any redness, swelling or ulcer. Lift the scrotum to inspect its posterior surface. Tiny dark-red papules of *angiokeratoma*, or round, firm, whitish nodules of *sebaceous cysts* can sometimes be seen. *Scabies* causes erythematous nodular lesions on the scrotum and glans penis. If intrascrotal swelling is present, observe whether it appears to extend into the groin and note whether both testes are in the scrotum. *Ulceration* can result from Behçet's disease, fungation of an underlying tumour of the testis, or from a gumma.

THE TESTES   (Fig. 27.2)
Place both hands below the scrotum, the right hand being inferior, and palpate both testes. Arrange the

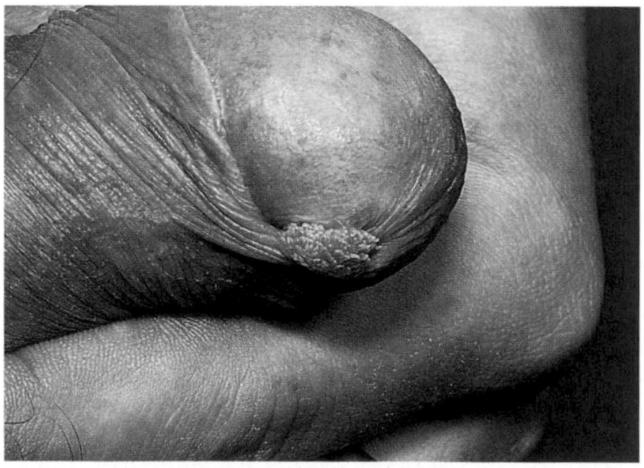

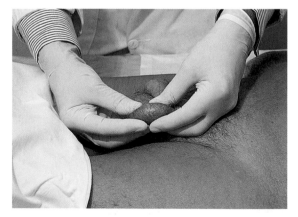

Figure 27.1 Genital wart on the frenum of the penis.

Figure 27.2 Palpation of the testis. Gloves should be worn.

hands and fingers as shown in Figure 27.2: this 'fixes' the testis so that it cannot slip away from the examining fingers. The posterior aspect of the testis is supported by the middle, ring and little fingers of each hand, leaving the index finger and thumb free to palpate. Gently palpate the anterior surface of the body of the testis; feel the lateral border with the index finger and the medial border with the pulp of each thumb. Note the size and consistency of the testis and any nodules or other irregularities. Now very gently approximate the fingers and thumb of the left hand (the effect of this is to move the testis inferiorly, which is easily and painlessly done because of its great mobility inside the tunica vaginalis). In this way the upper pole of the testis can be readily felt between the approximated index finger and thumb of the left hand. Next move the testis upwards by reversing the movements of the hands and gently approximating the index finger and thumb of the right hand, so enabling the lower pole to be palpated. The normal testes are equal in size, varying between 3.5 and 4 cm in length.

THE EPIDIDYMIS

The head of the epididymis is found at the upper pole of the testis on its posterior aspect. It is a soft nodular structure about 1 cm in length. The tail lies on the posterolateral aspect of the inferior pole of the testis. The tail is also soft, but unlike the head it has a coiled tubular form. Occasionally the epididymis is situated anterior to the testis.

THE SPERMATIC CORD

Finally palpate the spermatic cord (Fig. 27.3) with the right hand. Then exert gentle downward traction on the testis, place the fingers behind the neck of the scrotum, and with the thumb placed anteriorly press forward with fingers of the right hand. The spermatic cord will be felt between the fingers and thumb; it is about 1 cm in width. The only structure that can be positively identified

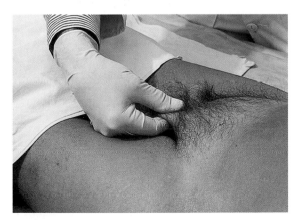

Figure 27.3 Palpation of the spermatic cord. Gloves should be worn.

within it is the vas deferens, which feels like a thick piece of string.

Repeat the examination on the other side. Remember that the patient should also be examined standing up to look for *varicocele* – dilated tortuous veins like a bag of worms in the scrotum. Hydrocele of the tunica vaginalis or a cyst of the epididymis are common causes of a painless scrotal swelling. *Hydrocele* can be demonstrated by transillumination, using a bright light source held in contact with the enlarged testicle, preferably in a darkened room. A *painless, unilateral, hard enlarged testis* must be considered malignant. Other painless enlargements include testicular gumma and tuberculous involvement. Acute epididymo-orchitis, torsion of the testis, strangulated inguinal hernia and some cases of testicular neoplasm cause a painful swelling. In torsion, the epididymis cannot be differentiated from the swollen testis, which lies at a higher level than the normal testis. In old age the testes may become atrophic. In younger men testicular atrophy often indicates chronic liver disease, usually alcoholic in aetiology, or it may be associated with previous torsion or varicocele. In swellings of uncertain origin ultrasound is useful.

ANORECTAL EXAMINATION

The anorectal region is particularly important in homosexual and bisexual men. Ask the patient to lie in the standard left lateral position with the knees drawn up, or in the knee–elbow position. Examine the anal and perianal skin for *inflammation, ulceration, fissures* and *tags*. Primary syphilis and herpes simplex virus infection can mimic an anal fissure. Anal tags should not be confused with anal warts (*condylomata acuminata*), which are sessile or pedunculated papillomata. Anal warts in turn should not be confused with the flat warty lesions of *condylomata lata*, which are the highly infectious lesions of secondary syphilis.

Gently insert a lubricated proctoscope and examine the rectal mucosa for pus, inflammation, ulceration, warts and threadworms. Take rectal tests. In patients who practise frequent receptive penoanal intercourse the anus may be lax.

FEMALE GENITALIA

It is best to examine women in the lithotomy position. Examine the perineum, vulva, and labia majora and minora for discharge, redness, swelling, excoriation, ulcers, warts and other lesions. In rape and sexual abuse cases, look for evidence of trauma. In such cases, forensic and genital examination by specially trained personnel may be required. Redness and swelling of the vulva with excoriations may be seen in thrush and trichomoniasis. Separate the labia and palpate Bartholin's glands: normally they are not felt. Bartholin's abscess may result from gonococcal

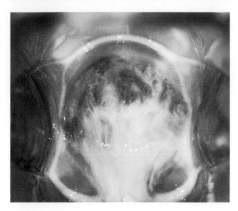

Figure 27.4 Mucopurulent cervicitis caused by *Chlamydia trachomatis*.

or chlamydial infection, and purulent discharge may be observed from Bartholin's duct, which is between the upper two-thirds and lower one-third of the labia. Wipe away any contaminating vaginal discharge from the urethral meatus and insert a bivalve Cusco speculum moistened with water. Paraffin jelly should not be used if a cervical cytological smear is to be performed. Note any inflammation of the vaginal wall (vaginitis) and the colour, consistency and odour of any discharge. A curd-like or cheesy white discharge suggests *thrush*, a frothy greenish-yellow discharge *trichomoniasis*, and an off-white homogenous discharge *bacterial vaginosis*. The last two conditions also have a fishy odour. Take tests (see below) from the posterior fornix of the vagina.

Wipe the cervix with a swab and examine it for *discharge* from the external cervical os, for *ectopy* or *ectropion* (ectopic columnar epithelium), and for *cervicitis, warts* and *ulcers*. Nabothian follicles may present as yellowish cysts, which may have prominent vessels on their surface, and are normal. Mucopurulent cervicitis may be caused by gonococcal or chlamydial infections (Fig. 27.4). Warts on the cervix appear as either flat or papilliferous lesions. Take tests, including a smear for *cervical cytology*, if indicated, to detect dysplasia and cancer of the cervix. This is particularly important because of the association of cervical cancer with oncogenic *human papilloma virus* infections. Then remove the speculum. Next examine the *urethral orifice* for discharge, inflammation and warts, and take endourethral tests (see below). Examine the *anal region* for lesions, as in homosexual men. If indicated, insert a lubricated proctoscope and examine the rectal mucosa for discharge or inflammation, and take tests.

BIMANUAL EXAMINATION
Use a bimanual examination technique to detect pelvic inflammatory disease and abnormalities of the upper genital tract. Uterine and fallopian tube tenderness with a positive cervical excitation test may indicate pelvic inflammatory disease. Tubo-ovarian abscess may be present.

COLPOSCOPY
If there are cervical warts, or the cervical cytology is dyskaryotic, the cervix should be examined under magnification using a colposcope. White areas after the application of 5% acetic acid suggest cervical wart virus infection or dysplasia, which can be confirmed by biopsy. Chlamydial follicular cervicitis may also be observed.

PUBIC REGIONS AND GROINS
Look for *pediculosis pubis* ('crabs') and nits. *Molluscum contagiosum* lesions appear as pearly or pinkish umbilicated papules. Look at the groins for *tinea cruris, thrush* and *erythrasma*. Tinea cruris and erythrasma give rise to a rash with a well-defined border, whereas in thrush the border is less well defined, often with erythematous satellite papules outside it. Erythrasma lesions show a coral-red fluorescence with Wood's light.

Swelling in the groin is usually due to hernia, lymphadenopathy or undescended testis. Genital ulceration with tender suppurative inguinal lymph nodes (*buboes*) will suggest chancroid and lymphogranuloma venereum. In *lymphogranuloma venereum* the ulcer may be transient and the buboes may have a grooved appearance resulting from lymphadenopathy above and below the inguinal ligament – 'sign of the groove'. In *primary syphilis* lymphadenopathy is painless, with mobile and rubbery nodes, although they can be painful if there is pyogenic secondary infection. *Anal, penile* and *vulval carcinoma* may metastasize to the inguinal lymph nodes. Inguinal lymphadenopathy may be part of a generalized disorder, as in lymphoma, secondary syphilis or viral infections, e.g. infectious mononucleosis and that due to HIV infection. Donovanosis may give rise to pseudobuboes, which are inguinal subcutaneous granulomata.

HIV INFECTIONS

The worldwide spread of human immunodeficiency virus (HIV) infection has resulted in a dramatic lowering of life expectancy in some countries, especially in Africa. HIV infection is categorized into A, B and C (Box 27.3), based broadly on the clinical evolution of the immunodeficiency state that leads to the development of the acquired immune deficiency syndrome (AIDS), on average some 8–15 years after infection if untreated.

- **Acute primary illness** – with fever, malaise, lymphadenopathy, muscle pain and sore throat, often with an erythematous, maculopapular rash and headache. Night sweats, weight loss,

Box 27.3 Centre for Disease Control (CDC) HIV clinical categories

Category A: Asymptomatic
- Acute infection
- Persistent generalized lymphadenopathy

Category B: Symptomatic infection excluding category A
- Bacteria: Bacillary angiomatosis
- Listeriosis
- Fungal: Candidiasis – oropharyngeal, vulvovaginal (persistent, frequent or poorly responsive to therapy)
- Viral: Herpes zoster (>1 episode or >1 dermatome)
  - Oral hairy leukoplakia
  - Constitutional symptoms: Fever (>38.5°C), diarrhoea 1 month
- Other: Cervical dysplasia – moderate or severe
  - Idiopathic thrombocytopenic purpura
  - Pelvic inflammatory disease
  - Peripheral neuropathy

Category C: AIDS-defining illness
- Bacteria: *Mycobacterium tuberculosis* – pulmonary, extrapulmonary
  - *Mycobacterium avium* complex or other mycobacterial infection with disseminated disease
  - Pneumonia – recurrent within 12-month period
  - *Salmonella* septicaemia, recurrent
  - Bacterial infections (multiple) in a child <13 years
- Fungal: Candidiasis – oesophagus, trachea, bronchi, lungs
  - Coccidioidomycosis – extrapulmonary
  - Cryptococcosis – extrapulmonary
  - Histoplasmosis – disseminated or extrapulmonary
  - *Pneumocystis jiroveci* pneumonia
- Helminth: Strongyloidosis – extraintestinal
- Protozoal: Cryptosporidiosis
  - Isosporiasis
  - Toxoplasmosis of brain
- Viral: Cytomegalovirus infection other than liver, spleen or lymph node
  - HIV encephalopathy, wasting syndrome
  - Herpes simplex – mucocutaneous ulcer 1 month, bronchitis, pneumonitis, oesophagitis
  - Progressive multifocal leukoencephalopathy
- Tumours: Cervical carcinoma, invasive
  - Kaposi's sarcoma
  - Lymphoma – brain, Burkitt's, immunoblastic or equivalent

diarrhoea, meningism, neuropathy and oral thrush may occur. There is HIV viraemia and severe immunosuppression, indicated by a high plasma HIV-RNA and a low CD4 T-lymphocyte count.

- **Asymptomatic phase** – following the acute infection the patient may be asymptomatic, or there may be persistent lymphadenopathy; the HIV-RNA decreases and the CD4 lymphocyte count increases and stabilizes (Fig. 27.5) to a baseline level.
- **Symptomatic phase** (category B).
- **AIDS-defining illnesses** (category C) – especially opportunistic infections such as tuberculosis and *Pneumocystis jiroveci* pneumonia, and neoplasms such as Kaposi's sarcoma (Fig. 27.6) and lymphoma.

Assessment of the patient with HIV infection should assess the extent of the disease and its complications. *Multisystem involvement is common, and in each system there may be multiple causes.* Examination of the mouth and the skin may provide clues that a patient is immunosuppressed. Common chest infections include tuberculosis, *Pneumocystis* and other bacterial pneumonias. Common cerebral lesions include toxoplasmosis, tuberculoma and lymphoma. Diarrhoea may be caused by HIV, drug treatment or opportunistic infections. Antiretroviral drug therapy may itself cause serious complications (Fig. 27.7).

Other retroviral infections, especially with HTLV-1, also cause human disease. HTLV-1 infection may be acquired by sexual contact. It is associated with the later development of T-cell lymphoma and leukaemia, often with hypercalcaemia, and with a slowly progressive neurological syndrome characterized by a progressive spastic paraparesis (tropical spastic paraparesis). These syndromes occur in regions where HTLV-1 infection is endemic, such as central Africa, the Caribbean and parts of Asia.

SYSTEMIC EXAMINATION

Particular attention should be paid to the skin, mouth, eyes, joints and, in late syphilis, the cardiovascular and nervous systems.

THE SKIN

A generalized rash occurs in drug allergy and in acute viral infections such as HIV seroconversion illness, acute hepatitis, cytomegalovirus infection, infectious mononucleosis and acute toxoplasmosis. The generalized rash of secondary syphilis can be itchy or non-itchy, and commonly involves the palms and soles. Gummata of the skin may be present in late syphilis. In disseminated gonococcal infection pustules with an erythematous base are seen mainly on the limbs, particularly near joints. Excoriated papules and burrows are features of scabies; generalized or crusted scabies may present as widespread crusted lesions. A psoriasis-like rash and keratoderma of the feet may be present in Reiter's disease. Behçet's disease causes recurrent painful orogenital ulcers. Stevens–Johnson syndrome

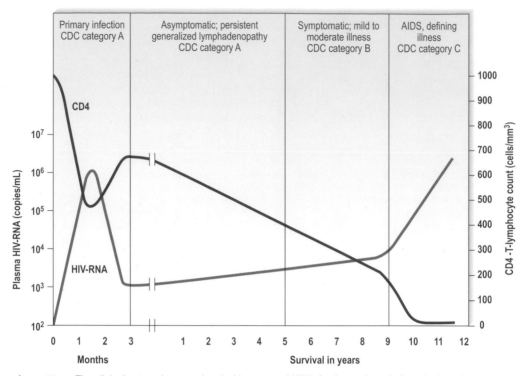

| Primary infection CDC category A | Asymptomatic; persistent generalized lymphadenopathy CDC category A | Symptomatic; mild to moderate illness CDC category B | AIDS, defining illness CDC category C |

Figure 27.5 The clinical categories associated with untreated HIV infection and survival can be loosely correlated with the plasma HIV-RNA and circulating CD4 T-lymphocyte count. Treatment with antiretrovirals and prophylaxis for opportunistic infections increases survival and can prevent or delay the progression to AIDS.

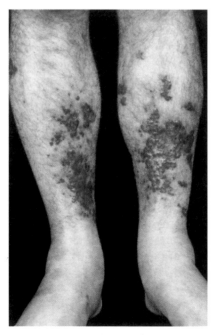

Figure 27.6 Kaposi's sarcoma of the lower legs with ankle oedema in a patient with AIDS.

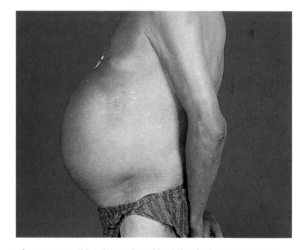

Figure 27.7 Lipodystrophy with abdominal adiposity and thin arm resulting from protease inhibitor treatment. Hyperlipidaemia and insulin resistance may be present.

can also present with painful orogenital ulceration and target lesions on the skin. In HIV infection, acute herpes zoster or scars of previous shingles, seborrhoeic dermatitis, severe fungal and bacterial infections, facial molluscum contagiosum and warts, bacillary angiomatosis and Kaposi's sarcoma may be present. The last may present with purplish nodules or plaques.

THE MOUTH

The mouth is a common site for syphilitic lesions: extragenital chancres in primary syphilis, mucous patches and snailtrack ulcers in secondary syphilis, and leukoplakia, chronic superficial glossitis and

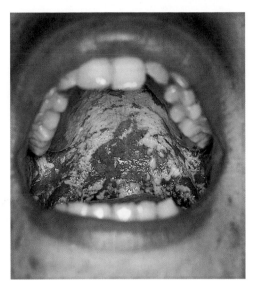

Figure 27.8 White plaques of oral candidiasis (which can be scraped off to reveal an erythematous base) in an HIV-positive patient.

gummatous perforation of the palate in late syphilis. In congenital syphilis, linear scars radiating from the mouth, known as rhagades, and Hutchinson's incisors – dome-shaped incisor teeth with a central notch – or Moon's/mulberry molars may be present. Genital herpes can spread to the mouth and vice versa if the patient practises orogenital intercourse. In HIV infection, oral hairy leukoplakia, consisting of persistent white hairy patches on the side of the tongue, and oral thrush, consisting of curdy white patches which can be removed, leaving behind a raw surface (Fig. 27.8) or erythematous areas, may be seen. Other oral manifestations of HIV include aphthoid ulcers, oral warts, gingivitis, severe peridontal disease, Kaposi's sarcoma and lymphoma.

THE EYES

Pediculosis pubis may be seen on the eyelashes. Conjunctivitis can be due to direct infection by *Chlamydia*, gonococcus, herpes simplex virus or molluscum, or can arise indirectly, as in Reiter's disease. Iritis can be seen in Reiter's disease, secondary and late syphilis, Behçet's disease and HIV infection. Congenital syphilis can present with interstitial keratitis, iritis and choroidoretinitis. *Argyll Robertson pupils* are small irregular pupils seen in neurosyphilis, particularly tabes dorsalis. They are non-reactive to light, but the *accommodation reflex* is present. In HIV infection there may be retinal exudates and haemorrhages due to retinal infarcts, and cytomegalovirus infection may cause a segmental or diffuse retinitis with exudates and haemorrhage.

THE JOINTS

Painful joint swelling may be present in Reiter's disease or disseminated gonococcal infection. Charcot's joints in tabes dorsalis are generally painless, deformed and hypermobile; Clutton's joints in congenital syphilis are painless bilateral joint effusions. HIV infection increases the risk of acquiring Reiter's disease.

THE ABDOMEN

Gonococcal and chlamydial infection can cause lower abdominal pain and tenderness if endometritis or salpingitis supervenes, and right hypochondrial pain and tenderness if perihepatitis (FitzHugh–Curtis syndrome) is present. Sexually transmitted hepatitis includes secondary syphilis and viral hepatitis. Hepatosplenomegaly may be present in secondary syphilis, acute viral hepatitis, HIV infection and associated opportunistic infections, or lymphoma. In HIV infection, retrosternal pain on swallowing indicates oesophageal infection by candida, herpes simplex virus and cytomegalovirus infection. Acute pancreatitis may complicate treatment with drugs such as didanosine. Renal colic may result from indinavir-induced stones.

SPECIAL INVESTIGATIONS

Cleanse the urethral meatus with a swab. If there is no visible discharge, gently milk the urethra forward from the bulb and note any discharge. A platinum or plastic bacteriological loop is inserted 1–2 cm into the urethra, proximal to the fossa navicularis, and the urethral material obtained is spread thinly on a glass slide for Gram staining. Endourethral material for gonococcal culture is placed directly on to a suitable culture plate or sent to the laboratory in modified Stuart's transport medium. Positive cultures are tested for antimicrobial sensitivities and β-lactamase production.

   Direct immunofluorescent antibody (DIF) staining can be performed for chlamydia using monoclonal antibodies, or an enzyme immunoassay (EIA) test for chlamydial antigen from endourethral material using a cotton-tipped wire swab. Nucleic acid amplification tests (NAAT) using polymerase chain reaction (PCR), strand displacement assay (SDA) or transcription mediated amplification (TMA) assay for chlamydia are more sensitive and can use urine instead of an endourethral specimen. NAAT can also be used to detect gonorrhoea.

GRAM STAINING   (Box 27.4)

If the patient has passed urine just before the test, the urethral smear may show no polymorphonuclear leukocytes because the urine will have washed out the accumulated urethral material. In such cases the patient should be asked to reattend for an

Box 27.4   Procedure for Gram staining

- Fix the smear on the slide by passing it through a flame twice.
- Stain with 2% crystal violet for 30 seconds, then wash with tap water.
- Stain with Gram's iodine for a further 30 seconds and wash with water.
- Decolorize with acetone for a few seconds.
- Wash with water and counterstain with 1% safranin for 10 seconds.
- After a final wash with water, dry by pressing between filter paper.

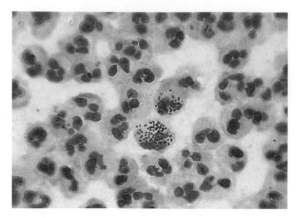

Figure 27.9   Gram-stained smear showing Gram-negative intracellular diplococci typical of *Neisseria gonorrhoeae*.

Box 27.5   Causes of non-gonococcal urethritis

Sexually transmitted diseases
- *Chlamydia trachomatis* D-K serovars
- *Mycoplasma genitalium*
- Unknown/ureaplasma?
- *Trichomonas vaginalis*
- *Herpes simplex virus*
- Intrameatal warts
- Meatal chancre

Non-sexually transmitted diseases
- Bacterial urinary tract infection
- Tuberculosis
- Urethral stricture
- Stevens–Johnson syndrome
- Benign mucous membrane pemphigoid
- Chemical
- Trauma
- Others

overnight or late afternoon urethral smear after holding urine for 8 or more hours. Gram-negative intracellular diplococci, which appear as opposing bean-shaped cocci within polymorphonuclear leukocytes under the microscope (Fig. 27.9), suggest gonococcal urethritis. The presence of five or more polymorphonuclear leukocytes per high-power field (×1000 magnification) with a negative test for gonococci indicates non-gonococcal urethritis (Box 27.5). The term non-specific urethritis is used to describe urethritis when specific causes, including *Chlamydia trachomatis*, *Mycoplasma genitalium*, trichomoniasis and non-sexually transmitted diseases such as bacterial urinary tract infection, have been excluded. However, the exclusion of *C. trachomatis* or *M. genitalium* infection may require specific and sensitive tests. A *wet preparation*, made by mixing urethral material using a loop with a drop of normal saline on a slide, can be examined by bright or dark field illumination for *Trichomonas*, which appear as ovoid protozoa with beating flagellae and in jerky motion.

'TWO-GLASS' TEST

Ask the patient to pass urine into two clear plastic cups, approximately 50 mL in the first glass and 100 mL in the second. The presence of several specks or threads that sink to the bottom in the first glass, with a clear second glass, indicates *anterior urethritis*; if there are threads in both glasses, *posterior urethritis* is indicated. Phosphaturia causes hazy urine in both glasses that clears with the addition of acetic acid. If the urine still remains hazy and there is pus in the urethral smear, this suggests either sexually transmitted urethritis with ascending infection in the bladder, or bacterial urinary tract infection with descending non-sexual infection to the urethra. The latter can be tested by a midstream urine culture. The urine must always be checked for sugar, protein, blood, cells and casts. Continuing symptomatic urethritis a week or more after successful treatment for gonorrhoea indicates that the patient has postgonococcal urethritis, a non-gonococcal urethritis unmasked following treatment for gonorrhoea.

VAGINAL DISCHARGE

Make a smear of the discharge for Gram staining to look for the spores and pseudomycelia of thrush, and for the absence of lactobacilli and the presence of mixed flora and 'clue cells' (Ison–Hay criteria), which are indicative of bacterial vaginosis. 'Clue cells' are vaginal epithelial cells covered with *Gardnerella vaginalis*, which are Gram-variable but mainly Gram-negative coccobacilli. A vaginal pH >4.5 using a litmus paper or strip is present in bacterial vaginosis and trichomoniasis. A wet-film preparation is examined for *Trichomonas*. Cultures for *Candida* and *Trichomonas* may also be per-

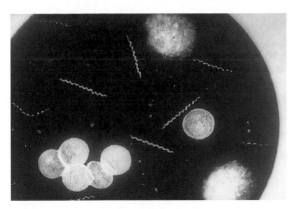

Figure 27.10 *Treponema pallidum* seen under the dark-field microscope. The spiral-like treponema can be seen, together with red blood cells.

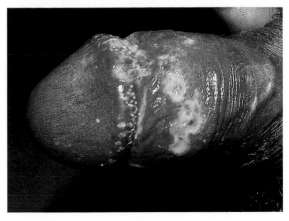

Figure 27.11 Acute ulcers of primary genital herpes. Both herpes simplex virus types I and II can cause genital herpes.

formed. A Gram-stained smear and culture, or NAAT of cervical, urethral and rectal secretions for gonorrhoea and a cervical and urethral diagnostic test for *Chlamydia trachomatis* should also be performed.

In those who practise peno-oral intercourse, a pharyngeal swab should be taken for culture for gonorrhoea and *Chlamydia*. A Gram-stained smear from the throat for gonorrhoea is useless because of the presence of other non-gonococcal *Neisseria*.

GENITAL ULCER

To investigate the cause of a genital ulcer, first cleanse the base of the ulcer with normal saline, then gently squeeze it until a drop of serum exudes. Catch the exudate on the edge of a coverslip. Place this on a glass slide and press down firmly between filter paper. Examine the slide under *dark-field microscopy* for the characteristic morphology and movements of *Treponema pallidum* (Fig. 27.10) – bending itself at an angle, rotating forward on its long axis, or alternating between contraction and expansion of its coils. Dark-field examination should be repeated for several days if syphilis is suspected.

Sometimes dark-field microscopy of suspected syphilitic ulcers may be negative, particularly if the patient has used a topical antiseptic or antibiotic cream. If regional lymph nodes are enlarged, a *lymph node aspiration* can be performed. After infiltration of the skin with 1% lignocaine, 0.2 mL of normal saline is injected into the node, the needle-tip moved around in the node, and then the saline aspirated. A drop is placed between a glass slide and coverslip, pressed between filter paper and examined under the dark-field microscope. In oral chancres, commensal treponemes from the gum margins may be confused with *Treponema pallidum*: because of this, immunofluorescent staining for pathogenic treponemes of serum from the ulcer, air-dried on a slide, is advisable. However, dark-field examination can be performed from oral ulcers away from the gum margin.

If anogenital herpes (Fig. 27.11) is suspected, the base of the blister or ulcer is swabbed and the swab sent for herpes simplex virus PCR, or placed in a viral transport medium for herpes culture. The diagnosis of donovanosis is based upon the demonstration of Donovan bodies, which stain in a bipolar fashion giving a 'safety pin' appearance within the cytoplasm of mononuclear cells in a Giemsa-stained tissue smear. Tissue is obtained by infiltrating the edge of the ulcer with 1% lignocaine and removing a small piece from the edge, which is then smeared on to a glass slide or crushed between two glass slides. If chancroid or lymphogranuloma venereum is suspected, culture or NAAT for *Haemophilus ducreyi* and *Chlamydia trachomatis* of the lymphogranuloma venereum serovars, respectively, may be indicated using material obtained from the ulcer or bubo.

SEROLOGICAL TESTS FOR SYPHILIS

There are two groups of serological tests for syphilis.

NON-SPECIFIC
- Anticardiolipin antibody, such as Venereal Disease Research Laboratories (VDRL) and Rapid plasma reagin (RPR).

SPECIFIC ANTITREPONEMAL ANTIBODY TESTS
- Treponemal enzyme immunoassay (EIA)
- *T. pallidum* haemagglutination (TPHA)
- *T. pallidum* particle agglutination (TPPA)
- Fluorescent treponemal antibody absorption (FTA-Abs).

The titre of the non-specific tests indicates disease activity and is useful for following up patients, particularly those who have been treated for primary, secondary or early latent syphilis, when the test should become negative or sustain a greater than twofold dilution or fourfold decrease in antibody titre within 6–12 months. After successful treatment of all stages of syphilis, the specific tests usually remain positive whereas the VDRL or RPR test may slowly revert to negative, but commonly remains positive in lower titre in late syphilis. *A greater than twofold dilution or fourfold increase in antibody titre following treatment indicates recrudescence or reinfection.*

The presence of a positive VDRL or RPR test on two occasions with negative specific tests and the absence of any evidence of treponemal disease indicates a *biological false positive* reaction. Acute false positive reactions may be due to acute febrile infections such as pneumonia, malaria, HIV infection and infective endocarditis, pregnancy and vaccination; they last less than 6 months. Chronic false positive reactions may indicate autoimmune diseases such as systemic lupus erythematosus, but can also occur in antiphospholipid syndrome, intravenous drug abusers, lepromatous leprosy and old age.

All patients should be screened for syphilis with serological tests using either the treponemal EIA, or combination of the VDRL or RPR and TPHA or TPPA. If syphilis is endemic, these tests should be repeated after 3 months if initial tests are negative. If primary syphilis is suspected, the EIA-IgM or FTA-Abs IgM test is also performed, as this is usually the first serological test to be positive. In babies with suspected congenital syphilis the EIA-IgM or FTA-Abs tests using an IgM conjugate should be requested because of passive transfer of maternal IgG antibodies across the placenta. When treponemes cannot be demonstrated, positive serological results must be confirmed by a second set of tests, but treatment should be started immediately in early infectious syphilis, or in pregnant women while awaiting confirmation.

Endemic treponematoses, such as yaws, bejel and pinta, may result in positive serological tests for syphilis. It is not possible to differentiate the treponematoses by serological tests. Patients may recall having such infection, or there may be a history of being brought up in the countryside in endemic areas, with evidence of signs of such infection, such as 'tissue-paper' scarring of the shins in yaws, which may suggest non-venereal treponematoses. However, there may be coinfection with syphilis, and it would be prudent to treat all positive treponemal serology as for syphilis.

INVESTIGATIONS FOR HIV INFECTIONS

Screening for antibody to HIV, the causal agent for AIDS, is advisable for patients at risk of infection because of the possibility of early intervention with anti-HIV agents, preventative treatment against opportunistic infections such as *Pneumocystis* pneumonia, and the prevention of transmission from mother to child. The latter is achieved by treating both mother (antepartum, during labour and at delivery) and baby at birth with antiretrovirals, caesarean section, and avoidance of breastfeeding. The test may also be indicated to confirm or exclude HIV infection as a cause of immunosuppression or problematic medical illness. Consent from the patient for the test to be carried out, with information regarding the test, is desirable. The test should be repeated at 3 months to cover the 'window' period for incubating infection. HIV-RNA viral load testing can also be performed for patients suspected of acute HIV infection, as the HIV antibody test may initially be negative. Immunological assessment must include analysis of lymphocyte subtypes, especially CD4 and CD8 counts: a selective reduction in the numbers of circulating CD4 cells is characteristic of the disturbed immune state. The HIV-RNA test and the CD4 T-lymphocyte count are prognostic indicators of HIV infection and can be used to monitor progression as well as treatment efficacy. Other investigations will depend on the suspected systems involved. Patients with headache or neurological signs should first have a CT or MRI brain scan to exclude intracerebral lesions before a lumbar puncture is performed. HIV genotypic or phenotypic resistance tests are helpful in deciding on the choice of antiretroviral regimen in treatment-naïve patients, or in those who are failing treatment.

INVESTIGATIONS IN HOMOSEXUAL AND BISEXUAL MEN

Gram-stained smears from the rectum and cultures from the rectum and throat of homosexual and bisexual men should also be obtained to exclude gonorrhoea, in addition to routine tests as for heterosexual men. In cases of proctitis, cultures or NAAT for herpes simplex and *Chlamydia trachomatis* of both D-K and LGV serovars may be indicated.

All homosexual and bisexual men should also be screened for hepatitis B surface antigen (HBsAg) and hepatitis B core antibody (anti-HBc). The presence of anti-HBc indicates that the patient has been exposed to the infection, whereas HBsAg indicates active infection. If both tests are negative, vaccination against hepatitis B should be offered. In HBsAg-positive patients the presence of hepatitis B e antigen (HBeAg) indicates high infectivity. If hepatitis is present, other infective causes, such as secondary syphilis, hepatitis A and C, as well as non-infective causes should be excluded.

Homosexual and bisexual men with diarrhoea should have their stools examined for *Giardia*, *Amoeba*, *Shigella* and *Salmonella*, and if HIV infection is suspected other causes of HIV-related diar-rhoea should be looked for. Threadworms may also be present.

OPHTHALMIA NEONATORUM

Ophthalmia neonatorum is defined as purulent con-junctivitis in the first 4 weeks of life. It should be differentiated from 'sticky eyes', which frequently result from blocked lacrimal ducts.

Ophthalmia neonatorum is commonly due to gonorrhoea, *Chlamydia* or non-sexually transmitted bacteria. A Gram-stained conjunctival smear can be a useful guide. The presence of polymorphonuclear leukocytes with Gram-negative intracellular diplo-cocci is presumptive evidence of gonorrhoea, but rarely may indicate *Moraxella catarrhalis* infection; culture must be carried out for full identification. The presence of pus cells with bacteria indicates bacterial ophthalmia, whereas the presence of pus alone suggests chlamydial ophthalmia. Chlamydial DIF, EIA, PCR, SDA or TMA tests, cultures for gon-orrhoea and other bacteria should be performed. Mixed infections may occur.

Chest symptoms such as a staccato cough and rapid breathing with poor feeding in the absence of fever may indicate chlamydial pneumonia. Auscul-tation of the chest may be normal but the chest X-ray may show consolidation.

If the ophthalmia is due to gonococcal or chlamy-dial infection, it is important to check the parents and their sexual partners.

SECTION 5

Ethics

Section contents

Ethical issues in medicine

M. Swash

28

INTRODUCTION

Successful medical practice requires a relationship of trust between doctor and patient. In family practice this relationship may be built up over several years, but in hospital practice or in an emergency the patient and the doctor may be meeting for the first time. A strict code of behaviour on the part of the doctor is required in order to set the scene for a trusting relationship. The code of medical ethics provides a suitable framework defining this relationship in professional, social and legal contexts. Patients expect a high standard of care when they seek help. This includes the expectation that:

- They will be consulted about decisions bearing on their treatment.
- They will be informed about their illness.
- They will be informed about the likely outcome of any treatment offered.
- Their right to confidentiality will be respected.

The capacity of a patient to take part in clinical decisions should never be underestimated. Always assume that a patient is able fully to understand the nature of the medical problem and its implications, whatever their educational level. Very often, it will be up to the doctor to introduce this topic at a suitable moment in the consultation. Some patients like to discuss the limits of what they would like to know early in a consultation, and many will define clearly the appropriate limits for dissemination of information to the family. These wishes must be respected.

Other influences are often brought to bear when considering how and what to tell a patient during diagnosis and treatment. The family may feel that the patient would not be able to comprehend medical information, or that this information will be too terrible a burden for them bear. Patients may insist that they do not wish the family to know about their medical problems or, sometimes, that they themselves do not wish to know the diagnosis. In all such instances the needs and rights of each individual patient should be considered paramount. Should there be any conflict in the relationships, the patient's interests are, first and foremost, always more important than those of the family. Fortunately, such conflicts of interest are very rare, and are often more apparent than real. With discussion they can usually be resolved.

HISTORICAL ASPECTS

In ancient Egypt rules of conduct for physicians included adherence to established methods of treatment. Later, the Code of Hammurabi formalized scales of payment for medical services, including penalties for negligence. In ancient Greece the Hippocratic Oath, a code of medical behaviour that underlies all modern clinical practice, required proper instruction of physicians, recognized that the physician's duty was to his patient – a duty that included an injunction to do no harm – and proscribed euthanasia and abortion, together with certain other risky or unacceptable procedures, such as lithotomy or castration. In addition, this Oath recognized the special nature of the doctor–patient relationship and stressed that it should not be abused. In both the Christian and the Muslim worlds the influence of Judaism in medical ethics has been strong, particularly in clarifying the responsibilities of individuals in relation to groups, as in the case of isolation of patients with serious infective conditions. This is an example of a special policy that puts the needs of the group temporarily on a level with those of the individual patient. Similar attitudes prevail in other religious environments.

AUTONOMY

The fundamental principle underlying the concept of a medical ethic is the autonomy of the patient. This means that the patient has the right to decide his or her own medical destiny: the physician may advise, but the patient decides. It is unacceptable for one individual – including the physician and relatives – to attempt to exert unconstrained power over the fate of another. Upon this notion rests the concept of seeking consent for medical interventions, for research, and for teaching, from the patient. Only in the case of a minor or a mentally disturbed person may consent be sought from the patient's lawful parents or guardians. Assent – but not consent – may be sought from relatives, for example in

497

the case of an unconscious patient in an intensive care unit. The physician or surgeon therefore has a duty not only to advise, but also to explain.

The origin of this ethic antedates the Christian era and is common to both Judaism and the Muslim world, in addition to all countries whose governance has been influenced by Christianity. It can thus be separated from any apparent religious background, itself an important aspect of the universality of the concept of a medical ethic.

CONSENT

The patient's consent should be sought for any treatment, however minor. In many instances consent is implied, as when a patient presents to a doctor with an injury and asks for treatment. In other circumstances a minor symptom may lead to the discovery of a serious illness requiring complex investigations and treatment. In this example consent will be required for each stage of the investigation and treatment, as part of the unfolding of the diagnosis and the management proposed.

For a patient to give consent sufficient accurate information about the illness must be given to enable them to decide whether the proposed treatment is both acceptable and in their own interests. There are four requirements on the doctor discussing an intervention with a patient:

- The procedure itself must be described, including the technique and its implications.
- Information about the risks and complications must be given – this usually means *all* risks.
- Associated risks (e.g. from anaesthesia or from other drugs that may be necessary) should be described.
- Alternative medical or surgical investigations or treatments should be discussed, so that the reasons for the specific advice given are clear. In addition, the implications of the 'do nothing' option should be discussed.

THE PROCEDURE FOR OBTAINING CONSENT

The amount of information divulged will vary according to the context of the discussion and according to the needs of the patient as they emerge in the consultation. For example, an operation on the knee of a sportsperson has far greater implications than the same operation in the case of a sedentary office worker. It is not appropriate to burden the patient with a textbook approach to medical knowledge. The objective is not to place the patient in the situation of having to decide between conflicting medical data, but to explain why the recommended mode of management is regarded as the

best in the circumstances. It may of course happen that during the discussion other factors come to light that result in the advice being altered. Clearly, this should be accepted as a happy outcome, as it implies agreement as to the best course.

SETTING THE SCENE

Discussions regarding consent for investigation and treatment are emotionally charged for the patient, and often for the doctor as well. Therefore, try to arrange a suitably quiet and pleasant environment for the discussion, one that is free of interruptions and away from unnecessary observers, such as other patients or unfamiliar nurses or students. Make time for the discussion – *never* appear rushed. Use simple language that the patient can understand. Be patient. If necessary, and with the patient's permission, involve relatives. If there is likely to be a language problem, make sure that an interpreter is available. At the end of the discussion check that the patient has actually understood. If there is any doubt, be prepared to have a further discussion; it is often better, in the case of really serious news, to have a discussion about management on several occasions, even after the treatment schedule has commenced. A written summary of the information supplied should be given to the patient for later consideration.

IMPLICATIONS OF CONSENT OR REFUSAL

In the event that the patient declines the recommended investigation or treatment, remember that not only is this their right, but also that the objective of the process of discussion is to allow the patient to understand the management proposed and to reach a decision about whether or not to proceed with it. Therefore, refusal is *not* a signal for the doctor to disengage from management of the patient but, rather, to continue to provide care to as high a level as is possible within the limits of what has been agreed and, if necessary, to continue discussions about future management.

If explicit consent is given, the patient and doctor should both sign an appropriate consent form. This procedure should be followed for all serious interventions. In hospital this will be a standardized form, and a similar form should be used in family or private practice to verify that the discussion took place. The mere act of both parties signing the form does not constitute proof that consent has been lawfully given: it simply documents that a discussion took place. Generally, however, it will be taken to mean that consent was obtained. It is wise, therefore, to make a separate, contemporaneous note describing what was discussed.

LEGAL REQUIREMENTS FOR CONSENT

There are three aspects of consent that are required in law:

- The patient must be mentally and legally competent to give consent.
- The patient must have been sufficiently well informed to be able to give consent.
- Consent must have been given voluntarily, and not under duress.

COMPETENCE FOR CONSENT

Competence is difficult to define. The patient must be able to understand the discussion. If there is doubt as to the patient's competence to give consent, consent should be obtained not only from the patient but also from a responsible relative. If necessary, enlist help from senior nursing staff, or even from a psychiatrist.

Special difficulties with consent arise when the patient is unconscious. If treatment is necessary in order to save life, it can and must be given without waiting for consent. If relatives are available they should be consulted, but their wishes are not necessarily paramount in the decision to initiate life-saving therapy. In the UK no adult can act as a proxy for another. The relatives may thus assent to treatment, but cannot legally consent to it. This limitation also means that relatives cannot legally refuse treatment that is medically in the best interests of the patient, although a conflict of this kind should be reason to consider, carefully and in detail with the relatives, the reasons for disagreement. In some countries relatives can be given powers of guardianship that allow them to give consent for the adult for whom they act as guardian.

Consent for the treatment of children is a matter that must be considered with care. In the UK, a minor (i.e. someone under the age of 16 years) can be treated without parental consent, provided that care has been taken to make sure that the child understands the nature of the treatment proposed and its possible risks, adverse effects and consequences. However, this should be a most exceptional decision. In practice, the parents' agreement should almost always be sought. An obvious exception would be in an emergency, for example after a life-threatening head injury, or when non-accidental injury is suspected. Difficult decisions sometimes arise, for example when the prescription of contraceptive drugs to a young girl is requested in circumstances where the young person does not wish her parents to know.

APPROPRIATELY INFORMED

The point at which a patient can be considered to be appropriately informed is a matter of judgement. Some patients make it clear that they do not wish for long and involved discussions, but others are comfortable with the process only when very full explanations have been given. It is often necessary to strike a balance. It is easy to frighten a patient by reciting unwelcome, but rare, possible complications of a procedure to such an extent that they refuse treatment. This should not be the objective of discussing treatment. If a procedure is so risky that the doctor feels it is not justified – i.e. it is futile – the patient should be advised accordingly rather than being asked to decide for themselves.

NOT UNDER DURESS

That consent was given without duress should be self-evident to both the patient and the doctor. If necessary, the patient should be given the opportunity to consider the decision after the initial discussion. The personal, religious and social beliefs of the doctor must not be allowed to intrude. If this is likely – for example in the case of a doctor required to advise on therapeutic abortion whose religious beliefs forbid this procedure – another doctor should be asked to take over the care of the patient. Remember that duress can arise unexpectedly. A patient may feel that he or she must embark on treatment in order to prevent stress at home. The right course here is to explore the nature of this stressful situation and take steps to alleviate it, in addition to considering medical treatment. Duress may be financial. There must be no financial advantage, in the form of either bribery or inducement, either to the patient or to the doctor in the management proposed. Political or social duress is an issue that has confronted physicians in many parts of the world in their relations with their patients, and constitutes a particularly difficult problem for an individual to resolve. It is clearly unethical.

CONSENT FOR RESEARCH

Similar rules of conduct apply to the obtaining of consent for research as for a patient's entry into a clinical trial of a new drug and for teaching. It should be a condition of all research that the question addressed is relevant and that the protocol is capable of answering the question proposed. These matters are the special concern of the clinical investigators and should have been thoroughly considered by the Research Ethics Committee (see below).

CONFIDENTIALITY

All aspects of the medical consultation are confidential. This common law duty is recognized by the public and is an essential part of the background to the consultation, as it allows the patient freedom of expression in the knowledge that disclosures made within the confines of the consulting room will not be made available to others. Indeed, in some aspects of medical practice, especially in the treatment of sexually transmitted diseases, and in much of psychiatric practice, confidentiality is fundamental.

The principle of confidentiality applies also to the medical records. These are held by the doctor or the group practice or, in the case of hospital records, by the hospital itself. Hospital records are not available to anyone other than the medical and nursing staff treating the patient, and are immune from police powers of search. They are made available, however, with the permission of the patient, and, once disclosed, can be used in evidence in court in both civil and criminal cases. Patients have the right to inspect their own medical records after seeking access in writing. The principle of confidentiality of medical information was recognized by Hippocrates, and has been affirmed subsequently – in modern times, for example, in the Declaration of Geneva of 1968. Although in the modern hospital medical information is far more widely available to a number of different health professionals and administrators, the principle of confidentiality must be strictly followed. In the UK, it is rigorously supported by the General Medical Council and its breach is regarded as a serious matter. In certain other European countries, for example France, medical confidentiality is protected by the criminal code.

The situations in which confidentiality can be relaxed include:

- When the patient or his or her legal adviser allows it
- When it is in the patient's interests
- If there is an overriding duty to society as a whole
- In cases of statutory disclosure
- In certain situations where inspection of medical records is allowed
- Sometimes after death.

WITH PERMISSION

A common example of relaxation of confidentiality with the patient's permission is when a doctor discusses the patient's problems or takes a history with others present (e.g. medical students or a nurse). The patient should be given the opportunity to ask that others leave.

IN THE PATIENT'S INTERESTS

When it is necessary that another family member be informed about the nature of a patient's illness, for example in order to obtain information essential for effective treatment, it may be judged in the patient's best interests to break confidentiality. Another example might arise if a patient was judged mentally incompetent and it became necessary to involve a legal adviser to handle their financial and legal

affairs during a severe illness. This generally requires permission from a court.

AN OVERRIDING DUTY TO SOCIETY

Occasionally confidentiality may be relaxed in the context of a known or possibly pending violent crime. In the case of an illness such as epilepsy or coronary heart disease that might impair the ability to control a vehicle, the responsibility to inform the authorities rests with the patient. In such instances it is generally thought to be in the interests of society to encourage voluntary disclosure, thereby maintaining the principle of confidentiality between doctor and patient. The clinician does have discretion, however, to break this principle in circumstances that entail serious public risk.

STATUTORY DISCLOSURE

Confidentiality is breached in the case of certain infectious diseases, such as tuberculosis, that are statutorily notifiable to the public health authorities. There is also a statutory duty for a doctor to help in the identification of a driver involved in a road traffic accident who, for example, might have attended a surgery or accident and emergency department after the accident. The doctor in the witness box is in a state of privilege, and is protected against any action for breach of confidentiality when instructed by a court to disclose potentially confidential information. Similarly, a court can ask that medical documents be released to it if they are regarded as necessary for the completion of a fair trial of an accused person.

INSPECTION OF MEDICAL RECORDS

In the UK the case notes themselves belong to the hospital or the health authority, and not to the patient or the doctor. Private patient notes belong to the doctor concerned. Patients themselves have a lawful right to inspect their own medical records, and can see any reports concerning their own medical condition that have been prepared before they are released to another party. Such reports can only be prepared with the permission of the patient or at the request of a statutory body, as in the context of an order under the Mental Health Act, or in the jurisdiction of a recognized court. Generally, persons other than the patient have no right to inspect the medical records of an individual unless permission is given in writing by the patient, or the records are subject to a subpoena from a recognized court. The inspection of medical records for epidemiological purposes and for medical audit is currently allowed, as these activities are clearly necessary, but there is a need for distinct guidelines to be established relating to these activities in order to protect confidentiality.

This right of access by the patient clearly makes it important to write in the records only statements that can later be justified or defended. Value judgements about a patient are not matters for comment in medical records.

AFTER DEATH

Generally the principle of confidentiality should extend to patients who have died. In the cases of a number of deceased public figures of recent years (e.g. Winston Churchill and John F. Kennedy) this principle was not adhered to on the grounds that there were matters of public interest involved. Whether this was really the case the reader can decide.

ORGAN DONATION

When a tissue that can be replaced by the donor's own tissues, such as blood or bone marrow, is given to another patient, no special ethical problem arises. When a living donor gives an irreplaceable organ, such as a kidney, difficulties arise. The donor must be of sound mind, not under duress, and must not be placed in a position to gain financially by the gift. In other words, the ordinary principles of consent apply. The sale of organs for transplantation is forbidden in all developed countries, and is rapidly becoming illegal in all countries. Similar considerations apply to the acquisition of donor organs from a minor, a practice about which it is particularly difficult to issue sound guidelines.

Because deceased persons have only limited rights over their organs, statutes have been introduced to regulate the practice of cadaver organ donation. This regulation is still evolving, and varies from country to country. In general, in the UK an organ can be removed from a deceased person if it is known that this was the wish of that person in life, whether for purposes of therapy, research or education, provided that the next of kin agrees. An organ can also be removed with the authorization of the next of kin, without knowledge of the deceased's wishes. However, this requirement has generally not led to the easy acquisition of organs such as kidneys for transplantation in the UK, as the next of kin are often distressed during the crucial and short period when it is possible to use cadaver organs for successful transplantation. In addition, the next of kin are often concerned to follow the supposed wishes of the deceased, or to contact other relatives for a decision, and by the time a decision is made it is too late. In some countries of the European Union there is a presumption, in the absence of any explicit statement to the contrary, that a deceased person would have wished to donate organs. However, this attitude is not general and it seems unlikely that it will become so, as clinicians are unlikely to take

organs if they believe this will cause distress to relatives. Voluntary schemes requiring a decision to consent to organ donation after death are generally preferred in most countries, even though there is a shortage of suitable organs for transplantation.

Certain religious constraints should be remembered. People of the Muslim faith are forbidden to accept organ donations from animals other than humans, and will not accept porcine products, for example pig valve grafts. However, porcine insulin is acceptable because it is a product of the animal and not one of its organs. Donations of organs from a living patient – for example the gift of a kidney from a relative – may be subject to the agreement of two wise men from the community, in addition to the usual ethical procedures required by any hospital in the western world.

ABORTION AND THE RIGHTS OF THE FETUS

The passage of the Abortion Act in the UK in 1967 marked a change in society's attitudes and, broadly, an acceptance by the medical profession of this change, illustrating that concepts of what is ethically acceptable change. None the less, there are still those who, for religious or other reasons find the legality of abortion unacceptable. Abortion was forbidden in the Oath of Hippocrates.

Much of the current controversy about abortion concerns the age of fetal viability. This has become a particular issue since fetal tissues have begun to be used in the treatment of certain diseases, and perhaps as a source of stem cells for organ growth and the production of neural and other cells for transplantation. Fetal viability is partly determined by medical science and medical skill in keeping small premature babies alive, and partly by biological factors. If the age of viability becomes a matter for legal definition by statute, it must be recognized that this statute will need to change with advances in medical science. There is a long-standing difficulty in resolving the logical description of the appropriate medical behaviour when the rights of an unborn fetus are seen as being in conflict with those of the mother herself.

The issue of fetal viability therefore differs from the more philosophical issue defining the stage of development at which the fetus becomes a person, imbued with human characteristics and subject to the same ethical considerations as a child or an adult. This issue can be resolved on religious grounds, by defining – as does the Roman Catholic Church – the onset of human life as the moment of conception, or by recognizing the onset of fetal movement or the external recognition of pregnancy. A simpler definition is that the fetus is invested with human status at the moment that independent existence begins, i.e. after birth. This approach, however, denies the fetus the ordinary ethical considerations of the right to life, or the protection from deliberate or negligent harm, that are accorded to persons, and therefore is likely to be rejected by many thoughtful observers. Because of the dependence of the fetus on its mother, the rights of the fetus are inevitably bound up with those of the pregnant woman.

In recent years there has been an emphasis on the rights of the fetus as a person-in-embryo. It is averred that the fetus has the same rights in common law and in society as a competent adult. In this approach the issue of medical viability becomes less relevant, as the fetus has rights whether or not it is medically viable.

RESUSCITATION

Resuscitation is generally available in hospitals in the event that cardiopulmonary arrest occurs unexpectedly. However, this is not always successful, and many patients, recognizing the terminal nature of their illness, may request that resuscitation not be attempted. This is an entirely valid request, which should be respected once it is certain that the options are clearly understood by the patient.

NOT FOR RESUSCITATION

Sometimes a patient is so seriously ill that there is doubt among medical and nursing attendants that it would be appropriate to resuscitate them in the event that they suffered a cardiac arrest. It should be recognized at the outset that this implies a judgement on the part of those charged with the responsibility of caring for the patient that, in some way, the patient's life is not worth saving. It should be asked whether any physician or surgeon is ever in a position to make such a judgement. Many would think that this is not a matter that one human should decide about another.

However, the question of whether or not resuscitation is to be attempted arises with increasing frequency in clinical practice, as medical technology becomes more complex and more effective, thus prolonging life into situations that would not occur but for the efforts of medical science. The situation most frequently arises when a patient has terminal cancer, and one of the medical or nursing team asks whether the 'crash team' should be called if the patient suffers circulatory or ventilatory collapse. Resuscitation for a few hours or days of further pain and discomfort might be regarded as an unnecessary prolongation of the terminal illness.

The decision to withhold resuscitation is a matter for which it is proper always to seek the patient's full, informed consent. Indeed, the patient's views are paramount, and should be respected whatever the views of the clinicians, nurses, or even the rela-

tives. Relatives have no legal rights in a decision about the possible resuscitation of another individual. Although they may be consulted, and their views noted, they should not be allowed to influence a decision once it has been made by the individual, unless it is decided that the patient is not competent by reason of dementia, or some other impairment of judgement, to reach a decision. Overt depression, for example, might be a reason for not accepting a patient's expressed wish not to be resuscitated.

Although it might be thought not helpful to a patient to discuss this issue openly, in fact the reverse is usually the case. Most patients near to death are aware of their situation and welcome the opportunity for full discussion of the issues. Indeed, it may give them the opportunity to discuss matters with their family more openly than would otherwise be possible. The agreement of the patient and medical staff should be signed in the case record; most hospitals now use a formal protocol to document this procedure.

As a general matter of policy it is wise to involve the most senior clinician concerned with the patient's care in discussions about 'do not resuscitate' orders. Many large hospitals have a resuscitation officer, part of whose duties it is to review such decisions as the resuscitation resource needs to be applied uniformly across the hospital, and not be more available to some patients than to others. In many hospitals policies for resuscitation and for withholding resuscitation, taking into account the issues outlined above, have been agreed by medical and nursing staff. These should be sufficiently flexible to allow change with evolving medical technologies, and with increasing levels of knowledge and involvement of the general public in such issues. Of course a patient should always be resuscitated when cardiopulmonary collapse is unexpected and their wishes are unknown.

CONSENT FOR AUTOPSY

It is nowadays necessary to be explicit in asking for consent for autopsy. As part of the autopsy, tissue samples will be taken and examined, and some may be retained for future use. If this is intended, or is likely to occur, permission to retain the samples must be obtained as part of the consent for autopsy. This process of consent implies that the family will be given some idea of what studies might be undertaken on the retained samples in the future. It may be considered appropriate to consider whether any circumstances might develop in which the family might reasonably expect to be informed of the results of any such studies. For example, if information of a predictive or genetic nature were to be obtained in relation to the risk of vascular disease, or of specific cancers, then the family might wish to know of this. This concept of extended consent involving future actions is as yet still developing. However, it is of considerable importance in the future of pathological research, not only on autopsies, but also in the context of biopsies and blood samples obtained during ordinary medical practice.

ETHICS COMMITTEES

There are two kinds of ethics committee, the *Clinical Ethics Committee* and the *Research Ethics Committee*. In the UK the Research Ethics Committee is concerned only with research. It will ascertain that proper arrangements exist to safeguard the patient's interests at all times, especially with regard to consent and to the recognition of any possible risks associated with a research protocol. Confidentiality must be maintained, and this must include the security of any computer-held records. Research involving human subjects, whether patients or controls, generated by medical staff, students, nurses or other paramedical staff is all properly within the remit of the Research Ethics Committee. No research is ethical that is not scientifically valid. Particular care is required in considering research in the intensive care unit and in paediatric practice, because of the difficulties of ensuring that consent can adequately be established and the level of dependence of the patients.

It is the role of the Research Ethics Committee to be impartial and authoritative. Research Ethics Committees in the UK are organized so as to be independent of local practice. The Research Ethics Committee functions as an autonomous committee of the health authority (the local component of the Department of Health). It consists of lay members, experienced medical and nursing researchers, and other relevant professionals who understand the wide variety of ethical and legal problems that can arise in research proposals involving human subjects. Research Ethics Committees insist that records related to research should be maintained in a state such that they are available to scrutiny by others for some years after the conclusion of the research, as part of the effort to prevent fraud. Adequate safeguards, and agreements for restitution for any harm inadvertently caused to a patient during participation in an approved research protocol, must be in place in the institution concerned. This will often involve an agreement with a sponsoring pharmaceutical company or other responsible organization. There are European and American guidelines and arrangements in force that cover these eventualities; these must be adhered to as appropriate for the country concerned.

Review by the established Research Ethics Committee is a requirement of the process of obtaining permission to commence a research protocol in Europe, and is a federal legal requirement in the USA. Indeed, the results of any research not complying with these requirements is not acceptable to the new products licensing bodies in these two parts of the world. Similar rules pertain in many other countries.

The Clinical Ethics Committee is concerned with practical clinical matters. It may be asked to consider the ethics of the application of scarce resources – for example in the selection of people for organ transplantation, the process of consent for 'do not resuscitate' decisions, decisions related to in vitro fertilization, and other matters arising in hospital clinical practice. This committee is constituted to be representative of staff and patients' interests and, like the Research Ethics Committee, will have lay as well as professional medical and nursing membership.

VOLUNTEERS IN RESEARCH

Particularly stringent rules relate to the selection of volunteers for research who are not themselves patients. Volunteers – like patients and the investigators themselves – should not accept inducements to take part in research. Indeed, such inducements should not in any way form part of a research protocol, except insofar as provision is made to cover incidental expenses and inconvenience. Any financial interest that the investigator or the employing department may have must be clearly acknowledged. Some agreed process of compensation for patients or volunteers in research programmes to whom harm is done, whether inadvertently or as a result of negligence, is a requirement for acceptance by the Research Ethics Committee. This usually involves the need for some form of insurance.

OTHER ETHICAL PROBLEMS

There are several other problems that arise in medical practice, many of which are likely to become more important in the coming years.

MEDICAL NEGLIGENCE

Court actions alleging medical negligence against doctors have become more common in many western countries in recent years. Medical accidents – meaning inadvertent adverse events – are common in clinical practice, occurring in perhaps as many as 4% of all medical interventions. Few of these result in any legal action. An accusation of negligence often implies that a doctor–patient relationship has broken down. For the doctor such an action is distressing and sometimes professionally damaging, even when shown to be unjustified.

In considering whether there has been negligence it is necessary to establish *causation*, *harm*, and *breach of professional duty*. The breach of professional duty or care is addressed by asking whether the standard of care afforded the patient fell below what was expected. The standard expected is that of the ordinary skilled practitioner in the field in question, practising in the circumstances pertaining. It is not that of the greatest expert in the land. Thus, in assessing possible negligence a court will need to establish:

- What the ordinary practice is
- That the doctor did not follow this practice
- That the doctor undertook a course of clinical management that no ordinarily skilled doctor in that specialty would have undertaken if acting with ordinary care.

A mistake in diagnosis is not necessarily negligent, and the test of the standard of care applicable to the ordinary practitioner in the specialty will be applied by the court in considering this. In the UK this is termed the Bolam test, after a particular case that led to the enunciation of the principle.

Doctors are expected to keep up to date in their expertise by *continuing medical education*, and this is an aspect that is relevant to this judgement. Doctors in training are expected, by and large, to exercise an appropriate standard of care, and no patient should expect a lower standard of care simply because they are cared for by a junior doctor with less experience. This would clearly be wrong. It is imperative, therefore, that in treating a patient advice and help should be sought from senior colleagues whenever relevant.

RESOURCE ALLOCATION

In every country, even the richest, there is a limitation on the availability of medical resources, the distribution of which is decided in different ways. In some countries it is decided by the capacity of any individual to pay for private medical care. In others it is made available more generally, but to a level decided by the limits of the resources devoted to it by a benevolent (or otherwise) government. The doctor is therefore often confronted by a limitation on the capacity to offer a treatment, for various possible reasons.

Because the doctor's responsibility is always first and foremost to the patient as an individual, and not to that group of potential patients in the general population who have not yet presented for treatment, this potential limitation of resources is relevant only in the general context of the politics of resource allocation for medicine. The individual patient's rights and the doctor's responsibilities in this matter are clear. The duty to the individual must always take precedence, and every effort must always be made to treat each patient to the best of the doctor's ability and in the best interests of that patient, utilizing such resources as are available, from whatever source.

Notwithstanding this duty of care to the individual patient, the doctor does have a duty to society to improve treatments whenever possible, and to make as widely available as possible treatments to those that will benefit from them. Currently much effort is being expended in trying to establish methods for measuring the benefits of treatments, in order that resource allocation decisions – themselves a problem in medical economics rather than in medical ethics – can be formulated more rationally.

HIV

Testing for HIV requires the consent of the patient or individual. It is usual to counsel the individual before testing, as there are implications for lifestyle, future health, and even employment hinging on the result of the test. Life insurance companies usually require HIV testing only for large insured liabilities.

GENETICS

The rapidly evolving availability of relatively accurate genetic testing for susceptibility to inherited diseases, based on the modern understanding of DNA and the genetic code, has raised a number of ethical problems for which most societies are not well prepared. For example:

- Who should have genetic tests done?
- What should be done with the results?
- Who – if anyone – should have access to the information, other than the patient?
- How should expensive treatments that may be possible for genetically determined disorders be made available?
- Is it socially and economically appropriate to prevent such disorders?

The application of genetic information to medical practice is a current major area of change. It can be expected to have profound implications for the management of most aspects of disease, and for the ways in which all societies view the acquisition and availability of medical information.

GENETIC COUNSELLING

Genetic counselling is relatively long-established. The clinical geneticist will usually be asked to assess the risks of genetically determined disease in the context of a known familial occurrence of a disease, for example Down's syndrome, Duchenne muscular dystrophy or cystic fibrosis. There is knowledge about the genetic causation of each of these conditions, and certain tests with various probabilities of accuracy are available to assess the risk for individuals in a family, and for the risk that a planned pregnancy might result in an affected offspring.

Major difficulties arise in deciding whether to inform someone who has been shown by genetic testing to be certain to develop a disease in later life, for example Huntington's disease. Such decisions should ideally be made before testing is undertaken at all. Even when offering counselling about the risks for planned pregnancies similar difficulties arise. The social costs in terms of unresolved problems to individuals and their families of offering treatment or prevention for genetic disorders are largely undetermined at present. Practice in this context will change as knowledge and experience accumulate.

LIFE INSURANCE AND GENETIC INFORMATION

There has been concern about the implications of genetic knowledge for life insurance, a problem that is similar to that related to occult HIV infection. An affected person might obtain insurance knowing of their own risk, thereby selecting against the insurance company. Life insurance is a business, and not a form of social security. Clearly it is in the best interests of the insurance company, which has a responsibility towards all its insured clients, to have knowledge of all relevant medical problems affecting a client so that an appropriate risk can be assigned to an individual policy. However, this concept may need to be adjusted in order to provide insurance to those affected by this genetic information. Of course, information about an individual should never be divulged to an insurance company – or to any other organization – without the written permission of the individual, and only after the implications have been discussed with the person.

PRINCIPLES OF MEDICAL ETHICS

Several modern attempts have been made to encapsulate the principles of ethical medical behaviour in a series of simple statements. The *Declaration of Geneva* (Box 28.1) represents a modern attempt to restate the Hippocratic Oath in terms acceptable to contemporary students and medical practitioners. *The International Code of Medical Ethics* (Box 28.2) was derived from these principles, and restates them in more direct terms. The *Declaration of Helsinki* (1975) sets out recommendations for the guidance of doctors wishing to undertake biomedical research involving human subjects. The recommendations of the Declaration of Helsinki are generally recognized as relevant to the design of research protocols.

The problems raised by the interaction of modern medical practice with government and with society as a whole are important, and will require much thought and analysis in the future. This chapter cannot pretend to raise all the issues, but should be taken as an introduction to what should be a daily consideration, both in learning about and in practising medicine.

Appendices

A guide to reference ranges used in pathology

M. Browne

A 'reference range' may be defined as the range of values obtained for a particular test in a defined group of individuals. The term 'normal range', which has frequently been used in the past, is roughly equivalent in meaning to 'the range of values obtained from a group of healthy individuals'. The concept of reference ranges was introduced to avoid the ambiguities inherent in the term normal ranges, and it was deliberately introduced as a vague term to force definition of the reference group.

The interpretation of medical laboratory data is a process of decision-making by comparing a test result with 'reference values', usually for age- and sex-matched healthy individuals, but sometimes with reference values for individuals with defined disease processes.

The values given in Tables A1.1 and A1.2 generally relate to the adult reference ranges for healthy individuals used by the laboratories in the Royal London Hospital and St Bartholomew's Hospital. For therapeutic drugs, the values in Table A1.1 refer to therapeutic target levels.

Reference ranges for infants and children sometimes differ greatly from those seen in adults; in addition, for a number of tests they are gender specific. It is also important to recognize that different laboratories may quote markedly different reference ranges for some tests, depending on the methods they use. The main differences in results will generally be seen with enzyme and hormone assays; interpretation of results must always be performed using the local reference ranges.

Each local laboratory publishes reference ranges for the tests it offers, and if there are doubts about interpretation, advice should be sought from the laboratory. It may be useful to ask for assay imprecisions, as these are relevant in determining a significant change in the results for an individual patient.

The ranges given in the tables are expressed in the *Système International d'Unités* (SI units), a system which has been accepted internationally since 1960. SI units are used in most recent publications, although you may also find values in older works in 'traditional units'. For this reason some of the analytes in the tables are also expressed in traditional units.

REFERENCE RANGES IN CLINICAL BIOCHEMISTRY

Table A1.1 Clinical biochemistry adult reference ranges

Tests	Reference range	SI units	Reference range	Traditional units
Serum				
Adrenocorticotrophic hormone, ACTH (09.00 h)	10–50	ng/L	10–50	pg/mL
Adrenocorticotrophic hormone, ACTH (24.00 h)	<10	ng/L	<10	pg/mL
Alanine aminotransferase, ALT	<40	U/L		
Albumin	35–50	g/L	3.5–5.0	g/dL
Aldosterone (lying)	135–400	pmol/L	4.9–14.4	ng/dL
Aldosterone (standing)	330–830	pmol/L	11.9–30.0	ng/dL
Alkaline phosphatase, ALP	39–117	U/L		
α_1-Antitrypsin	1.1–2.1	g/L	110–210	mg/dL
α-Fetoprotein (non-pregnant)	<10	kiu/L		
Aluminium	<0.4	μmol/L	<10	μg/L
Ammonia	<40	μmol/L	<68	μg/dL
Amylase	25–125	U/L		
Androstenedione	3–8	nmol/L	86–230	ng/dL
Androstenedione (prepubertal)	<1.0	nmol/L	<29	ng/dL
Angiotensin-converting enzyme, ACE	10–70	U/L		
Aspartate aminotransferase, AST	12–39	U/L		

Tests	Reference range	SI units	Reference range	Traditional units
Serum *(cont'd)*				
β₂-Microglobulin (<60 years)	<2.4	mg/L		
β₂-Microglobulin (>60 years)	<3.0	mg/L		
Bicarbonate	22–29	mmol/L	22–29	mEq/L
Bilirubin (total)	<17	µmol/L	<1.0	mg/dL
Bilirubin (direct)	<4	µmol/L	<0.2	mg/dL
C1 esterase inhibitor antigen	150–350	mg/L	15–35	mg/dL
C1 esterase inhibitor function	>68%			
C3	0.75–1.65	g/L	75–165	mg/dL
C4	0.20–0.60	g/L	200–600	mg/dL
C-reactive protein	<10	mg/L		
CA 125	<37	kU/L		
CA 15–3	<30	kU/L		
CA 19–9	<35	kU/L		
Caeruloplasmin	0.20–0.60	g/L	200–600	mg/dL
Calcitonin (male)	<11.5	ng/L		
Calcitonin (female)	<4.6	ng/L		
Calcium	2.15–2.65	mmol/L	8.6–10.6	mg/dL
Carbamazepine (trough)	4–12	mg/L		
Carcinoembrionic antigen, CEA	<5	µg/L		
Catecholamines – norepinephrine (noradrenaline)	<4.14	nmol/L	<0.70	ng/mL
Catecholamines – epinephrine (adrenaline)	<1.31	nmol/L	<0.23	ng/mL
Chloride	98–106	mmol/L	98–106	mEq/L
Cholesterol (recommended)	<5.2	mmol/L	<200	mg/dL
Cholesterol (population range)	3.5–6.7	mmol/L	135–259	mg/dL
Cholesterol, HDL (male)	0.8–1.8	mmol/L	30.0–70	mg/dL
Cholesterol, HDL (female)	1.0–2.3	mmol/L	39–90	mg/dL
Copper	11–20	µmol/L	70–127	µg/dL
Cortisol (midnight)	<50	nmol/L	<18	µg/dL
Cortisol (09.00 h)	200–600	nmol/L	7–22	µg/dL
Creatine kinase (CK), male	<195	U/L		
Creatine kinase (CK), female	<170	U/L		
Creatinine (male)	79–118	µmol/L	0.9–1.3	mg/dL
Creatinine (female)	58–93	µmol/L	0.7–1.1	mg/dL
Creatinine clearance (male)	95–140	mL/min		
Creatinine clearance (female)	85–125	mL/min		
Dehydroepiandrosterone, DHEAS (male)	2.8–12.0	µmol/L	103–442	µg/dL
Dehydroepiandrosterone, DHEAS (female)	1.9–9.4	µmol/L	70–346	µg/dL
Dehydroepiandrosterone (DHEAS), preadrenarche	<0.5	µmol/L	<18	µg/dL
Digoxin (6–8 h after dose)	1.0–2.0	mg/L		
Dihydrotestosterone, DHT (male)	1.0–2.6	nmol/L	29–76	ng/dL
Dihydrotestosterone, DHT (female)	0.3–0.93	nmol/L	9–27	ng/dL
Ferritin	10–160	µg/L	10–160	ng/mL
Follicle-stimulating hormone (male)	1–10	IU/L	1–10	mIU/mL
Follicle-stimulating hormone (follicular)	1–10	IU/L	1–10	mIU/mL
Follicle-stimulating hormone (mid–cycle)	<50	IU/L	<50	mIU/mL
Follicle-stimulating hormone (luteal)	1–8	IU/L	1–8	mIU/mL
Follicle-stimulating hormone (postmenopausal)	>25	IU/L	>25	mIU/mL
γ-Glutamyltransferase, GGT (male)	<58	U/L		
γ-Glutamyltransferase, GGT (female)	<31	U/L		
Gastrin (fasting)	<40	pmol/L	<180	pg/mL
Glucose (fasting)	3.5–6.0	mmol/L	63–108	mg/dL
Haemoglobin A1c (DCCT aligned – target)	<7%			
Human chorionic gonadotrophin, HCG (non-pregnant)	<3	IU/L	<3	mIU/mL
17-Hydroxyprogesterone (male)	1.0–10.0	nmol/L	33–333	ng/dL
17-Hydroxyprogesterone (female follicular)	1.0–10.0	nmol/L	33–333	ng/dL
17-Hydroxyprogesterone (female luteal)	1.0–20.0	nmol/L	33–667	ng/dL
17-Hydroxyprogesterone (neonatal)	<80	nmol/L	<2667	ng/dL
IGF-1 (0–3 years)	49–289	µg/L		
IGF-1 (4–6 years)	52–297	µg/L		
IGF-1 (7–9 years)	53–300	µg/L		
IGF-1 (10–12 years)	90–637	µg/L		
IGF-1 (13–16 years)	172–675	µg/L		
IGF-1 (17–20 years)	94–506	µg/L		
IGF-1 (21–49 years)	94–358	µg/L		
IGF-1 (>50 years)	69–225	µg/L		

Tests	Reference range	SI units	Reference range	Traditional units
Serum (cont'd)				
Immunoglobulin A	0.8–4.0	g/L	80–400	mg/dL
Immunoglobulin G	5.5–16.5	g/L	550–1650	mg/dL
Immunoglobulin M	0.4–2.0	g/L	40–200	mg/dL
Immunoglobulin E	0–81	KU/L	<0.81	U/mL
Insulin – fasting	4–20	mU/L	4–20	µU/mL
Iron (male)	11–32	µmol/L	60–180	µg/dL
Iron (female)	7–30	µmol/L	40–170	µg/dL
Lactate (venous plasma)	0.5–2.2	mmol/L	0.5–2.2	mEq/L
Lactate dehydrogenase	240–480	U/L		
Lithium (target)	0.5–1.0	mmol/L	0.5–1.0	mEq/L
Luteinizing hormone (males)	1.0–8.0	U/L	1.0–8.0	mIU/mL
Luteinizing hormone (follicular)	1.0–10.0	U/L	1.0–10.0	mIU/mL
Luteinizing hormone (midcycle)	<75	IU/L	<75	mIU/mL
Luteinizing hormone (luteal)	1–13	IU/L	1–13	mIU/mL
Luteinizing hormone (postmenopausal)	>16	IU/L	>16	mIU/mL
Magnesium	0.70–1.00	mmol/L	1.70–2.43	mg/dL
Oestradiol (male)	28–56	pmol/L	8–43	pg/mL
Oestradiol (follicular)	40–407	pmol/L	11–111	pg/mL
Oestradiol (midcycle)	315–1828	pmol/L	85–498	pg/mL
Oestradiol (luteal)	161–774	pmol/L	44–211	pg/mL
Oestradiol (postmenopausal)	<201	pmol/L	<55	pg/mL
Osmolality	275–295	mmol/kg		
Paracetamol	None detectable	mg/L		
Parathyroid hormone (adult)	1.1–6.8	pmol/L		
Parathyroid hormone (2–15 years)	1.1–3.6	pmol/L		
Phenobarbitone (trough)	15–40	mg/L		
Phenytoin (trough)	5–20	mg/L		
Phosphate	0.8–1.5	mmol/L	2.5–4.6	mg/dL
Potassium	3.5–5.1	mmol/L	3.5–5.1	mEq/L
Progesterone (follicular)	<8	nmol/L	<250	ng/dL
Progesterone (luteal)	>30	nmol/L	>943	ng/dL
Prolactin	<450	mIU/L		
Prostate-specific antigen (<40 years)	<1.4	µg/L		
Prostate-specific antigen (40–49 years)	<2.0	µg/L		
Prostate-specific antigen (50–59 years)	<3.0	µg/L		
Prostate-specific antigen (60–69 years)	<4.0	µg/L		
Prostate-specific antigen (>70 years)	<4.4	µg/L		
Protein (total)	62–77	g/L	6.2–7.7	g/dL
Renin activity (lying)	150–2100	pmol/L/h		
Renin activity (standing)	1150–4370	pmol/L/h		
Salicylate	None detectable	mg/L		
Sex hormone-binding globulin, SHBG (male)	17–50	nmol/L	0.49–1.44	µg/dL
Sex hormone-binding globulin, SHBG (female)	22–126	nmol/L	0.63–3.63	µg/dL
Sodium	136–146	mmol/L	136–146	mEq/L
Testosterone (male)	9–27	nmol/L	259–778	ng/dL
Testosterone (female)	<2.9	nmol/L	<84	ng/dL
Testosterone (prepubertal)	<0.8	nmol/L	<23	ng/dL
Theophylline (trough)	10–20	mg/L		
Thyroid-stimulating hormone	0.3–4.0	mU/L	0.3–4.0	µU/mL
Thyroxine (free), fT_4	11–25	pmol/L	0.8–2.0	ng/dL
Thyroxine (free), fT_4 (first trimester)	11.6–19.2	pmol/l	0.9–1.5	ng/dL
Thyroxine (free), fT_4 (second trimester)	9.3–16.3	pmol/L	0.7–1.3	ng/dL
Thyroxine (free), fT_4 (third trimester)	8.0–15.2	pmol/L	0.6–1.2	ng/dL
Tri-iodothyronine (total), tT_3	1.00–2.70	nmol/L	64–175	ng/dL
Triglycerides (fasting)	<2.1	mmol/L	<186	mg/dL
Urate (males)	202–416	µmol/L	3.4–7.0	mg/dL
Urate (females)	142–339	µmol/L	2.4–5.7	mg/dL
Urea (<70 years)	2.5–6.4	mmol/L	7.0–18.0	mg/dL
Urea (>70 years)	3.7–10.0	mmol/L	10.4–28.0	mg/dL
Vitamin D, 25 Hydroxy- (summer)	15–100	nmol/L	6–38	ng/mL
Zinc	11–24	µmol/L	72–157	µg/dL
CSF				
Glucose	70% of serum	mmol/L	70% of serum	mg/dL
Immunoglobulin G	<40	mg/L		
Lactate	1.1–2.8	mmol/L		
Protein	<400	mg/L	<40	mg/dL

Tests	Reference range	SI units	Reference range	Traditional units
CSF *(cont'd)*				
Protein (newborn)	400–1200	mg/L	40–120	mg/dL
Protein (up to 1 month)	200–800	mg/L	20–80	mg/dL
Urine				
Albumin	<20	mg/24 h		
Bilirubin	Negative			
Calcium	2.5–7.5	mmol/24 h	100–300	mg/24 h
Catecholamines – noradrenaline (adult)	<560	nmol/24 h	<95	µg/24 h
Catecholamines – adrenaline (adult)	<144	nmol/24 h	<26	µg/24 h
Catecholamines – dopamine (adult)	<3194	nmol/24 h	<489	µg/24 h
Chloride	60–180	mmol/24 h	60–189	mEq/24 h
Cortisol (free)	40–340	nmol/24 h	14–123	µg/24 h
Creatinine	9–18	mmol/24 h	1.01–2.04	g/24 h
Cystine	No excess detected			
Homovanillic acid, HVA (adult)	<45	µmol/24 h	<8	mg/24 h
5–Hydroxyindoleacetic acid, 5HIAA	<50	µmol/24 h	<10	mg/24 h
Magnesium	3.0–5.0	mmol/24 h		
Osmolality	50–1200	mmol/kg		
Oxalate (male)	0.08–0.49	mmol/24 h	7–44	mg/24 h
Oxalate (female)	0.04–0.32	mmol/24 h	4–30	mg/24 h
Oxalate (children)	0.14–0.42	mmol/24 h	12–38	mg/24 h
Phosphate (diet dependent)	13–42	mmol/24 h	0.5–1.3	g/24 h
Porphobilinogen	No excess			
Porphyrins	No excess			
Potassium (diet dependent)	35–90	mmol/24 h	35–90	mEq/24 h
Protein (total)	<0.15	g/24 h	<150	mg/24 h
Sodium (diet dependent)	60–180	mmol/24 h	60–180	mEq/24 h
Urate (diet dependent)	3.5–4.2	mmol/24 h	0.6–0.7	g/24 h
Urea (diet dependent)	166–581	mmol/24 h	4.6–16.5	g/24 h
Urobilinogen	No excess			
Zinc	4.5–9.0	mmol/24 h	294–588	µg/24 h
Faeces				
Elastase	>200	µg/g		
Laxative screen	None detectable			
Occult blood	None detectable			
Porphyrins	No excess			
Reducing substances	None detectable			
Total fat	<18	mmol/24 h	<5	g/24 h
Weight	<200	g/24 h		
Sweat				
Sodium	<60	mmol/L	<60	mEq/L
Chloride	<70	mmol/L	<70	mEq/L

REFERENCE RANGES IN HAEMATOLOGY

Table A1.2   Haematology adult reference ranges

Tests	Reference range	Units
Blood		
Activated partial thromboplastin time, APPT	23–31	s
Basophils	$<0.01–0.10 \times 10^9$	cells/L
Bleeding time	2.5–9.5	min
Eosinophils	$0.04–0.40 \times 10^9$	cells/L
Erythrocyte sedimentation rate, ESR (male)	1–10	mm/h
Erythrocyte sedimentation rate, ESR (female)	3–15	mm/h
Factor VIIIc	0.50–1.25	IU/mL
Factor IX	0.50–1.29	IU/mL
Fibrinogen	1.5–4.5	g/L
Folate (serum)	3.1–12.4	µg/L
Folate (red cell)	149–640	µg/L
G6PD (WHO)	10.1–18.5	IU/gHb
Haematocrit (males)	0.400–0.540	
Haematocrit (females)	0.370–0.470	
Haemoglobin (male)	13.5–17.5	g/dL
Haemoglobin (female)	11.5–16.5	g/dL
Haemoglobin A2	1.5–3.3	%
Haemoglobin F	<1.0	%
Haptoglobins	90–380	mg/dL
Lymphocytes	$1.50–4.00 \times 10^9$	cells/L
Mean cell haemoglobin, MCH	27.0–32.0	pg
Mean cell haemoglobin concentration, MCHC	32.0–36.0	g/dL
Mean cell volume, MCV	80–96	fL
Methaemoglobin	<1	%
Monocytes	$0.20–0.80 \times 10^9$	cells/L
Neutrophils	$2.00–7.50 \times 10^9$	cells/L
6PGD	5.6–11.6	IU/gHb
Platelets	$150–400 \times 10^9$	cells/L
Prothrombin time, INR	1.00–1.30	ratio
Pyruvate kinase	11–21	IU/gHb
Red blood cell count, RBC (male)	$4.5–6.5 \times 10^{12}$	cells/L
Red blood cell count, RBC (female)	$3.8–5.8 \times 10^{12}$	cells/L
Reticulocytes	0.2–2.0	%
Thrombin time	12–16	s
Viscosity (plasma)	1.50–1.72	mPa/s
Vitamin B_{12}	179–1132	ng/L
White blood cell count, WBC	$4.0–11.0 \times 10^9$	cells/L

Collecting specimens for laboratory analysis

M. Millar

VENEPUNCTURE

Check the identity of the patient and explain the procedure to them. The taking of a blood sample from a non-consenting patient might be construed in law as battery, and the cooperation of the patient can generally be taken to imply consent. Use the non-dominant arm if possible. Apply a tourniquet around the upper arm over the middle of the biceps so as to impede the venous but not the arterial flow. Wash or use an alcohol gel to decontaminate your hands. Wear gloves because it is not always possible to avoid contaminating the skin with blood, and there is always the potential for bloodborne viruses to spread to you through abrasions and other skin lesions. Clean the skin over the vein using alcohol. The skin is rendered tense by the operator's left hand; the hub of the needle, attached to a blood collection device (such as a vacuum tube holder), is held parallel to the patient's arm; the patient is asked to 'make a fist' and then the needle, with the bevel upwards, is inserted into a prominent vein. The median basilic vein is usually convenient, with the needle pointed in the direction of blood flow. A vein that can be felt is generally easier to enter than one that can only be seen. The required amount of blood is collected into the appropriate container for the test(s) requested, and the tourniquet is removed before the needle is withdrawn, as otherwise a haematoma may form. As soon as the needle is withdrawn a gauze swab is placed on the puncture site and the patient is asked to press this against the site for 1–2 minutes (flexing the elbow may increase the risk of a haematoma). Occasionally a vein in the forearm or wrist may prove more convenient than one at the elbow, but the procedure is then usually more painful. Needles must be disposed of into a 'sharps' container. To avoid the possibility of a needle-stick injury, minimize manipulations with needles as far as possible.

Most biochemical and immunological tests require serum samples and these sample tubes do not contain anticoagulant. Plasma samples require anticoagulation, usually with heparin, citrate or EDTA. EDTA is used for most haematological investigations and heparin for most simple chemical tests, with the exception of blood glucose, for which bottles containing sodium fluoride are necessary. For blood group and serological investigations blood should be taken into a dry sterile bottle or tube.

MICROBIOLOGY AND VIROLOGY SPECIMENS

Special care is necessary both in the collection and the transport of specimens for microbiological examination to the laboratory because:

- Successful detection and antimicrobial susceptibility testing often depends on the viability of the organisms.
- Overgrowth of the normal flora present in the specimen can hinder detection of the pathogen, which is often present only in small numbers.
- Careless collection techniques can lead to cross-contamination with organisms present on the patient's or operator's skin, or in the environment.
- Some tests (such as urine culture, HIV viral load) are quantitative. Sample collection and transport arrangements can have a significant impact on the numbers of microorganisms present in the sample.

The majority of bacteria and fungi that cause disease are free-living and so can be cultured under appropriate conditions. Viruses are obligate intracellular parasites and can only be cultured using tissue culture systems. The advantage of culture is that it is a general method which allows both the expected and the unexpected to be detected. Culture also allows isolates to be tested for susceptibility to antimicrobial compounds using growth inhibition tests. In addition to culture, agents of infection can be detected using a variety of microscopy techniques, including conventional light microscopy (Gram stain), immunofluorescence (*Pneumocystis carinii* detection in sputum), and electron microscopy (norovirus). There are also antigen detection systems that detect microbial components in clinical samples, such as those used to detect capsular components from the yeast *Cryptococcus neoformans* in the cerebrospinal fluid of immunocompromised patients.

Many different types of antibody test are available to detect the specific antibodies associated with various phases of infection. Traditionally, antibodies have been detected and assayed in serum. Antibody responses can also be detected in other body fluids, including CSF and saliva. The prevalence of antibodies in a population can give an indication of how common a disease is in that population. To identify active current infection it is generally necessary to demonstrate either the presence of IgM or a four-fold increase in the titre of total antibody during the course of the illness.

Increasingly, nucleic acid detection systems are being used. The nucleic acid detection systems may be linked with microscopy (in situ hybridization) or involve target or probe amplification linked with an amplified product detection system. The polymerase chain reaction (PCR) is one example of a target amplification method. These methods may be quantitative and so can be used to indicate how well an infection such as HIV has been controlled by treatment. There is increasing use being made of broad-range nucleic acid detection methods, such as eubacterial PCR, in which sequences of the bacterial 16S rDNA, which are conserved in all bacteria, are amplified. The exact sequence amplified can allow identification of the infecting agent.

TISSUE DISCHARGES, PUS, CSF AND OTHER FLUIDS (Figs A2.1–3)

It is important always to send a sufficient quantity of material to the laboratory. Generally, about 10–15 g of tissue or discharge and up to 25 mL of fluid are necessary. If possible it is better to send fluid and tissue rather than swabs. Some types of bacteria do not survive well on swabs, for example bacteria killed by oxygen (anaerobes), because of the large air–fluid interface of a swab. The chances of isolating a pathogen can be improved by inoculation of culture media in the clinic, as is common practice in genitourinary medicine clinics. The use of swabs with a charcoal-containing transport medium improves the chance of pathogen recovery on culture. Swab samples for viral studies require special viral transport media.

BLOOD CULTURES

The numbers of bacteria in blood varies from fewer than 10 colony-forming units (CFU)/mL in immunocompetent individuals with transient bacteraemia to thousands of CFU/mL in immunocompromised individuals with overwhelming sepsis. Bacteraemia is usually transient. Conditions giving a persistent bacteraemia include brucellosis and endocarditis. This means that if a sufficient blood volume is collected at the time of presentation of patients with suspected endocarditis, then the initiation of

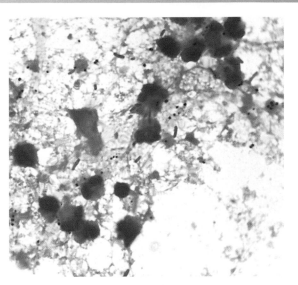

Figure A2.1 Pus from abscess, containing Gram-positive cocci and Gram-negative rods.

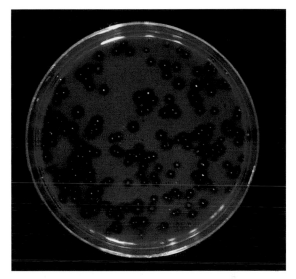

Figure A2.2 β-Haemolytic streptococci cultured from a throat swab on a blood agar medium.

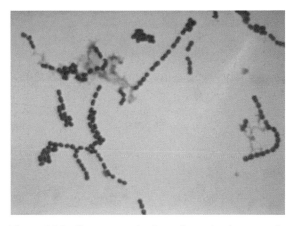

Figure A2.3 Gram smear of culture of pus showing a growth of streptococci.

antibiotic therapy should not be delayed. Bacterial viability and growth in blood cultures may be inhibited by antibiotic treatment. Special media may be required for the growth of some types of bacteria, such as *Mycobacterium* spp. Samples for blood cultures require particular care to avoid contaminating the sample or inoculating the culture bottle with skin bacteria. The collection of blood for culture usually requires a needle and syringe, rather than a vacuum tube. To avoid needlestick injury it is acceptable *not* to use a fresh needle to inoculate the culture bottle. The optimum blood volume to be collected from an adult to maximize the chance of a positive culture result without oversampling is 20–30 mL. Commercial blood culture bottles should give clear indications of the maximum amount of blood for each bottle. Before you withdraw blood, the patient's skin and the bottle cap should be cleansed with 70% alcohol or alcohol chlorhexidine, and allowed to dry. Modern laboratory blood culture systems monitor the bottles continuously, usually by direct or indirect measurement of the concentration of product(s) of microbial metabolism, such as CO_2. Continuous monitoring allows the time to positivity to be determined, and this gives a measure of the bacterial load in the original sample. Time to positivity can help with excluding or including a central venous catheter (CVC) as a source of bloodstream infection. Blood collected through a colonized CVC often contains very large numbers of bacteria and gives a shorter time to positivity than does peripheral blood collected at the same time.

URINE

Interpretation of the results of urine culture depends on the quantification of CFU/mL. It is most important that samples are appropriately collected and transported to the laboratory, so that bacteria do not proliferate or die off in the sample. Urine specimens should reach the laboratory within 4 hours of voiding, unless specific precautions are taken to prevent bacterial multiplication before cultures are set up. Urine specimens may be stored overnight at 4°C. Urine samples can be tested using a commercially available stick for the presence of leukocyte esterase and/or nitrites. Urinary tract infection can be reliably excluded in most outpatient and some inpatient groups when the urine is visually clear and such tests are negative. Samples collected through the urethra, such as an appropriately collected midstream specimen of urine (MSU) always contain bacteria, but usually in numbers $<10^3$ CFU/mL. Urinary tract infection can only be diagnosed when the numbers exceed a threshold value (10^5 CFU/mL in an immunocompetent adult). In the absence of urinary tract infection suprapubic samples should be sterile. For tuberculosis three early morning urine

(EMU) specimens should be submitted to the laboratory. For the diagnosis of schistosomiasis the terminal 5 mL of a freshly voided specimen is required.

URINE COLLECTION METHODS
- **Catheter specimen of urine (CSU)** Aspirate the urine, via a 21-gauge needle and syringe, from the rubberized part of the tubing connecting the catheter to the collection bag. *Do not collect urine from the tap outlet of the bag.*
- **Early morning urine (EMU)** Send the entire first-voided specimen – usually about 250 mL – to the laboratory in the large sterile container provided. Three consecutive morning specimens should be taken.
- **Midstream urine (MSU)** A urine specimen is collected by the patient mid-micturition, after instruction or with the assistance of a nurse, after the labia or penile orifice has been cleaned with water.

EXAMINATION OF FAECES

Human faeces contain $>10^{12}$ organisms/g wet weight as normal flora, whereas gut bacterial pathogens rarely exceed 10^5 organisms/g. Because of the relative scarcity of pathogens in faecal specimens, Gram-stained smears of faeces are not usually examined. However, occasionally in infections caused by *Campylobacter* spp. the typical seagull-shaped Gram-negative bacteria are present in sufficient numbers to be identifiable in a directly stained smear of a faecal specimen. The mainstay of diagnosis of bacterial infections of the gut is by culture. Correct collection and transportation of the specimen to the laboratory is particularly important, as incorrect technique can lead to the death of the pathogen or to overgrowth by normal gut flora. Recently antigen and nucleic acid detection tests have been developed for the diagnosis of enteric infections, such as sensitive and specific antigen detection of *Helicobacter pylori* in stool samples. For the detection of *Entamoeba histolytica* infestation the faecal specimen must be kept at body temperature until it can be examined. Other cysts and ova can be detected by examination of stool sent in a plain sterile container.

COLLECTION OF FAECAL SPECIMENS
Approximately 20 mL of stool should be collected on three separate occasions as early as possible in the illness, and placed in three separate sterile containers. For immediate transfer to the laboratory dry sterile containers are suitable. As there are a large number of bacterial species that can cause diarrhoea, the laboratory will use many different selective culture media to increase the isolation rate. It is essential to note on the accompanying request form any

relevant clinical details to enable the laboratory staff to seek the most likely pathogens. Important information includes a history of travel to potentially endemic areas, prior antibiotic therapy, any known outbreak of sporadic disease, possible contamination of food, and any immune susceptibilities.

Many of the viruses that cause diarrhoea cannot be cultured. Diagnosis is therefore often by immunological techniques, or by electron microscopic identification of the virus. When viral pathogens are suspected, specimens should be placed in a dry sterile container and sent to the laboratory promptly, or frozen at −20°C (−70°C is optimal, but rarely available). For direct detection of viral particles by electron microscopy many particles must be present. Electron microscopy is a specific but not very sensitive technique.

THE RESPIRATORY TRACT

Material may be taken for the detection of bacterial or viral infections. Specimens can be taken from the throat, the nasopharynx, the sputum, or by bronchoalveolar lavage. A tracheal aspirate can be obtained by a skilled operator by sampling through the cricothyroid membrane.

THROAT SWABS

Vigorously swab the tonsillar areas, the posterior pharynx, and any areas of visible inflammation, exudation, ulceration or membrane formation. For bacterial cultures, use a plain swab with transport medium. For viral detection, use a plain swab with virus transport medium. The specimen should be sent immediately to the laboratory or stored at 4°C; it should not be frozen. Rapid bedside antigen tests are available for the diagnosis of streptococcal sore throat, and these may require the use of swabs supplied by the manufacturer of the commercial kit.

NASOPHARYNX

Specimens of nasopharyngeal secretions are used principally for diagnosis of whooping cough (caused by *Bordetella pertussis*). The specimen is obtained using a wire pernasal swab, which is passed gently along the base of the nostril into the nasopharynx, rotated, removed, and placed in transport medium. The laboratory may need prior warning of the arrival of the specimen so that appropriate culture media can be prepared.

For the detection of viral pathogens from the nasopharynx an aspirated specimen is obtained using a suction catheter.

SPUTUM

Samples collected through the upper respiratory tract become contaminated with very large numbers of upper respiratory tract microorganisms. If a microorganism that does not usually colonize the upper respiratory tract is isolated from sputum it is reasonable to assume that it has a pathogenic role, but many of the agents of lower respiratory tract infection may be found in the healthy upper respiratory tract. It is therefore important to consider other diagnostic methods (apart from sputum culture) for the identification of agents of lower respiratory tract infection, such as blood culture, serology, and antigen and DNA detection systems. For the best results an early-morning freshly expectorated sputum specimen should be collected in a dry, sterile bottle. A physiotherapist can assist with the collection of a sample, through both chest percussion and the use of nebulized saline, but care must be taken when highly infectious and potentially lethal infections, such as severe acute respiratory syndrome (SARS), are considered in the differential diagnosis. In this type of situation the risks of infecting staff must be balanced against the risks associated with failure to make a specific diagnosis as a result of poor sample collection. For isolation of mycobacteria three consecutive morning specimens should be obtained.

BRONCHOALVEOLAR LAVAGE

This technique involves invasive sampling of the lower respiratory tract, either directed through a rigid or flexible endoscope or non-directed (usually through a tracheal tube). In patients mechanically ventilated for more than a few days ventilator-associated pneumonia (VAP) is a common complication. The cause of VAP may be inferred from microbiological analysis of the tracheal aspirates, although a bronchoalveolar lavage (BAL) (directed or non-directed) may give results that are more representative of the microbiology of the lung parenchyma. In immunocompromised patients there is a wide range of potential pathogens, including bacteria, fungi, viruses, protozoa and parasites. Bronchoalveolar lavage allows the lower respiratory tract to be sampled and a wide range of potential pathogens to be identified.

THE GENITAL TRACT

A variety of techniques are used to diagnose genital tract infection. These may require the use of a speculum in females to allow sampling of the endocervix, and special processing and transport methods to optimize the chances of pathogen identification. Suboptimal diagnostic methods not only allow untreated infection to spread to others, but may also have serious implications for future fertility and for the newborn infant. Therefore, whenever possible the patient should be referred to a genitourinary medicine clinic for diagnosis. Empirical treatment of sexually transmitted diseases with antibiotics is increasingly unreliable because of the increasing number of antibiotic-resistant strains.

Pathogens may be identified using microscopy, culture or serology. Nucleic acid detection methods are increasingly used for the diagnosis of infection with *Chlamydia trachomatis* and *Neisseria gonorrhoeae*. These methods can by applied to urine samples, facilitating the screening of patients in an outpatient or community context.

THE SKIN

Fungal pathogens such as dermatophytes and *Candida albicans* can be detected in skin scrapings, hair or nail cuttings, usually transported in black paper so that they can be easily identified.

THE EYES

Bacterial pathogens can be isolated using conjunctival swabs. Using a firm action, thoroughly swab the inner surface of the lower and then the upper eyelid, using a separate swab for each eye. Use a plain swab and charcoal transport medium. Viral pathogens can be detected using a swab moistened with sterile saline to collect secretions from the palpebral conjunctiva and using viral transport medium. Corneal ulcers and intraocular infections may require the use of specialized diagnostic methods and therefore referral of the patient to an ophthalmologist.

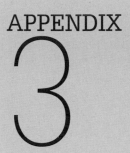
Blood and intestinal parasites

M. Glynn

Parasitic diseases remain extremely widespread across the world, especially in tropical countries where clean water is in short supply. Some, especially intestinal parasites, are also endemic in developed countries. They can be broadly divided into blood parasites (Box A3.1) and intestinal parasites (Box A3.2).

In general these diseases are suspected when assessing a patient who lives or has lived in an endemic area, or who has travelled to such an area. There can be a very wide range of symptoms, but for the bloodborne parasites there is often fever, lymphadenopathy, rash and hepatosplenomegaly, and for the intestinal parasites there are often specific GI symptoms.

For blood parasites the diagnosis may depend on actually finding the parasite itself (Fig. A3.1), finding antibodies to it, or observing pathological changes typical of it. Malaria is very widespread, and infection due to *Plasmodium falciparum* can be particularly severe, with rapid worsening. A blood film should be examined urgently, with several repeat films if clinical suspicion is high and the first film is negative. Occasionally empirical treatment without confirmation is sensible.

For faecal parasites the diagnosis is usually made by finding the parasite itself, or cysts and eggs, in the stool (Fig. A3.2). Because excretion can be intermittent at least three separate stool samples should be examined (and sometimes as many as six). For some parasites (particularly *Entamoeba histolytica*) the stool should be examined fresh (usually within 1 hour of passing) and preferably still warm.

The most important method of reducing the burden of parasitic disease across the world is to make clean water universally available and to reduce infection by biting insects and other vectors. As yet few vaccinations are available. Most of these diseases have some treatment and many are curable, although in developing countries lack of access to health services with adequate diagnostic facilities limits the scope of treatment, and morbidity and mortality remain high.

Box A3.1 Common blood parasites

Bacteria
- *Borrelia burgdorferi*, causing Lyme disease
- *Borrelia duttoni*, causing tickborne relapsing fever

Protozoa
- *Plasmodium* species, causing malaria
- *Trypanosoma* species
- *Leishmania* species

Helminths
- *Wuchereria bancrofti*, causing lymphatic filariasis (elephantiasis)
- Loa loa

Trematodes
- Schistosoma

Box A3.2 Common intestinal parasites

Protozoa
- Amoebae
- *Giardia*

Helminths
- Hookworms
- *Ascaris*
- *Trichuris*
- *Strongyloides*
- Tapeworms

Cestodes
- *Taenia*, causing cysticercosis
- Echinococcosis, causing hydatid disease

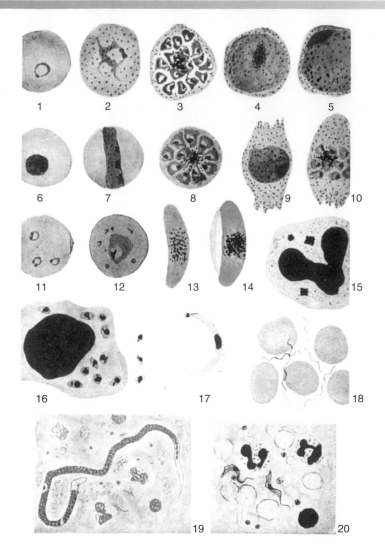

Figure A3.1   Blood parasites.

1   *Plasmodium vivax*. Ring stage. ×2000.
2   *Plasmodium vivax*. Amoeboid form. ×2000.
3   *Plasmodium vivax*. Fully developed schizont. ×2000.
4   *Plasmodium vivax*. Male gametocyte. ×2000.
5   *Plasmodium vivax*. Female gametocyte. ×2000.
6   *Plasmodium malariae*. 'Compact' form. ×2000.
7   *Plasmodium malariae*. 'Band' form. ×2000.
8   *Plasmodium malariae*. Fully developed schizont. ×2000.
9   *Plasmodium ovale*. Female gametocyte. ×2000.
10 *Plasmodium ovale*. Fully developed schizont. ×2000.
11 *Plasmodium falciparum*. Red blood corpuscle containing various types of young ring. ×2000.
12 *Plasmodium falciparum*. 'Old' ring, showing altered staining reaction and Maurer's dots. ×2000.
13 *Plasmodium falciparum*. Male gametocyte (or crescent). ×2000.
14 *Plasmodium falciparum*. Female gametocyte or crescent. ×2000.
15 *Plasmodium falciparum*. Pigment in polymorphonuclear leukocyte. ×2000.
16 *Leishmania donovani* from a spleen smear. Some lying free, and others within the cytoplasm of an endothelial cell. ×2000.
17 *Trypanosoma cruzi*. Adult form as seen occasionally in the blood of patients suffering from Chagas' disease (South American trypanosomiasis). ×2000.
18 *Borrelia recurrentis*. ×2000.
19 *Loa-loa*. ×600.
20 *Trypanosoma rhodesiense* as seen in a thick blood film of patient suffering from African trypanosomiasis. ×1000.

All magnifications approximate.
Drawings by W. Cooper.

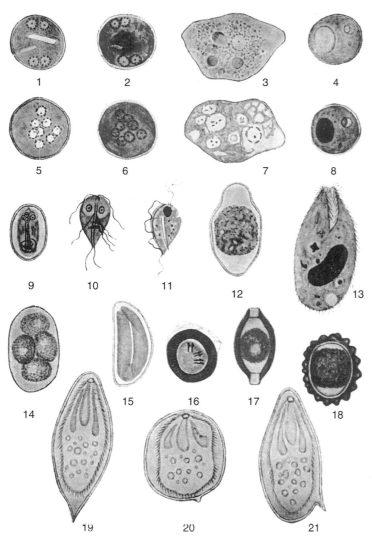

Figure A3.2 Intestinal parasites.

1   *Entamoeba histolytica.* Fully developed four-nucleated cyst containing chromatid bodies, as seen in a saline preparation. ×1500.
2   *Entamoeba histolytica.* Four-nucleated cyst as seen in iodine preparation. ×1500.
3   *Entamoeba histolytica.* Active form, containing ingested red blood cells, as seen in a saline preparation. ×1500.
4   *Iodamoeba bütschlii.* Cyst, as seen in a saline preparation. Note the unstained glycogen vacuole. ×1500.
5   *Entamoeba coli.* (Non-pathogenic) fully developed eight-nucleated cyst, as seen in a saline preparation. ×1500.
6   *Entamoeba coli.* (Non-pathogenic) eight-nucleated cyst stained by Lugol's iodine solution. ×1500.
7   *Entamoeba coli.* (Non-pathogenic) active form, as seen in a saline preparation. ×1500.
8   *Iodamoeba bütschlii.* (Non-pathogenic) cyst stained by Lugol's iodine solution. ×1500.
9   *Giardia lamblia.* Cyst form, stained by Heidenhain's haematoxylin. ×1500.
10 *Giardia lamblia.* Active (trophozoite) form, stained by Heidenhain's haematoxylin. ×1500.
11 *Trichomonas hominis.* Stained by Giemsa's method. ×1500.
12 *Isospora belli (I. hominis).* Undeveloped oocyst as passed in human faeces. ×500.
13 *Balantidium coli.* Active form stained by Heidenhain's haematoxylin. ×350.
14 Ovum of *Ankylostoma duodenale* (hookworm). ×500.
15 Ovum of *Enterobius vermicularis* (threadworm). ×500.
16 Ovum of *Taenia solium or T. saginata* (tapeworms). ×500.
17 Ovum of *Trichuris trichiura* (whipworm). ×500.
18 Ovum of *Ascaris lumbricoides* (roundworm). ×500.
19 Ovum of *Schistosoma haematobium.* ×300.
20 Ovum of *Schistosoma japonicum.* ×300.
21 Ovum of *Schistosoma mansoni.* ×300.

All magnifications approximate.
Drawings by W. Cooper.

Index

C

D